Medicine and surgery

A concise textbook

Giles Kendall

MBBS, BSc (Hons), MRCPCH
Research Fellow
Centre for Perinatal Brain Protection and Repair
University College London

Kin Yee Shiu

MBBS, BA Hons (Cantab), MRCP
Specialist Registrar in Nephrology Imperial College of Science,
Technology and Medicine Hammersmith Hospital London

Contributing editor

Sebastian L Johnston

MBBS, PhD, FRCP
Professor of Respiratory Medicine
National Heart and Lung Institute & Wright Fleming Institute
of Infection and Immunity
Imperial College London & St Mary's NHS Trust

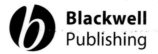

Blackwell
Publishing

Dedication:

To our families, our students and our teachers.

© 2005 G. Kendall, K.Y. Shiu and S.L. Johnston
Published by Blackwell Publishing Ltd
Blackwell Publishing, Inc., 350 Main Street, Malden, Massachusetts 02148-5020, USA
Blackwell Publishing Ltd, 9600 Garsington Road, Oxford OX4 2DQ, UK
Blackwell Publishing Asia Pty Ltd, 550 Swanston Street, Carlton, Victoria 3053, Australia

First published 2005

Library of Congress Cataloging-in-Publication Data

Kendall, Giles.
 Medicine and surgery : a concise textbook / Giles Kendall, Kin Yee Shiu, with contributing editor Sebastian L Johnston.
    p. ; cm.
  Includes index.
  ISBN-13: 978-0-632-06492-2 (alk. paper)
  ISBN-10: 0-632-06492-7 (alk. paper)
1.   Internal medicine. 2.   Surgery.
  [DNLM: 1.   Internal Medicine. 2.   Physiological Processes. 3.   Surgical Procedures, Operative. WB 115 K51m 2005]   I. Shiu, Kin Yee.   II. Johnston, Sebastian L.   III. Title.
  RC46.K52 2005
  616–dc22

  ISBN-13: 978-0-632-06492-2   2005003363
  ISBN-10: 0-632-06492-7

A catalogue record for this title is available from the British Library

Set in 9.5/12 Minion & Frutiger by TechBooks, New Delhi, India
Printed and bound in India by Replika Press Pvt. Ltd

Commissioning Editor: Fiona Goodgame, Vicki Noyes and Martin Sugden
Development Editor: Geraldine Jeffers
Production Controller: Kate Charman

For further information on Blackwell Publishing, visit our website:
http://www.blackwellpublishing.com

Contents

Preface

The concept of this book arose in part from a frustration with traditional textbooks, which address medicine, surgery and pathology as separate disciplines. This separation is frequently artificial, as patients often do not present to the doctor with an isolated medical or surgical problem. *Medicine and Surgery: A concise textbook* is a new textbook in which the pathophysiology and epidemiology of disease is presented alongside medical and surgical aspects to provide a truly integrated text. This unique approach allows the book to be used as a comprehensive undergraduate reference book.

Another driving force behind this book was the lack of a comprehensive text that students could turn to for the essential knowledge required to pass their final exams. *Medicine and Surgery: A concise textbook* is also a book that can be used by final year students to enable them to quickly and efficiently revise their knowledge. Whilst covering the core syllabus of undergraduate medicine and surgery we have kept the information to that which is essential to the undergraduate.

Diseases have been arranged by system and have been presented under consistent subheadings to aid understanding and revision. This is also the manner in which students are often expected to present in exams. At the beginning of each chapter the system is considered from a clinical perspective with a discussion of the symptoms and signs relevant to that system. Investigations and procedures that are used in multiple conditions are also considered in the clinical sections. Specific topics that have been excluded include diseases of childhood, orthopaedic, ENT and ophthalmology. These have had to be excluded to maintain the book at a manageable size.

This book has evolved over the last few years with the help of students and specialists who have reviewed and revised individual chapters or sections. We hope you find the final product useful and we encourage you as readers to help us revise future editions by sending your comments and suggestions for improvement.

Acknowledgements

We would like to thank all the anonymous specialists for their review and revision of the individual chapters; without this input the book would have not been as up to date and comprehensive as it is. We would also like to thank our families, friends and colleagues for their support and encouragement, especially Dr Man Fai Shiu and Dr Téa Johnston for their inspiration, guidance and encouragement throughout the project. Finally we would like to thank all at Blackwell Publishing, including Fiona Goodgame, Martin Sugden and especially Geraldine Jeffers for her tireless work and support.

Principles and practice of medicine and surgery

1

Fluid and electrolyte balance

Water and sodium balance

Approximately 60% of the body weight in men and 55% in women consists of water. Most of this exists within two physiological fluid 'spaces' or compartments: about two-thirds within the intracellular compartment and one-third in the extracellular compartment. The extracellular compartment consists of both intravascular fluid (blood cells and plasma) and interstitial fluid (fluid in tissues, which surrounds the cells). Additionally a small amount of fluid is described as in the 'third space', e.g. fluid in the gastrointestinal tract, pleural space and peritoneal cavity. Pathological third space fluid is seen with gastrointestinal obstruction or ileus and pleural effusion or ascites.

Water remains in physiological balance between these compartments because of the concentration of osmotically active solutes. Osmosis is the passage of water from a low concentration of solute through a semipermeable membrane to a more concentrated solution. A proportion of the total osmotic pressure is due to the presence of large protein molecules; this is known as the colloidal osmotic pressure or oncotic pressure.

- *Intracellular–extracellular fluid balance:* The cell membrane acts as semipermeable to sodium and potassium because the Na^+-K^+-ATPase pump keeps moving sodium out of the cell into the interstitial fluid and moving potassium into the cell. Sodium is the main determinant of extracellular fluid volume.

- *Intravascular–interstitial fluid balance:* The capillary wall is semi-impermeable to plasma proteins, whereas sodium passes freely across the capillary wall. This means that proteins (through oncotic pressure), rather than sodium, exert the osmotic effect to keep fluid in the intravascular space. The hydrostatic pressure generated across the capillaries offsets this, driving intravascular fluid out into the interstitial fluid. If there is a reduction in plasma protein levels (hypoalbuminaemia), the low oncotic pressure can lead to oedema; this is where there is excess interstitial fluid at the expense of intravascular fluid.

Water is continually lost from the body in urine, stool and through insensible losses (the lungs and skin). This water is replaced through oral fluids, food and some is derived from oxidative metabolism. Sodium is remarkably conserved by normal kidneys, which can make virtually sodium-free urine, e.g. in hypovolaemia. Obligatory losses of sodium occur in sweat and faeces, but account for <10 mmol. The average dietary intake of sodium in the United Kingdom is ~140 mmol/day, which is the equivalent of 8 g of salt. The recommended sodium intake for a healthy diet is 70 mmol/day. Normal kidneys can easily excrete this sodium load, and in a healthy person the body is able to maintain normal fluid balance by sensing the concentration of sodium and the extracellular volume. This process is under the control of both local sensing mechanisms and more distant neurohormonal mechanisms. These drive thirst and water intake on the one hand and renal excretion or conservation of sodium and water on the other. In disease states or due to an excess or lack of salt and/or water intake, this normal balance may be disturbed.

There are essentially four patterns of water and sodium imbalance:

- Sodium depletion is usually due to excess sodium loss, e.g. due to vomiting or diarrhoea, or burns. Water is lost with the sodium, so the serum sodium usually remains normal, but hypovolaemia results. If hypertonic fluid is lost or if there has been water replacement but insufficient sodium replacement (typically in a patient who is vomiting and only drinking water or only given intravenous 5% dextrose or dextrosaline), hyponatraemia results, which can lead to confusion, drowsiness, convulsions and coma (see page 4).
- Water deficiency due to inadequate intake of water leads to dehydration. The plasma osmolality rises and hypernatraemia occurs. This stimulates thirst and vasopressin release, which increases water reabsorption by the kidneys. Pure water depletion is rare, but many disorders mostly lead to water loss with some sodium loss. Initially water moves from the cells into the extracellular compartment, but then both the intracellular and extracellular compartments become volume depleted, causing symptoms and signs of fluid depletion (see section Assessing Fluid Balance below).
- Sodium excess rarely occurs in isolation. It is usually found in combination with water excess, causing fluid overload with peripheral oedema, pulmonary oedema and hypertension. The effect on serum sodium and fluid balance depends on the relative excess of sodium compared to water. Sodium excess > water excess causes hypernatraemia (see page 3) whereas water excess > sodium excess causes hyponatraemia.
- Water excess may be due to abnormal excretion e.g. in syndrome of inappropriate antidiuretic hormone (SIADH; see page 444) or excessive intake. In normal circumstances the kidney excretes any excessive water intake, but in renal disease or in SIADH, water is retained. This invariably causes hyponatraemia (see page 4). Patients often remain euvolaemic, but if there is also some degree of sodium excess there may be symptoms and signs of fluid overload.

Assessing fluid balance

This is an important part of the clinical evaluation of patients with a variety of illnesses, which may affect the circulating volume or sodium and water balance. Examples include patients with any history of cardiac, liver or renal failure, those with symptoms such as vomiting and diarrhoea, perioperative patients or any patient who has other losses, e.g. from bleeding or drains. Clinical evaluation of fluid balance requires the observation of several signs that together point to whether the patient is euvolaemic (normal fluid balance), fluid depleted (reduced extracellular fluid) or fluid overloaded (increased extracellular fluid). In most cases when the patient is fluid depleted, there is decreased circulating volume; however in fluid overload, there may either be increased circulating volume or decreased circulating volume depending on the mechanism.

- Fluid depletion may be suggested by an appropriate history of losses or reduced intake, but this can be unreliable. Symptoms of thirst and any postural dizziness should be enquired about. Signs of volume depletion include a mild tachycardia, reduced peripheral perfusion (cool dry hands and feet, increased capillary refill time >3 seconds), postural hypotension and/or hypotension, and reduced skin turgor (check over the anterior chest wall as the limbs are unreliable, particularly in the elderly). The jugular venous pressure is low and urine output reduced (oliguria, see later in this chapter).
- Fluid overload is more likely to occur in patients with cardiac, liver or renal failure, particularly if there has been over-enthusiastic fluid replacement. Breathlessness is an early symptom. Tachypnoea is common and there may be crackles heard bilaterally at the bases of the chest because of pulmonary oedema. The jugular venous pressure is raised and sacral and/or ankle oedema may be present (bedbound patients often have little ankle oedema, but have sacral oedema). The blood pressure is usually normal (occasionally high), but blood pressure and heart rate are often unreliable because of underlying cardiac disease: in heart failure the blood pressure often falls with worsening fluid overload. Pleural effusions and ascites suggest fluid overload, but in some cases there may be increased interstitial or third space fluid with reduced intravascular fluid so that the patient has decreased circulating volume with signs of intravascular hypovolaemia.

Urine output monitoring and 24-hour fluid balance charts are essential in unwell patients. Daily weights are useful in patients with fluid overload particularly those with renal or cardiac failure. Oliguria (urine output below 0.5 mL/kg/h) requires urgent assessment and intervention. A low urine output may be due to prerenal (decreased renal perfusion due to volume depletion or poor cardiac function), renal (acute tubular necrosis or other causes of renal failure) or postrenal (urinary or catheter obstruction) failure.

In fluid depletion, the management is fluid resuscitation. In previously fit patients, particularly if there is hypotension, more than 1 L/h of colloids or crystalloids (usually saline) may be needed and several litres may be required to correct losses. However, the management is very different in fluid overload or in oliguria due to other causes. In most cases, clinical assessment is able to distinguish between these causes. In cases of doubt (and where appropriate following exclusion of urinary obstruction) a fluid challenge of ~500 mL of normal saline or a colloid (see page 9) over 10–20 minutes may be given. However, care is required in patients at risk of cardiac failure (e.g. previous history of cardiac disease, elderly or with renal failure), when smaller initial volumes and more invasive monitoring (such as a central line to allow central venous pressure monitoring) and frequent assessment is needed. Patients should be reassessed regularly (initially usually within 1–2 hours) as to the effect of treatment on fluid status, urine output and particularly for evidence of cardiac failure:

- If urine output has improved and there is no evidence of cardiac failure, further fluid replacement should be prescribed as necessary.
- If the urine output does not improve and the patient continues to appear fluid depleted, more fluid should be given. However, in patients who are difficult to assess, clinically more invasive monitoring such as central venous pressure (CVP) monitoring may be required. This is performed via a central line, usually placed in the internal jugular vein. A normal CVP is 5–10 cm of water above the right atrium. The CVP is either monitored continuously or hourly and fluids are titrated according to the results. However, CVP measurements should only form part of the clinical assessment and in practice they can be unreliable.
- If there is any evidence of cardiac failure, fluid administration should be restricted and diuretics may be required.
- If hypotension persists despite adequate fluid replacement, this indicates poor perfusion due to sepsis or

cardiac failure, and these patients may require inotropic support.

Further investigations and management depend on the underlying cause. Baseline and serial U&Es to look for renal impairment (see page 230) should be performed. Where there is suspected bleeding, the initial FBC may be normal, but this will fall after fluid replacement is given due to the dilutional effect of fluids. Chest X-ray may show cardiomegaly and pulmonary oedema. Arterial blood gases can be helpful in identifying any acid–base disturbance due to renal failure or degree of hypoxia due to underlying lung disease or pulmonary oedema.

Hypernatraemia

Definition
A serum sodium concentration >145 mmol/L.

Incidence
This occurs much less commonly than hyponatraemia.

Age
Any. Infants and elderly at greatest risk.

Sex
M = F

Aetiology
This is usually due to water loss in excess of sodium loss, often in combination with reduced fluid intake. Those at most risk of reduced intake include the elderly, infants and confused or unconscious patients.

- Causes of water loss include burns, sweat, hyperventilation, vomiting and diarrhoea, diabetes insipidus (see page 445) and hyperosmolar non-ketotic coma (see page 461).
- Hypernatraemia may be iatrogenic due to osmotic diuretics which cause more water than sodium loss or excessive administration of sodium, usually in intravenous fluids.
- A rarer cause of hypernatraemia is Conn's syndrome (see page 442) or ectopic ACTH syndrome.

Pathophysiology
The normal physiological response to a rise in extracellular fluid osmolality is for water to move out of cells. Patients become thirsty and there is increased vasopressin

release stimulating water reabsorption by the kidneys. Water moving out of cells causes the cells to shrink. In response to this, electrolytes are transported across the cell membrane, changing the membrane potential. Changes in the membrane potential in the brain leads to impaired neuronal function and if there is severe shrinkage, bridging veins are stretched leading to intracranial haemorrhage. Cells also begin to produce organic solutes after about 24 hours to draw fluid back into the cell.

Clinical features

The symptoms of hypernatraemia include thirst, nausea and vomiting. Patients may be irritable or tired, progressing to confusion and finally coma. On examination there may be features of fluid depletion including reduced skin turgor, hypotension, tachycardia, peripheral shutdown and reduced urine output. Signs of fluid overload suggest excessive administration of salt or Conn's syndrome. Polyuria and polydipsia suggest diabetes insipidus or hyperglycaemia. There may be neurological signs such as tremor, hyperreflexia or seizures.

Complications

Hypernatraemic encephalopathy and intracranial haemorrhage (may be cerebral, subdural or subarachnoid) may occur in severe cases. Too rapid rehydration can cause cerebral oedema as the cells cannot clear the organic solutes rapidly.

Investigations

- The diagnosis is confirmed by the finding of high serum sodium on U&Es. Serum glucose and urine sodium, potassium and osmolality should also be requested. If there is raised urine osmolality, this is a sign that the kidneys are responding normally to hypernatraemia by producing low volume, high concentration urine. The underlying cause is therefore due to non-renal fluid losses.
- Conn's syndrome or ectopic ACTH syndrome is suggested by a mild hypernatraemia, hypertension, hypokalaemia (in the absence of diuretic drugs used to treat hypertension) and a raised urinary potassium.
- CT scan of the head is indicated if there are neurological symptoms or signs, and in severe hypernatraemia to look for an underlying cause (such as head trauma) or complications such as haemorrhage.

Management

- The aim is to gradually reduce the serum sodium concentration by no more than 0.5–1 mmol/L/h in order to avoid cerebral oedema. Urine output and plasma sodium should be monitored frequently. The underlying cause should also be looked for and treated.
- If the patient is alert and conscious he/she should be allowed to drink freely as this is the safest way to correct hypernatraemia.
- If the patient is fluid depleted, intravenous replacement should be with 0.9% saline to restore intravascular volume. In severe hypernatraemia even 0.9% saline is less hypertonic than the plasma so this will help to correct the high sodium.
- If the patient is not fluid depleted but is unable to drink, 5% dextrose is given slowly.
- In hyperosmolar non-ketotic coma saline or half-normal saline (0.45% saline) should be used until glucose concentrations are near normal. This is to prevent worsening hyperglycaemia which can alter the osmolality further.

Prognosis

The mortality rate of severe hypernatraemia is as high as 60% often due to coexistent disease, and there is a high risk of permanent neurological deficit.

Hyponatraemia

Definition

A serum sodium concentration <135 mmol/L.

Incidence

Occurs relatively commonly, with 1% of hospitalised patients affected.

Age

Any. Young and old are at greater risk.

Sex

M = F

Aetiology

The causes of hyponatraemia are given in Table 1.1. It is most useful to consider the causes according to whether

Table 1.1 Important causes of hyponatraemia

Hyponatraemia with fluid depletion	Vomiting, diarrhoea, drains, burns, pancreatitis, sweat
	Renal failure and salt-losing renal disease
	Addison's disease
Euvolaemic hyponatraemia	Psychogenic polydipsia
	Alcohol excess with malnutrition
	Syndrome of inappropriate antidiuretic hormone (SIADH)
	Postoperative patients, particularly after inappropriate fluids
Hyponatraemia with fluid overload	Congestive cardiac failure, cirrhosis, nephrotic syndrome
	Renal failure
	Severe hypothyroidism
Drugs	Diuretics (e.g. thiazide diuretics, amiloride, loop diuretics)
	Nonsteroidal anti-inflammatory drugs
	Many psychiatric medications (e.g. haloperidol, selective serotonin reuptake inhibitors)
	Opiates, ecstasy

it is acute or chronic and whether there is fluid depletion, euvolaemia or fluid overload.

- Acute hyponatraemia is usually due to vomiting and diarrhoea and/or inappropriate intravenous fluids such as dextrose or dextrosaline.
- Common causes of chronic hyponatraemia include SIADH, Addison's disease, congestive cardiac failure and drugs.

Pathophysiology

Normally when serum osmolality falls, ADH production ceases and the kidneys rapidly excrete the excess water (up to 10–20 L/day). In order for the kidneys to excrete water there needs to be the following:

- Adequate filtrate reaching the thick ascending loop of Henle (where sodium is extracted to produce a dilute urine). This is impaired in renal failure and hypovolaemia (reduced glomerular filtration rate) or reduced effective circulating volume such as in cardiac failure.
- Adequate active reabsorption of sodium at the loop of Henle and distal convoluted tubule, this is impaired by all diuretics.

- A collecting duct that is impermeable to water, so that dilute urine is excreted. ADH acts on the collecting duct to make it permeable. Any cause of raised ADH will increase water reabsorption and hence tend to cause hyponatraemia. ADH is increased in SIADH, hypovolaemia, reduced effective circulating volume (e.g. cardiac failure, nephrotic syndrome), postoperatively (pain and stress), and increased ADH activity is caused by certain drugs. Lack of glucocorticoid can also cause increased permeability of the collecting duct, because cortisol inhibits ADH.
- In psychogenic polydipsia, patients drink such large volumes of water that the ability of the kidney to excrete it is exceeded. In chronic alcoholics who are malnourished, the renal ability to excrete free water may be markedly impaired due to lack of dietary solutes to as little as 4 L a day and any excess fluid may cause hyponatraemia.

As serum sodium levels fall, water moves from the extracellular compartment into cells. The brain is most sensitive to this and if hyponatraemia occurs rapidly oedema develops, leading to raised intracranial pressure, brainstem herniation and death. If hyponatraemia develops more slowly, the cells can offset the change in osmolality by extrusion of organic solutes. This reduces the degree of water movement and there is less cerebral oedema. When treatment is initiated, if serum sodium levels are corrected too rapidly in a patient who has had chronic hyponatraemia, cell shrinkage can occur due to movement of water out of the cells, causing more damage.

Clinical features

Symptoms of hyponatraemia include lethargy, anorexia, nausea, vomiting, fatigue, headache, confusion and a decreased conscious state. The severity depends on the degree of hyponatraemia and the rapidity at which it develops. In severe cases, the patient may have seizures or become comatose. It is important to take a careful drug history, including the use of any illicit drugs such as heroin or ecstasy. There may be symptoms and signs of fluid depletion or fluid overload (see page 2).

Investigations

To determine the cause of hyponatraemia the following tests are needed: the plasma osmolality, urine osmolality and urine sodium concentration.

- Plasma osmolality is low in most cases of hyponatraemia. If it is normal or high, this is pseudohyponatraemia, which may be due to abnormally high lipid levels or the presence of other osmotically active agents in the blood such as glucose (hyperglycaemia). In these cases treatment is aimed at the underlying cause.
- Urine osmolality helps to differentiate the causes of hyponatraemia with a low plasma osmolality. If there is raised ADH secretion (as in most cases) the urine remains concentrated at $\geq$300 mosmol/kg. If the urine is dilute, this suggests psychogenic polydipsia or excessive inappropriate intravenous dextrose or dextrosaline.
- Urine sodium concentration is low ($\leq$20 mmol/L) in hypovolaemia (although it is falsely raised by diuretic therapy or if there is renal salt-wasting). Fluid repletion should lead to the production of dilute urine (low osmolality) with higher sodium concentrations. However, in SIADH, the urine remains concentrated despite a low plasma osmolality.

In addition, thyroid function tests and cortisol should be checked as there are often multifactorial causes in hyponatraemia and leaving these conditions undetected and untreated is potentially life-threatening. A short Synacthen test (see page 441) may also be indicated.

Management

In all cases, treating the underlying cause successfully will lead to a return to normal values.
- Fluid depletion is treated with saline or colloid replacement.
- Water overload is best treated by fluid restriction to as little as <1 L/day but in severe cases diuretics with hypertonic saline may be given. Mannitol can be used to reduce cerebral oedema. Anticonvulsants may be necessary to treat fits.
- In salt and water overload, continued diuretics with water restriction are used. Intravenous saline should be avoided and patients must adhere to a low-sodium diet. In severe nephrotic syndrome with oedema, intravenous albumin may be required together with diuretics.

Prognosis

Acute severe symptomatic hyponatraemia has a mortality as high as 50%. Chronic symptomatic hyponatraemia has a mortality of up to 12%, but asymptomatic hyponatraemia has a good outcome.

Potassium balance

Almost all of the body's potassium stores are intracellular, with a high concentration of potassium maintained in the intracellular fluid by the Na^+-K^+-ATPase pump exchanging it for sodium. This is important in maintaining cellular membrane potential and small changes in the extracellular potassium level affect the normal function of cells, particularly of muscle cells, e.g. myocardium and skeletal muscle.

Various factors can act to change total body stores of potassium:
- Intake can be increased by a potassium-rich diet or by oral or intravenous supplements.
- Potassium is found in high levels in gastric juice and most of this is reabsorbed in the small intestine. A small amount of potassium is lost in the stool. Vomiting or diarrhoea can reduce total body potassium.
- The kidneys are the main route of excretion of potassium, excreting 90% of the intake. Potassium excretion by the kidneys is controlled by aldosterone, which acts on the distal tubules and collecting ducts to increase sodium reabsorption and potassium excretion. Disturbances of the renin–angiotensin–aldosterone system can therefore cause alterations in the potassium level. In severe renal failure, when 90% of the renal function is lost, the kidneys become unable to excrete sufficient potassium.

The normal intracellular to extracellular ratio of potassium is affected by acid–base status, insulin, catecholamines, aldosterone and drugs.

In most tissues, including the kidney, potassium and hydrogen ions compete with each other at the cell membrane to be exchanged for sodium. If the hydrogen concentration is high (acidotic conditions), the kidney excretes hydrogen ions in preference to potassium; in the tissues, hydrogen ions compete with potassium to be taken up by the cells, so extracellular potassium concentration rises (hyperkalaemia). As the acidosis is corrected, potassium is taken up by the cells and may cause hypokalaemia. Conversely, in metabolic alkalosis potassium is excreted in exchange for hydrogen ions, leading to hypokalaemia.

Insulin and activation of β_2 receptors tend to drive potassium into cells, lowering the serum potassium concentration.

Hyperkalaemia

Definition
A serum potassium level of >5.5 mmol/L is defined as hyperkalaemia. Hyperkalaemia of >6.0 mmol/L can cause cardiac arrhythmias and sudden death without warning.

Incidence
This is a common problem, affecting as many as 1 in 10 inpatients.

Aetiology
The causes are given in Table 1.2.

Pathophysiology
Hyperkalaemia lowers the resting potential, shortens the cardiac action potential and speeds up repolarisation, therefore predisposing to cardiac arrhythmias. The rapidity of onset of hyperkalaemia often influences the risk of cardiac arrhythmias, such that patients with a chronically high potassium level are asymptomatic at much greater levels.

Clinical features
Hyperkalaemia is almost always asymptomatic and only diagnosed on blood testing. There may be a history of conditions that predispose to hyperkalaemia and it is important to take a careful drug history. Foods high in potassium include bananas, citrus fruits, tomatoes and salt substitutes. The first indication of hyperkalaemia

Table 1.2 Causes of hyperkalaemia*

Increased intake	Transcellular movement	Decreased output
Excess K⁺ therapy: (oral or i.v.)	Acidosis	Renal failure
Diet	Insulin deficiency	Drugs e.g. K⁺
Massive	β-blockers	sparing
transfusion of	Haemolysis	diuretics, ACE
stored blood	Rhabdomyolysis	inhibitors
	Digoxin toxicity	Addison's disease

*Artefactual hyperkalaemia may occur in old or haemolysed blood samples.

may be a cardiac arrhythmia or sudden cardiac arrest. Uncommonly there may be reduced tendon reflexes and muscle power.

Investigations
U&Es, calcium, magnesium to look for evidence of renal impairment and any associated abnormality in sodium, calcium and magnesium. Low calcium can increase the risk of arrhythmia. An arterial blood gas to look for acidosis may be indicated and diabetics should have their glucose checked.

An ECG should be performed immediately in all cases. Abnormalities occur in the following order: tall, tented T-waves, small P-wave and a widened, abnormal QRS complex. Patients may develop bradycardia or complete heart block, and if left untreated may die from ventricular standstill or fibrillation. Continuous ECG monitoring should occur until the hyperkalaemia is treated and ECG abnormalities resolve.

Management
Ideally hyperkalaemia should be prevented in at-risk patients by regular monitoring of serum levels and care with medication and intravenous supplements. Once hyperkalaemia is diagnosed, withdraw any potassium supplements or causative drugs.

If the hyperkalaemia is mild (<6.0 mmol/L) and the ECG is normal, withdrawal of causative drugs or treatment of the underlying cause may be sufficient. Moderate asymptomatic hyperkalaemia (6.0–6.9 mmol/L) needs early specific treatment. If there are ECG changes, severe muscle weakness or the potassium level is >7 mmol/L, it is a medical emergency:

- Calcium gluconate is given intravenously. The calcium provides some immediate cardio-protection by reducing myocardial excitability, even in a patient with normal serum calcium levels. It can be repeated after a few minutes if the abnormalities on ECG persist.
- Until treatment of the underlying cause can take place, a glucose and insulin infusion promotes intracellular K⁺ uptake. Salbutamol nebulisers have a similar effect through β receptor stimulation. These can be repeated whilst the underlying cause is addressed, but have only a temporary effect.
- Diuretics, e.g. loop diuretics can be used to increase renal excretion. Oral ion-exchange resins or enemas

may be used to increase gastrointestinal elimination of potassium. Oral resins can cause severe constipation, so these should be given with laxatives and are not a long-term solution.

- Any acidosis should be corrected.
- Refer to a renal physician or intensive care unit for haemofiltration or haemodialysis if the hyperkalaemia is refractory to treatment or if there is severe renal failure.

Hypokalaemia

Definition

A serum potassium level of <3.5 mmol/L. Moderate hypokalemia is defined as a level of 2.5–3 mmol/L and severe as <2.5 mmol/L.

Incidence

This is a very common problem, occurring in up to 20% of inpatients.

Aetiology

The most common cause is diuretics. Other causes are given in Table 1.3.

Pathophysiology

Hypokalaemia causes disturbance of neuromuscular function by altering the resting potential and slowing

Table 1.3 Causes of hypokalaemia

Decreased intake	Transcellular movement	Increased output
Usually iatrogenic: lack of oral intake or i.v. replacement	Alkalosis Insulin treatment	Renal losses: diuretics, low serum magnesium, renal tubular acidosis
		GI losses: vomiting, diarrhoea, purgative abuse, intestinal fistula, ileal loop
Malnutrition		Conn's/Cushing's syndrome and 2° hyperaldosteronism
		Ectopic ACTH (e.g. small lung carcinoma)
		Liquorice abuse, carbenoxolone
		Drugs: β agonists, steroids, theophylline

repolarisation. This causes muscle weakness including the respiratory muscles and ECG changes (see below) predisposing to atrial and ventricular arrhythmias. In severe hypokalaemia sudden cardiac or respiratory arrest may occur. Other effects include the following:

- Metabolic alkalosis: In hypokalaemia there is reduced potassium secretion into the renal tubules and increased reabsorption at the H^+/K^+ ATPase pump so more H^+ ions are lost. Hypokalaemia can both cause and maintain a metabolic alkalosis. Alkalosis also tends to promote the movement of K^+ into cells, worsening the effective hypokalaemia.
- Increased digoxin toxicity: Digoxin acts by inhibition of the Na^+/K^+ ATPase pump. In low-potassium states the effect of digoxin is increased, thereby increasing the risk of toxicity even at normal digoxin levels.

Clinical features

Hypokalaemia is often asymptomatic even when severe and is therefore frequently diagnosed on incidental blood testing. Symptoms include skeletal muscle weakness, muscle cramps, constipation, nausea or vomiting and polyuria. Neuropsychiatric symptoms include confusion, hallucinations, depression and even psychotic features. It is important to take a careful drug history. On examination the patient may be hypotensive and there may be evidence of cardiac arrhythmias such as bradycardia, tachycardia or ectopic beats. There may be reduced muscle strength, fasciculations or tetany. The first sign may be cardiorespiratory arrest.

Investigations

Apart from checking the serum potassium, U&Es, calcium and magnesium should be sent to look for other electrolyte abnormalities. An arterial blood gas may be indicated to look for alkalosis. The ECG shows prolonged PR interval, depressed ST segment, flattened or inverted T-wave and rarely a prominent U-wave (which appears as a long QT interval). Ventricular/atrial premature contractions or fibrillation may be seen or torsades de pointes.

Management

If severe hypokalaemia or cardiac arrhythmias are present, urgent treatment is required. Treat any life-threatening arrhythmias appropriately and give intravenous potassium with continuous cardiac monitoring.

The highest rate of administration of potassium recommended in severe hypokalaemia is 20 mmol/h: this is higher than the usual rate of 10 mmol/h recommended in mild to moderate hypokalaemia. In asymptomatic patients with mild-to-moderate hypokalaemia oral or intravenous potassium supplements are given. The serum potassium must be rechecked frequently, e.g. every 4 hours. Any underlying cause should be looked for and managed appropriately.

Intravenous fluids

Intravenous fluids may be necessary for rapid fluid replacement, e.g. in a shocked patient, or for maintenance in patients who are unable to eat and drink or who are unable to maintain adequate intake in the face of large losses, e.g. due to diarrhoea. When prescribing intravenous fluids certain points should be remembered:

- Are intravenous fluids the best form of fluid replacement? If possible, oral fluids are preferable or if swallow is impaired consider nasogastric administration, which has the advantage of allowing nasogastric feed to be given to provide nutrition.
- Which intravenous fluid should be given? Ideally this should be the one that matches any fluid and electrolyte deficit or losses most closely. For example, blood loss should be replaced with a blood transfusion and salt and water loss (e.g. vomiting, diarrhoea) with normal saline. Additional potassium replacement is often needed in bowel obstruction, but may be dangerous in renal failure.
- In calculating the volume required for maintenance check if is there increased insensible loss, e.g. due to sweating in pyrexial patients, or are there other fluids being administered which need to be taken into account? For example, some patients are on intravenous drugs or intravenous nutritional supplements (total parenteral nutrition).
- Patients at risk of cardiac failure (elderly, cardiac disease, liver or renal impairment) require special caution as they are more prone to develop fluid overload.

There is no universally applicable fluid regimen. The choice of fluid given and the rate of administration depend on the patient, any continued losses and all patients must have continued assessment of their fluid balance using fluid balance charts, observations and clinical examination as well as monitoring of serum electrolytes by serial blood tests.

Fluid preparations: Intravenous fluid has to be isotonic to lysis of red blood cells. The administration of water alone would lead to water moving across cell membranes by osmosis, such that the cells would swell up and burst. Giving hypertonic fluid is equally dangerous, as it causes water to move out of cells.

- Most intravenous fluids used are crystalloids (saline, dextrose, combined dextrose/saline, Hartmann's solution). It should be remembered that dextrose is rapidly metabolised by the liver; hence giving dextrose solution is the equivalent of giving water to the extracellular fluid compartment. If insufficient sodium is given in conjunction, or the kidneys do not excrete the free water, hyponatraemia results. This is a common problem, often because of inappropriate use of dextrose or dextrosaline and because stress from trauma or surgery as well as diseases such as cardiac failure promote antidiuretic hormone (ADH) release. This leads to a mild form of syndrome of inappropriate antidiuretic hormone (SIADH; see page 444) where there is water retention by the kidneys with resulting hyponatraemia.
- Colloids (albumin, dextran or gelatin-based fluids) contain high-molecular-weight components that tend to be retained in the intravascular compartment. This increases the colloid osmotic pressure (oncotic pressure) of the circulation and draws fluid back into the vascular compartment from the extracellular space. A smaller volume of colloid compared to crystalloid is needed to have the same haemodynamic effect. Theoretically they are of benefit for rapid expansion of the intravascular compartment; however, they have anticoagulant, antiplatelet and fibrinolytic effects, which may be undesirable. There has been no consistent demonstrable benefit of using colloid over crystalloid in most circumstances. In addition, the use of albumin solution in hypoalbuminaemic patients (which seems logical) has been associated with increased pulmonary oedema, possibly due to rapid haemodynamic changes or capillary leakage of albumin.

Fluid regimens: These should consist of maintenance fluids (which covers normal urinary, stool and insensible losses) and replacement fluids for additional losses and to correct any pre-existing dehydration. Fluid regimens must also take into account that patients of differing

Table 1.4 Maintenance fluid requirements

Fluid requirement	30–35 mL/kg/day
Sodium requirement	1.5–2 mmol/kg/day
Potassium requirement	1 mmol/kg/day

weight have different fluid and electrolyte requirements (see Table 1.4). Potassium is added to intravenous fluids in patients who are not being fed, although this should be done with care. Both hypokalaemia and hyperkalaemia (see page 7) are potentially life-threatening and serum potassium must be checked daily in patients who are given potassium replacement. Patients with acute or chronic renal failure should not have potassium added routinely to fluid replacement (although hypokalaemia should of course be treated). Rapid administration of potassium is dangerous, so even in hypokalaemia no more than 10 mmol/h is recommended (except in severe hypokalaemia within an intensive care setting) and the potassium must be uniformly mixed in the bag.

A typical daily maintenance regime for a 70 kg man with normal cardiac and renal function consists of 8 hourly bags of:
- 1 L of 0.9% saline with 20 mmol KCl added,
- 1 L of 5% dextrose with 20 mmol KCl added and
- 1 L of 5% dextrose with 20 mmol KCl added.

In general, dextrosaline is not suitable for maintenance, as it provides insufficient sodium and tends to cause hyponatraemia. Postoperative patients are also more prone to hyponatraemia due to mild SIADH, so may require proportionally more sodium, e.g. 2 L of 0.9% saline to 1 L of 5% dextrose. Replacement fluids generally need to be 0.9% saline, as losses tend to have a high sodium concentration, e.g. drain fluid, blood, vomitus and diarrhoea.

Fluids should not be prescribed without taking into account the patient's current fluid balance, continued losses and underlying coexistent diseases. It should also be remembered that intravenous fluids do not provide any significant nutrition.

Acid–base balance

The normal pH of arterial blood is 7.35–7.45. Normally hydrogen (H^+) ions are buffered by two main systems:
- Proteins including haemoglobin comprise a fixed buffering system.

- Bicarbonate is a very important buffer, as it has both a gaseous and an aqueous phase:

$$CO_2 \leftrightarrow CO_2 + H_2O \leftrightarrow H_2CO_3 \leftrightarrow H^+ + HCO_3{}^-$$

This means that bicarbonate buffering is a very powerful way of maintaining the body's pH through both rapid and slow compensation:
- Rapid compensation takes place at the lungs, where CO_2 can be blown off in response to acidosis. This reduces the amount of H_2CO_3 (carbonic acid) in the blood as shown by the equation and so acutely compensates for acidosis. Conversely, if pCO_2 concentrations rise, e.g. in hypoventilation, then acidosis can result (respiratory acidosis).
- In long-term abnormalities of pH balance, this mechanism is inadequate because the body's stores of bicarbonate become depleted. The kidney is able to compensate for this, by increasing its reabsorption of bicarbonate in the proximal tubule.

The arterial blood gas is used to assess acid–base status. The pH is first examined to see if the patient is acidotic or alkalotic. The pCO_2 and bicarbonate are then examined to identify the cause of any acid–base disturbance and any compensation that may have occurred. Most arterial blood gas machines also provide the base excess. This is a calculated figure, which provides an estimate of the metabolic component of the acid–base balance. The base excess is defined as the amount of H^+ ions that would be required to return the pH of the blood to 7.35, if the pCO_2 were adjusted to normal. A normal base excess is –2 to +2. A more negative base excess signifies a metabolic acidosis (hydrogen ions need to be removed) and a more positive base excess signifies a metabolic alkalosis (hydrogen ions need to be added). The pO_2 is examined separately to determine if there is respiratory failure.

There are four main patterns:
- Acidosis with high pCO_2 defines a respiratory acidosis. If this is acute, there is no compensation (i.e. the bicarbonate levels are normal). In chronic respiratory acidosis renal reabsorption of bicarbonate will reduce the acidosis (partial metabolic compensation) or return the pH to a normal level (complete metabolic compensation). Causes include respiratory failure (see page 127).
- Acidosis with low bicarbonate and negative base excess defines a metabolic acidosis. If the patient is able the respiration will increase to reduce carbon dioxide and hence return the pH to normal (partial or complete

respiratory compensation). Causes of metabolic acidosis include salicylate poisoning (see page 528), lactic acidosis or diabetic ketoacidosis (see page 460). Alternatively failure to excrete acid or increased loss of HCO_3^-, such as renal tubular disease (see page 251) and diarrhoea. Hyperkalaemia may occur as an important complication (see page 7) particularly if there is also acute renal failure.

- Alkalosis with a low carbon dioxide defines respiratory alkalosis. This may result from any cause of hyperventilation including stroke, subarachnoid haemorrhage, meningitis, pyrexia, hyperthryoidism, pregnancy or anxiety. It is generally an acute condition and so little compensation occurs.
- Alkalosis with a high bicarbonate and a positive base excess defines metabolic alkalosis. It is rare and may be caused by loss of acid from the gastrointestinal tract (e.g. vomiting) or from the kidney (e.g. Cushing or Conn's syndrome). Hypokalaemia may occur (see page 8).

Hypercalcaemia

Definition
A serum calcium level of >2.6 mmol/L.

Incidence
Relatively common.

Aetiology
Important causes of hypercalcaemia are given in Table 1.5. More than 80% of cases are due to malignancy or primary hyperparathyroidism (see page 446).

Pathophysiology
Hypercalcaemia prevents membrane depolarisation leading to central nervous system effects, decreased muscle power and reduced gut mobility. It also has multiple effects on the kidney: it reduces the glomerular filtration rate; it can cause acute or chronic renal failure; it can also cause nephrogenic diabetes insipidus (see page 445), urinary stones (see page 270) and calcium deposition in the kidney and other tissues. Hypercalcaemia causes shortening of the Q–T interval but this is not associated with an increased risk of cardiac arrhythmias.

Clinical features
The condition may be asymptomatic and diagnosed incidentally on calcium measurement. Early symptoms are often insidious, including loss of appetite, fatigue, lethargy, weakness, constipation and thirst. The symptoms of hypercalcaemia can be summarised as bones, stones, moans and groans:

- Bone pain may be due to metastases, multiple myeloma or bone disease as a complication of hyperparathyroidism.
- Urinary stones.
- Moans due to confusion and drowsiness. Depression and acute psychosis can also occur.
- Groans due to abdominal symptoms such as nausea, vomiting, pain and constipation.

Deposition of calcium in heart valves, coronary arteries and other blood vessels may occur. Hypertension is relatively common, possibly due to renal impairment and also related to calcium-induced vasoconstriction.

Table 1.5 Important causes of hypercalcaemia

Increased bone resorption	Increased GI absorption	Decreased output
Hyperparathyroidism	Excess calcium intake (milk-alkali syndrome):	Renal failure
	Calcium supplements	Thiazide diuretics
Malignancy (3 mechanisms):	Antacids	Familial hypocalciuric
Osteolytic metastases	Excess vitamin D:	hypercalcaemia (FHH)
PTH-like peptide	Vitamin D supplements	
Osteoclast activating factors	Increased production of active Vitamin D	
(multiple myeloma, lymphoma)	metabolites occurs in granulomatosis	
Paget's disease	disorders (e.g. sarcoidosis, TB) and in	
Immobilisation	lymphoma	

Investigations

These are aimed at assessing the severity of hypercalcaemia to guide management and to look for the underlying cause. The serum calcium should be checked and corrected for serum albumin because only the ionised calcium (not bound to protein) is active. The total serum calcium is corrected as follows:

$$\text{Corrected calcium} = \text{Measured calcium} + 0.02(40 - \text{serum albumin})$$

- Mild hypercalcaemia (2.6–2.8 mmol/L) is suggestive of primary hyperparathyroidism.
- Moderate to severe hypercalcaemia is more commonly due to malignancy.

Blood should be sent for U&Es (to look for renal impairment), serum protein electrophoresis and Bence Jones protein (to look for myeloma) and a PTH (parathyroid hormone) level. If the PTH level is normal or high, this is diagnostic of hyperparathyroidism because it should be suppressed in hypercalcaemia. A chest X-ray may demonstrate malignancy or sarcoidosis. Serum phosphate may be helpful, as it tends to be low in malignancy or primary hyperparathyroidism but high in other causes. If PTH is low, PTH-like peptide can be measured.

Other tests which may be useful include the following:
- Urinary calcium, which is raised in most causes of hypercalcaemia, but relatively low (<100 mg or 2.5 mmol/day) in milk–alkali syndrome, thiazide diuretic use and FHH.
- Vitamin D and its active metabolites.
- Serum angiotensin converting enzyme (ACE), which may be raised in pulmonary sarcoidosis.

Management

This depends on the severity, whether acute or chronic and the underlying cause. Any causative drugs should be withdrawn.
- Patients should be assessed for fluid status and any dehydration corrected. Rehydration reduces calcium levels by a dilutional effect and by increasing renal clearance. Intravenous saline is often needed because many patients feel too nauseous to tolerate sufficient oral fluids and polyuria is common due to nephrogenic diabetes insipidus.
- Loop diuretics such as furosemide can be used in conjunction with fluids to increase renal excretion of calcium and prevent fluid overload.
- Bisphosphonates can be used, which inhibit bone turnover and therefore reduce serum calcium. Steroids may be used if the underlying diagnosis is a known malignancy, but is less useful if there is ectopic PTH production.
- If there is renal failure, early consultation with a nephrologist is needed, as increased renal excretion of calcium is often impossible or difficult to achieve and dialysis may be required.
- Further management depends on the underlying cause.

Hypocalcaemia

Definition

A serum calcium level of <2.2 mmol/L.

Aetiology

Hypocalcaemia may be caused by
- vitamin D deficiency,
- hypoparathyroidism (after parathyroidectomy, thyroid or other neck surgery),
- pseudohypoparathyroidism,
- magnesium depletion by inducing end-organ PTH resistance or deficiency (causes include diuretics, alcoholism and malnutrition),
- hyperphosphataemia,
- acute pancreatitis and severe sepsis,
- acute respiratory alkalosis,
- drugs, e.g. chemotherapy especially cisplatin, bisphosphonates and
- calcium chelators, e.g. citrate following large transfusions of blood.

Pathophysiology

Hypocalcaemia causes increased membrane potentials, which means that cells are more easily depolarised and therefore causes prolongation of the Q–T interval, which predisposes to cardiac arrhythmias. It may also cause refractory hypotension and neuromuscular problems include tetany, seizures and emotional lability or depression.

Clinical features

The condition may be asymptomatic and diagnosed incidentally on calcium measurement.

Neuromuscular manifestations

Early symptoms include circumoral numbness, paraesthesiae of the extremities and muscle cramps. Common but less specific symptoms include fatigue, irritability, confusion and depression. Myopathy with muscle weakness and wasting may be present. Carpopedal spasm and seizures are signs of severe hypocalcaemia. Elicitation of Trousseau's sign and Chvostek's signs should be attempted, although it can be negative even in severe hypocalcaemia:

- Trousseau's sign: Carpal spasm induced by inflation of a sphygmomanometer above systolic BP for 3 minutes.
- Chvostek's sign: Contraction of the ipsilateral facial muscles (including the eye, nose and corner of the mouth) after tapping the facial nerve anterior to the ear.

The BP may be low despite fluids or inotropes. Cardiac failure may occur.

Other findings may include papilloedema and in chronic cases cataracts, dry puffy coarse skin with brittle and thinned hair and nails.

Investigations

These are aimed at assessing the severity of hypocalcaemia to guide management and to look for the underlying cause. The serum calcium should be checked and corrected for serum albumin (see above). Blood should also be sent for magnesium, phosphate, U&Es and for PTH level. An ECG should be done to look for ECG changes (increased QT interval, cardiac arrhythmias). Other investigations depend on the suspected cause.

Management

This depends on the severity, whether acute or chronic and the underlying cause. Mild hypocalcaemia is treated with oral supplements of calcium and magnesium where appropriate. Severe hypocalcaemia may be life-threatening and the first priority is resuscitation as needed (e.g. management of seizures or cardiac arrhythmias), followed by the administration of intravenous calcium. Calcium gluconate contains only a third of the amount of calcium as calcium chloride but is less irritating to the peripheral veins.

Perioperative care

The preoperative assessment

Underlying any decision to perform surgery is a recognition of the balance between the risk of the procedure and the potential benefits to the patient. All patients undergo a preoperative assessment (history, examination and appropriate investigations) both to review the diagnosis and need for surgery, and to identify any coexisting disease that may increase the likelihood of perioperative complications. In general any concerns regarding coexisting disease or fitness for surgery should be discussed with the anaesthetist who makes the final decision regarding fitness for anaesthesia.

Cardiac disease

Ischaemic heart disease remains the most important risk factor for patients undergoing surgery. It is vital as part of a preoperative assessment to identify underlying cardiac disease by history, examination and, where appropriate, investigations. An ECG should be performed in any patient with a history suggestive of cardiac disease and in all patients over 50 years of age.

- Following a myocardial infarction the risk of re-infarction is maximal over subsequent 6 weeks, if surgery is performed the re-infarction rate increases dramatically. Elective surgery should be deferred by at least 6 months wherever possible.
- Hypertension should be controlled prior to any elective surgery to reduce the risk of myocardial infarction or stroke. Specialist cardiac advice may be required prior to emergency surgery in severely hypertensive patients.
- Arrhythmias should ideally be corrected prior to surgery. Chronic or complex arrhythmias should be discussed with a cardiologist prior to surgery wherever possible.
- Patients with signs and symptoms of cardiac failure should have their therapy optimised prior to surgery and require special attention to perioperative fluid balance.
- Patients with abnormal or prosthetic heart valves, patent ductus arteriosus or septal defects, and patients with a history of bacterial endocarditis should have prophylactic oral or intravenous antibiotic cover for any surgical procedures.

Respiratory disease

- The preoperative assessment should identify coexisting respiratory conditions. Patients must be asked about smoking and where possible should be encouraged to stop smoking at least 6 weeks prior to surgery. Although chest X-rays are often performed as part of the routine assessment of preoperative patients, they should not be relied on to identify underlying respiratory diseases. In general, a chest x-ray is not indicated unless there are acute respiratory signs or severe chronic respiratory disease with no film in the last 12 months.
- Patients with chronic obstructive pulmonary disease (COPD) are at significant risk of postoperative respiratory complications. Patients with severe disease may benefit from a preoperative respiratory opinion and formal respiratory function testing. Preoperatively all therapy should be optimised; pre- and postoperative physiotherapy is essential. Postoperative analgesia should allow pain free ventilation and coughing, to maximise ventilation and reduce the risk of postoperative pneumonia.

Diabetes mellitus

Patients with diabetes are at increased risk perioperatively both from the diabetes itself (hypoglycaemia and ketoacidosis) and from the complications of diabetes (ischaemic heart disease, vascular insufficiency, renal failure and increased risk of infection).

- Diet-controlled diabetics often require no specific intervention, but should have perioperative blood glucose monitoring.
- Patients on oral hypoglycaemic agents should omit their drugs on the morning of surgery (unless undergoing a short day case procedure) and restart when oral diet recommences. Perioperative blood sugar levels should be monitored. In more major surgery, or when patients are to remain nil by mouth for a prolonged period, intravenous dextrose and variable dose intravenous short acting insulin should be considered.
- Insulin-controlled diabetics normally require conversion to intravenous dextrose and variable dose intravenous short acting insulin prior to surgery. Close monitoring of blood sugar and urine for ketones is essential. Once oral diet is recommenced the patient should convert back to regular subcutaneous insulin therapy.

Coagulation disorders

- Deep vein thrombosis, which may be complicated by pulmonary embolism, is a significant postoperative risk. Risk factors include previous history of thromboembolic disease, specific thrombophilic disorders (protein C deficiency, protein S deficiency, factor V Leiden mutations), smoking, obesity, prolonged postoperative immobility, malignancy and drugs such as the combined oral contraceptive pill. Wherever possible, risk factors should be identified and modified (including stopping the combined oral contraceptive pill 4 weeks prior to major surgery). Specific prophylaxis includes subcutaneous low-molecular-weight heparin injections and compression stockings, which should be considered for at-risk patients.
- Bleeding disorders such as haemophilia, use of anticoagulant or antiplatelet medication and chronic liver disease may cause perioperative bleeding. Patients with known coagulation factor or vitamin K deficiencies may require perioperative replacement therapy. Anti-coagulant medication may be reduced, changed or stopped depending on the underlying indication for anticoagulation.

Liver disease

Patients with chronic liver disease may have impaired coagulation (vitamin K and coagulation factor deficiencies), altered metabolism of drugs, increased susceptibility to infection and hypoalbuminaemic oedema. Coagulation deficiencies should be corrected prior to surgery and careful fluid balance is essential. The patient's alcohol intake should be elicited; symptoms of withdrawal from alcohol may occur during a hospital admission.

Renal disease

Pre-existing renal impairment predisposes to the development of acute tubular necrosis. Hypotension should be avoided and urinary output should be monitored so that oliguria can be recognised early and treated.

Emergency surgery

In patients requiring emergency surgery there may not be enough time to identify and correct all coexistent diseases. It is however essential to identify any cardiac, respiratory, metabolic or endocrine disease, which may affect anaesthesia. An ECG, chest X-ray and where appropriate, arterial blood gas analysis should be obtained without additional delay. Any anaemia, fluid and electrolyte imbalance or cardiac failure should be corrected prior to surgery wherever possible.

Prophylactic antibiotics in surgery

Specific guidelines regarding the use of perioperative antibiotic prophylaxis vary between hospitals but these are generally used if there is a significant risk of surgical site infection. They are indicated in most gastrointestinal surgery, neurosurgery, surgery involving insertion of a prosthesis (including joint replacement), transurethral prostate resection, coronary artery bypass surgery and lower limb vascular surgery. Prophylaxis for immunodeficient patients requires expert microbiological advice.

However, it is important to note that antibiotic use is associated with acute hypersensitivity reactions, increasing antibiotic resistance and the development of pseudomembranous colitis (see page 150).

Nutritional support in surgical patients

Significant nutritional deficiency impairs healing, lowers resistance to infection and prolongs the recovery period. Malnutrition may be present preoperatively particularly in the elderly and patients with malignancy. Perioperative nutritional support may be necessary if the patient is unable to maintain sufficient intake to balance the increased postoperative nutritional requirement.

Enteral nutrition is the treatment of choice in all patients with a normal, functioning gastrointestinal tract. It is generally safer than intravenous nutrition and it helps to maintain the integrity of gastrointestinal mucosa. Liquid feeds either as a supplement or replacement may be taken orally, via a nasogastric tube or via a gastrostomy. Liquid feeds may be whole protein, oligopeptide or amino acid based. These also provide glucose, essential fats, electrolytes and minerals.

Parenteral nutrition is indicated when patients cannot maintain a sufficient calorie intake via the enteral route. Indications include intestinal resection, fistulae, motility disorders and extensive small bowel disease. Mixed preparations of amino acid, glucose and lipid are used with trace elements, vitamins and electrolytes also added.

Parenteral nutrition is hypertonic, irritant and thrombogenic. They should ideally be infused through some form of central venous access. Peripheral parenteral nutrition may cause significant injury if extravasation occurs. Other complications of parenteral nutrition include line infection and septicaemia, thrombosis and embolism, liver damage and metabolic disturbance (osmotic diuresis, acute hyperosmolar syndrome and electrolyte imbalances).

Postoperative complications

Postoperative complications may occur at any time post-surgery and include general surgical complications (bleeding, infection, deep vein thrombosis), those specific to the procedure (anastomotic leaks, fistulae, adhesions, wound dehiscence) and complications secondary to coexisting disease (ischaemic heart disease, chronic obstructive airways disease, diabetes mellitus).

Immediate complications arise during the first postoperative day:
- Haemorrhage: Primary haemorrhage refers to continuation of bleeding from surgery. It requires aggressive management and may necessitate return to theatre. Reactive haemorrhage occurs from small vessels, which only begin to bleed as the blood pressure rises postoperatively. Blood replacement may be required and in severe cases the patient may need to return to theatre.
- Myocardial infarction is a significant risk in patients with ischaemic heart disease. Surgery may contraindicate the use of thrombolytic agents.
- A low-grade pyrexia is normal in the immediate postoperative period but may also arise due to infection, collections or deep vein thrombosis.
- Low urine output may occur as a result of volume depletion, renal failure, poor cardiac output or urinary obstruction. The patient may require urinary catheterisation (or flushing of the catheter if already in situ) and a clinical assessment of cardiovascular status including heart rate, blood pressure (including assessment of postural drop), inspection of the JVP, evidence of pulmonary oedema and where needed CVP measurement (see page 3).

Early postoperative complications occur in the subsequent days.
- Deep vein thrombosis and risk of thromboembolism. High-risk patients should receive prophylaxis (see section The Preoperative Assessment). Patients may

present with painful swelling of the legs, low-grade pyrexia or with signs and symptoms of a pulmonary embolism.

- Confusion due to hypoxia, metabolic disturbance, infection, drugs, or withdrawal syndromes.
- General infections include pneumonia secondary to pooling of secretions, urinary tract infections and cannula site infections.
- Surgical site complications include paralytic ileus, anastomotic leaks, surgical site infections (with secondary haemorrhage as a result of the infection), fistula formation and wound dehiscence (total wound breakdown). Intestinal fistulae may be managed conservatively with skin protection, replacement of fluid and electrolytes and parenteral nutrition. If such conservative therapy fails the fistula may be closed surgically.
- Postoperative hypoxia is almost always initially due to perioperative atelectasis unless a respiratory infection was present preoperatively. Prophylaxis and treatment involves adequate analgesia, physiotherapy and humidification of administered gases. Respiratory failure may occur secondary to airway obstruction. Laryngeal spasm/oedema may occur in epiglottitis or following traumatic intubation. Tracheal compression may complicate operations in the head and neck. In the absence of obstruction hypoxia may result from drugs causing respiratory depression, infection, pulmonary embolism or exacerbation of pre-existing respiratory disease. Respiratory support may be necessary.
- Acute renal failure may result from inadequate perfusion, drugs, or pre-existing renal or liver disease. Once hypovolaemia has been corrected any remaining renal impairment requires specialist renal support.
- Prolonged immobility increases the risk of pressure sores especially in patients with diabetes or vascular insufficiency. Skin care, hygiene, turning of the patient and the use of specialised mattresses should prevent pressure sores. Treatment involves debridement, treatment of any infection, application of zinc paste and in severe cases, plastic surgery.

Late postoperative complications, which may occur weeks or years after surgery, include adhesions, strictures and incisional hernias.

Surgical site infection

Definition
Surgical site infections include superficial site infections (skin and subcutaneous tissues), deep site infections (involving fascia and muscle layers) and organ or space infections (such as abscess, bone infections, etc).

Aetiology
Superficial and deep site infections occur due to *Staphylococcus aureus* (including MRSA), *Staphylococcus epidermidis* (specific association with prosthetic material including cannulae) and *Streptococci* or mixed organisms. The organisms responsible for organ or space infections are dependent on the site and the nature of the surgical condition, e.g. anaerobic organisms in bowel perforation or anastomotic leaks, *Streptococci* and *Staphylococci* in bone infections. The risk of surgical site infection is dependent on the procedure performed. Contaminated wounds such as in emergency treatment for bowel perforation carry a very high risk of infection.

Patients at particular risk include the elderly, malnourished, immunodeficient and those with diabetes mellitus.

Clinical features
Superficial infections appear as a cellulitis (redness, warmth, swelling and tenderness) around the wound margin, there may be associated lymphadenopathy. It may be of value to draw round the area of erythema to monitor progression and response to treatment. Deeper infections and collections may present as pyrexia with few external signs. Specific presentations depend on the site, e.g. peritonitis or pus discharging from surgical drains.

Complications
Localised infections, especially in high-risk patients may spread to cause generalised septicaemia and septic shock. Wound dehiscence (total wound breakdown) is rare. It is preceded by a high volume serous discharge from the wound site and necessitates surgical repair.

Investigations
Pyrexial patients require investigations. Paired aerobic and anaerobic blood cultures should be taken (preferably

during pyrexial episodes) and any pus or wound discharge sent for microscopy and culture. Patients with pyrexia and no obvious localising signs or symptoms may require imaging such as ultrasound, CT scanning or isotope bone scanning to identify the source of infection.

Management
- Prophylaxis against infection includes meticulous surgical technique and the use of prophylactic antibiotics. Severely contaminated wounds may be closed by delayed primary suture. Contaminated cavities, such as the abdomen, require the placement of surgical drains.
- Where possible the underlying cause of the infection should be treated, e.g. removal of infected material, closure of anastomotic leaks.
- Superficial surgical site infections may respond to antibiotics (penicillin and flucloxacillin, depending on local policy). Deeper surgical site infections may require the removal of one or more skin sutures to allow drainage of infected material. Abscesses generally require drainage either by surgery or radiologically guided aspiration alongside the use of appropriate antibiotics.

Pain control

Many medical and surgical patients experience pain. Surgery causes tissue damage leading to the release of local chemical mediators that stimulate pain fibres. In addition direct damage to nerves can cause pain. Ischaemia, obstruction, infections, inflammation and joint disease also cause pain. Cancer is an important cause of pain. Pain may be induced by movement, which is sometimes unavoidable, e.g. the thorax and abdominal wall when breathing. In contrast, immobility can cause pain due to pressure sores and joint stiffness. In addition, a patient's perception of pain is altered by many factors, including the patient's overall physical and emotional well-being, cultural background, age, sex and ability to sleep adequately. Depression and fear often worsen the perception of pain.

Types of pain
Tissue damage causes a nociceptive pain, which can be further divided into a sharp, stabbing pain, which is conveyed by the finely myelinated Aδ fibres, and a dull,

throbbing, 'slow' pain, which is conveyed by the larger non-myelinated C fibres. Nociceptive pain is usually acute, tends to resolve as tissue heals and responds well to opioid analgesia (see below). Injury or abnormal function within the nervous system causes neuropathic pain. It is felt as an area of burning or a shooting pain. It may be triggered by non-painful stimuli such as light touch, so-called allodynia. Examples of causes include postherpetic neuralgia, peripheral neuropathy, e.g. due to diabetes, and phantom limb pain. Neuropathic pain is often difficult to treat, partly because of its chronic but episodic nature and it is less responsive to opiates. Most of the time, pain has both nociceptive and neuropathic components.

Benefits of treating pain
The principal reason for treating pain is to relieve suffering. It improves patients' ability to sleep and their overall emotional health. However, good pain control can also have other benefits: postoperatively it can improve respiratory function, increase the ability to cough and clear secretions, improve mobility and hence reduce the risk of complications such as pneumonia and deep vein thromboses. This allows a faster recovery.

Assessing pain
To diagnose and then treat pain first requires asking the patients about their pain. Often, if pain is treated aggressively and early, it is easier to control than when the patient becomes distressed and exhausted. Patients should be asked to score their pain on a scale from none to very severe (sometimes a 10-point scale is useful, where 0 represents no pain and 10 the worst imaginable pain). In some cases where verbal communication is not possible or difficult, a visual scale of 1–10 or pictures of faces representing degrees of pain is useful. They should be asked what precipitates pain, such as movement or breathing, and whether the pain prevents or interrupts sleep. It is important to establish whether the pain is nociceptive, neuropathic or both. Often there is more than one pain and these may require separate treatment plans.

In a patient who is already taking analgesia, it is useful to assess their current use, the effect on pain and any side-effects. The patient should also be asked about his or her beliefs about drugs they have been given before. The patients should be involved as far as possible in the management of their pain. Adverse effects such as nausea and constipation are predictable, patients should be alerted to these and provided with means by which these can be treated early.

The WHO ladder of analgesia

The World Health Organisation analgesia ladder is a method for choosing appropriate analgesia depending on the severity of pain. It was originally developed for cancer patients but is useful for many types of pain. Initially, analgesia may be given on an as needed basis, but if frequent doses are required, regular doses should be given, so that each dose is given before the effect of the previous dose wears off. A combination of different drugs often improves the pain relief with fewer adverse effects. After analgesia is initiated, if it is ineffective at maximal dose, the next step on the ladder is tried. Certain drugs are contraindicated or used with caution in patients with co-morbidities. Postoperative patients may descend the ladder, as severe pain is expected immediately after tissue damage and this pain reduces as healing takes place.

STEP 1 (Mild pain): Non-opioid analgesia is used, such as paracetamol or an NSAID. These may be given orally or rectally.

STEP 2 (Mild to moderate pain): Weak opioids such as codeine, dihydrocodeine or tramadol orally or intramuscularly are added to regular paracetamol or an NSAID.

STEP 3 (Moderate to severe pain): Strong opioid analgesia such as morphine or diamorphine is used.

Modes of delivery of opioids

The oral route is preferred for most patients, but for patients unable to take oral medication or for rapid relief of acute pain, intramuscular or intravenous boluses are faster acting and more suitable. The disadvantage of boluses for continued pain is that often there is a delay between the patient experiencing pain and analgesia being given. In intensive care settings or terminal care a continuous infusion by a syringe driver may be appropriate, but with any continuous delivery system there is a risk of accidental overdose, so regular monitoring of pain score, sedation score and respiratory rate is needed. In stable patients with severe ongoing pain, a transdermal patch may be suitable. These release opioid in a controlled manner, usually over 72 hours.

Patient-controlled analgesia (PCA) is a system by which the patients can determine the frequency of dosing of their analgesia. A loading dose is given first, then the patient presses a button to deliver subsequent small boluses of intravenous opioid. The PCA pump has a lockout time usually set at 5–10 minutes, which allows time for each dose to take effect before another dose can be given. This prevents respiratory depression due to accidental overdose by the patient repeatedly pressing the button. If the patient becomes overly sedated, the delivery of opioid ceases. If patients are not adequately analgesed, the bolus dose is increased. This system is not suitable for patients who are too unwell or confused to understand the system and be able to press the button.

Local and regional anaesthetic

Local anaesthetic is useful perioperatively. It is often given around the wound or as a regional nerve block to provide several hours of pain relief. Spinal anaesthesia is useful for surgery of the lower half of the body. Postoperatively, continued analgesia using an epidural catheter to administer boluses or a continuous infusion is useful. Usually a combination of local anaesthetic with an opioid is used. The advantage of epidural analgesia is that there is good pain control with a lesser risk of the systemic side-effects of opioids. However, complications include hypotension due to sympathetic block, urinary retention and motor weakness. Patients require specialist care and monitoring on a ward accustomed to the management of patients with epidurals.

Co-analgesics

These are other drugs that are not primarily analgesics, but can help to relieve pain. In particular, neuropathic pain is relatively insensitive to opioids; drugs such as antidepressants and anticonvulsants are more effective, e.g. amitryptiline or gabapentin. Tramadol is a weak opioid that has some action at adrenergic and serotonin receptors and so may be useful for combination nociceptive and neuropathic pain. Muscle spasm often responds to benzodiazepines.

Non-pharmacological treatment

In addition to prescribing analgesia, it is important to consider other methods that relieve pain, such as treating the underlying cause, immobilising a painful joint with a splint, mobilising joints for stiffness and treating concomitant depression. Acupuncture, local heat or ice, massage and transcutaneous electrical nerve stimulation (TENS) can often help with pain.

Infections

Nosocomial infections

Infections acquired during a hospital stay are called nosocomial infections. Usually an infection is considered to be nosocomial if it arises >72 hours after admission, as earlier infections are usually presumed to have been acquired in the community. For patients who are only briefly admitted the infection may only become manifest after discharge.

Approximately 10% of patients admitted to a hospital in the United Kingdom acquire a nosocomial infection. Infections may be spread by droplet inhalation or direct hand contact from hospital staff or equipment. The patients most at risk are those at extremes of age, those with significant co-morbidity, the immunosuppressed and those with recent surgery. Risk factors also depend on the site, for example pneumonia is more common in patients who are ventilated, who are bedbound or who have had thoracic or abdominal surgery. Instrumentation such as urinary catheterisation or central lines can introduce infections.

The commonest sites of nosocomial infections are
- urinary tract infections,
- respiratory tract infections,
- surgical site infections (see page 16),
- bacteraemia,
- skin infections, e.g. of burns and
- gastrointestinal infections.

Nosocomial infections are most commonly bacterial, particularly *Staph. aureus, Pseudomonas* and *Escherichia coli. Clostridium difficile* is a common cause of diarrhoea in patients given broad-spectrum antibiotics (see page 150). Viruses are also important, e.g. small round structured viruses (SRSV), which have caused outbreaks of diarrhoea in some hospitals, influenza and other respiratory infections can affect patients and staff alike (as dramatically highlighted by the outbreak of SARS in 2003). Fungi, particularly *Candida* and *Aspergillus*, are also becoming more important.

Many of the pathogens that cause nosocomial infections have a high level of antibiotic resistance, which is a major cause of concern. Some examples include the following:

- Methicillin resistant *Staph. aureus* (MRSA) is resistant to flucloxacillin and most other commonly used anti *Staphylococcal* agents. It is treated by vancomycin or teicoplanin. Nasal colonisation and skin clearance is achieved by topical cream and antiseptic washes.
- Vancomycin resistant *Enterococcus* (VRE) is increasingly common.
- Vancomycin-intermediate/resistant *Staph. aureus* (VISA/VRSA) emerged with cases of VISA in the late 1990s and VRSA in 2002. It is still rare, but of concern. It is also called GISA (glycopeptide-intermediate SA) because vancomycin is a glycopeptide.

Prevention of nosocomial infections

The principles are to avoid transmission by always washing hands after examining a patient, strict aseptic care of central lines and isolation of cases in a side-room or even by ward. Certain patients are given prophylactic antibiotics, e.g. preoperatively, where possible indwelling urinary catheters or central lines should be avoided or the duration of use minimised. Early mobilisation and discharge also help to reduce the period of risk. Once patients are identified as having diarrhoea or being infected with resistant organisms they should be barrier nursed in a separate room. Staff and visitors should wear gloves, aprons and where appropriate masks whilst in the room, and disinfect their hands following the visit with alcohol gel. Patients at high risk because of neutropenia are also isolated and reverse barrier nursed to try to protect them from exposure to infections.

In addition, overuse of antibiotics particularly broad-spectrum antibiotics should be avoided. Where the development of resistance is likely, combination antibiotics are used.

Pyrexia of unknown origin (PUO)

Definition

An intermittent or continuous fever >38°C lasting more than 3 weeks and without diagnosis despite initial investigations.

Aetiology

See Table 1.6.

Table 1.6 Causes of pyrexia of unknown origin

Cause	%	Examples
Infection	30–40	*Bacterial infections* – bacterial endocarditis, abscess (e.g. intra-abdominal), hepatobiliary infection, urinary tract infection, osteomyelitis, typhoid fever, tuberculosis, brucellosis, Lyme disease, syphilis *Viral infections* – cytomegalovirus infection, Epstein–Barr virus, HIV infection Fungal infections – *Candida albicans,* Cryptococcus *Protozoal infections* – malaria, toxoplasmosis
Neoplasia	20–30	Renal cell carcinoma, hepatocellular carcinoma, disseminated carcinoma, lymphomas, atrial myxoma
Rheumatological Disorders	10–20	Rheumatoid arthritis, SLE, vasculitis (polymyalgia rheumatica, temporal arteritis, polyarteritis nodosum)
Miscellaneous	15–20	Drugs, thyrotoxicosis, Crohn's disease, sarcoidosis, occult haematoma
No diagnosis	5–15	

Clinical features

A careful history, including systematic review is essential.

- Pattern and duration of fever (although the correlation between fever patterns and specific diseases is weak), weight loss, night sweats, headaches, rashes and any other symptoms.
- Previous illnesses including operations and psychiatric illnesses.
- Specific factors including family history, immunisation status, occupational history, travel history, history of consumption of unusual foods (e.g. unpasteurised milk), drug history (including over-the-counter medications, homeopathic preparations, drugs of abuse), sexual history, infectious contacts and animal contacts (including possible exposure to ticks and other vectors).

A full systematic examination is required including the following:

- Documentation of pattern and duration of fever.
- Specific features include rashes, lymphadenopathy, genitoperitoneal lesions, organomegaly, new or changing cardiac murmurs, signs of arthritis, abdominal tenderness or rigidity and a neurological evaluation including fundoscopy.

Investigations

1 Initial investigations: close monitoring of temperature; chest X-ray; urine for urinalysis, microscopy, culture and sensitivity; full blood count and peripheral blood film; repeated blood cultures taken at times of fever; culture of wounds, intravenous lines and other relevant sites, e.g. CSF; urea, creatinine, electrolytes and blood sugar; creatine kinase and liver function tests; C-reactive protein, ESR and immunoglobulins.

2 Specific blood tests and microbiology may be required for certain indications:
- Malarial exposure: Repeated thick and thin blood films, antigen testing.
- Intravenous drug use or at risk: Hepatitis serology, HIV testing.
- Suspected thyrotoxicosis: Thyroid function testing.
- Suspected rheumatological disorder: ANA, anti-DNA antibody, ANCA.
- Specific agent suspected: Serial titres for EBV, CMV, influenza, Toxoplasma, Lyme disease, chlamydia, salmonella, *Borrelia recurrentis*, Q fever, leptospirosis.

3 Other procedures that may also be considered are
- abdominal ultrasound for intra-hepatic, subphrenic or paracolic abscesses.
- white cell scan for demonstration of an abscess, empyema or osteomyelitis.
- bone scan for osteomyelitis or metastatic bone disease.
- CT and MRI for lymphoma, tumours or abscesses.
- transoesophageal echocardiography for infective endocarditis or atrial myxoma.
- bone marrow biopsy for leukaemia or culture for miliary TB.
- biopsy either endoscopically or percutaneously of suspected area.

Management

Blind treatment should be avoided unless the patient is septicaemic or deteriorating. In such cases a best guess of the cause and hence the antibiotic cover has to be made depending on the results of history, examination and investigations available. It is essential to continue regular reassessment for new symptoms or signs and to stop all other drugs wherever possible.

Septicaemia and septic shock

Definitions
Bacteria in the blood can produce a wide spectrum of clinical entities from mild physiological abnormalities to septic shock.
- Bacteraemia is a transient asymptomatic presence of organisms in the blood.
- Septicaemia is used to describe organisms multiplying in blood causing symptoms. There is a systemic inflammatory response syndrome (SIRS) clinically defined by pyrexia, tachycardia, and leucocytosis. The term sepsis syndrome refers to the additional presence of inadequate organ function/perfusion (confusion, hypoxaemia, raised lactate or oliguria).
- Septic shock refers to the presence of severe sepsis with associated hypotension and organ dysfunction despite adequate fluid resuscitation.

Aetiology
Risk factors for development of sepsis include increasing age, immunodeficiency, liver damage and malignancy. Specific causes include
- direct introduction of bacteria into the blood stream via peripheral or central intravenous line (*Staph. epidermidis*),
- gastrointestinal perforation, rupture or ischaemia leading to bacterial translocation (*E. coli, Streptococcus faecalis*, anaerobic organisms),
- bacteraemia arising from the urinary tract including pyelonephritis, renal abscess, acute prostatitis (*E. coli, Klebsiella aerogenes, Proteus mirabilis*),
- overwhelming pneumococcal infection in patients with impaired or absent splenic function (*Streptococcus pneumoniae*),
- meningococcaemia from a respiratory source may also result in sepsis with or without associated meningitis (*Neisseria meningitidis*),
- patients with surgical site infections (*Staph. aureus, E. coli*, anaerobes) and
- burns (*Staph. aureus, Streptococci, Pseudomonas*).

Pathophysiology
The normal mechanisms involved in overcoming infection become detrimental when the infection is generalised. Bacteria cell wall components such as lipopolysaccharide (gram-negative bacteria), peptidoglycan (gram-positive and gram-negative bacteria) and lipoteichoic acid (gram-positive bacteria) cause the production and release of proinflammatory cytokines from macrophages, monocytes and neutrophils. These include interleukin (IL)-1, IL-5, IL-6, IL-8, IL-11, IL-15 and tumour necrosis factor (TNF)-α. Complement activation causes further tissue damage and widespread activation of the coagulation cascade results in disseminated intravascular coagulation (DIC). Hypotension results from widespread induction of nitric oxide causing a generalised vasodilation. Cellular damage may occur through a combination of ischaemia, direct cytopathic damage and apoptosis.

Clinical features
The systemic inflammatory response syndrome is defined as follows:
- Temperature over 38°C or less than 36°C.
- Heart rate over 90 beats per minute.
- Respiratory rate over 20 breaths per minute or $PaCO_2$ more than 4.3 kPa.
- WBC over 12×10^9/L or less than 4×10^9/L, or >10% immature (band) forms.

Organ hypoperfusion may manifest as altered mental state, lactic acidosis or oliguria. Systemic hypotension is defined as a systolic blood pressure below 90 mmHg or a reduction of more than 40 mmHg from baseline. Patients may go on to develop multiorgan dysfunction including acute respiratory distress syndrome, disseminated intravascular coagulation, hepatic failure, renal failure and confusion or coma.

Investigations
Blood and where appropriate, urine, stool, pus and CSF should be sent for culture prior to starting treatment whenever possible. Full blood count, glucose, urea and electrolytes, liver function tests, arterial blood gases and coagulation screen should be sent and repeated regularly until the patient is stable.

Management
- Aggressive resuscitation is essential. Airway patency and oxygenation must be maintained and may require the use of an oropharyngeal airway or endotracheal intubation. Blood pressure support involves aggressive fluid replacement via wide bore canulae with careful monitoring. CVP measurement allows assessment of fluid resuscitation, and the response of the CVP to fluid challenge helps guide further resuscitation.

Refractory hypotension despite adequate volume replacement requires the use of inotropic agents such as adrenaline, noradrenaline, dopamine or dobutamine in an intensive care setting.

- Identification and management of underlying causes may require surgical intervention or the removal of indwelling catheters or lines.
- Antibiotic therapy should be based on local guidelines and chosen on the basis of presumed infection source until the results of microbiological investigations are known. Septicaemia originating in skin and soft tissue infections requires flucloxacillin and benzylpenicillin. If methicillin resistant *Staph. aureus* (MRSA) is suspected vancomycin or teicoplanin should be used. Septicaemia following intestinal perforation should be treated with cefuroxime, gentamicin and metronidazole. Septicaemia from the urinary tract should be treated with a cephalosporin and gentamicin. If *Pseudomonas* infection is suspected piperacillin or ciprofloxacin are effective.

- Other treatments such as immunoglobulin, anticytokine antibodies, recombinant protein C and nitric oxide synthetase inhibitors are under investigation. Steroids and nonsteroidal anti-inflammatory agents have not been shown to be of benefit.

Prognosis

The reported mortality from septicaemia ranges from 15 to 50% depending on the severity of sepsis and the general status of the patient prior to the illness.

Cardiovascular system

2

Clinical

Symptoms

Cardiovascular chest pain

Chest pain can arise from the cardiovascular system, the respiratory system, the oesophagus or the musculoskeletal system. The major causes of chest pain in the cardiovascular system include ischaemia, pericarditis and aortic dissection.

Enquire about chest pain ask about the site, nature (constricting, sharp, burning, tearing), radiation, precipitating/relieving factors and any associated symptoms. Ask also about the time course, i.e. onset, duration, constant or episodic. SOCRATES may be used as a mnemonic:

- Site
- Onset
- Character
- Radiation
- Alleviating factors
- Time course
- Exacerbating factors
- Symptoms associated with the pain

Ischaemic heart pain is classically a central aching chest pain, often described as a tightness or heaviness, constricting or crushing in nature, radiating into the arms (particularly the left) and jaw. However, this varies between individuals and therefore the pattern of pain is very significant.

- The pain of chronic stable angina is brought on by exercise or emotion, and it is usually relieved within 2–3 minutes by rest and relaxation. It tends to be worse in cold weather or after meals. It may be associated with shortness of breath. Sublingual glyceryl trinitrate (GTN), which dilates the coronary arteries, should also rapidly relieve it.
- Angina that occurs at rest or is provoked more easily than usual for the patient is due to acute coronary syndrome (see page 36). It often persists for longer and although it may respond to GTN, it tends to recur. In acute coronary syndrome it is not possible to differentiate angina from myocardial infarction without further investigations.
- In myocardial infarction the pain bears no relationship to exertion. Typically the pain has the same character, but it is more severe and unrelieved except by opiate analgesia. Features suggestive of myocardial infarction rather than angina include pain, which lasts longer than 30 minutes, associated symptoms due to the release of catecholamines including sweating, dizziness, nausea and vomiting. Some patients describe a feeling of impending doom (angor animi).

Pericarditis causes a sharp or aching pain. It is a retrosternal or epigastric pain that radiates to the neck, back or upper abdomen. The pain is usually altered in severity in relation to posture, typically exacerbated by deep inspiration or lying flat and relieved by leaning forwards. The pain of pericarditis may last days or even 2–3 weeks.

Aortic dissection causes a very severe central tearing chest or abdominal pain that radiates through to the back. Its onset is abrupt and of greatest intensity at the time of onset.

Chest pain associated with tenderness is suggestive of musculoskeletal pain. Pleuritic pain (e.g. pneumonia, pulmonary embolism) is usually sharp and made worse by inspiration and coughing. Oesophageal pain is a retrosternal sensation often related to eating and may be associated with dysphagia. Oesophageal reflux causes a retrosternal burning pain, often exacerbated by bending forwards. Pain from the gallbladder or stomach can often mimic cardiac pain. Equally, pain arising from structures in the chest may present as abdominal pain, e.g. myocardial infarction, pneumonia.

Dyspnoea

Dyspnoea is defined as difficulty in breathing. In general dyspnoea arises from either the respiratory or cardiovascular system and it is often difficult to distinguish between them.

- Cardiac dyspnoea is generally the result of left ventricular failure when fluid accumulates in the interstitium of the lungs. The patient may notice it on strenuous exertion initially, with gradually reducing 'exercise tolerance' (the distance a patient can walk before having to stop for a rest). In severe failure, patients are breathless at rest. In any acute exacerbation of cardiac dyspnoea an underlying cause should be sought, such as ischaemia, arrhythmias or a worsening heart valve lesion.
- Orthopnoea is defined as breathlessness on lying flat. This symptom normally arises when a patient's exercise tolerance is already reduced. It is thought that two mechanisms are responsible for this phenomenon: a redistribution of fluid through gravity in the lungs and a pressing of the abdominal contents on the diaphragm, which reduces the vital capacity of the lungs. Many patients avoid the sensation of breathlessness by propping themselves up on pillows at night, or, in severe cases, sleeping in a chair. Orthopnoea is highly suggestive of a cardiac cause of dyspnoea, although it may also occur in severe respiratory disease due to the second mechanism.
- Paroxysmal nocturnal dyspnoea is waking from sleep suddenly breathless. It is thought to occur by a similar mechanism to orthopnoea coupled to a decreased sensory response whilst asleep. Patients awake breathless and anxious, they often describe having to sit up

and may hang their legs over the side of the bed or go to the window to relieve the dyspnoea.

- Cheyne–Stokes respiration is alternate cyclical hyperventilation and hypoventilation (or even apnoea). This occurs in patients with very severe left ventricular failure, in some normal individuals (often elderly), in patients with cerebrovascular disease and patients receiving opiate analgesia. It is thought that this pattern of breathing results from depression of the respiratory drive centre within the brain.
- Patients with severe acute left ventricular failure often have a cough productive of frothy sputum, which may be blood stained. Frank haemoptysis may occur in mitral stenosis or following a pulmonary embolus. However, the major causes of frank haemoptysis are from the respiratory system.

Palpitations

A palpitation is an increased awareness of the heartbeat. It may be a fluttering, rapid sensation or a slow, sometimes heavy thumping sensation. The patient may feel 'a missed beat', or their heart beating irregularly.

It is important to try to elicit from the patient when the palpitations occur, precipitating factors, duration, rate and rhythm (ask the patient to tap out the beat with their hand). Associated symptoms may include breathlessness, dizziness, syncope and/or chest pain.

- Palpitations during or just after exercise, or caused by anxiety are often simply awareness of a normal heart rate.
- Palpitations lasting just a few seconds are often due to premature beats. The patient becomes aware of the pause that occurs in the normal rhythm after a premature beat and may sense the following stronger beat.
- Post-palpitation polyuria is a feature of supraventricular tachycardia due to the release of atrial natriuretic peptide. Some patients may know how to terminate their rapid palpitations with manoeuvres such as squatting, straining or splashing ice-cold water on the face. These features are very suggestive of a distinct tachyarrhythmia rather than general anxiety or premature beats.

Syncope

Syncope is defined as a transient loss of consciousness due to inadequate cerebral blood flow. Cerebral perfusion is dependent on the heart rate, the arterial blood pressure as well as the resistance of the whole vasculature. Changes in any of these may result in syncope. There may be no warning, or patients may describe feeling faint, cold and clammy prior to the onset. They may have blurred vision, tinnitus and appear very pale prior to the loss of consciousness. Whilst unconscious they are hypotonic with a very slow or difficult to feel pulse. Within a few seconds they spontaneously recover, they tend to be flushed and sweaty but not confused (unless prolonged hypoxia leads to a tonic-clonic seizure).

- Vasovagal syncope is very common and occurs in the absence of cardiac pathology. Predisposing factors include prolonged standing, fear, venesection, micturition or pain. There is peripheral vasodilation causing a reduced ventricular filling. The heart contracts forcefully, which may lead to a reflex bradycardia via vagal stimulation and hence a loss of consciousness.
- Postural syncope (fainting on standing) is seen in patients with autonomic disorders, salt and water depletion, hypovolaemia or due to certain drugs especially antianginal and antihypertensive medication.
- Cardiac arrhythmias may result in syncope if there is a sudden reduction of the cardiac output. This may occur in bradycardias or tachycardias (inadequate ventricular filling time). The loss of consciousness occurs irrespective of the patient's posture. A Stokes–Adams attack is a loss of consciousness related to a sudden loss of ventricular contraction particularly seen during the progression from second to third degree heart block.
- Carotid sinus syncope is a rare condition mainly seen in the elderly. As a result of hypersensitivity of the carotid sinus, light pressure, such as that exerted by a tight collar, causes a severe reflex bradycardia and hence syncope.
- Exertional syncope occurs in aortic valve or subvalve stenosis. The syncope results from an inability of the heart to increase cardiac output in response to increased demand.

The immediate management of syncope or impending syncope is to lie the patient down and raise their legs increasing cerebral blood flow.

Intermittent claudication

Claudication describes a cramp-like pain felt in one or both calves, thighs or buttocks on exertion. In severe cases the pain causes the patient to limp, hence the term claudication and the pain characteristically disappears when exertion is stopped, hence the term intermittent. The distance a patient can usually walk on the flat before onset of pain is termed the claudication distance. Intermittent claudication is caused by peripheral vascular insufficiency to the muscles of the legs. The disease is in proximal large and medium-sized arteries to the lower limbs, i.e. the iliac and femoral arteries. As the narrowing of the arteries becomes more significant, the claudication distance decreases. Eventually rest pain may occur, this often precedes ischaemia and gangrene of the affected limb.

Signs

Oedema

Oedema is defined as an abnormal accumulation of fluid within the interstitial spaces. A number of mechanisms are thought to be involved in the development of oedema. Normally tissue fluid is formed by a balance of hydrostatic and osmotic pressure.

Hydrostatic pressure is the pressure within the blood vessel (high in arteries, low in veins). Oncotic pressure is produced by the large molecules within the blood (albumin, haemoglobin) and draws water osmotically back into the vessel. The hydrostatic pressure is high at the arterial end of a capillary bed hence fluid is forced out of the vasculature (see Fig. 2.1).

The colloid osmotic pressure then draws fluid back in at the venous end of the capillary bed as the hydrostatic

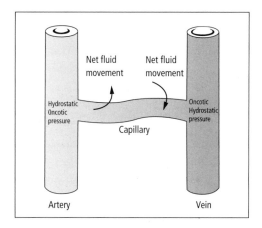

Figure 2.1 Mechanism of oedema.

pressure of the venules is low. Any remaining interstitial fluid is then returned to the circulation via the lymphatic system.

Mechanisms of cardiovascular oedema include the following:

- Raised venous pressure raising the hydrostatic pressure at the venous end of the capillary bed (right ventricular failure, pericardial constriction, vena caval obstruction).
- Salt and water retention occurring in heart failure, which increases the circulating blood volume with pooling on the venous side again raising the hydrostatic pressure.
- The liver congestion that occurs in right-sided heart failure may reduce hepatic function, including albumin production. Albumin is the major factor responsible for the generation of the colloid osmotic pressure that returns the tissue fluid to the vasculature. A drop in albumin therefore results in an accumulation of oedema.

Oedema is described as pitting (an indentation or pit is left after pressing with a thumb for several seconds) or nonpitting. Cardiac oedema is pitting unless long standing when secondary changes in the lymphatics may cause a nonpitting oedema. Distribution is dependent on the patient. Patients who are confined to bed develop oedema around the sacral area rather than the classical ankle and lower leg distribution. Pleural effusions and ascites may develop in severe failure.

Cyanosis

Cyanosis is a blue discolouration of the skin and mucous membranes. It is due to the presence of desaturated haemoglobin and becomes visible when levels rise above 5 g/dL. Cyanosis is not present in very anaemic patients due to the low haemoglobin levels. Cyanosis is divided into two categories:

- Peripheral cyanosis, which is seen in the fingertips and peripheries. When occurring without central cyanosis it is due to poor perfusion, as the sluggish circulation leads to increased desaturation of haemoglobin. This may be as a result of normal vasoconstriction in the cold, poor peripheral circulation or a poor cardiac output.
- Central cyanosis also affects the warm mucous membranes such as the tongue. It is a result of failure of

oxygenation. This may be a result of blood bypassing the lungs (right to left shunting) or due to severe lung disease.

The arterial pulse

The pulse should be palpated at the radial and carotid artery looking for the following features:

- The rate is normally counted over 15 seconds and multiplied by 4. The normal pulse is defined as a rate between 60 and 100 beats per minute. Outside this range it is described as either a bradycardia or a tachycardia.
- The rhythm is either regular, regularly irregular, i.e. irregular but with a pattern, or irregularly irregular, which is suggestive of atrial fibrillation.
- The character and volume of the pulse are normally assessed at the brachial or carotid artery. Character and volume felt at the carotid may be described according to the waveform palpated (see Fig. 2.2).
- Pulse delay is a delay in the pulsation felt between two pulses. Radio-femoral delay is suggestive of coarctation of the aorta, the lesion being just distal to the origin of the subclavian artery (at the point where the ductus arteriosus joined the aorta). Radio-radial delay suggests arterial occlusion due to an aneurysm or atherosclerotic plaque.

Jugular venous pressure

The internal jugular vein is most easily seen with the patient reclining (usually at 45°), with the head supported and the neck muscles relaxed and in good lighting conditions. The jugular vein runs medial to the sternomastoid muscle in the upper third of the neck, behind it in the middle third and between the two heads of sternocleidomastoid in the lower third. It is differentiated from the carotid pulse by its double waveform, it is nonpalpable, it is occluded by pressure and pressure on the liver causes a rise in the level of the pulsation (hepatojugular reflex). The jugular waveform and pressure give information about the pressures within the right atrium as there are no valves separating the atrium and the internal jugular vein (see Fig. 2.3).

The height of the jugular venous pressure (JVP) is assessed as the vertical height from the sternal angle to the point at which the JVP is seen. A height of greater than 3 cm represents an abnormal increase in filling pressure

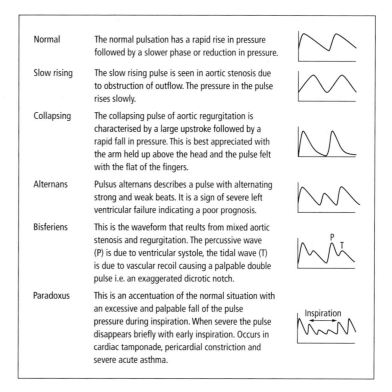

Normal	The normal pulsation has a rapid rise in pressure followed by a slower phase or reduction in pressure.	
Slow rising	The slow rising pulse is seen in aortic stenosis due to obstruction of outflow. The pressure in the pulse rises slowly.	
Collapsing	The collapsing pulse of aortic regurgitation is characterised by a large upstroke followed by a rapid fall in pressure. This is best appreciated with the arm held up above the head and the pulse felt with the flat of the fingers.	
Alternans	Pulsus alternans describes a pulse with alternating strong and weak beats. It is a sign of severe left ventricular failure indicating a poor prognosis.	
Bisferiens	This is the waveform that reults from mixed aortic stenosis and regurgitation. The percussive wave (P) is due to ventricular systole, the tidal wave (T) is due to vascular recoil causing a palpable double pulse i.e. an exaggerated dicrotic notch.	
Paradoxus	This is an accentuation of the normal situation with an excessive and palpable fall of the pulse pressure during inspiration. When severe the pulse disappears briefly with early inspiration. Occurs in cardiac tamponade, pericardial constriction and severe acute asthma.	

Figure 2.2 Arterial pulse waveforms.

Once the atrium is filled with blood it contracts to give the 'a' wave
- The 'a' wave is lost in atrial fibrillation.
- The 'a' wave is increased in pulmonary stenosis, pulmonary hypertension and tricuspid stenosis (as a consequence of right atrial or right ventricular hypertrophy).

The atrium relaxes to give the 'x' descent; however, the start of ventricular contraction causes ballooning of the tricuspid valve as it closes, resulting in the 'c' wave. The further 'x' descent is due to descent of the closed valve towards the cardiac apex.

With the tricuspid valve closed the return of venous blood fills the atrium giving the 'v' wave.
- Tricuspid regurgitation gives a 'cv' wave.

The tricuspid valve opens at the end of ventricular systole giving the 'y' descent.

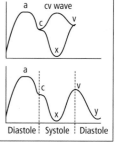

Figure 2.3 The jugular venous pressure waveform.

of the right atrium. This may occur in right-sided heart failure, congestive cardiac failure and pulmonary embolism.

Precordial heaves, thrills and pulsation

- A parasternal heave is a cardiac impulse palpated by placing the flat of the hand on the costal cartilages, to the left of the patient's sternum. It may be due to right ventricular hypertrophy when the impulse is at the same time as the apex beat and carotid pulsation. Less commonly it is due to left atrial enlargement when the pulsation occurs before the apex beat or carotid pulsation.
- A thrill is a palpable murmur and is due to turbulent blood flow. A thrill is indicative of a loud murmur. The flat of the hand should be placed at the base and apex of the heart. For example, a diastolic thrill at the apex is suggestive of severe mitral stenosis (aortic regurgitation rarely produces a thrill).
- The apex beat is defined as the most inferior and lateral cardiac pulsation. It should be identified and its position defined according the intercostal space (count down from the sternal angle which is at the second intercostal space) and the relationship to the chest (midclavicular line, anterior axillary line, etc). The normal position is the fourth or fifth intercostal space in the left midclavicular line. The character of the pulsation should also be palpated, but these may be subtle (see Table 2.1).

Heart murmurs

Heart murmurs are the result of turbulent blood flow. Certain features of any murmur should be noted.

Table 2.1 Character of an abnormal apex beat

Description	Character	Typical underlying lesion
Tapping	Sudden but brief pulsation	Mitral stenosis
Thrusting	Vigorous, nonsustained	Mitral or aortic regurgitation
Heaving	Vigorous and sustained	Aortic stenosis, systemic hypertension

Timing to systole or diastole is achieved by palpation of the carotid pulse whilst auscultating. A systolic murmur occurs at the same time as the carotid pulse, whereas a diastolic murmur occurs in the pause between carotid pulses. Murmurs are further described according to their relationship to the cardiac cycle.

- A systolic murmur may be pansystolic when the first and second heart sounds cannot be heard separate from the murmur. This occurs in mitral regurgitation, tricuspid regurgitation and with a ventricular septal defect.
- An ejection systolic murmur is a crescendo–decrescendo murmur and the second heart sound can be heard distinct from the end of the murmur. It is heard with aortic stenosis, pulmonary stenosis and with an atrial septal defect (the sound being produced by increased flow across the pulmonary valve).
- A late systolic murmur is heard in mitral valve prolapse.
- An early diastolic murmur is heard with aortic regurgitation, and a mid-late diastolic murmur is heard with mitral stenosis.

The area in which the murmur is heard at the greatest intensity and any radiation should be noted. This is most helpful when the flow of blood is considered according to the lesion, for example aortic stenosis radiates to the neck, mitral regurgitation radiates to the axilla. The intensity of the murmur may be graded (see Table 2.2) and the pitch also noted.

Investigations and procedures

Coronary angioplasty

Coronary angioplasty is a technique used to dilate stenosed coronary arteries in patients with ischaemic heart disease. The indications for use of angioplasty have changed over the years with the technique now used for

Table 2.2 Simple grading of the intensity of a heart murmur

Grade	Description
1/4	Just audible with concentration
2/4	Easily audible, but not loud
3/4	Loud
4/4	Loud and audible over a wide area

many stenoses previously thought to be treatable only by bypass grafting. Current practice is for left main stem disease or triple vessel disease to be treated by bypass grafting for prognostic reasons with almost all other lesions being considered for angioplasty for symptom control. In addition, patients with concomitant conditions precluding bypass surgery, e.g. lung disease, may be considered for angioplasty even for left main stem or advanced multivessel disease.

Early angiography and angioplasty is now being increasingly used immediately following a myocardial infarction, in order to reduce the risk of further infarction. This is especially where the acute event is a limited or non-ST elevation myocardial infarction.

PTCA (percutaneous transluminal coronary angioplasty) is performed under local anaesthetic. A small balloon is passed up the aorta via peripheral arterial access under radiographic guidance. Once within the affected coronary artery, the balloon is inflated to dilate the stenosis, compressing the atheromatous plaque and stretching the layers of the vessel wall to the sides. A stent is often used to reduce recurrence. Some stenoses cannot be dilated due to calcification of the vessel, small vessel or the position or length of stenosis. During the procedure there is a risk of thrombosis, so patients are given intravenous heparin and aspirin. If stents are used, another antiplatelet agent (clopidogrel) is also used to prevent in-stent thrombosis in the first few days/weeks and the patient remains on lifelong aspirin.

Complications

The main immediate complication of balloon angioplasty is intimal/medial dissection leading to abrupt vessel occlusion. This, and the problem of late restenosis, has been largely resolved with the routine implantation of a stent. There is a risk of complications, including emergency coronary artery bypass surgery, myocardial infarction and stroke (due to thrombosis and plaque, or haemorrhage) but these tend to be lower than for coronary artery bypass surgery. More commonly, local haematoma at the site of arterial puncture may occur. Overall mortality is approximately 0.5%.

Prognosis

Depending on the anatomy of the lesion, significant restenosis occurs between 30 and 60% after balloon angioplasty without stenting. Stent implants generally reduce this to approximately 15–20% and this has been further reduced with drug-eluting stents. These slowly release a drug (e.g. sirolimus) over 2–4 weeks to modify the healing response.

Coronary artery bypass surgery

Surgery for coronary artery disease is useful in patients with severe symptoms despite medical treatment. It has also been shown to improve outcome in patients with triple vessel disease or left main stem coronary artery disease.

Cardiopulmonary bypass

In order to operate safely in a bloodless, immobile field whilst maintaining an adequate circulation to the rest of the body cardiopulmonary bypass is most commonly used. A cannula is placed in the right atrium in order to divert blood away from the heart. The blood is then oxygenated by one of two methods:
- Bubble oxygenators work by bubbling 95% oxygen through a column of blood.
- Membrane oxygenators work by bringing the blood and oxygen together via a gas permeable membrane.

Bubbles are then removed by passing the blood through a sponge. The blood is then heated or cooled as required. A roller pump compresses the tubing driving the blood back into the systemic side of the circulation at an arterial perfusion pressure of between 50 and 100 mmHg. If the myocardium is to be opened, cross-clamping the aorta gives a bloodless field; the heart is protected from ischaemia by cooling to between 20 and 30°C. Systemic cooling also lowers metabolic requirements of other organs during surgery. Beating heart bypass grafting is now possible using a mechanical device to stabilise the target surface area of the heart, but access to the posterior surface of the heart can be difficult.

Coronary artery surgery

The internal mammary artery is the graft of choice as 50% of saphenous grafts become occluded within 10 years. The coronary arteries are opened distal to the obstruction and the grafts are placed. If the saphenous vein is used, its proximal end is sewn to the ascending aorta. The surgery takes approximately 1–2 hours. Once the heart is reperfused, it rapidly regains activity. Ventricular fibrillation is deliberately induced during cardiopulmonary bypass to reduce heart movement and avoid additional ischaemia and internal defibrillating paddles are used to restore sinus rhythm.

Complications

Aspirin is usually continued for the procedure, but other antiplatelet drugs such as clopidogrel are stopped up to 5 days in advance. During the procedure patients are heparinised to prevent thrombosis. Antibiotic cover is provided using a broad spectrum antibiotic to prevent bacteraemia. Operative mortality depends on many factors including age and concomitant disease, it usually varies from 1 to 5%. There is a similar, age-related risk of stroke.

Prognosis

Approximately 90% of patients have no angina postoperatively, with almost all patients experiencing a significant improvement. Over time symptoms may gradually return due to progression of atheroma in the arteries or occlusion of vein grafts. Less than half are symptom-free at 10 years. Outcome is improved by risk factor modification (stopping smoking, lowering high blood pressure, treating hyperlipidaemia and diabetes effectively, etc).

Angioplasty or re-do coronary artery surgery may be possible if medication is insufficient to control symptoms; however, repeat surgery has a higher mortality. Angioplasty using stent implantation is suitable for grafts or native vessels.

Valve surgery

Valve surgery is used to treat stenosed or regurgitant valves, which cause compromise of cardiac function.

Conservative surgery is performed whenever possible. The aortic valve is not usually amenable to conservative surgery and usually requires replacement if significantly diseased. A stenosed mitral valve may be treated by following procedures:

- Percutaneous mitral balloon valvuloplasty in which a balloon is used to separate the mitral valve leaflets. This is now the preferred technique unless there is coexisting mitral regurgitation.
- Closed valvotomy uses a dilator that is passed through a left sub-mammary incision into the left atrial appendage.

- Open valvotomy and valve repair is performed under cardiopulmonary bypass. The valve leaflets are separated under direct vision. This is used for patients with coexisting mitral regurgitation.

Valvular regurgitation when due to dilation of the valve ring may be treated by sewing a rigid or semi-rigid ring around the valve annulus to maintain size (annuloplasty). If regurgitation is due to areas of flail leaflets, e.g. due to infective endocarditis or chordal rupture, part of the leaflet may be resected or even repaired with a piece of pericardium to restore valve competence.

Valve replacement: Using cardiopulmonary bypass the diseased valve is excised and a replacement is sutured into place. Valves may be divided into mechanical and biological types:

- Early mechanical valves were ball and cage type such as the Starr–Edwards valve. Current designs all have some form of tilting disc such as the single disc Björk–Shiley valve or the double disc St Jude valve. They are durable, but require lifelong anticoagulation therapy to prevent thrombosis of the valve and risk of embolism.
- Biological valves may be xenografts (from animals) or homografts (cadaveric). Xenografts are made from porcine valves or from pericardium mounted on a supportive frame. They are treated with glutaraldehyde to prevent rejection and are used to replace aortic or mitral valves. They do not require anticoagulation unless the patient is in atrial fibrillation but have a durability of approximately 10 years. Valve failure may result from leaflet shrinkage or weakening of the valve competence causing regurgitation, or calcification causing valve stenosis.

Valve replacements are prone to infective endocarditis, which is difficult to treat (and may require removal of a mechanical valve).

Valve replacement provides marked symptomatic relief and improvement in survival. Operative mortality is approximately 2%, but this is increased in patients with ischaemic heart disease (when it is usually combined with coronary artery bypass grafting), lung disease and the elderly. Perioperative complications include haemorrhage and infection. Late complications include haemolysis and valve failure. Arrhythmias also occur. All prosthetic valves require antibiotic prophylaxis against infective endocarditis during non-sterile procedures, e.g. dental treatment, lower gastrointestinal or urogenital procedures and they may also become infected from any source of bacteraemia.

Permanent pacemakers

Cardiac pacemakers are used to maintain a regular rhythm, by providing an electrical stimulus to the heart through one or more electrodes that are passed to the right atrium and/or ventricle.

Common indications for a permanent pacemaker:
- Complete heart block.
- Sick sinus syndrome with symptomatic bradycardia.

Types of permanent pacemaker

There are several types of pacemaker, most pacemakers are programmable through the skin by radio transmission. Pacemakers may be single chamber, i.e. single electrode usually to the right ventricle, or dual chamber, i.e. one electrode to the right ventricle and one to the right atrium. The descriptive code for the most commonly used pacemakers consists of up to four letters (see Table 2.3).

Common types of pacemakers are as follows:
- VVI is a single chamber pacemaker that senses and paces the ventricle. If it senses a beat, the paced beat is Inhibited. It is often used in patients with atrial fibrillation with AV block.
- DDD is a dual chamber pacemaker that is capable of sensing and pacing both the atrium and ventricle. It is used in complete heart block in the absence of atrial fibrillation. It can sense if an atrial beat is not followed by a ventricular beat (due to lack of AV node conduction), in which case it will trigger a ventricular beat. It can also trigger an atrial beat followed at a

suitable interval by a ventricular beat if the atrium does not contract spontaneously.

Procedure

The pacemaker is inserted under local anaesthetic normally taking 45 minutes to 1 hour. A small diagonal incision is made a few centimetres below the clavicle and the electrodes are passed transvenously to the heart. The pacemaker box is then attached to the leads and implanted subcutaneously. The procedure is covered with antibiotics to reduce the risk of infection.

Complications

The procedure is generally low-risk. The most important complications are pneumothorax due to the venous access and surgical site infection. As long as aspirin and anti-coagulants are stopped prior to the procedure, significant haematoma or bleeding is unusual.

The pacemaker function is checked within 24 hours of implantation. Annual follow-up is required to ensure that the battery life is adequate and that there has not been lead displacement. Patients are allowed to drive after 1 month (current DVLA rules), i.e. after the 4-week pacemaker check. Most pacemakers last 5–10 years.

In electromagnetic fields such as in airport security most pacemakers are now programmed to go into a default pacing mode so as not to fail. Even so patients are advised to avoid close proximity to strong electromagnetic fields. MRI scanning is contraindicated and pacemakers must be removed postmortem, if the patient is to be cremated.

Echocardiography

Echocardiography essentially means ultrasonography of the heart. It is a very useful, non-invasive method by which the heart and surrounding structures can be

Table 2.3 Descriptive codes for pacemakers

	Code position			
	1	**2**	**3**	**4**
Category	Paced chamber	Sensed chamber	Pacemaker response	Program functions
	V (Ventricle)	V (Ventricle)	T (Triggered)	P (Programmable)
	A (Atrium)	A (Atrium)	I (Inhibited)	M (Multi-programmable)
	D (Dual)	D (Dual)	D (Dual)	0 (none)
		0 (none)	R (Reverse)	R (Rate responsive)

imaged. It requires technical expertise to obtain images and clinical expertise to interpret the results appropriately. The following features are typically assessed:

- Anatomical features such as cardiac chamber size, myocardial wall thickness and valve structure or lesions. Ventricular aneurysms or defects such as atrial or ventricular septal defects can be seen.
- Functional features including wall motion (any localised wall motion abnormality as well as a general assessment of the overall contractility of the ventricles, often measured as fractional shortening or ejection fraction) and valve motion. Doppler ultrasound is used to measure the velocity of jets of blood, e.g. to assess severity in valve stenosis.
- The aortic root may be examined for dilatation or dissection.
- Pericardial fluid appears as an echo-free space between the myocardium and the parietal pericardium.
- Mass lesions such as thrombus or tumour may be seen within the heart.

The principles of echocardiography are the same as those of ultrasound. A transducer is used to generate ultrasound waves that are directed at the heart. When a wave encounters an interface of differing echogenicity, some of it is reflected and some absorbed. Any reflected waves (echoes) that reach the transducer are sensed and processed into an image. The time taken for the wave to bounce back measures the distance of the interface. Tissues or interfaces that reflect the waves strongly such as bone/tissue or air/tissue will appear very white (echogenic) and also prevent any tissues underneath from being imaged well. Fluid is anechoic, so appears black. The ribs and lungs limit the ability to visualise the heart because they cast acoustic shadows. Transoesophageal echocardiography (TOE) is a more invasive method used when poor views are obtained on transthoracic echocardiography, or when more detailed views are required particularly of structures near the oesophagus such as the atria and great vessels, the mitral valve or prosthetic valves. A transducer probe is mounted on the tip of a flexible tube that is passed into the oesophagus. The patient needs to be nil by mouth prior to the procedure, local anaesthetic spray is used on the pharynx, and intravenous sedation may be required for the procedure to be tolerated.

There are three types of echocardiography: two dimensional, M-mode and Doppler.

Two dimensional is useful for evaluating the anatomical features. Standard views are obtained.

- Left parasternal: With the transducer rotated appropriately through a window in the third or fourth intercostal space, long and short axis views can be obtained.
- Apical: This is a view upwards from the position of the apex beat and gives a long axis view of the heart, where all four chambers can be seen simultaneously.

M-mode is a way by which the motion of individual structures along a narrow path can be carefully studied. It is a one-dimensional view (depth) with time as the second dimension on the image produced. Structures that do not move appear as a horizontal line, whereas structures that move, e.g. valves, are seen as zigzag lines, which move in time with the cardiac cycle. The distances between structures, or the thickness of structures, can therefore be carefully measured at different times of the cardiac cycle.

Doppler allows the analysis of the direction and velocity of blood flow, and therefore is particularly useful in the evaluation of valve lesions. It is used to calculate pressure gradients, e.g. in aortic stenosis. It can also be used to generate 2-D images with simultaneous imaging of flow direction and velocity.

Common indications for echocardiography:

- Suspected valvular heart disease, including infective endocarditis.
- Heart failure, to assess left ventricular function and look for any valve lesions or regurgitation, and any evidence of a cardiomyopathy.
- Postmyocardial infarction for suspected complications, such as ventricular septal rupture or papillary muscle rupture. It will also identify areas of ischaemic myocardium or previous myocardial infarction as areas of hypokinetic or akinetic myocardium, as well as an overall assessment of left ventricular function.

Ischaemic heart disease

Ischaemic heart disease

Definition

In the normal heart there is a balance between the oxygen supply and demand of the myocardium. A supply of oxygen insufficient for the myocardial demand results in ischaemia of the myocardial tissue. The predominant cause of cardiac ischaemia is reduction or interruption of coronary blood flow, which in turn is due to atherosclerosis $+/-$ thrombosis causing coronary artery narrowing.

Incidence
Ischaemic heart disease results in 30% of all male deaths and 23% of all female deaths in the Western world.

Age
Increases with age.

Sex
M > F

Geography
More common in the Western world where it is the commonest cause of death.

Aetiology/pathophysiology
Risk factors can be divided into those that are fixed and those that are modifiable:
- Fixed: Age, sex, positive family history.
- Modifiable: Smoking (direct relationship to the number of cigarettes smoked), hypertension, diabetes mellitus, LDL and total cholesterol levels (HDL cholesterol is protective).

Ischaemic heart disease is essentially synonymous with coronary artery disease. Rarely cardiac ischaemia may result from hypotension (reduced perfusion pressure), severe anaemia, carboxyhaemoglobinaemia or myocardial hypertrophy.

Four main syndromes are associated with coronary artery disease:
- Chronic stable angina results from the presence of atherosclerotic plaques within the coronary arteries reducing the vessel lumen and limiting the blood flow. Symptoms are only present on exertion (see below).
- Acute coronary syndrome encompasses unstable angina, non-ST elevation myocardial infarction and acute myocardial infarction with ST elevation. It results from rupture of an atherosclerotic plaque and subsequent thrombosis (see page 36).
- Variant/Prinzmetal's angina (see page 40).
- Ischaemic heart failure/cardiomyopathy, which may occur without overt acute symptoms.

Chronic stable angina

Definition
Chest pain occurring during periods of increased myocardial work because of reduced coronary perfusion.

Incidence
Angina is common reflecting the incidence of ischaemic heart disease.

Age
Incidence increases with age.

Sex
M > F. Premenopausal women are relatively protected.

Geography
Predominantly a disease of the Western world, but this pattern is changing with the increasing affluence of the developing world.

Aetiology
Angina is most commonly associated with atheroma, although exertional chest pain can occur with other conditions, such as aortic stenosis and hypertrophic cardiomyopathy. In 'stable angina', pain is precipitated by physical exertion, meals, cold weather and high emotion (anger, excitement), and it is relieved by rest.

Pathophysiology
The pathology of stable angina is the presence of high-grade stenosis of at least one coronary artery resulting in a reduction of at least 50% of the lumen diameter or 75% of the lumen area. The underlying mechanism is atheroma, which affects large and medium-sized arteries. The true pathogenesis of atheroma is not fully understood but the following factors are thought to play a role:
- Stage I: Damage to the endothelium of the arteries allows the entry of cholesterol rich LDLs into the intima. At this stage the cholesterol is extracellular.
- Stage II: Normally macrophages are unable to phagocytose cholesterol as they lack the required receptor; however, once the LDLs are oxidised they are taken up by macrophages by a receptor-independent pathway. The resultant lipid-laden macrophages are

termed foam cells, an accumulation of which causes a visible pale bulge called a fatty streak.

Fatty streaks are often visible within the first year of life, and these occur worldwide, even in areas where atheroma is uncommon. This suggests that the initiation of fatty streak may not be due to the risk factors for atherosclerosis.

- Stage III: The macrophages release lipid and cytokines into the intima, resulting in the stimulation of intimal cell proliferation. These cells secrete collagen and the plaque becomes fibrotic. The result is a raised yellow lipid plaque.
- Stage IV: The secreted collagen forms a dense fibrous cap. The lesion, now termed a fibrolipid plaque, contains free lipid as well as foam cells with an overlying fragile endothelium.

Clinical features

The classical description of angina pectoris is of a heavy chest pain, often described as like a tight band around the chest. It may range from a mild dull ache or mild chest tightness to a crushing, severe pain. It may radiate to the jaw or arms (especially the left), sometimes it is only in the jaw, neck, arm or hand. The nature of pain and its severity do not necessarily indicate the severity of disease. The pattern of pain is often more consistent. It is brought on by exertion or emotion and relieved within a few minutes of rest. A grading system exists based on the level of activity provoking pain (see Table 2.4). It is important to elicit whether there has recently been a reduction in the exercise tolerance (crescendo angina), or angina at rest (see section Acute Coronary Syndrome, page 36).

Macroscopy

Atheroma tends to affect large and medium-sized arteries and is confined to the systemic circulation. There are

Table 2.4 New York Heart Association classification of angina

Grade I	Pain as a result of strenuous physical activity only
Grade II	Slight limitation of ordinary physical activity (pain on walking up a hill)
Grade III	Marked limitation of ordinary activity (pain on walking on the flat)
Grade IV	Inability to carry on physical activity

four patterns of plaque depending on its position and the ratio of the lipid pool to the fibrous cap:

Concentric fibrous: 48% of plaques
Eccentric fibrous: 12% of plaques
Concentric lipid rich: 28% of plaques
Eccentric lipid rich: 12% of plaques

The eccentric lipid rich plaques are the most likely to ulcerate due to the markedly abnormal flow pattern through the vessel and the relatively thin fibrous cap.

Microscopy

Plaques are located in the intima of the arterial wall. They consist of a pale lipid rich area and a pink stained fibrous cap. They contain varying amounts of free lipid, collagen and foam cells. Late in the evolution of a plaque the underlying media becomes thinned by pressure atrophy.

Investigations

- The ECG is often normal, although there may be signs of hypertrophy and old infarction.
- Exercise ECG can determine exercise tolerance and usually shows ST depression or T wave changes in the distribution of the lesion (see Fig. 2.4).
- Thallium-201 uptake scan may show areas of infarction and reversible ischaemia.
- Echocardiogram both during resting and under stress (dobutamine) may show abnormal ventricular wall function.
- Coronary angiography can be used but carries a small morbidity and mortality risk.
- MRI angiography is non-invasive and may prove a useful alternative.

Management

Acute attack: stop exercise, use glyceryl trinitrate (GTN) sublingually.

General management includes identification and treatment of any exacerbating cause such as anaemia or thyrotoxicosis. Risk factor modification is crucial, in particular stopping smoking, treatment of hypertension, improving diabetic control and lowering cholesterol.

Medical management: aspirin or other antiplatelet agents such as clopidogrel reduce the risk of myocardial infarction. HMGCoA reductase inhibitors (statins), which lower cholesterol, are effective for primary and secondary prevention of myocardial infarction.

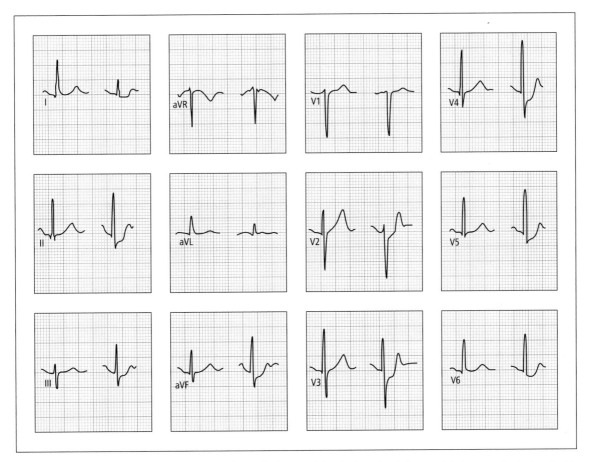

Figure 2.4 Exercise test. The figure shows a cardiac cycle from each lead taken at rest (left) and during exercise (right). In this example exercise results in widespread ST depression (ischaemic changes) in the inferior (II, III, aVF) and anterolateral chest leads (V2–V6).

Symptomatic treatment may involve one or a combination of the following:

- β-blockers reduce the oxygen demand of the heart by reducing the heart rate and the force of ventricular contraction. They are particularly useful after a myocardial infarction to reduce the risk of a subsequent cardiac event.
- Long acting nitrates (oral or transcutaneous) are coronary artery dilators and are useful in patients who respond to sublingual GTN.
- Calcium channel blockers such as diltiazem and amlodipine reduce coronary artery tone. Diltiazem and verapamil also reduce the heart rate and the force of ventricular contraction resulting in a decreased myocardial oxygen demand. They should be used with

care in conjunction with β-blockers or in patients with heart failure.
- Potassium channel openers such as nicorandil are third line agents.

If symptoms cannot be controlled by medication, the main choices for coronary intervention are between coronary angioplasty (see page 28) and coronary artery bypass surgery (see page 29).

- Coronary artery bypass grafting is indicated where it may improve prognosis or when symptoms persist to an extent that interferes with normal life despite medical treatment. In patients with triple vessel disease or left main stem coronary artery disease, surgery improves outcome. Operative mortality depends on several factors including age and concomitant disease.

- Percutaneous transluminal coronary angioplasty (PTCA) is carried out under local anaesthetic. A balloon is inflated in the coronary artery to reduce the stenosis.

Prognosis

Prognosis is dependent on severity of disease, number of coronary arteries affected, left ventricular function and coexistent disease such as diabetes mellitus, peripheral vascular disease, hypertension and renal impairment.

Acute coronary syndrome

Definition

Acute coronary syndrome (ACS) encompasses ischaemic cardiac chest pain of recent origin. It includes the following:

- Unstable angina describes clinical states between stable angina and acute myocardial infarction. Unstable angina is considered to be present in patients with ischaemic chest pain and symptoms suggestive of ACS without elevation of markers of cardiac damage. It includes angina at rest lasting more than 20 minutes, crescendo angina and angina occurring more than 24 hours after an acute myocardial infarction.
- Non-ST elevation myocardial infarction (previously known as non-Q wave MI) differs primarily in that the myocardial ischaemia is severe enough to cause myocardial damage sufficient to produce a detectable rise in markers of cardiac damage (troponins and creatine kinase).
- An acute, evolving or recent myocardial infarction is defined as a rise and fall of biochemical markers of myocardial damage (e.g. troponin or CK-MB) with at least one of the following:
  - Ischaemic symptoms.
  - Development of pathologic Q waves on the ECG.
  - ECG changes indicative of ischaemia (ST segment elevation or depression).
  - Following coronary artery intervention (e.g. angioplasty).

Pathophysiology

As with stable angina, the underlying pathological lesion is the atheromatous plaque. In ACS there is fissuring of an atheromatous plaque, which initiates thrombosis with a subsequent risk of total occlusion of the vessel. Eccentric plaques with a lipid-rich morphology are at greatest risk of fissuring. Over the course of minutes, hours or days the plaque may fissure, thrombose over and reseal several times, causing recurrent episodes of pain at rest or markedly reduced exercise tolerance. Depending on the severity and duration of occlusion, the vessel affected and the presence of any collateral blood supply, this process may result in unstable angina, NSTEMI or myocardial infarction with ST elevation.

Clinical features

Patients present with severe ischaemic chest pain, which is identical to that of angina pectoris (central crushing chest pain, radiating to jaw and left arm) but occurs at rest or is provoked more easily, persists for longer and often fails to respond to medical treatment. Patients require emergency assessment and investigation to allow rapid thrombolytic therapy for those with an acute myocardial infarction with ST elevation. It is essential to identify risk factors for and previous history of ischaemic heart disease (see page 33).

Investigations

The initial emergency investigation is a 12-lead ECG. If there is ST segment elevation or new left bundle branch block, the diagnosis is acute myocardial infarction (STEMI, see page 37). If there is no ST segment elevation, the patient may have unstable angina or NSTEMI (see below).

Unstable angina and non-ST elevation myocardial infarction (NSTEMI)

Definition

Acute coronary syndrome without ST elevation (see above).

Incidence

120,000 cases in England and Wales per annum.

Clinical features

Patients present with the acute ischaemic chest pain of ACS.

Investigations
- Serial ECGs are essential to exclude the development of an acute myocardial infarction (ST segment elevation or new left bundle branch block). In non-ST elevation ACS, the ECG may be normal or show ST depression and/or T wave changes corresponding to the area of the lesion. There may also be signs of hypertrophy or previous infarction (Q waves). The evolution of ECG changes is also useful for prognostic information and planning of management. Additional ECGs should also be performed during subsequent episodes of chest pain.
- Twelve hours after the onset of chest pain, a troponin T or I level should be checked. If this is raised, this is diagnostic of a NSTEMI. If the level is normal patients are defined as having unstable angina.

Management
Once diagnosed with non-ST elevation ACS, all patients should be commenced on aspirin and subcutaneous low-molecular-weight heparin. Coexisting arrhythmias should be treated and oxygen given as appropriate. Continuing chest pain is treated with intravenous glyceryl trinitrate infusion. Patients should be commenced on a β-blocker (unless contraindicated) and an oral nitrate once the intravenous infusion is not required. In patients with contraindications to β-blockers, a non-dihydropyridine calcium channel antagonist, e.g. diltiazem should be used.

Patients can be stratified as to acute ischaemic risk depending on symptoms and investigations (see Table 2.5).

Table 2.5 Risk stratification of unstable angina and NSTEMI

Low risk	Clinically stable, normal ECG, negative 12-hour troponin
Intermediate risk	Recurrent symptoms without new ECG changes or persistence of previous abnormal ECG
High risk	Raised 12-hour troponin level without ST elevation or new Q waves
Highest risk	Refractory or recurrent symptoms with ischaemic ECG changes
	Ischaemia with haemodynamic compromise or arrhythmia. Elevated troponin with recurrent ECG changes

- Low-risk patients should be discharged with an elective exercise/stress test pre- or post-discharge.
- Intermediate-risk patients should have an inpatient stress or exercise test. If this shows reversible ischaemia angiography and revascularisation should be considered.
- High-risk patients may benefit from a glycoprotein IIb/IIIa inhibitor (which prevents platelet aggregation) together with unfractionated intravenous heparin in place of low-molecular-weight heparin. They should undergo inpatient angiography and revascularisation as appropriate.
- Very high risk patients should be given a glycoprotein IIb/IIIa inhibitor together with unfractionated intravenous heparin in place of low-molecular-weight heparin and where possible undergo emergency angiography with revascularisation unless contraindicated.

Prognosis
Unless aggressively treated, approximately 10% of patients (excluding those with a normal ECG) will proceed to myocardial infarction or death within 1 month.

Acute myocardial infarction (STEMI)

Definition
Myocardial infarction (MI) is death of myocardial tissue as an end stage to ischaemia. An acute, evolving or recent myocardial is diagnosed by a rise and fall of biochemical markers of myocardial damage (e.g. troponin or CK-MB) with at least one of the following:
- Ischaemic symptoms.
- Development of pathologic Q waves on the ECG.
- ECG changes indicative of ischaemia (ST segment elevation or depression).
- Following coronary artery intervention (e.g. angioplasty).

Incidence
240,000 cases per year in England and Wales.

Aetiology
Myocardial infarction almost always occurs in patients with atherosclerosis of the coronary arteries (see page 33).

Table 2.6 Patterns of acute myocardial infarction

Artery occluded	Pattern of infarction
Right coronary artery	Inferior MI (and posterior MI, if the circumflex artery is small)
Left anterior descending (LAD)	Anteroseptal MI
Left circumflex artery	Posterior MI (sometimes inferior, if the right coronary artery is small)
Left main stem	Extensive anterolateral MI

Pathophysiology

Acute myocardial infarction is caused by the occlusion of a coronary artery, usually as the result of rupture of an atherosclerotic plaque with subsequent development of thrombus. The myocardium supplied by that artery initially becomes ischaemic and if the occlusion does not resolve leads to infarction. Myocardial infarctions occur more commonly in the early morning possibly due to increased coronary artery tone, increased platelet aggregatability and decreased fibrinolytic activity. The extent and distribution of the infarct is dependent on the coronary artery affected, but also on individual variation due to variable anatomy and presence of collaterals (see Table 2.6).

Clinical features

Patients typically present with central crushing chest pain worse than stable angina, radiating to the jaw and arms (especially the left), which occurs at rest and lasts for some hours. It may provoke fear of imminent death (angor animi), but it may be less severe or even asymptomatic (especially diabetics, hypertensives and in the elderly). It is often associated with restlessness, breathlessness, sweating, nausea and vomiting. Signs may include pallor, sweating, hypotension, tachycardia, raised venous pressure and bibasal crepitations.

Macroscopy/microscopy

In the infarct-related artery, there is nearly always evidence of plaque rupture/erosion and thrombotic occlusion. In the infarct zone a sequence of changes occurs:

- 0–12 hours: Not visible macroscopically, there is loss of oxidative enzymes shown with nitroblue tetrazolium (NBT) stain.
- 12–24 hours: Infarcted area appears pale with intercellular oedema.
- 24–72 hours: Cellular inflammation visible.
- Weeks to months: White scar tissue develops through the process of repair.

Immediate complications

Sudden death, one third of patients who suffer an MI die within the first hour, most before admission to hospital.

Early complications (1 day to 2 weeks)

- Cardiac arrhythmias: Particularly ventricular fibrillation and ventricular tachycardia. If the atrioventricular node is involved bradyarrhythmias are common, although any arrhythmia is possible.
- Left ventricular failure is common with very large areas of infarction, which cause contractile dysfunction. Cardiogenic shock may result from low cardiac output due to extensive myocardial damage, rupture of the ventricular septum or papillary muscle leading to mitral regurgitation. The latter present with worsening refractory heart failure and a loud pansystolic murmur. If left untreated this has a very poor prognosis, and early surgical correction should be considered.
- Ventricular wall rupture usually occurs 2–10 days after a large transmural infarct. A haemopericardium develops due to exsanguination into the pericardial cavity resulting in tamponade and rapid death. This complication tends to affect older hypertensive patients, females more than males and the left ventricle more than the right.
- Thrombosis may occur on the inflamed endocardium over the infarction with resulting risk of embolism.

Long-term complications

- Recurrent ischaemia or myocardial infarction may occur due to thrombus formation within the same or other coronary arteries.
- Impaired left ventricular function leading to chronic cardiac failure.
- Ventricular aneurysms may form as the collagen scar that replaces the infarcted tissue formation does not contract and is non-elastic. Ventricular aneurysms are frequently complicated by thrombus formation but embolism is rare. They may worsen cardiac failure.
- Dressler's syndrome is a form of autoimmune-mediated pericarditis and pericardial effusion associated

Table 2.7 Distribution of ECG abnormalities in myocardial infarction

Infarct site	Leads	Artery
Anteroseptal	V1–V3	Septal
Anterior	V2–V5	LAD
Anterolateral	V1–V6, I, aVL	Left main stem
Lateral	I, II, aVL	Diagonal (branch of LAD)
Inferior	II, III, aVF	Right or circumflex
Posterior	V1, V2 (reciprocal i.e. ST depression)	Circumflex

with a high ESR; anti-inflammatory and steroid therapy may be necessary. It occurs 1–4 weeks after an infarction and presents with fever, chest pain and a pericardial rub on auscultation.

Investigations

ECG: The earliest change seen is ST segment elevation, the T wave then becomes inverted. The development of persistent Q waves usually denotes a more substantial infarct. The site of ischaemia and which artery is affected may be deduced from the site of ECG changes (see Table 2.7).

Biochemical markers of myocardial damage (see Fig. 2.5):

- Cardiac troponin is highly sensitive and specific; it is released early and persists for 7–10 days. It is also raised in NSTEMI (see page 36). It is now available as a bedside test.

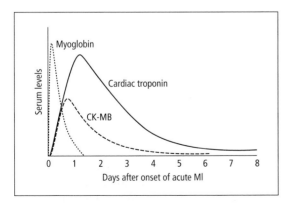

Figure 2.5 Biochemical markers of myocardial damage.

- Creatine kinase peaks within 24 hours; it is also produced by skeletal muscle and brain. CKMB is an isoenzyme that is specific for myocardial damage.
- Myoglobin levels rise within 2–3 hours of muscle injury, reach their highest levels by about 8–12 hours and fall back to normal by about 1 day.

Management

- Oral aspirin (300 mg) should be given as quickly as possible, followed by lifelong low-dose daily aspirin.
- The pain of a myocardial infarction should be controlled using diamorphine (with metoclopramide or cyclizine as an antiemetic).
- High flow oxygen should be given unless contraindicated.
- Thrombolytic therapy is routinely given as soon as possible after confirmation of the diagnosis and usually up to 12 hours after the onset of symptoms. Streptokinase is used in most patients. Recombinant tissue plasminogen activator (tPA) is used in young patients (<50 years), patients with anterior myocardial infarction, hypotension or in patients previously exposed to streptokinase. Contraindications to thrombolysis must be excluded, e.g. pregnancy, recent surgery, active bleeding or uncontrolled hypertension. Intravenous heparin is given in conjunction with all forms of tPA.
- β-blockers reduce myocardial demand and may limit the extent of infarction if given early; however, they can increase the risk of cardiac failure and hypotension. These should be given to all patients without evidence of heart failure unless contraindicated.
- ACE inhibitors should be given to patients following infarction, even without evidence of cardiac failure. They reduce mortality, reduce the number who develop cardiac failure and slow progression of the infarct, by improving the remodelling of myocardium postinfarct. Therapy is usually commenced the following day.
- Post-MI all patients should be commenced on a statin lipid lowering drug.
- Diabetic patients should be treated with an intravenous insulin sliding scale to ensure good glycaemic control, avoiding hypo- and hyperglycaemia. All diabetic patients should be treated with subcutaneous insulin for 3 months after discharge rather than oral agents.

- New developments include pre-hospital diagnosis and thrombolysis by trained paramedics. Primary percutaneous coronary intervention (i.e. angioplasty and stenting) has been shown to achieve lower mortality and earlier discharge following myocardial infarction. It is of particular value in patients with contraindications to thrombolysis. It is not currently available in most hospitals in the United Kingdom. Glycoprotein IIb/IIIa inhibitors are currently under evaluation.

Full mobilisation should be achieved after about 3 days and discharge at 5 days, if there are no complications. Risk factors for coronary disease should be identified and modified where possible (stop smoking, lower serum cholesterol, control hypertension, diabetics should be treated with insulin for 3 months). All patients should be offered rehabilitation for physical and psychological preparation for return to normal activities. The patient may return to work after 2–3 months, depending on the type of work. Car driving is not permitted for 4 weeks and HGV and public service licences are withdrawn pending evaluation.

If symptoms recur post-MI, or exercise tolerance testing shows continued myocardial ischaemia patients may be referred for angiography with a view to angioplasty or coronary artery bypass grafting.

Prognosis
50% 30-day mortality; 25% die before reaching hospital. Of those who leave hospital alive, 15–25% die within the first year. Subsequent mortality is highly dependent on age and comorbidity.

Variant/Prinzmetal's angina

Definition
Angina of no obvious provocation not as a direct result of atheroma.

Aetiology/pathophysiology
Caused by spasm of a coronary artery most often without atheroma or in association with a mild eccentric lesion. The reason for spasm occurring is unknown.

Clinical features
Pain is usually more severe and more prolonged than classical angina occurring at rest particularly in the early morning.

Complications
Arrhythmias may occur in the ischaemic episode (usually heart block and ventricular tachycardia), and very rarely the ischaemia may result in myocardial infarction.

Investigations
ECG shows characteristic ST elevation during an attack.

Management
- Nitrates and calcium antagonists are useful as prophylaxis and as acute treatment. β-blockers tend to increase coronary tone and hence exacerbate the angina. It may be necessary to treat the arrhythmias provoked by the spasm.
- Surgical treatment is rarely necessary or possible.

Prognosis
The prognosis in patients with angina without underlying heart or metabolic disease is very good.

Rheumatic fever and valve disease

Rheumatic fever

Definition
Recurrent inflammatory disease affecting the heart; it occurs following a streptococcal infection.

Incidence
1 in 100,000 United Kingdom/United States population per year; incidence has declined over the last 100 years.

Age
First attack usually 5–15 years.

Sex
M = F

Geography
Common in Middle and Far East, South America and Central Africa, declining in the West.

Aetiology
Cell-mediated autoimmune reaction following a pharyngeal infection with β-haemolytic streptococcus of

Lancefield group A (*Streptococcus pyogenes*). Risk factors for streptococcal infection include poverty and overcrowded conditions, the reduction of which, together with the increased use of antibiotics, may well explain the decline in developed countries.

Pathophysiology

It appears that antistreptococcal antibodies crossreact with antigens in connective tissues, particularly of endothelial-lined tissues such as blood vessels, endocardium, pericardium and synovial membranes. All three layers of the heart may be affected (pancarditis); the characteristic lesion is the Aschoff's nodule (see in section Microscopy below).

- Pericarditis: Nodules are seen within the pericardium associated with an inflammatory pericardial effusion.
- Myocarditis: Nodules develop within the myocardium associated with inflammation. This may result in decreased myocardial function and left ventricular failure.
- Endocarditis: Nodules may form anywhere on the endocardium, but tend to cause more damage and erosion when they occur within the heart valves as vegetations. These may result in an acute disturbance of valve function.

Recurrent attacks may occur over many years.

Clinical features

There may be a history of pharyngitis in up to 50% of patients. The diagnosis is made on two or more major manifestations or one major plus two or more minor manifestations (Duckett Jones criteria).

Major manifestations may be remembered as PACES:

- Pancarditis presents with new or changed cardiac murmurs (due to endocarditis) and the ECG changes of myocarditis and pericarditis. A pericardial friction rub may be audible due to pericarditis.
- Arthritis affecting multiple large joints that ranges in severity from mild aches to severe non-destructive arthritis, which may occur sequentially in different joints (flitting arthritis).
- Chorea (Sydenham's chorea) is characterised by jerky non-repetitive movements associated with reduced muscle tone. Postpuberty this manifestation is confined to females.
- Erythema marginatum is an erythematous rash composed of red, well-circumscribed lesions with a pale

centre over the trunk and limbs, which appear and disappear over a matter of hours.

- Subcutaneous painless nodules may be palpated over the extensor surfaces, tendons, joints and bony prominences.

Minor manifestations: pyrexia, raised ESR/CRP, arthralgia, previous rheumatic fever, long PR interval on ECG and a leucocytosis. Non-specific symptoms include malaise and loss of appetite.

Evidence of a preceding streptococcal infection such as positive throat culture, elevated antistreptolysin O titre or other streptococcal antibodies is suggestive.

Macroscopy

Fibrinous vegetations form on the edges of the valve leaflets with associated oedema. Valve leaflets may fuse and scar, particularly affecting the mitral and aortic valves.

Microscopy

Aschoff's nodules are granulomatous lesions composed of a necrotic core of degenerated collagen surrounded initially by macrophages and lymphocytes. Over time these cells are replaced by histiocytes, which may be multinucleated. Nodules heal by scarring.

Complications

More than 50% of patients with acute rheumatic carditis will develop chronic rheumatic valve disease 10–20 years later, particularly mitral and aortic stenosis. These may be complicated by atrial fibrillation, heart failure, infective endocarditis and mural thrombus formation.

Investigations

- Cultures of blood and tissues are sterile by the time rheumatic fever manifests, but throat swabs may be positive and there may be serological evidence (raised antistreptolysin O titre or other antistreptococcal antibodies).
- Non-specific indicators of inflammation, such as a raised ESR and leucocytosis.
- ECG shows prolonged PR interval and non-specific T wave changes. Pericarditis may initially result in widespread ST elevation, concave upwards. After a few days ST returns to the isoelectric point and there is T wave inversion.

- Echocardiography is used to examine the function of the cardiac valves and may be helpful in diagnosing pancarditis.

Management
- Patients with a clinical diagnosis of rheumatic fever should be treated with benzylpenicillin regardless of culture results.
- Pain, fever and inflammation are treated with high-dose aspirin. Carditis may be treated with a course of high-dose corticosteroids.
- Patients may require treatment for heart failure (see page 63) and chorea may respond to haloperidol.
- Following recovery patients should receive prophylactic penicillin for at least 5 years after the last attack or until the age of 20 years, whichever is the later.

Prognosis
Although symptomatic improvement occurs with treatment, therapy does not appear to prevent subsequent valve damage.

Mitral regurgitation

Definition
Flow of blood from the left ventricle to the left atrium during systole through an incompetent mitral valve.

Aetiology
In developing countries rheumatic disease accounts for the majority of cases of mitral regurgitation, often accompanied by mitral stenosis as a form of mixed mitral disease. In developed countries other causes predominate:
- Prolapsing mitral valve.
- Myocardial infarction may lead to papillary muscle dysfunction or rupture.
- Any disease that causes dilation of the left ventricle, such as dilated cardiomyopathy. Congestive heart failure may also cause mitral regurgitation due to downward displacement of the papillary muscle. This leads to a failure of the valve cusps to meet and regurgitation ranging in severity according to the degree of left ventricular enlargement.

- Infective endocarditis may cause destruction of the valve cusps.
- Idiopathic rupture of chordae tendinae.

Pathophysiology
In acute mitral regurgitation, retrograde blood flow from the left ventricle into the left atrium causes the left atrial pressure to increase. There is an increase in the pulmonary venous pressure and there may be pulmonary oedema. In longstanding mitral regurgitation there is a gradual enlargement of the left atrium. This allows the increased volume of atrial blood to be compensated for without a rise in the atrial pressure. The left ventricular stroke volume increases due to volume overload and over time this results in left ventricular hypertrophy.

Clinical features
Acute mitral regurgitation (e.g. following rupture of the chordae or papillary muscle dysfunction) presents with acute left-sided heart failure and pulmonary oedema. In most cases mitral regurgitation is chronic and is asymptomatic for many years. Patients may present with palpitations or symptoms of left ventricular failure (dyspnoea, orthopnoea, paroxysmal nocturnal dyspnoea). On examination the pulse is normal volume, but may be irregular due to atrial fibrillation. The apex is thrusting and becomes displaced downward and laterally. On auscultation the first heart sound is soft due to incomplete apposition of the valve cusps and there is a pansystolic murmur best heard at the apex radiating to the axilla. There may be a prominent third heart sound due to the sudden rush of blood back into the dilated left ventricle in early diastole.

Complications
Patients develop left ventricular failure due to chronic volume overload. Atrial fibrillation is common due to atrial dilation, with an increased risk of thromboembolism. Other complications include pulmonary oedema and infective endocarditis.

Investigations
- The chest X-ray shows cardiomegaly due to left atrial and left ventricular enlargement. Valve calcification may be seen in cases due to rheumatic fever. There may be evidence of pulmonary oedema.

- ECG is initially normal, but may show left atrial delay (bifid P waves, p mitrale), left ventricular hypertrophy or atrial fibrillation.
- Echocardiography is diagnostic allowing demonstration and quantification of the retrograde blood flow. The clinical effect of the valve lesion is however best assessed by measurement of the left ventricular dimensions (an end systolic dimension of over 5 cm indicates ventricular decompensation).

Management

- Mild mitral regurgitation in the absence of symptoms is managed conservatively, more severe disease with evidence of progressive cardiac enlargement is treated surgically. Valve repair is increasingly the operation of choice, but valve replacement may be required for severely diseased valves. Papillary muscle dysfunction and chordal rupture may require emergency valve replacement.
- Patients not undergoing surgery may require treatment of any complications such as cardiac failure or atrial fibrillation.
- Prophylaxis against infective endocarditis is required.

Mitral valve prolase

Definition
Prolapsing mitral valve is a condition in which the valve cusps prolapse into the left atrium during systole. It is also known as floppy mitral valve. A particular form of prolapse may result from myxomatous degeneration of the leaflets named Barlow's syndrome.

Incidence
Echocardiography reveals prolapsing mitral valve in 5% of the normal population; however, not all are clinically significant, especially in the absence of any mitral incompetence.

Age
Young adulthood.

Sex
F > M

Aetiology
Often there is no obvious underlying cause. Associated with Marfan's syndrome, thyrotoxicosis, rheumatic or ischaemic heart disease. There is also a familial element. It is thought to be due to progressive stretching of the valve leaflets.

Pathophysiology
The normal anatomy of the mitral valve prevents prolapse thus one or more anomalies must be present: excessively large mitral valve leaflets, an enlarged mitral annulus, abnormally long chordae or disordered papillary muscle contraction. During systole one of the valve leaflets (usually the posterior) balloons up into the atrium. In some cases this causes retraction at the normal point of contact of the valve cusps and hence mitral regurgitation. The condition does not often cause significant regurgitation.

Clinical features
Most patients are asymptomatic but some complain of left submammary stabbing chest pain. On auscultation there may be a mid-systolic click, with a late systolic (or occasionally pansystolic) murmur if regurgitation occurs.

Complications
Rupture of one of the chordae may occur leading to severe acute valve regurgitation. Arrhythmias including supraventricular tachycardia and complex ventricular ectopy may occur. There is an increased risk of thromboembolism and infective endocarditis.

Investigations
- ECG may be normal or show minor ST abnormalities.
- Echocardiography shows the mid-systolic bulging of the valve leaflets.

Management
β-blockers are used in patients with chest pain or palpitations. Patients with mitral valve regurgitation require prophylaxis against infective endocarditis. Patients with coexisting atrial fibrillation should be anticoagulated. Rarely severe cases may require valve repair or replacement.

Mitral stenosis

Definition
An abnormal narrowing of the mitral valve.

Incidence
Declining in the Western world due to the decline of rheumatic fever.

Sex
2F : 1M

Aetiology
Almost all mitral stenosis is secondary to rheumatic heart disease; it is also the most common valve to be affected by rheumatic fever. All other causes are rare, but include rheumatoid arthritis, systemic lupus erythematosus and congenital valve narrowing.

Pathophysiology
The pathological process of rheumatic fever results in fibrous scarring and fusion of the valve cusps with calcium deposition. The valve becomes stiff, failing to open fully. When the normal opening of 5 cm^2 is reduced to 1 cm^2 the mitral stenosis is severe. The pressure within the left atrium rises and left atrial hypertrophy occurs. As a consequence of this the pressure in the pulmonary circulation rises and eventually right atrial pressure will rise leading to right-sided heart failure. The cardiac output falls with little increase possible on exertion.

Clinical features
The condition is asymptomatic until the valve is narrowed by around 50%. The initial symptoms are due to pulmonary venous hypertension and the resultant oedema, with dyspnoea, orthopnoea and paroxysmal nocturnal dyspnoea. Atrial arrhythmias are common and may cause palpatations. A cough productive of frothy, blood-tinged sputum may occur (frank haemoptysis is rare). Progression leads to symptoms of right-sided heart failure (weakness, fatigue and peripheral oedema). On examination the patient may have mitral facies (bilateral, dusky cyanotic discoloration of the face). In severe mitral stenosis atrial fibrillation is very common. The apex beat is tapping in nature due to a palpable first heart sound.

On auscultation there is a loud S$_1$ as the mitral valve only closes when the ventricle contracts. There is an opening snap after S$_2$ caused by the stiff mitral valve, followed by a mid to late diastolic rumbling murmur due to turbulent flow through the stenosed valve. If the patient is in sinus rhythm there is a pre-systolic increase in the volume of the murmur due to increased flow during atrial contraction. Pulmonary hypertension may result in pulmonary regurgitation with an early-diastolic murmur (Graham–Steell murmur).

Complications
Complications are frequent:
- Atrial fibrillation (AF) due to atrial dilation and hypertrophy.
- Risk of stroke or systemic embolisation with mitral stenosis and AF is high.
- Pulmonary hypertension and right-sided heart failure.
- If the stiff valve also fails to close properly, mixed mitral stenosis and regurgitation.

Investigations
- Chest X-ray shows selective enlargement of the left atrium (bulge on the left heart border). Calcification within the mitral valve may be visible and there may be signs of pulmonary hypertension and oedema.
- In sinus rhythm, the ECG may show a bifid P wave due to delayed left atrial activation; however, atrial fibrillation is common. Signs of right ventricular hypertrophy such as right axis deviation, right ventricular hypertrophy or right bundle branch block may also be seen.
- Echocardiography is diagnostic showing the narrowing and immobility of the valve. Doppler studies can assess the degree of stenosis and any concomitant mitral regurgitation. If there is tricuspid regurgitation pulmonary pressures can also be calculated.
- Cardiac catheterisation is used if Doppler is inconclusive and to assess for coronary artery disease if valve replacement is contemplated.

Management
The course of mitral stenosis is gradual with intervention based on symptomatology. Associated atrial fibrillation is treated with digoxin and anticoagulation. Cardiac failure may also require treatment. Prophylaxis against

infective endocarditis is required. Patients with refractory pulmonary venous congestion or pulmonary hypertension are treated surgically by conservative surgery or valve replacement (see page 30).

Aortic regurgitation

Definition
Retrograde blood flow through the aortic valve from the aorta into the left ventricle during diastole.

Aetiology/pathophysiology
Aortic regurgitation is caused by incompetence of the valve in diastole, allowing blood to leak back into the left ventricle. This may result from:
- Inability of the valve cusps to close properly due to thickening, shrinkage, perforation or a tear in the cusp. Causes include rheumatic heart disease (now rare in the United Kingdom), infective endocarditis occurring on a previously damaged or bicuspid aortic valve, and various arthritides such as Reiter's syndrome, ankylosing spondylitis or rheumatoid arthritis.
- Significant dilation of the aortic annulus such that the cusps are separated at the edges. Causes include severe hypertension, dissecting aneurysm and Marfan's syndrome.

As a result of the volume overload, the left ventricle gradually enlarges and the ejection fraction is increased (Starling's mechanism). It is only when volume overload is excessive and chronic that the left ventricle fails. The first sign of this decompensation is a reduction in the ejection fraction, leading to an increased end systolic volume. There is also reduced coronary artery perfusion with associated increased risk of myocardial ischaemia.

Clinical features
Aortic regurgitation is asymptomatic until left ventricular failure develops. Patients usually present with dyspnoea, a pounding heart beat and angina. On examination there is a large volume pulse, which is collapsing in character (see page 27). The blood pressure has a wide pulse pressure (high systolic and low diastolic pressure). The apex is displaced laterally and downwards and is heaving in nature. Various signs of the high-velocity blood flow have been described but are rare.

On auscultation there is a high pitched early diastolic murmur running from the aortic component of the second heart sound. There may be an accompanying mid-systolic ejection murmur due to volume overload. An Austin Flint murmur may also be heard. This is a mid-diastolic rumbling murmur due to back flow of blood during diastole causing a partial closure of the mitral valve.

Investigations
- Chest X-ray shows an enlarged left ventricle and possibly dilation of the ascending aorta.
- ECG may show signs of progressive left ventricular hypertrophy.
- Echocardiogram is diagnostic demonstrating abnormal valve movement. Doppler studies demonstrate and quantify the regurgitation. The best way to monitor the clinical effect of the valve lesion is to measure the left ventricular dimension. An end systolic dimension of over 5 cm indicates decompensation.

Management
- Any underlying causes such as infective endocarditis should be treated. Antibiotic prophylaxis against infective endocarditis should be administered when appropriate.
- Symptomatic relief can be given by treatment of any associated heart failure.
- Refractory symptoms with evidence of increasing heart size or diminishing left ventricular function are indications for surgical intervention usually by valve replacement.

Prognosis
Mild or moderate aortic regurgitation has a relatively good prognosis and thus surgical intervention is not required. However, it is important to perform surgical correction before irreversible left ventricular failure develops.

Aortic stenosis

Definition
Aortic stenosis is a pathological narrowing of the aortic valve.

Aetiology

- Congenital bicuspid aortic valves can initially open with little obstruction. There is however turbulent flow across these valves, which become thickened and calcified. Severe stenosis may develop over a period of 20–30 years.
- Congenital aortic valve narrowing leads to presentation in infancy or childhood.
- Rheumatic fever results in progressive cusp adherence, thickening and calcification. It is often associated with aortic incompetence and mitral valve disease.
- Sclerotic aortic stenosis is due to degenerative changes in the cusps seen in the elderly. It may lead to thickening and calcification of the aortic valve, which is often mild and asymptomatic.

Pathophysiology

The outflow of the left ventricle is obstructed causing the pressure within the left ventricle to rise. This pressure overload results in left ventricular hypertrophy and a relative ischaemia of the myocardium with associated angina. As the stenosis becomes more severe, reduced coronary artery perfusion exacerbates myocardial ischaemia even if the coronary arteries are normal. Impaired left ventricular emptying is most apparent during times of increased cardiac demand such as exercise. Ischaemia and hypertrophy of the left ventricle may lead to arrhythmias and left ventricular failure.

Clinical features

Patients are asymptomatic until there is severe stenosis when they present with exercise-induced syncope, angina or dyspnoea. Sudden cardiac death may also occur. Late symptoms include orthopnoea and paroxysmal nocturnal dyspnoea.

On examination the pulse is low volume and slow rising (see page 27). On palpation there may be an aortic systolic thrill felt in the right second intercostal space. The apex is slow and thrusting in nature but not displaced. On auscultation there may be a systolic ejection click, followed by a mid-systolic ejection murmur heard best in the right second intercostal space and radiating to carotids. The murmur is best heard with the patient leaning forward with breath held in expiration.

Investigations

- Chest X-ray may show a post-stenotic dilation of the ascending aorta and left ventricular hypertrophy.

- ECG shows left ventricular strain or hypertrophy related to the degree of stenosis.
- Echocardiography is diagnostic, often showing cusp thickening and calcification. Doppler studies quantify the degree of stenosis and can measure left ventricular function.
- Cardiac catheterisation can demonstrate the pressure difference between the left ventricle and aorta, and is required to examine the coronary arteries prior to surgery.

Management

- Treatment includes management of angina and cardiac failure. Vasodilators such as nitrates must be avoided in severe aortic stenosis as they can cause syncope due to a fall in systolic blood pressure. ACE inhibitors are also relatively contraindicated. β-blockers are often the drug of choice.
- Severe stenosis (pressure gradient over 60 mmHg) or symptomatic stenosis are indications for surgery (see page 30). Operative mortality is approximately 2%, but this is increased if coronary artery bypass is also required. Balloon valvuloplasty may be used in patients unfit for surgery or to improve cardiac function prior to surgery.

Prognosis

When symptomatic, death occurs within a few years without surgical intervention.

Pulmonary stenosis

Definition

Narrowing of the pulmonary valve, resulting in pressure overload of the right ventricle.

Aetiology

This is almost invariably a congenital lesion either as an isolated lesion or as part of the tetralogy of Fallot. Rarely it may be an acquired lesion secondary to rheumatic fever or the carcinoid syndrome.

Pathophysiology

The obstruction to right ventricular emptying results in right ventricular hypertrophy and hence decreased ventricular compliance, which leads to right atrial hypertrophy. If severe, the condition leads to right ventricular failure, often with accompanying regurgitation of the tricuspid valve and signs of right-sided heart failure.

Clinical features

Severe pulmonary obstruction leads to right-sided heart failure in the first few weeks of life. Patients with mild pulmonary stenosis are asymptomatic (diagnosed incidentally from the presence of a murmur or the presence of right ventricular hypertrophy on the ECG). Patients may have non-specific symptoms such as fatigue or dyspnoea. Syncope is a sign of critical stenosis, which requires urgent treatment.

On examination a large 'a' wave may be seen in the JVP (see page 27). Auscultation reveals a click and harsh mid-systolic ejection murmur heard best on inspiration in the left second intercostal space often associated with a thrill. A left parasternal heave may also be felt due to right ventricular hypertrophy.

Investigations

- Chest X-ray may show a prominent pulmonary artery due to post-stenotic dilation.
- ECG may reveal right ventricular strain or hypertrophy indicating the degree of stenosis.
- Echocardiography is used to examine and quantify the flow across the stenosed valve. It is also essential to identify any associated cardiac lesions such as tetralogy of Fallot. Assessment of right ventricular function is essential.
- Cardiac catheterisation may be used to assess the level and degree of the stenosis.

Management

Mild stenosis does not require treatment. In more severe cases intervention is required before decompensation of the right ventricle occurs. Balloon dilatation has more or less replaced the need for surgery except in the context of more complex congenital heart disease.

Tricuspid regurgitation

Definition

Retrograde blood flow from the right ventricle to the right atrium during systole.

Aetiology

Tricuspid regurgitation can be divided into functional, i.e. secondary to dilation of the right ventricle, and organic tricuspid regurgitation:

- Functional tricuspid regurgitation occurs with cor pulmonale, right-sided myocardial infarction or pulmonary hypertension.
- Organic tricuspid regurgitation occurs with rheumatic mitral valve disease, infective endocarditis and the carcinoid syndrome. Infective endocarditis affecting the tricuspid valve is seen particularly in intravenous drug abusers. Ebstein's anomaly is a congenital dysplasia of the tricuspid valve with abnormal valve cusps and a downward malpositioning of the valve.

Pathophysiology

Regurgitation of blood into the right atrium during systole results in high right atrial pressures and hence right atrial hypertrophy and dilatation. Volume overload results in an initial increase in right ventricular stroke volume (Starling's mechanism) until decompensation occurs, after which there is a reduction in cardiac output and signs of right-sided heart failure.

Clinical features

Patients may present with symptoms and signs of right-sided heart failure such as ankle oedema, fatigue and ascites. On examination a prominent V (systolic) wave may be seen in the JVP (see page 27) and a pulsatile enlarged liver may be palpable. A right ventricular heave may be felt at the left sternal edge. On auscultation there is a pansystolic murmur, which unlike mitral regurgitation is accentuated by inspiration heard best at the left lower sternal edge.

Complications

Atrial fibrillation is very common. In the chronic untreated patient there can be hepatic cirrhosis from the pressure effect on the liver.

Investigations

The chest X-ray may show right atrial and ventricular enlargement. Echocardiography is diagnostic and is also essential to assess right ventricular function.

Management

Functional tricuspid regurgitation usually resolves with management of heart failure. Severe organic tricuspid regurgitation or refractory functional regurgitation may require operative repair (or rarely replacement).

Cardiac arrhythmias

A cardiac arrhythmia is a disturbance of the normal rhythm of the heart. Many arrhythmias are asymptomatic unless myocardial function is compromised. Normal sinus rhythm is not exactly regular as there are fluctuations in autonomic tone with respiration. On inspiration the parasympathetic tone falls and the heart rate increases, conversely on expiration parasympathetic tone rises and the heart rate decreases. This variation is normal and is referred to as sinus arrhythmia.

Cardiac arrhythmias can be classified according to whether they are bradycardias (<60 bpm) or tachycardias (>100 bpm).

Bradycardias may be due to disorders of the sinus node or the atrioventricular (AV) node:

- Sinus bradycardia and sinus node disease (also called sick sinus syndrome).
- Atrioventricular block where the atria may be acting normally, but the AV node does not conduct the impulses normally to the ventricles.

Tachycardias are also subdivided according to their origin:

- Sinus tachycardia.
- Supraventricular tachycardia including atrial or junctional (AV nodal) tachycardias.
- Ventricular tachyarrhythmias such as ventricular tachycardia and ventricular fibrillation are often secondary to ischaemic myocardial damage. Torsades de pointes is a distinctive type of ventricular tachycardia associated with a long Q–T interval with a characteristic ECG (see page 55).

A useful clinical division is between narrow complex tachycardias, which are due to supraventricular (atrial or junctional) tachycardias, and broad complex tachycardias, which are most often ventricular in origin. However, in patients with bundle branch block and in cases where the rapid rate of supraventricular tachycardias causes transient bundle branch block, broad complex tachycardias can be supraventricular in origin.

Sinus nodal arrhythmias

Sinus bradycardia

Definition
A sinus rate of less than 60 bpm.

Aetiology
- It is a normal finding in athletes.
- Sinus node damage, e.g. myocardial infarction or degeneration in old age.
- Hypothermia, hypothyroidism.
- Drug therapy, e.g. β-blockers (including eye drops) or anti-arrhythmic drugs.
- Raised intra-cranial pressure due to increased vagal discharge.
- Severe cholestatic jaundice due to deposition of bilirubin in the conducting system.

Pathophysiology
The cardiac output is a function of not only the heart rate but also the stroke volume and hence in mild cases of sinus bradycardia there is no compromise of the cardiac output as a result of increased stroke volume.

Clinical features
Most patients are asymptomatic but occasionally post-MI or in the elderly, cardiac failure or hypotension may arise, as the stroke volume is unable to maintain cardiac output. If bradycardia is episodic and severe, syncope may occur.

Investigations
Sinus bradycardia is diagnosed on ECG. Investigations of causes include temperature, thyroid function tests and liver function tests if the patient is jaundiced.

Management
Most cases do not require treatment other than withdrawal of drugs or treatment of any underlying cause. In acute symptomatic sinus bradycardia intravenous atropine may be required. Chronic symptomatic bradycardia may require a permanent cardiac pacemaker.

Sinus tachycardia

Definition
Sinus rate above 100 bpm.

Aetiology/pathophysiology
Sinus tachycardia is a physiological response to maintain tissue perfusion and oxygenation. Causes include exercise, fever, anaemia, hypovolaemia, hypoxia, heart failure, hyperthyroidism, pulmonary embolism, drugs and emotion.

Clinical features
Palpitations with an associated rapid, regular pulse rate. Features of any underlying cause often predominate.

Investigations
The ECG confirms sinus rhythm and demonstrates the tachycardia. Appropriate investigations of the underlying cause may be required.

Management
Treatment is aimed at the underlying cause. β-blockers can slow the rate, but this is rarely of clinical benefit.

Sinus node disease

Definition
Sinus node disease or sick sinus syndrome is a tachycardia/bradycardia resulting from damage to the sinus node.

Aetiology/pathophysiology
Sinus node disease is relatively common in the elderly due to ischaemia, infarction or degeneration of the sinus node. The condition is characterised by prolonged intervals between consecutive P waves (sinus arrest) and periods of sinus bradycardia. Pauses in the sinus rhythm may allow tachycardias (typically atrial fibrillation) from other foci to emerge. This combination of fast and slow supraventricular rhythms is known as tachy-brady syndrome.

Clinical features
Tachycardia may cause palpitations, and long pauses may cause dizziness and syncope. On examination the pulse rate may be regular, bradycardic, tachycardic or variable with pauses. Carotid sinus massage typically leads to a sudden and sometimes prolonged sinus pause. It should therefore only be attempted where there is monitoring and resuscitation equipment.

Complications
The most important complication is cardiac syncope, as in other forms of bradycardia. It may develop associated AV nodal block and Increased risk of thromboembolism.

Investigations
The diagnosis is usually made with a 24-hour ECG. Twelve-lead ECG may show evidence of underlying ischaemia or previous myocardial infarction.

Management
Permanent pacing is required for symptomatic patients. In addition anti-arrhythmic drugs may be required to control any tachycardia. Patients require anticoagulation to reduce the risk of thromboembolism.

Atrial arrhythmias

Atrial ectopic beats

Definition
Atrial ectopic beats include extrasystoles and premature beats.

Aetiology
Atrial ectopics are common in normal individuals. All cardiac cells have intrinsic pacemaker ability. They gradually depolarise until a threshold is reached at which point rapid depolarisation occurs and a cardiac action potential is fired. This is most rapid in the sinoatrial node, the normal pacemaker of the heart. If in a single or group of cells the gradual depolarisation is more rapid than usual, or if the voltage threshold for rapid depolarisation is reduced they may stimulate a cardiac depolarisation resulting in an ectopic beat. This process is termed enhanced automaticity. Common causes are electrolyte abnormalities, alcohol or nicotine excess, anaemia, medications such as β-agonists, and hypoxaemia.

Pathophysiology

As the depolarisation of the heart arises from within the atria, the QRS complex of the ECG is preceded by a P wave which may be of different configuration as atrial depolarisation has a different origin to normal. The QRS complex is the same as normal because the depolarisation of the ventricles begins from the AV node.

Clinical features

Patients are often asymptomatic but may complain of an irregular or thumping heartbeat. The patient may complain of a skipped beat, as there is a compensatory pause after an extrasystole.

Investigations

ECG shows early, abnormal P waves followed by a normal QRS complex and a compensatory pause. Ectopic P waves are often best seen in lead V1.

Management

Atrial ectopic beats do not require treatment, although underlying causes of increased automaticity should be identified and managed. If atrial ectopic beats are frequent they may progress to other atrial arrhythmias.

Atrial flutter

Definition

Atrial flutter is a rapid atrial rate between 280 and 350 bpm, most commonly 300 bpm.

Aetiology

Atrial flutter is almost always a complication of myocardial disease such as ischaemic, hypertensive and rheumatic heart disease, cardiomyopathies, myocarditis and constrictive pericarditis. It may be caused by thyrotoxicosis.

Pathophysiology

Normally once a cardiac cell has been depolarised it is refractory to re-stimulation for a short period. This prevents waves of cardiac depolarisation flowing in a retrograde direction. If, however, the conduction through the myocardium is slow (usually due to myocardial damage), adjacent cells may have recovered from their refractory period allowing restimulation and hence the formation of a recurrent cycle of depolarisation or circus movement (also termed re-entry).

In atrial flutter the circuit is single and has a characteristic location in the right atrium involving an area close to the entrance of the vena cavae. This relatively fixed physical characteristic explains the typical ECG appearance and consistent cycle length between individual patients.

Whilst the atrial rate is between 280 and 350 beats, the normal atrioventricular delay in the AV node limits the ventricular rate. This usually produces a 2:1, 3:1 or 4:1 atrioventricular block.

Clinical features

Atrial flutter presents with palpitations, dizziness, syncope or cardiac failure. It may occur persistently or in episodes (paroxysmal atrial flutter) that last minutes or hours to days. The pulse rate is dependent on the degree to which the AV node blocks the rate but is most commonly around 150 bpm (2:1 block). Massage of the carotid sinus causes a transient increase in block with consequent slowing of the ventricular rate.

Investigations

Atrial flutter produces a characteristic regular sawtooth 'flutter' waves at a rate of 300 bpm seen best in lead V1. If there is 2:1 block, the QRS complexes often obscure the flutter waves, but carotid sinus massage should reveal them (see Fig. 2.6).

Management

DC cardioversion is the best treatment to restore sinus rhythm rapidly. Drug treatment is used to control the ventricular rate, prevent recurrence and may occasionally restore sinus rhythm. Following electrophysiological assessment, recurrence may be prevented by radiofrequency ablation of atrial flutter circuits. Digoxin increases AV block and reduces the ventricular rate, amiodorone may restore sinus rhythm and reduce the frequency of paroxysms.

Atrial fibrillation

Definition

Atrial fibrillation is a quivering of atrial myocardium resulting from disordered electrical and muscle activity.

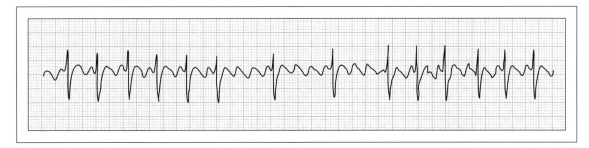

Figure 2.6 ECG in atrial flutter showing flutter waves revealed by carotid sinus massage.

Incidence
Common

Age
Increases with age: 1% in people aged 60 years and 5% over 70 years.

Sex
M > F

Aetiology
Causes may be divided into cardiac and systemic. Lone atrial fibrillation is when no structural or organic cause can be found.
- Cardiac: Atrial enlargement is a common mechanism for the onset of atrial fibrillation. Various cardiac and systemic conditions cause a chronic rise in atrial pressure and in time lead to atrial enlargement, e.g. ischaemic, hypertensive and rheumatic heart disease, mitral valve disease, cardiomyopathies and pulmonary disease.
- Systemic causes include thyrotoxicosis, alcohol and acute infections especially pneumonia.

Pathophysiology
Atrial fibrillation is the result of multiple re-entrant circuits in the atria (see above). Since each of these numerous circuits have different cycle times, the result is a constant train of irregular impulses of various amplitude reaching the AV node, resulting in a very irregular ventricular response. The AV node blocks some of the transmissions, but an irregularly irregular pulse of between 100 and 160 per minute usually results. Atrial fibrillation may be paroxysmal with attacks lasting minutes to hours. Symptoms may arise if there is a high ventricular

rate, in the elderly who depend on atrial function to achieve sufficient ventricular filling, or if there is associated significant cardiac damage. Abnormal atrial blood flow predisposes to thromboembolism.

Clinical features
Atrial fibrillation is often asymptomatic. Patients may present with palpitations, acute cardiac failure or the gradual onset of increasing shortness of breath. On examination there is an irregularly irregular pulse with varying pulse volume. There is also loss of the 'a' wave of the JVP.

Investigations
- ECG shows fine irregular oscillations of the base line, with a QRS totally irregular in timing normally at a rate of between 100 and 160 bpm (see Fig. 2.7).
- Thyroid function tests should be performed in all patients. In acute atrial fibrillation, underlying ischaemia such as a recent myocardial infarction or unstable angina should be excluded.

Management
- Restoration of sinus rhythm may be achieved with synchronised DC cardioversion or by use of amiodarone or other drugs. DC cardioversion has a high relapse rate. The longer the atrial fibrillation has been present, the less the likelihood of restoring sinus rhythm.
- Maintenance of sinus rhythm may be achieved with anti-arrhythmic drugs, but long-term use of amiodarone has significant side effects. Digoxin does not prevent recurrence.
- Control of the ventricular rate is achieved with drugs such as digoxin, calcium channel blockers and/or β-blockers.

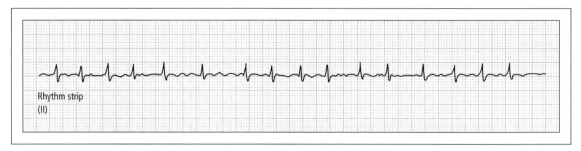

Rhythm strip
(II)

Figure 2.7 ECG in atrial fibrillation showing irregularly irregular QRS complexes and fine oscillations in the baseline.

- Warfarin anticoagulation is used in patients over the age of 65 years and in those at increased risk of thromboembolism including presence of hypertension, valve disease and left ventricular dysfunction. In younger patients without other risk factors aspirin may be used as an alternative. Anticoagulation is also indicated for at least 1 month preceding and post-DC cardioversion.

Junctional arrhythmias

Junctional tachycardia

Definition
Tachycardia with the source being at or involving the AV node (also called AV nodal tachycardias) usually with rates 140–220 bpm.

Aetiology/pathophysiology
The majority of junctional tachycardias are due to re-entry circuits.

- These may be confined to the AV node (AV nodal re-entry tachycardia – AVNRT). The abnormal AV node consists of both slow and fast conducting pathways. Usually there is a slow anterograde pathway from atria to ventricles and a fast retrograde pathway back to the atria, which forms the re-entry circuit. The ECG during normal sinus rhythm is unremarkable. The re-entrant circuit is concealed as it slow, close to the node and does not interfere with normal AV node activity.
- Alternatively there may be an aberrant conduction pathway at a distance from the AV node (AV re-entry tachycardia AVRT). The most well-recognised condi-

tion of tachycardia due to aberrant pathway is Wolff–Parkinson–White syndrome (see page 53). The AV node acts as a fast or slow anterograde pathway and the accessory pathway conducts back to the atria to form the re-entry circuit.

Junctional tachycardias may occur spontaneously or may be triggered by exertion, tobacco, coffee or alcohol. They last for minutes to hours or rarely days. The frequency of occurrence is very variable even in a single individual.

Clinical features
The characteristic clinical picture is of sudden onset of palpitations sometimes accompanied by chest pain, dyspnoea and polyuria due to high circulating levels of atrial naturetic peptide. During an attack the pulse is between 140 and 220 bpm, and in severe cases, the rapid rate impairs cardiac filling and may result in hypotension.

Investigations/management
- During a paroxysm patients require a 12-lead ECG and continuous ECG monitoring. Normal rapid regular QRS complexes are seen. In AV nodal tachycardia P waves are usually hidden within the QRS complex. If the retrograde pathway is slow with delayed atrial contraction, inverted P waves appear between complexes. Carotid sinus massage or bolus injection of adenosine may produce an immediate cessation of the arrhythmia. In contrast, atrial tachycardia and atrial flutter will produce only transient slowing of the ventricular rate due to the increase in AV node block.
- Between paroxysms diagnosis is often difficult. Exercise testing, 24-hour Holter monitors or patient activated recorders may be useful.

- Prophylaxis involves identification and avoidance of trigger factors where possible. Pharmacological prophylaxis may be achieved using anti-arrhythmic drugs (e.g. flecainide). Radiofrequency ablation of the AV node or accessory pathway is being increasingly used as an effective method to prevent recurrence.

Wolff–Parkinson–White syndrome

Definition
Congenital predisposition to recurrent supraventricular tachycardia due to the presence of an extra accessory pathway between the atria and the ventricles.

Aetiology
Abnormal connection between atrium and ventricle (e.g. bundle of Kent) that allows quick conduction from the atria to the ventricles bypassing the AV node. Half of patients have a tachycardia either due to re-entry or atrial fibrillation.

Pathophysiology
Normally the fast conduction through the bundle of Kent allows the adjacent area of ventricle to be rapidly depolarised (preexcitation), whilst the remainder of the ventricle is depolarised by the normal route. However, the two pathways may form a re-entry circuit with the fast accessory pathway causing a retrograde stimulation of the atria and hence the AV node. The result is a form of paroxysmal supraventricular tachycardia.

Clinical features
In sinus rhythm Wolff–Parkinson–White syndrome is asymptomatic. Patients may experience paroxysms of palpitations sometimes accompanied by chest pain and dyspnoea, which may last minutes, hours or days.

Investigations
- During sinus rhythm the rapid conduction through the accessory pathway causes a short PR interval (<0.12 seconds) and a wide QRS complex beginning with a slurred part known as a δ wave (see Fig. 2.8).
- During a tachycardic episode, the conduction enters the ventricle through the AV node thus the PR interval and QRS morphology return to normal. Retrograde excitation of the atria causes abnormal P waves following the QRS complex.

Complications
Sudden cardiac death may rarely occur if atrial fibrillation occurs. This leads to ventricular fibrillation because the accessory pathway can conduct rapid impulses without the usual blocking effect of the AV node, leading to sudden death.

Management
- Re-entrant tachycardias are treated with drugs that block retrograde conduction through the accessory pathway, e.g. disopyramide, propanolol or amiodarone. Verapamil and digoxin are contraindicated as they accelerate anterograde conduction through the accessory pathway.
- Symptomatic patients should be offered a specialist evaluation for radioablation of the accessory pathway.

Prognosis
With age the pathway may fibrose and so some patients 'grow out of' the condition.

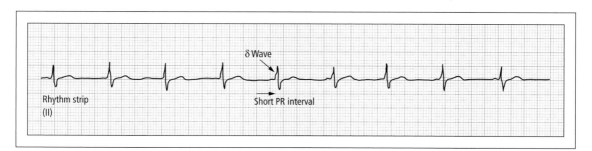

Figure 2.8 Resting ECG in Wolff–Parkinson–White syndrome.

Ventricular arrhythmias

Ventricular ectopic beats

Definition

A ventricular ectopic/extrasystole/premature beat is an extra myocardial depolarisation triggered by a focus in the ventricle.

Aetiology/pathophysiology

Ventricular ectopics are not uncommon in normal individuals and increase in incidence with advancing age. Common causes include ischaemic heart disease and hypertension. Ectopic beats may arise due to any of the mechanisms of arrhythmias, such as a re-entry circuit or due to enhanced automaticity (which may occur with electrolyte abnormalities, alcohol or nicotine excess, anaemia, medications such as β agonists or hypoxaemia). When ventricular ectopic beats occur regularly after each sinus beat, it is termed bigeminy, which is frequently due to digoxin.

Clinical features

Patients are usually asymptomatic but may feel uncomfortable or beaware of an irregular heart or missed beats. On examination the pulse may be irregular if ectopics are frequent.

Investigations

- ECG shows broad bizarre QRS complexes without preceding P, followed by an inverted T wave and then a pause before the next sinus beat (see Fig. 2.9).
- Echocardiography and exercise testing may be used to look for underlying structural or ischaemic heart disease.

Management

Ventricular ectopic beats do not require treatment although any underlying cause should be identified and managed.

Prognosis

Ventricular ectopics worsen the prognosis in patients with underlying ischaemic heart disease but there is no evidence that anti-arrhythmic drugs improve this.

Ventricular tachycardia

Definition

Tachycardia of ventricular origin at a rate of 120–220 bpm.

Aetiology

Ventricular tachycardia is normally associated with underlying coronary, ischaemic or hypertensive heart disease, or cardiomyopathies.

Pathophysiology

The underlying mechanism is thought to be enhanced automaticity, leading to re-entry circuit as in other tachycardias. In ventricular tachycardia there is a small (or sometimes large) group of ischaemic or electrically non-homogeneous cells, typically resulting from an acute myocardial infarction.

Clinical features

The condition is episodic with attacks usually lasting minutes. Patients may experience palpitations, shortness of breath, chest pain and if there is a resultant

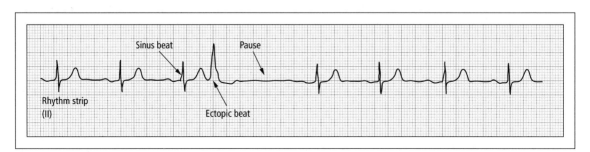

Figure 2.9 Ventricular ectopic beat.

compromise of cardiac output overt cardiac failure or loss of consciousness may occur. The presenting picture is dependent on the rapidity of the tachycardia and the function of the left ventricle, as well as general condition of the patient (e.g. hypovolaemia, anaemia, ischaemic heart disease, etc). On examination during an acute episode the rapid regular pulse is felt and as the atria are dissociated from the ventricles they may contract against a closed AV valve resulting in cannon 'a' waves in the JVP. Carotid sinus massage may help to distinguish ventricular tachycardia, which does not respond, from supraventricular tachycardia with bundle branch block, which may respond.

Investigations
The ECG shows a broad complex tachycardia, AV dissociation (independent P wave activity). Low serum potassium or magnesium may predispose to arrhythmias, so levels should be checked.

Complications
Cardiac arrest due to pulseless ventricular tachycardia or ventricular fibrillation. Pulmonary oedema or syncope may also occur.

Management
- Any underlying electrolyte disturbance should be identified and managed.
- If the patient has low cardiac output and is hypotensive, intravenous amiodarone or emergency synchronised DC cardioversion is used.
- Anti-arrhythmic drugs such as amiodarone and β-blockers often in combination with other drugs are used to prevent further episodes. Implantable cardioverter defibrillators, which automatically detect VT and VF and terminate the arrhythmia with overdrive pacing or DC shock, may be used.
- Patients require treatment of any underlying condition such as ischaemic heart disease.
- Pulseless VT is treated as per cardiac arrest with basic and advanced life support. Early defibrillation is needed to restore sinus rhythm.

Prognosis
Recurrent VT has a worse prognosis, particularly in the context of myocardial infarction.

Torsades de pointes

Definition
Torsades de pointes or 'twisting of the points' is a condition in which there is episodic tachycardia and a prolonged Q–T interval when in sinus rhythm.

Aetiology
It arises when ventricular repolarisation is prolonged due to congenital cause, hypokalaemia, hypocalcaemia, anti-arrhythmic drugs, tricyclic antidepressants or bradycardia from the sick sinus syndrome. It may also occur in overdose of drugs that prolong the Q–T interval.

Pathophysiology
It is thought that the long Q–T interval allows adjacent cells, which are repolarising at slightly different rates, to trigger one another in a knock-on effect. The Q–T interval is prolonged by biochemical abnormalities and drugs, and is also prolonged in bradycardic states.

Clinical features
It typically recurs in frequent short attacks, causing presyncope, syncope or heart failure.

Investigations
Repetitive bursts of rapid regular, polymorphic, QRS complexes, the axis of which undergoes cyclical change. During periods of sinus rhythm a prolonged Q–T interval is seen.

Complications
The major risk of torsades de pointes is progression to ventricular fibrillation.

Management
Any underlying cause should be identified and corrected. Overdrive pacing at 90–100 bpm may terminate the arrhythmia and is the best method for preventing recurrences, alternatively an infusion of isoprenaline may be used. If cardiac output is compromised synchronised DC cardioversion is used.

Ventricular fibrillation

Definition
Chaotic electromechanical activity of the ventricles causing a loss of cardiac output.

Incidence
The most common cause of sudden death and the most common primary arrhythmia in cardiac arrest.

Aetiology
May occur de novo, as a sequelae to a myocardial infarction, post-electrocution or as a result of other arrhythmias or drug overdose including digoxin and adrenaline. It may be preceded by another arrhythmia such as torsades de pointes or develop in the context of complete heart block. Hypokalaemia and hypomagnesaemia may also result in ventricular fibrillation.

Pathophysiology
The underlying electrical activity consists of multiple ectopic foci and small re-entry circuits with resulting uncoordinated contractions such that cardiac ventricular filling and cardiac output fall to zero.

Clinical features
The clinical picture is of cardiac arrest with loss of arterial pulsation, loss of consciousness and cessation of breathing.

Investigations
ECG shows the chaotic rhythm with ventricular complexes of varying amplitude, rate and form distinguishing it from pulseless electrical activity and asystole (the other causes of cardiac arrest).

Management
- Early defibrillation is the most important treatment, as the longer it is delayed the less likely reversion to sinus rhythm is possible. Cardiopulmonary resuscitation should be initiated to maintain organ perfusion until defibrillation can be given.
- Prevention of recurrent of ventricular fibrillation is with antiarrhythmics usually amiodarone.
- Increasingly automatic implantable cardiac defibrillators (AICDs) are implanted to prevent sudden death. The most common indication is for 'failed sudden

death' where a subject is fortunate to survive such an event. It is now customary to use these in patients known to have a high risk of sudden cardiac death.

Conduction disturbances

Atrioventricular block

Atrioventricular or heart block describes an alteration in the normal pattern of transmission of action potentials between the atria and the ventricles. The normal function of the AV node is to delay the transmission of action potentials and hence protect the ventricles from transmission of atrial rates fast enough to impair cardiac filling. Block at the AV node may result in (see Fig. 2.10)
- a prolongation of the time required for transmission (first degree block).
- intermittent failure of transmission (second degree block).
- complete failure of transmission (third-degree heart block).

First degree atrioventricular block

Definition
Atrioventricular block describes an alteration in the transmission of action potentials between the atria and the ventricles. First degree block is a prolongation of the time required for AV transmission.

Aetiology
First degree block occurs occasionally in normal individuals but may follow rheumatic fever, ischaemic heart disease or digoxin toxicity. In the young it is often caused by high vagal tone. First degree block may progress onto other forms of heart block.

Clinical features
First degree atrioventricular block is asymptomatic.

Investigations
- ECG shows a prolongation of the PR interval >0.2 seconds (one large square on a standard ECG) with QRS complexes following every P wave (see Fig. 2.11).
- Digoxin level in patients on digoxin to exclude overdose.

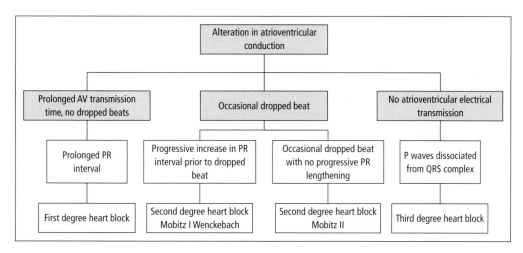

Figure 2.10 Atrioventricular block.

Management
No treatment is required.

Second degree atrioventricular block – Mobitz type I (Wenckebach phenomenon)

Definition
Second degree atrioventricular block is intermittent failure of AV transmission. In Mobitz type I (Wenckebach phenomenon) the missed beat is preceded by a progressive lengthening of the PR interval.

Aetiology
Occurs most commonly in association with underlying acute coronary pathology such as post-MI. Wenckebach phenomenon may result from digoxin, verapamil or β-blocker overdose and a benign form exists in the young and athletes due to high vagal tone.

Pathophysiology
The site of pathology of Mobitz type I is the AV node itself (in contrast to Mobitz II where infra nodal pathology is thought to be the cause). Complete AV block may develop, when a ventricular escape rhythm must occur for cardiac output to be maintained.

Clinical features
Patients are usually asymptomatic; however, an irregular pulse is detected on examination.

Investigations
The ECG reveals the progressive lengthening of the PR interval until a beat is missed after which the PR interval returns to normal and the cycle recurs (see Fig. 2.12).

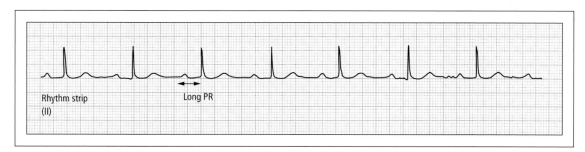

Figure 2.11 First degree atrioventricular block.

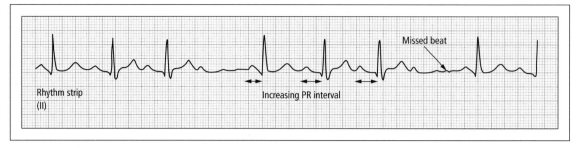

Figure 2.12 Second degree atrioventricular block — Mobitz type I (Wenckebach Phenomenon).

Complications

With the exception of cases occurring in the young and athletes, Wenckebach carries similar risks to Mobitz II with increased risk of ventricular bradycardia and sudden death. The greatest risk is at time of progression from second to third degree block as the ventricular escape rhythm is most unreliable at this time.

Management

- Post-MI atropine may be used intravenously to reduce AV block and increase ventricular rate. Cardiac pacing may be required either as a temporary measure or permanently in persistent cases.
- Other symptomatic patients should be paced permanently.

Second degree atrioventricular block – Mobitz type II

Definition

In Mobitz type II second degree atrioventricular block there is intermittent failure of AV transmission with a normal PR interval.

Incidence

Rare, less common than Mobitz type I.

Aetiology

Second degree block occurs most commonly in association with underlying acute coronary pathology such as post-MI.

Pathophysiology

The site of pathology of Mobitz type II is low in the conducting system – infra nodal in the His–Purkinje system.

Clinical features

A low ventricular rate may result in symptoms and signs of heart failure or may be asymptomatic.

Investigations

The ECG shows regular P waves with a normal PR interval, with missed beats not preceded by increasing PR interval. Most commonly every third or fourth atrial beat fails to conduct to the ventricle. In 2:1 block it is not possible to categorise as type I or type II as there is no opportunity to see PR prolongation. Ventricular escape beats may be seen.

Complications

Patients are at risk of progression to third degree heart block, which may present as cardiac syncope. If the ventricular rhythm fails totally, sudden death results.

Management

- Atropine may be used intravenously to reduce AV block and increase ventricular rate.
- Post-MI prophylactic temporary pacing may be required. If patients do not return to sinus rhythm or if not associated with myocardial infarction permanent pacing is indicated.

Third degree atrioventricular block (complete heart block)

Definition

Third degree heart block is complete electrical dissociation of the atria from the ventricles.

Aetiology

- Acute third degree heart block is almost always as a result of inferior myocardial infarction due to occlusion of the right coronary artery, which supplies the AV node and bundle of His. It may also occur following a massive anterior myocardial infarction and is a sign of poor prognosis.

- Chronic complete heart block is most commonly due to fibrosis of both bundle branches in the elderly. Rare causes include drugs, post-surgery, rheumatic fever and myocarditis.

Pathophysiology

With AV dissociation, an ectopic ventricular pacemaker is responsible for maintaining ventricular contractions. Depending on the site of this pacemaker the QRS complexes may be either narrow or wide:

- Narrow complex disease is due to disease of the AV node or proximal bundle of His. The ectopic pacemaker within the specialised conducting fibres distal to the lesion gives a reliable rate of 50–60 bpm and is associated with congenital heart disease, inferior infarction, rheumatic fever and cardiac drugs, e.g. β-blockers.
- Broad complex disease is due to more distal disease of the Purkinje system. The pacing thus arises within the myocardium giving an unreliable 15–40 bpm rate. In the elderly causes include fibrosis of the central bundle branches (Lenegre's disease). It may also be associated with ischaemic heart disease.

Clinical features

- Severity of symptoms is dependent on the rate and reliability of the ectopic pacemaker, and whether or not the myocardium can compensate for the bradycardia. Patients with underlying ischaemic heart disease, particularly recent myocardial infarction are most at risk of complications. Symptoms include those of cardiac failure, dizziness and Stokes–Adams attacks (syncopal episodes lasting 5–30 seconds due to failure of ventricular activity).
- On examination, there are occasional cannon waves in the JVP due to the atria contracting on a closed tricuspid valve, with a variable intensity of the first heart sound.

Investigations

The ECG is diagnostic revealing independent, unrelated atrial and ventricular activity.

Complications

Cardiac failure, Stokes–Adams attacks, asystole, sudden cardiac death.

Management

- In acute complete heart block, intravenous isoprenaline or a temporary pacing wire may be used. Post-MI it often resolves within a week.
- Identification and removal of any cause.
- Chronic complete AV block requires permanent pacing even in asymptomatic cases as this reduces mortality.

Prognosis

Untreated chronic AV block with Stokes–Adams episodes has a 1-year mortality of 35–50%.

Left bundle branch block

Definition

Block of conduction in the left branch of the bundle of His, which normally facilitates transmission of impulses to the left ventricle

Aetiology/pathophysiology

The most common cause is ischaemic heart disease. The block may be complete or partial.

Clinical features

Most patients are asymptomatic but reversed splitting of the second heart sound may be observed. Normally, the second heart sound splits during inspiration because the increased flow of blood into the right side of the heart delays the pulmonary component. In left bundle branch block the second heart sound is split on expiration, because left ventricular conduction delay causes the aortic valve to close after the pulmonary valve. On inspiration it occurs together with the pulmonary component because the pulmonary component is also delayed.

Investigations

ECG shows a characteristic RsR' M shape in seen in lead V5 or V6. There is a deep 'S' wave in leads V1–V3. Left bundle branch block results in a QRS complex of greater than 0.12 seconds. There is left axis deviation and the morphology of the QRS complex is abnormal

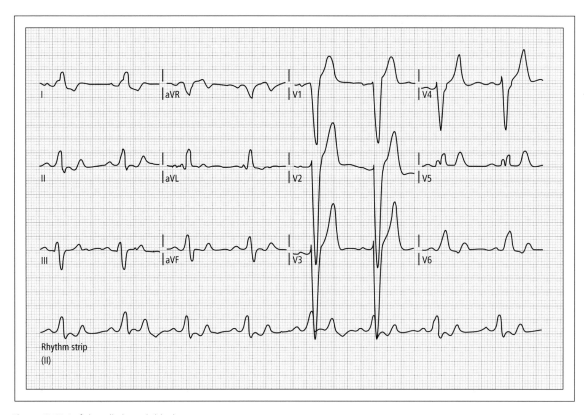

Figure 2.13 Left bundle branch block.

(see Fig. 2.13). Acute left bundle branch block may be a sign of acute myocardial infarction (see pages 37–39).

Complications
Syncope due to intermittent complete heart block.

Management
Treatment is not necessary.

Right bundle branch block

Definition
Block to the right branch of the bundle of His, which normally facilitates transmission of impulses to the right ventricle.

Aetiology/pathophysiology
Right bundle branch block is often due to a congenital abnormality of little significance, but may be associated with atrial septal defects. In older patients it is commonly caused by ischaemic heart disease, fibrosis of the bundles or pulmonary disease. Acute onset right bundle branch block may be associated with pulmonary embolism or a right ventricular infarct.

Clinical features
Right bundle branch block is asymptomatic and is often an incidental finding. There is widened splitting of the heart sounds with the pulmonary sound occurring later than normal.

Investigations
The characteristic RsR' is seen best in lead V1 and a late S wave is seen in V6. Complete block of the bundle results in a QRS complex of greater than 0.12 seconds (see Fig. 2.14).

Complications
Syncope due to intermittent complete heart block.

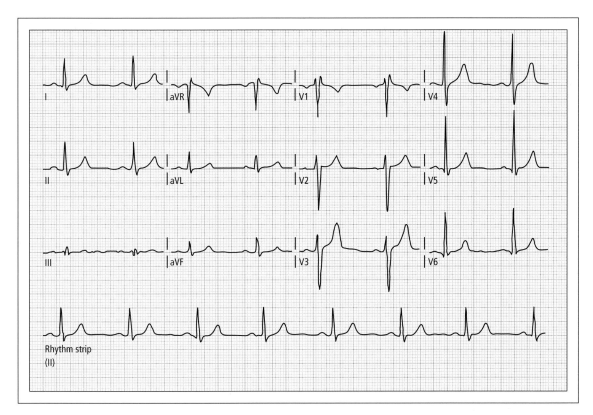

Figure 2.14 Partial right bundle branch block.

Management
Treatment is not necessary.

Prognosis
Isolated right bundle branch block, particularly in a young person is generally benign. Concomitant left or severe right axis deviation may indicate block in one of the fascicles of the left bundle, which can occur as a precursor to complete heart block which in turn carries a worse prognosis.

Cardiac failure

Heart failure

Definition
Heart failure is a complex syndrome that can result from any cardiac disorder (structural or functional) resulting in a failure to maintain sufficient cardiac output to meet the demands of the body. The clinical syndrome of heart failure is characterised by breathlessness, fatigue and fluid retention.

Prevalence/incidence
900,000 cases in the United Kingdom; 1–4 cases per 1000 population per annum.

Age
Average age at diagnosis 76 years.

Aetiology
The most common cause of heart failure in the United Kingdom is coronary artery disease (65%). Causes include
- myocardial dysfunction, e.g. ischaemic or hypertensive heart disease, cardiomyopathy.

- inadequate cardiac outflow, e.g. valvular regurgitation or aortic stenosis.
- cardiac arrhythmias, e.g. atrial fibrillation.
- inadequate ventricular filling, e.g. constrictive pericarditis, cardiac tamponade, tachycardias.
- increased demand, e.g. anaemia, thyrotoxicosis, Paget's disease, beriberi.

Pathophysiology

The mechanism by which the heart fails to deliver a sufficient cardiac output is dependent on the underlying cause.

In myocardial dysfunction there is an inability of the normal compensatory mechanisms to maintain cardiac output. These mechanisms include

- Frank–Starling mechanism in which increased preload results in an increase in contractility and hence cardiac output.
- myocardial hypertrophy with or without cardiac chamber dilatation, which increases the amount of contractile tissue.
- release of noradrenaline, which increases myocardial contractility and causes peripheral vasoconstriction.
- activation of the renin–angiotensin–aldosterone system causes sodium and water retention resulting in increased the blood volume and venous return to the heart (preload).

Other causes of heart failure including valvular heart disease and cardiac arrhythmias may cause heart failure in the absence of myocardial dysfunction, conversely a patient may have objective evidence of ventricular dysfunction with no clinical evidence of cardiac failure.

Chronic pulmonary oedema results from increased left atrial pressure, leading to increased interstitial fluid accumulation in the lungs and therefore reduced gas exchange, lung compliance and dyspnoea. It can be acutely symptomatic when lying flat (orthopnea) or at night (paroxysmal nocturnal dysnoea) due to redistribution of blood volume and resorption of dependent oedema.

Clinical features

Clinically it is usual to divide cardiac failure into symptoms and signs of left and right ventricular failure, although it is rare to see isolated right-sided heart failure except in chronic lung disease. Grading of the severity of symptoms of heart failure is by the New York Heart Association (NYHA) classification (see Table 2.8).

Table 2.8 NYHA classification of functional severity of heart failure

NYHA class	Classification
I	No limitations, ordinary activity does not result in fatigue or breathlessness
II	Slight limitation of physical activity, patients are comfortable at rest
III	Marked limitation of physical activity, comfortable at rest but physical activity causes symptoms
IV	Symptoms present at rest, inability to carry out physical activity without discomfort

Left-sided heart failure

- Causes include myocardial infarction, systemic hypertension, aortic stenosis/regurgitation, mitral regurgitation, cardiomyopathy.
- Symptoms: Fatigue, exertional dyspnoea, orthopnoea, paroxysmal nocturnal dyspnoea.
- Signs: Late inspiratory fine crepitations at lung bases, third heart sound due to rapid ventricular filling and cardiomegaly at a late stage.

Right-sided heart failure

- Causes include myocardial infarction, chronic lung disease (cor pulmonale), pulmonary embolism, pulmonary hypertension, pulmonary stenosis/regurgitation, tricuspid regurgitation and left-sided heart failure with resultant increase in pulmonary venous pressure.
- Symptoms: Fatigue, breathlessness, anorexia, nausea, ankle swelling.
- Signs: Raised jugular venous pressure, liver congestion causing hepatomegaly, pitting oedema of the ankles (or sacrum if patient is confined to bed).

Congestive cardiac failure is the term for a combination of the above, although it is often arbitrarily used for any symptomatic heart failure.

Investigations

- Chest X-ray may show cardiomegaly. Chronic pulmonary oedema results in dilation of the pulmonary veins particularly those draining the upper lobes (upper lobe vein diversion), pleural effusions and Kerley B lines (engorged pulmonary lymphatics). There may also be evidence of acute pulmonary oedema with 'bat wing' alveolar or ground glass shadowing.

- ECG may demonstrate strain patterns or hypertrophy and underlying pathology such as a previous myocardial infarct. Cardiac arrhythmias may be present.
- Echocardiography is used to assess ventricular function. It can demonstrate regional wall motion abnormalities, global dysfunction and overall left ventricular ejection fraction. Echocardiography can also show any underlying valvular lesions as well as demonstrating the presence of cardiomyopathy.
- Other investigations that may be useful include radionuclide ventriculography and measurement of B-type natriuretic peptide (BNP).

Management

Patients require correction or control of underlying causes or contributing factors where possible, such as anaemia, pulmonary disease, thyrotoxicosis, hypertension, cardiac arrhythmias and infection. Ischaemic or valve disease often requires specific treatment.

Patients should be advised to stop smoking and reduce alcohol and salt intake. Weight loss and regular aerobic exercise should be encouraged. Patients with evidence of fluid overload should restrict their fluid intake to 1.5–2 L/day.

Patients with left ventricular systolic dysfunction have been shown to benefit from

- angiotensin-converting enzyme (ACE) inhibitors, which should be given to all patients even if asymptomatic. These should be used in conjunction with a diuretic if there is any evidence of peripheral oedema. Angiotensin II receptor antagonists may be used in place of ACE inhibitors in intolerant patients. They can also be used in addition to a combination of ACE inhibitors, β-blockers and diuretics in patients who remain symptomatic.
- β-blockers (bisoprolol, carvedilol or metoprolol) have been shown to reduce mortality in all patients with heart failure. They should be started at low dose and increased gradually.
- low-dose spironolactone, which improves prognosis in patients with moderate to severe heart failure (NYHA class III and IV). Patients require careful monitoring of renal function and potassium levels.
- digoxin, which is currently recommended for patients who remain symptomatic despite maximal treatment with other agents; however, in patients without atrial fibrillation there is no evidence of improved prognosis.

- other treatments including high-dose diuretics, biventricular pacing, left ventricular assist devices and cardiac transplantation. Anticoagulation should be considered in atrial fibrillation or with left ventricular thrombus. Automatic implantable cardiac defibrillator (AICD) have been shown to improve survival in patients with severe left ventricular dysfunction secondary to ischaemic heart disease. Statin lipid lowering drugs may be of benefit even in patients without ischaemic heart disease.

Patients with right ventricular dysfunction are treated symptomatically with diuretics and may benefit from ACE inhibitors.

Prognosis

Overall mortality is 40% in the first year after diagnosis, thereafter it falls to 10% per year.

Acute pulmonary oedema

Definition

Fluid accumulation within the interstitial lung tissue and alveoli. Pulmonary oedema may be a sign of chronic heart failure (also termed pulmonary venous congestion) or may occur acutely.

Aetiology/pathophysiology

Acute pulmonary oedema is usually an acute deterioration in patients with cardiac failure who have chronic pulmonary oedema. There may be a provoking factor such as excessive fluid intake/administration, arrhythmias, negative inotropic drugs, angina, myocardial infarct or infection. There is an acute accumulation of fluid in the alveoli. Other causes include inhalation of toxic gases, drowning and renal failure.

Clinical features

Patients develop acute severe dyspnoea at rest, hypoxaemia and distress. There may be wheeze and cough productive of frothy pink sputum. On examination there may be poor peripheral perfusion resulting in moist, cold cyanosed skin. On auscultation crepitations may be heard throughout the lung fields.

Investigations

- Chest X-Ray: There may be signs of chronic pulmonary oedema such as upper lobe vein diversion, pleural effusions and Kerley B lines. In acute pulmonary oedema there may be 'bat wing' or ground glass pulmonary shadowing.

- Blood gases: There is an initial fall in arterial pO_2 and pCO_2 due to hyperventilation. As the patient tires or in severe cases the pCO_2 rises.
- Other investigations include ECG and an echocardiogram to look for the underlying cause.

Management

- The patient is placed in the sitting position and should be given high flow oxygen. Careful fluid balance is essential and may include urinary catheterisation.
- Additional ventilatory support may be required including continuous positive airway pressure.
- Intravenous diuretic gives immediate venodilatation and later increased renal fluid excretion.
- Intravenous diamorphine (with an antiemetic) reduces distress, venodilates and relieves dyspnoea.
- Intravenous glyceryl trinitrate is used to venodilate and thus reduce the cardiac preload.
- Aminophylline infusion can be considered if there is bronchoconstriction. It also increases vasodilatation and increases cardiac contractility.
- If patient is hypertensive hydralazine or diazoxide (arterial dilators) can be used to reduce cardiac afterload and hence increase stroke volume.
- Any underlying problem such as arrhythmia should be corrected.

Cardiogenic shock

Definition

Severe circulatory failure resulting from a low cardiac output usually characterised by severe hypotension.

Aetiology

This is an extreme type of acute cardiac failure the most common cause of which is myocardial infarction. Other causes include acute severe valve incompetence, or ventricular septal defect post-MI.

Pathophysiology

Cardiogenic shock is severe heart failure despite an adequate or elevated central venous pressure, distinguishing it from hypovolaemic or septic shock. Hypotension may result in a reduction in coronary blood flow, which

can aggravate myocardial ischaemia and cause further reduction in cardiac output.

Clinical features

The patient has cool peripheries with a rapid low volume pulse. There is tachypnoea, oligo/anuria and extreme distress. There may be associated symptoms of left ventricular failure, including pulmonary oedema.

Investigations

- ECG to look for evidence of myocardial infarction or any cardiac arrhythmias.
- Chest X-ray to look for evidence of cardiomegaly and cardiac failure (see page 62).
- Echocardiogram should ideally be performed urgently to identify any correctable valve lesions and assess cardiac structure and function.

Management

- Patients require intensive care, high flow oxygen and careful fluid management.
- Cardiac inotropes are usually necessary to maintain systemic blood pressure. Increasing skin temperature and oxygen saturation are a guide to improvement.
- Any cardiac arrhythmia should be corrected and angioplasty considered in patients with cardiogenic shock in the setting of acute myocardial infarction.
- Intra-aortic balloon pumping may be instituted but it does not improve mortality unless there is an underlying correctable cause.
- Surgical intervention may be life saving in cases of mitral valve incompetence, acquired ventricular septal defect or critical coronary artery disease.

Prognosis

Mortality of 80%.

Chronic cor pulmonale

Definition

Right-sided heart failure resulting from chronic lung disease.

Incidence

Commonest cause of pulmonary hypertensive heart disease.

Sex
M > F

Geography
Related to the extent of cigarette smoking.

Aetiology
The most common cause is chronic obstructive pulmonary disease.

- Chronic lung disease: Chronic bronchitis, emphysema, asthma, pulmonary fibrosis, bronchiectasis, cystic fibrosis.
- Pulmonary hypertension.
- Recurrent pulmonary emboli.
- Obstructive sleep apnoea.

Pathophysiology
Hypoxia is a potent cause of pulmonary arterial vasoconstriction, this coupled with an effective loss of lung tissue results in progressive pulmonary hypertension and hence increased pressure load on the right ventricle. With time there is compromise of right ventricular function and development of right ventricular failure, often with tricuspid regurgitation.

Clinical features
Pulmonary hypertension, right ventricular failure and the chest disease together produce the clinical picture. Dyspnoea, cyanosis, elevated jugular venous pressure, peripheral oedema and hepatic congestion may occur.

Investigations
The ECG may be normal or may show tall peaked P waves in lead II, right ventricular hypertrophy, right axis deviation or right bundle branch block. The use of chest X-ray, CT scan and lung function tests may help identify the underlying lung disease. Echocardiography is used to exclude left-sided heart failure.

Management
- Heart failure should be treated and the underlying lung pathology should be treated vigorously.
- Acute chest infections should be treated promptly with antibiotics and steroids where appropriate.
- Long-term oxygen therapy has been shown to improve prognosis in hypoxic chronic obstructive airways disease but must be maintained for > 18 hours per day.

- Atrial fibrillation is a common complication and should be treated appropriately.

Prognosis
This is related to the underlying lung pathology and extent of respiratory failure.

Disorders of pericardium, myocardium and endocardium

Disorders of the pericardium

Acute pericarditis

Definition
Acute pericarditis is an acute inflammation of the pericardial sac.

Aetiology
Multiple aetiologies but common causes are as follows:

- Myocardial infarction: 20% of patients develop acute pericarditis in the first few days following an infarction, although it is often asymptomatic and therefore goes undetected. Dressler's syndrome is an immune-mediated pericarditis occurring between 1 month and 1 year in < 1% of patients following myocardial infarction and is associated with a high ESR.
- Viruses: The specific agent is often unidentified but may include coxsackie B, influenza, measles, mumps, varicella and HIV.
- Other causes include uraemia, connective tissue disorders, trauma, rheumatic fever, tuberculosis and malignant infiltration. Acute bacterial pericarditis is unusual.

Pathophysiology
During acute pericarditis the pericardium is inflamed and covered in fibrin causing a loss of smoothness and an audible friction rub on auscultation.

Clinical features
Sharp substernal pain with radiation to the neck and shoulders and sometimes the back. Characteristically the pain is relieved by sitting forward and made worse by lying down, movement or deep inspiration. A pericardial

friction rub is pathognomonic but may be transient, best heard at the left sternal edge accentuated by leaning forward and held expiration.

Complications

Pericarditis is often complicated by pericardial effusion and occasionally tamponade. Where there is an associated myocarditis, features of heart failure may be present.

Macroscopy/microscopy

An acute inflammatory reaction with both pericardial surfaces coated in a fibrin-rich exudate.

Investigations

- ECG usually shows widespread ST elevation, concave upwards (as opposed to the convex upward configuration of a myocardial infarction).
- Other investigations are required to help identify an underlying cause, e.g. FBC (infection), U&Es (renal failure), ESR and cardiac enzymes (to exclude myocardial infarction).
- Chest X-ray may suggest a pericaridal effusion (globular looking heart with increased size of the cardiac shadow).
- Other investigations may be indicated, including echocardiogram, viral titres and blood cultures.
- Pericardial aspiration may be used to obtain fluid for diagnosis, but is only considered where there is either a significant fluid collection or an undetermined aetiology.

Management

Analgesia and anti-inflammatory treatment with aspirin or NSAIDs is usually effective. A small percentage of patients may have a later relapse when steroids may be required. Drainage is necessary for cardiac tamponade.

Prognosis

Most cases of acute pericarditis, particularly of viral origin, run a benign and self-limiting course.

Constrictive pericarditis

Definition

A condition in which reduced elasticity of the pericardium results in poor cardiac output.

Aetiology

Haemopericardium, tuberculous pericarditis and acute pericarditis may result in constrictive pericarditis. In many cases there is no identifiable cause.

Pathophysiology

Chronic inflammation, or healing after acute pericarditis may cause the pericardium to become thick, fibrous and calcified. This surrounds and constricts the ventricles such that the heart cannot fill properly, hence causing a reduction in cardiac output.

Clinical features

The predominant features are of right-sided heart failure:

- Raised jugular venous pressure, ascites, hepatomegaly, ankle and sacral oedema.
- The JVP has a steep y descent (Friedreich's sign). During inspiration there is an increase in pressure and hence neck vein distension (Kussmaul's sign).
- Pulsus paradoxus may occur, this is a greater than normal fall in pulse volume during inspiration. This is due to the transient reduction in left ventricular filling, which occurs as a result of reduction in pulmonary venous return to the left atrium during inspiration.
- There is initially sinus tachycardia and atrial fibrillation may develop. Auscultation reveals soft S1 and S2 with a loud diastolic (early third) heart sound or pericardial knock due to rapid but abbreviated ventricular filling.

Investigations

- Chest X-ray is frequently normal but may show a relatively small heart. There may be a shell of calcified pericardium particularly on the lateral film.
- ECG shows low QRS voltages with flat or inverted T waves.
- Echocardiogram can sometimes show thickening of the pericardium and an abnormal ventricular filling pattern. However, it may be normal even in the presence of the disease.
- MRI is the investigation of choice to define the location of pericardial thickening and also may evaluate ventricular and valvular function.

Management

Medical intervention is of little value except for digoxin to control atrial fibrillation. The treatment of choice is surgical removal of a substantial proportion of the pericardium (pericardectomy). This is also helpful diagnostically, particularly for tuberculosis.

Prognosis

The majority of patients respond well to surgery. The exceptions are if there is coexistent atrial fibrillation, valve disease or left ventricular dysfunction.

Pericardial effusion

Definition

A pericardial effusion is fluid in the pericardial sac.

Aetiology

Almost any cause of acute pericarditis induces the formation of an exudate. A pericardial transudate may occur as a result of cardiac failure.

Pathophysiology

Fluid accumulating within the closed pericardium may reduce ventricular filling and hence cause compromise of the cardiac output (cardiac tamponade).

Clinical features

Heart sounds are soft and apex beat is difficult to palpate. If the effusion accumulates quickly, features of low cardiac output failure usually appear. Slow accumulation of fluid is often well tolerated until very large due to distension of the pericardial sac.

Investigations

- Chest X-ray often shows an enlarged globular heart, which may have very clear borders (because cardiac movements occur within the fluid and so do not blur the X-ray).
- The ECG shows reduced voltages with varying voltages between successive beats.
- Echocardiogram is diagnostic with the demonstration of the echo free zone around the heart, usually posteriorly.

Management

This is determined by the size and haemodynamic effect of the effusion. Small effusions (i.e. less than 0.5 cm separation of pericardium) do not require specific treat-

ment, but follow-up observation is mandatory to identify developing tamponade. Pericardiocentesis (needle aspiration of the fluid) may be indicated to establish the cause and to relieve tamponade. In cases of recurrent effusion, surgical treatment with a pericardial window allows drainage to the pleural space.

Cardiac tamponade

Definition

Pericardial/cardiac tamponade is an acute condition in which fluid in the pericardial sac causes impaired ventricular filling.

Aetiology

The commonest cause of tamponade is malignancy. It may occur with other causes of pericarditis and effusion and also as a post-traumatic complication following cardiac catheterisation, cardiac perforation, cardiac surgery or chest injury.

Pathophysiology

The pericardium is a non-distensible bag around the heart. Once the space between the pericardium and the heart becomes full of fluid the ventricles are prevented from filling properly during diastole thus reducing the cardiac output.

Clinical features

Hypotension with sinus tachycardia and a raised JVP, which may increase further on inspiration (Kussmaul's sign). The pulse is of low volume and reduced on inspiration (pulsus paradoxus). Oliguria or anuria develops rapidly and eventually there is hypotension and shock.

Complications

If not identified and treated, cardiac tamponade may rapidly lead to death from low output state.

Investigations

Patients are investigated as for pericardial effusion. If the tamponade is haemodynamically compromising the diagnosis may have to be clinical, but ideally an echocardiogram is done immediately on suspicion. Echocardiogram is diagnostic, can estimate the volume of fluid present and assess the severity of cardiac compromise.

Management

If there is compromise of the cardiac output, needle aspiration of the pericardium should be performed via the xiphisternal route, preferably under radiographic guidance. The needle is inserted 1 cm below the xiphisternum and angled to point towards the left shoulder (45°). If the ECG is left in place, with the V lead attached to the needle, penetration of the myocardium shows up as ST elevation. The relief following pericardiocentesis is often temporary, so a fine catheter should be inserted for continuous drainage until the underlying condition is corrected. Definitive surgery is required if needle drainage is unsuccessful.

Disorders of the myocardium

Myocarditis

Definition
An acute or chronic inflammatory disorder of the myocardium.

Aetiology
Myocarditis is often a feature of a systemic infection but occasionally septicaemia may lead to focal suppurative lesions. Known causative factors:
- Viruses: Coxsackie, cytomegalovirus.
- Protozoa: *Trypanosoma cruzi* (Chagas' disease), *Toxoplasma gondii*.
- Radiation chemicals and drugs, e.g. cytotoxic agents.
- Bacterial infection, e.g. *Corynebacterium*, *Coxiella*.
- Myocarditis is an important feature of rheumatic fever.

Pathophysiology
Myocarditis may arise by direct effect, toxin or immunopathology.

Clinical features
Myocarditis is an acute illness characterised by fever and cardiac failure. Patients often experience chest pain due to an associated pericarditis. Signs include soft heart sounds, third sound, tachycardia and often a pericardial friction rub. Myocarditis may be complicated by arrhythmias.

Microscopy
The myocardium shows an acute inflammatory reaction with interstitial oedema and cellular infiltration.

Investigations
- Chest X-ray may show cardiac enlargement.
- ECG may show ST and T wave abnormalities and arrhythmias.
- Cardiac enzymes are elevated.
- Cardiac biopsy shows acute inflammation.
- Viral IgM antibody titres may be increased.

Management
Bed rest and eradication of the acute infection, i.e. supportive therapy. Cardiac failure and arrhythmias may need treatment.

Prognosis
Depending on the aetiology the prognosis is usually good, although a chronic cardiomyopathy may occasionally result.

Cardiomyopathies

These are diseases of the heart muscle, which may be primary (intrinsic to myocardium) or secondary (due to an external or systemic cause).
- Primary cardiomyopathies include dilated cardiomyopathy, hypertrophic cardiomyopathy and restrictive cardiomyopathy. They are classified according to the functional abnormality and are described below.
- Secondary cardiomyopathies occur when ventricular dysfunction results from ischaemia (ischaemic cardiomyopathy), poorly controlled hypertension (hypertensive cardiomyopathy), valvular disease (valvular cardiomyopathy) or other systemic diseases such as thyrotoxicosis, chronic anaemia, drugs or toxins, viruses and alcohol.

Dilated cardiomyopathy

Definition
Progressive ventricular dilatation with normal coronary arteries.

Aetiology
Most cases are idiopathic but are often assumed to follow an undiagnosed viral myocarditis. The commonest identifiable cause is high alcohol intake. Other factors:
- Genetic: Single gene mutations and skeletal muscular dystrophies.

- Familial: 30% of cases have relatives with left ventricular dysfunction or enlargement.
- There is an association with chronic infective, toxic or immune myocarditis.

Many systemic diseases may cause the clinical features of dilated cardiomyopathy, e.g. ischaemic heart disease, amyloidosis, metabolic diseases, haemochromatosis and systemic lupus erythematosus.

Pathophysiology

The dilatation of the heart results in impaired contraction especially affecting the left ventricle. Left ventricular failure causes an elevated end-diastolic pressure with resultant increase in pressure within the pulmonary circulation and eventually right-sided heart failure. The dilatation also results in a functional regurgitation at the tricuspid and/or mitral valves (valve ring dilation).

Clinical features

- Symptoms are dependent upon the degree of cardiac failure. Patients tend to present with dyspnoea and orthopnoea, which may be acute or of more insidious onset.
- On examination, the JVP is raised possibly with a systolic pressure wave (cv wave) due to tricuspid regurgitation, and the blood pressure is low. Tachycardia is common and low perfusion results in peripheral vascular shutdown (small thready pulse, cold extremities and peripheral cyanosis). Auscultation may reveal a gallop rhythm (tachycardia with third heart sound due to rapid ventricular filling) and the pansystolic murmurs of mitral and tricuspid regurgitation. Ankle and/or sacral oedema, mild hepatomegaly and jaundice, due to hepatic congestion or tricuspid regurgitation, and ascites are signs of right-sided heart failure.

Macroscopy/microscopy

The ventricles are dilated (left more than right), the chamber walls are thin and the muscle poorly contractile. Fibrosis tends to occur in the dilated myocardium with a cellular infiltration especially T lymphocytes.

Complications

Atrial fibrillation is common, particularly in alcoholic cardiomyopathy, and bouts of ventricular tachycardia may occur. Mural thrombosis may occur in either ventricle with the associated risk of systemic embolisation.

The impaired cardiac output leads to failure to perfuse the kidneys and hence secondary renal failure.

Investigations

- Chest X-ray shows cardiac enlargement with signs of pulmonary oedema including upper lobe vein diversion, Kerley B lines and may show pleural effusions.
- ECG usually shows sinus tachycardia or atrial fibrillation, there may be non-specific T wave changes.
- Echo reveals ventricular dilation, poor contractility and will demonstrate any valvular regurgitation.
- Cardiac catheterisation may be needed to exclude coronary artery disease, as this may present similarly without any history of angina or myocardial infarct.
- Patients should also have an ESR, creatine kinase, viral serology, U&Es, LFTs and calcium, iron studies and thyroid function tests to help identify the underlying cause.

Management

- General measures include bed rest, fluid restriction and quitting alcohol.
- Treat arrhythmias (digoxin especially useful in atrial fibrillation) and commence treatment for cardiac failure (see page 63) with care as it may cause hypotension.
- Patients with atrial fibrillation, a history of thromboembolic disease or a presence of intracardiac thrombous should be anti-coagulated. Severe cases may benefit from anti-coagulation without other risk factors.

Prognosis

The prognosis is very poor. Young patients may be treated with cardiac transplantation.

Hypertrophic cardiomyopathy

Definition

Hypertrophic or hypertrophic obstructive cardiomyopathy (HOCM) is a condition of the myocardium with massive hypertrophy of the ventricular walls.

Aetiology

- Half the cases are due to an autosomal dominant inherited point mutation of the β myosin heavy chain, which codes for a component of the cardiac muscle fibre.

- In families with a history of sudden cardiac death from HOCM, there is an association with the angiotensin converting enzyme (ACE) genotype DD.

Pathophysiology

There is marked hypertrophy of one or both ventricles particularly affecting the ventricular septum. This may result in obstruction to the outflow of the left ventricle, which is made worse on contraction of the ventricle. The muscle fibres relax poorly and as a result there is poor left ventricular filling and contraction, with disordered mitral valve movement.

Clinical features

Hypertrophic cardiomyopathy often presents similarly to aortic stenosis with dyspnoea, angina, syncope, or sudden death. Signs of heart failure are common but occur at a late stage. Initially the pulse is jerky with a rapid outflow due to hypertrophy, in the late stages obstruction results in a slow rising pulse. The JVP shows an increase in the size of the 'a' wave (atrial contraction). Palpation reveals a prominent thrusting apex, which may be double (palpable atrial contraction). There may be a systolic murmur (and thrill) due to ventricular outflow obstruction maximal at the left sternal edge. This may be varied by dynamic maneouvres or drugs that can alter the degree of functional obstruction. A fourth heart sound is often heard caused by ventricular filling due to atrial contraction.

Complications

Thrombosis and consequent systemic embolisation may occur requiring anticoagulation. Prophylaxis is required against infective endocarditis. It is associated with Wolff–Parkinson–White Syndrome. Ventricular arrhythmias are common and may lead to sudden cardiac death.

Macroscopy/microscopy

Hypertrophy is asymmetrically distributed. The increase in thickness occurs particularly of the interventricular septum. Disorganised branching of abnormal, short, thick muscle fibres, in which there are large nuclei.

Investigations

- ECG shows ST, and T wave changes with evidence of hypertrophy (anterior Q wave, T wave inversion and increased QRS voltage).

- Echocardiography shows a small left ventricular cavity with generalised or asymmetrical hypertrophy of the septum. Mitral valve movement is also characteristic. Twenty-five per cent of patients have outflow tract obstruction.
- MRI scanning is of particular value if echocardiography cannot obtain adequate views particularly in apical hypertrophy.
- 24-hour ECG monitoring is used to detect episodes of ventricular tachycardia.
- Exercise testing is helpful for risk assessment, i.e. loss of rise in blood pressure or onset of arrhythmia during exercise are high risk features for sudden cardiac death.

Management

- β-blockade is the mainstay of treatment as this lowers the pressures within the left ventricle.
- Arrhythmias: β-blockers and amiodarone are used to prevent ventricular arrhythmias and there is increasing use of automatic implantable cardiac defibrillators (AICD). Atrial fibrillation is preferably treated with DC synchronised cardioversion. Refractory atrial fibrillation is treated with digoxin.
- Surgical treatment: Occasionally resection of the hypertrophied septal wall (myotomy/myectomy) is indicated with, where necessary, a mitral valve replacement. Surgical intervention is usually reserved for severely symptomatic patients.
- Septal ablation by selective alcohol injection into a sizeable septal branch of the left anterior decending artery has been shown to achieve similar results to surgery.
- If patients have angina nitrates should be avoided, and diuretics should only be used with care as these increase the degree of functional obstruction.

Prognosis

Factors suggesting a worse prognosis include young age or syncope at presentation and a family history of sudden death due to HOCM.

Restrictive cardiomyopathy

Definition

Restrictive or infiltrative cardiomyopathy is a rare disorder of cardiac muscle resulting in restricted ventricular filling.

Aetiology

Amyloidosis, scleroderma, sarcoidosis, iron storage diseases (haemochromatosis) and eosinophilic heart disease (endomyocardial fibrosis and Loeffler's eosinophilic endocarditis).

Pathophysiology

Infiltrative disease causing a decrease in ventricular compliance (increase in stiffness) affecting the myocardium. The result is a failure of relaxation during diastole, impairment of ventricular filling and compromise of cardiac output. Valves may also be affected by the underlying disease.

Clinical features

Patients present in a similar way to constrictive pericarditis with a tachycardia, raised JVP with steep x and y descents. There may be a third heart sound due to abrupt ventricular filling. Enlarged liver, ascites and peripheral oedema may all be seen.

Complications

Thrombus formation is common, and arrhythmias and sudden death occur.

Investigations

Chest X-ray frequently shows cardiac enlargement, echo shows symmetrical myocardial thickening, normal ejection fraction but impaired filling. Differentiation from constrictive pericarditis using these methods can be difficult. Definitive diagnosis may require cardiac catheterisation and cardiac biopsy. Alternatively amyloid may be diagnosed in other organs or using a serum amyloid protein (SAP) scan.

Management

No specific treatment. Low-dose diuretics and vasodilators may provide some relief from symptoms. Patients with eosinophilic heart disease may benefit from treatment with steroids and cytotoxic drugs.

Prognosis

The condition is commonly progressive.

Disorders of the endocardium

Infective endocarditis

Definition

An infection of the endocardium (endothelial lining of the heart and valves).

Incidence

6 per 100,000 (1500 cases) per year in United Kingdom.

Aetiology

Although infective endocarditis may occur on normal endocardium, it is more common on a congenital or acquired cardiac abnormality. Patients most at risk include those with rheumatic valve disease, mitral valve prolapse, bicuspid aortic valve, coarctation, ventricular septal defect or persistent ductus arteriosus. Prosthetic valves may become infected either early (within 60 days of implantation) or late.

The clinical pattern is dependent on the infective organism:

- *Streptococcus viridans* (α-haemolytic group of *Streptococcus* which includes *Streptococcus milleri* and *Streptococcus mutans*) causes 50% of cases. It is an upper respiratory tract commensal.
- *Staphylococcus aureus* and *Staphylococcus epidermidis* (skin commensals) cause 25% of cases (in acute infective endocarditis, *Staph. aureus* is responsible for 50% of cases).
- *Enterococcus faecalis* causes 10% of cases.
- There are many other rarer bacterial causes and fungal causes include *Candida*, *Aspergillus* and *Histoplasma*.

The disease is also dependent on the portal of entry, and risk factors include

- Recent dental treatment (even descaling) or poor dental hygiene.
- Infections such as pneumonia, urinary tract infection or any form of chronic sepsis including skin infection.
- Carcinoma of the colon (*Enterococcus* endocarditis).
- Central lines and intravenous drug abuse (tricuspid valve particularly).
- Post-surgery.

Pathophysiology

The clinical picture of infective endocarditis is a balance between the virulence of the organism, the susceptibility and immunity of the individual. The result is either an acute infection or a more insidious (subacute) course. The bacteria proliferate on the endocardium, causing the development of friable vegetations containing bacteria, fibrin and platelets. This may result in destruction of valve leaflets, perforation and hence disturbance of function. The disease process predisposes to the formation of thrombus with the potential for emboli. Cytokine generation causes fever. There is a vasculitis and the formation of immune complexes.

- In acute endocarditis (particularly where *Staph. aureus* is the cause) the disease is rapid, progresses to cardiac failure and is often fatal.
- The majority of cases are subacute in which bacterial multiplication is slower and the cardiac lesion may be less obvious; however, systemic manifestations become more significant.

Clinical features

A fever and a new or changing murmur is endocarditis until proven otherwise, although these signs are not universal.

Typical presentations:

- Acute bacterial endocarditis presents with fever, new or changed heart murmurs, vasculitis and infective emboli. Severe acute heart failure may occur due to chordal rupture or acute valve destruction.
- Subacute endocarditis presents with general symptoms such as fever, night sweats, weight loss, malaise and symptoms of cardiac failure or thromboembolism.

General signs:

- Malaise, pyrexia, anaemia and splenomegaly, which may be tender.
- Clubbing of the nails is seen only in subacute forms as it takes months to develop.
- Arthralgia may occur as a result of immune complex deposition.

Cardiac lesions:

- New or changed murmurs are characteristic.
- Cardiac failure occurs as a result of the haemodynamic disturbance due to the valve lesion(s), e.g. aortic or mitral regurgitation.

Skin lesions:

- Osler's nodes are tender nodules palpated at the tips of fingers and toes; they are embolic or vasculitic lesions causing pulp infarcts.

- Splinter haemorrhages, linear dark streaks seen in the nail bed are due to vasculitis.
- Janeway lesions are small, flat, erythematous lesions on soles and palms, particularly the thenar and hypothenar eminences, caused by vasculitis.
- Petechiae may be embolic or vasculitic often seen on mucosa of pharynx and retinal haemorrhages may be seen (Roth's spots are haemorrhages with a pale centre).

Investigations

- Blood cultures are positive in 90% when three sets of cultures are taken from differing sites.
- Echocardiography is used to visualise vegetations and to assess the degree of valvular dysfunction. If the transthoracic echo is not diagnostic a transoesophageal echo is useful especially to show mitral valve disease, aortic root abscess and to visualise leaflet perforations.
- Full blood count shows an anaemia with neutrophilia. There is a high ESR and CRP.
- Microscopic haematuria results from the immune complexes. Urine cultures may be required to identify a urinary tract infection, and renal ultrasound may be indicated to demonstrate a renal abscess.
- Chest X-ray may show heart failure or pulmonary infarction/abscess.
- ECG may show a prolonged PR interval suggests aortic root abscess encroaching on the atrioventricular node.

Complications

- Cardiac failure is the most serious potential complication particularly when treatment is delayed.
- Virtually any organ system may be affected by mycotic emboli, which commonly develop into abscesses. For example cerebral, renal, splenic or mesenteric infarction and abscess formation in left-sided cardiac lesions, or pulmonary abscesses in right-sided cardiac lesions. Cerebral emboli may cause infarction or mycotic aneurysms resulting in convulsions, hemiplegia or other abnormal neurology. Emboli may even occur after treatment has been completed.
- Nephrotic syndrome or renal failure due to the glomerulonephritis that occurs following immune complex deposition within the kidneys.

Management

It is important to identify the organism responsible for the endocarditis; however, this should be balanced with the need to treat promptly. Once cultures are sent, intravenous antibiotics should be commenced based on the most likely pathogens if there is a high suspicion of bacterial endocarditis.

- Blind treatment includes benzylpenicillin or flucloxacillin, and gentamicin for its synergistic effect, as these will cover the most common organisms *Staphylococcus*, *Streptococcus* and *Enterococcus*. Oral fusidic acid is added if *Staphylococcus* is suspected.
- When the culture results are known endocarditis should be treated with the most appropriate antibiotics. It is best to have a multidisciplinary approach with early microbiological and surgical advice.
- It is usually necessary to continue antibiotic treatment for 6 weeks, but this may be converted to oral therapy after 2 weeks if the organism is sensitive.

Indications for surgical intervention in infective endocarditis to repair or replace valves:

- Sufficient valve damage to cause symptomatic heart failure.
- Persistent infection refractory to treatment, or relapse following end of treatment.
- Development of aortic root abscess (lengthening PR interval).
- Fungal infection (large vegetations) rarely responds to medical treatment alone.
- Multiple embolisation.
- Prosthetic valves commonly require surgery together with medical therapy.

The timing of surgery is a balance between the desire to eradicate bacteria prior to the procedure and the need for early surgery due to the compromised haemodynamic state. After surgery a full course of drug treatment should be given to eradicate the organisms.

Prophylactic treatment: Abnormal or prosthetic heart valves, patent ductus or septal defects and patients with previous endocarditis are advised to have prophylactic oral or intravenous antibiotic cover for non-sterile procedures. For example, amoxycillin for dental procedures, and amoxycillin and gentamicin for oropharyngeal, gastrointestinal or genitourinary procedures.

Prognosis

Despite advances in treatment, overall mortality is still 15% and as high as 40–60% in prosthetic valve endocarditis; this is due to changing patterns of the disease (elderly, drug addicts, prosthetic valves, antibiotic resistance).

Hypertension and vascular diseases

Systemic hypertension

Definition

Hypertension means high blood pressure (BP). The World Health Organisation latest guidelines define hypertension with three grades of severity that reflect the fact that systolic and diastolic hypertension are independent risk factors for complications of hypertension:

- Grade 1 (mild): A systolic BP of $\geq$140 mmHg or a diastolic BP of $\geq$90 mmHg.
- Grade 2 (moderate): A systolic BP of $\geq$160 mmHg or a diastolic BP of $\geq$100 mmHg.
- Grade 3 (severe): A systolic BP of $\geq$180 mmHg or a diastolic BP of $\geq$110 mmHg.

Incidence

Common. Up to 25% of the adult population is hypertensive by these criteria.

Age

Increases with age (>50% affected over the age of 65 years).

Sex

M > F

Geography

Rising prevalence of hypertension in the developing world, together with longer life expectancies, is increasing the morbidity of complications.

Aetiology

Divided into primary (essential) and secondary hypertension:

Essential hypertension (>90%)

- Non-modifiable: Genetic (racial and familial), gender (males higher).
- Modifiable: Obesity, alcohol intake, diet (especially high salt intake).

Secondary hypertension (<10%)

- Renal (80%): Most commonly glomerulonephritis, recurrent/chronic pyelonephritis, and polycystic kidneys. Hypertension is also a common cause of renal disease.
- Endocrine causes: Acromegaly, Cushing's syndrome, Conn's syndrome and phaechromocytoma.
- Cardiovascular (uncommon): Coarctation of the aorta, renal artery stenosis.
- Pregnancy (pre-eclampsia).
- Drugs: Oral contraceptives, NSAIDs, steroids. Carbenoxalone and liquorice mimic aldosterone.

Pathophysiology

- Hypertension accelerates the age-related process of arteriosclerosis 'hardening of the arteries' and predisposes to atherosclerosis in larger arteries. Arteriosclerosis, through smooth muscle hypertrophy and intimal thickening, reduces luminal diameter in smaller arteries and so increases peripheral vascular resistance and exacerbates hypertension.
- The chronic increased pressure load on the heart results in left ventricular hypertrophy and over time this leads to heart failure.
- Arteriosclerosis also reduces renal perfusion pressure, which activates the renin–angiotensin system. Salt and water retention occurs, which can itself worsen hypertension.

In some individuals the pressure rise is more rapid and such patients are said to have malignant hypertension (with rapidly worsening end-organ damage such as hypertensive retinopathy and renal impairment). Without treatment these patients die within 1–2 years.

Clinical features

As blood pressure varies considerably (e.g. diurnal variation, recent alcohol intake, stress and anxiety) the diagnosis should be based on multiple measurements taken on several different occasions. These should be taken with the patient relaxed and at rest. In cases of doubt, 24-hour blood pressure recordings may be helpful such as when 'white coat' hypertension is suspected.

A full history and examination should be performed to assess the extent, to look for any underlying cause or contributing factors and to look for complications. Often hypertension is asymptomatic and the history and examination are unremarkable.

Table 2.9 Risk factors for cardiovascular disease

Males >55 years; Females >65 years
Smoking
Total cholesterol >6.1 mmol/L or LDL-cholesterol >4.0 mmol/L
HDL-cholesterol: Males <1.0 mmol/L and Females <1.2 mmol/L
History of cardiovascular disease in first-degree relatives before age 50
Obesity, physical inactivity

Complications

Hypertension is a major risk factor for cerebrovascular disease (strokes), heart disease (coronary artery disease, left ventricular hypertrophy and heart failure) (see Table 2.9) and renal failure. Other important complications include peripheral vascular disease and dissecting aortic aneurysms.

In patients with malignant hypertension there is risk of cerebral oedema, left ventricular failure, renal impairment with proteinuria and microscopic haematuria. In severe hypertension, retinal haemorrhages, exudates and papilloedema are features of malignant hypertension.

Macroscopy/microscopy

- Benign hypertension and small arteries: There is hypertrophy of the muscular media, thickening of the elastic lamina, fibroelastic thickening of the intima and reduction in the size of the lumen.
- Malignant hypertension and small arteries: Loose myxomatous intimal proliferation with reduced lumen and normal media.
- Arterioles: There is hyaline wall thickening (hyaline arteriosclerosis), increased rigidity and reduced lumen size.
- Malignant hypertension and arterioles: Fibrinoid necrosis is seen in the walls of arterioles.

Investigations

- Routine investigations must include fasting plasma glucose, serum total cholesterol and lipid profile, U&Es, FBC, urinalysis (dipstick), ECG and serum uric acid.
- Other tests may include echocardiogram, carotid ultrasound, microalbuminuria (essential test in diabetics), quantitative proteinuria (if dipstick test positive) and fundoscopy in severe hypertension.

Table 2.10 Stratification of risk depending on blood pressure and risk factors

	Blood pressure (mmHg)				
	Normal **SBP 120–129 or** **DBP 80–84**	**High Normal** **SBP 130–139 or** **DBP 85–89**	**Grade 1** **SBP 140–159 or** **DBP 90–99**	**Grade 2** **SBP 160–179 or** **DBP 100–109**	**Grade 3** **SBP >179 or** **DBP >109**
No other risk factors	Average risk	Average risk	low risk	Moderate risk	High risk
1–2 risk factors	Low risk	Low risk	Moderate risk	Moderate risk	Very high risk
3+ factors, TOD*, ACC† or diabetes	Moderate risk	High risk	High risk	High risk	Very high risk

*Target Organ Damage (TOD) including left ventricular hypertrophy, microalbuminuria, hypertensive retinopathy grade III or IV, or radiological evidence of widespread atherosclerosis.
†Associated clinical conditions (ACC) include cerebrovascular disease, cardiac disease, renal disease or peripheral vascular disease.

- Specialist tests include further tests for end organ damage (cerebral, cardiac renal) and tests for the causes of secondary hypertension (renin, aldosterone, corticosteroids, catecholamines, arteriography, renal and adrenal ultrasound, MRI brain).

Management
Treatment is based on the total level of cardiovascular risk and the level of systolic and diastolic blood pressure (see Tables 2.9 and 2.10)
- All patients should be advised to have lifestyle changes, including weight reduction, alcohol limitation, salt restriction, reduced total and saturated fat intake and increased fruit and vegetable consumption and increased exercise. Stopping smoking as well as the actions mentioned above will also reduce overall cardiovascular risk.
- Patients with high or very high risk should begin treatment immediately. Patients with moderate risk should remain under close follow-up. If after 3 months their systolic blood pressure is above 139 or the diastolic above 89, treatment should be started. The remainder of patients and those with low or average risk should remain under long-term follow-up.
- Combination drug treatment is often required. A treatment algorithm is shown in Fig. 2.15.

Prognosis
Patients with untreated malignant hypertension have a 1-year mortality rate of 90%. In general the risks from hypertension are dependent on:
- The level of blood pressure,

- Presence of retinal changes, presence of renal or cardiac impairment,
- Being male is a greater risk than female,
- Age (young fare worse than old) and
- Coexistence of coronary disease and risk factors.

Peripheral arterial disease

Definition
Peripheral arterial disease describes a spectrum of pathological processes affecting either the larger arteries or small vessels.

Incidence
Very common.

Age
Mainly over 50 years

Sex
M > F

Geography
More common in the Western world.

Aetiology/pathophysiology
Atheromatous plaques form especially in larger vessels at areas of haemodynamic stress such as at the bifurcation of vessels and origins of branches. It may affect younger patients, particularly diabetics and smokers.

Arteriosclerosis, 'hardening of the arteries', is an age-related condition accelerated by hypertension. It often occurs in conjunction with atheroma.

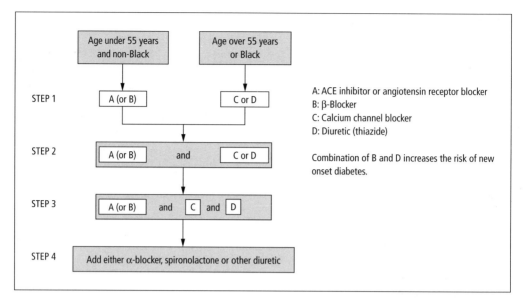

STEP 1   A (or B)   C or D

STEP 2   A (or B)   and   C or D

STEP 3   A (or B)   and   C   and   D

STEP 4   Add either α-blocker, spironolactone or other diuretic

Age under 55 years and non-Black   Age over 55 years or Black

A: ACE inhibitor or angiotensin receptor blocker
B: β-Blocker
C: Calcium channel blocker
D: Diuretic (thiazide)

Combination of B and D increases the risk of new onset diabetes.

Figure 2.15 Treatment algorithm for hypertension.

- In larger arteries fibrosis of the muscular or elastic media weakens the wall and the vessel lumen enlarges. This can lead to 'unfolding of the aorta' and aortic regurgitation.
- In smaller arteries and arterioles, the predominant effects are smooth muscle hypertrophy and intimal thickening forming concentric layers of collagen, causing luminal narrowing.

Clinical features

Chronic peripheral arterial disease in the lower limbs causes intermittent cramp-like pain in the muscles during exercise and is relieved by rest – so-called intermittent claudication. With increasing severity of ischaemia the claudication distance falls. Severe claudication may be associated with non-healing leg ulcers that progress to gangrene. Eventually the patient develops pain at rest and this indicates critical arterial insufficiency and is a surgical emergency.

On examination, signs include cool, dry skin with loss of hair, thready or absent pulses in the affected areas and a lack of venous filling. There is often discolouration, i.e. pallor or a dark hue due to slow circulation. In advanced cases there is ulceration (see Table 2.11) or even gangrene. There may be aneurysms (e.g. abdominal or popliteal) and bruits should be listened for.

Table 2.11 Comparison of arterial with venous ulcers

	Arterial	**Venous**
Position	Tips of toes and pressure areas	Gaiter area
Tenderness	Very tender	Painful at first but settles down
Temperature	Surrounding area is cold	Warm
Size	Any size	Any size or shape
Edge	Punched out edge	Sloping purple colour
Base	Grey/yellow sloughing tissue	Covered in pink granulation tissue

Hypertension may be the underlying cause or may be secondary to renal artery stenosis caused by atheroma.

The underlying processes are common to the entire arterial tree, therefore associated symptoms and signs should be elicited, e.g. chest pain, transient ischaemic attacks, impotence (due to internal iliac artery disease).

Complications

- Gangrene and loss of limbs. Diabetics are at particular risk due to diabetic neuropathy, which allows ulceration, trauma and infection to progress without pain.
- Acute arterial occlusion due to thrombus or emboli from the heart or a larger vessel may cause pain, pallor,

paraesthesia and paralysis, which is a surgical emergency (see page 80).

Investigations

- X-ray may show calcification of the vessels in the leg.
- Doppler ultrasound to measure ankle systolic blood pressure and assess blood flow.
- Arteriography or digital subtraction angiography allows visualisation of the arterial tree.

Management

- Risk factors should be modified where possible, stopping smoking in particular may prevent further deterioration and improves symptoms in many cases. Care should be taken to avoid trauma. Exercise should be encouraged as it improves collateral supply.
- Low-dose aspirin should be used to reduce risk of thromboembolism.
- In most patients clinical symptoms are static or fluctuate, so conservative care is sufficient. There are four options for persistently severe symptoms. Arteriosclerosis in older patients is difficult to treat surgically, as the vessels are small.
  1 Sympathectomy reduces vasospasm. It is useful to relieve rest pain in small vessel disease. It can be done percutaneously with an injection of phenol.
  2 Percutaneous angioplasty is most useful for short stenoses or occlusions in medium-sized arteries such as the iliac, femoral and renal arteries; however, as patients often present late the disease may be too widespread. A guide wire is inserted and then a balloon fed over the wire and inflated within the lesion. Stents are often used to improve patency. Complications include restenosis, dissection or thrombosis.
  3 Arterial reconstruction is preferably reserved for critical ischaemia or severely limiting intermittent claudication, because failed grafting worsens symptoms and repeat surgery is very difficult. In addition, most patients have other conditions such as ischaemic heart disease, diabetes and cerebrovascular disease, which increases peri- and postoperative morbidity and mortality. Procedures include
     - femoro-popliteal grafts using saphenous vein, or polytetrafluorethylene (PTFE) and
     - more distal disease is best treated with a bypass graft from the common femoral artery to the

popliteal or tibial artery as the stenosis or occlusion is usually long.
  4 Amputation: vascular disease causes more than 90% of all amputations; however, most vascular disease does not result in this. The level of amputation is dependent on blood supply, state of joints, general health and age. Conservation of the knee joint is important (possible in 50%) for prosthesis and walking. Normally the stump is closed by primary suture.

Prognosis

Five-year patency rates with femoro-distal bypass vary between 30 and 50%, aortoiliac reconstruction has a patency rate of 80%. The most common cause of death peri-operatively and during long-term follow-up is ischaemic heart disease.

Aneurysms

Definition

An aneurysm is defined as an abnormal focal dilation of an artery (see Table 2.12).

Pathophysiology

- An arterial aneurysm may be true or false. A true aneurysm is enclosed by all three layers of the arterial wall. A true aneurysm may be further subdivided into saccular in which there is a focal out-pouching or fusiform where there is dilation of the whole circumference of the vessel. A false (pseudo) aneurysm occurs following penetrating trauma when there is a pulsatile haematoma, which is in contact with the arterial lumen.
- Aneurysms tend to slowly enlarge, causing local pressure problems. They may dissect and cut off blood supply to tissue or rupture with resulting haemorrhage.
- Altered flow patterns predispose to thrombus formation, which may embolise to distal arteries or cause occlusion at the site of the aneurysm.

Investigations

CT and ultrasound scanning can demonstrate the position and type of aneurysm. Arteriography or 3-D reconstruction using MRI is used to outline the anatomy.

Table 2.12 Types of aneurysm

Aetiology	Site	Cause	Incidence
Atherosclerotic	Abdominal and thoracic aorta	Thinning and fibrous replacement of media	Most common
Syphilitic	Ascending aorta and arch	Inflammatory destruction of media and fibrous replacement	Now rare
Berry	Cerebral arteries	Congenital defects in elastic lamina/media	Common in patients with adult polycystic kidney disease
Infective (mycotic)	Any	Destruction of wall by bacteria in infected thrombus	Rare

Abdominal aortic aneurysm

Definition
Abnormal dilation of the abdominal aorta.

Incidence
Abdominal aortic aneurysms (AAA) are present in 2% of men aged 60–84 years and are an important cause of death, 6000 per annum in United Kingdom.

Age
Increases with age, rare under 50 years.

Sex
M > F (10–20:1)

Geography
Becoming more common in the developed world.

Aetiology
Risk factors are as for atherosclerosis, including smoking, hypercholesterolaemia, age, sex, diabetes. Hypertension in particular plays an important role in the enlargement and rupture. Patients with abdominal aortic aneurysms commonly have associated coronary artery disease, cerebrovascular disease and more extensive peripheral vascular disease.

Pathophysiology
The arterial wall becomes thinned and is replaced with fibrous tissue and stretches to form a dilated saccular or fusiform aneurysm. The majority (95%) are infrarenal, i.e. arise below the renal arteries, but they may extend down to the iliacs or there may be multiple separate aneurysms, e.g. femoral and popliteal. Suprarenal aneurysms may also involve the thoracic aorta.

As the aneurysms slowly enlarge at an average of 0.5 cm per year, they cause local pressure problems and have an increased risk of rupture. They may dissect and cut off blood supply to tissue (e.g. kidneys) or rupture with resulting haemorrhage.

Altered flow patterns predispose to thrombus formation, which may embolise to distal arteries or cause occlusion at the site of the aneurysm.

Clinical features
Abdominal aortic aneurysms may be found incidentally as a central expansile mass on examination or as calcification on an X-ray. A tender mass suggests a high risk of rupture.

Patients may present with a dull, aching chronic or intermittent epigastric or back pain due to expansion. Rupture causes a tearing epigastric pain that radiates through to the back or referred sciatic or loin to groin pain. Rupture through all three layers of the wall causes profound shock. Occasionally a small leak 'herald bleed' may cause a shorter, less severe episode of pain some days or weeks before rupture occurs.

Fistula formation into the bowel causes catastrophic fresh rectal bleeding.

Complications
Thirty per cent of aneurysms will eventually rupture. More than half of aneurysms over 6 cm will rupture within 2 years – thromboembolism.

Investigations
CT with contrast and ultrasound scans will demonstrate the position and wall thickness of the aneurysm. Angiography or 3-D MRI reconstruction may be used to

define the anatomy prior to deciding on surgical management.

Management
- Ruptured abdominal aortic aneurysm is a surgical emergency.
- Careful resuscitation is required, maximal systolic blood pressure should be 80–90 mmHg to maintain renal and cerebral perfusion without exacerbating the leakage. O negative blood may be required until blood is cross-matched, as blood loss can be massive.
- Surgery at a specialist centre gives the best outcome, but patients may not be fit for transfer.
- The aneurysm is cross-clamped, partially excised and replaced with a Dacron graft. If the aneurysm is too low, or when the iliac and femoral arteries are either aneurysmal or too diseased with atherosclerosis, a 'trouser' bifurcation graft is used to anastomose to the iliac or femoral arteries.
- Asymptomatic small aneurysms should be managed conservatively with aggressive management of hypertension and other risk factors for atherosclerosis and yearly ultrasound scans to monitor progress.
- Abdominal aortic aneurysms over 5 cm should be treated electively. Whilst surgical techniques remain the standard treatment, increasingly endovascular stenting techniques are being used that can be performed under local anaesthetic.

Prognosis
Mortality rate in elective surgery is 5% or less. In ruptured abdominal aortic aneurysms only 20% survive, even if patients survive to surgery mortality is 50%. Suprarenal aneurysms have a much poorer prognosis with a high risk of renal impairment. Many patients have concomitant ischaemic heart disease or cerebrovascular disease, which affects outcome.

Thoracic aortic aneurysms and aortic dissection

Definition
Aortic dissection is defined as splitting through the endothelium and intima allowing the passage of blood into the aortic media.

Aetiology
Predisposing factors to thoracic aortic aneurysms, which may dissect include hypertension, atherosclerosis, bicuspid aortic valve, pregnancy, increasing age and Marfan's syndrome. In all cases there is degeneration of collagen and elastic fibres of the media, known as 'cystic medial necrosis'. Trauma, including insertion of an arterial catheter, is also a cause.

Pathophysiology
There is an intimal tear, then blood forces into the aortic wall, it can then extend the split further along the wall of the vessel.
- Type A dissections involve the ascending aorta (see Fig. 2.16), and in these cases the major risk is of dissection tracking back towards the heart, causing haemopericardium and tamponade. These are further subdivided depending on whether the dissection extends

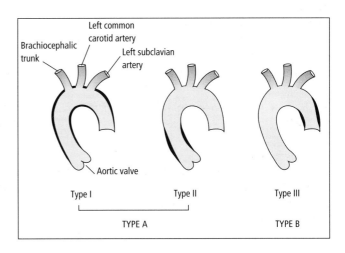

Figure 2.16 Types of aortic dissection.

beyond the brachiocephalic trunk (Type I) or not (Type II). Most thoracic aortic dissections are Type A, and these have the highest mortality.

- Less commonly the dissection is confined to the descending aorta (Type B or Type III). The most common site for these to start is at the point of the ductus arteriosus, i.e. opposite to the left subclavian artery. Type I and Type III aortic dissections threaten the spinal arteries as well as the arteries supplying the abdominal viscera, e.g. mesenteric and coeliac axes and the renal arteries. They may extend as far down as the iliac arteries.

Clinical features

Dissection classically presents with excruciating sudden onset central chest pain, which may be mistaken for an acute myocardial infarction. The pain tends to be tearing, most severe at the onset and radiates through to the back. Most patients are hypertensive at presentation. Hypotension suggests significant blood loss, acute haemopericardium or disruption of the aortic valve. A difference in the blood pressure between the arms suggests impaired flow to one of the subclavian arteries. There may be reduction in the pulses distal to the lesion.

Auscultation may reveal the early diastolic murmur of aortic regurgitation and occasionally a pericardial rub. Haemorrhage from descending aortic aneurysms may cause dullness and absent breath sounds at the left lung base due to a left pleural effusion (haemothorax).

Complications

Dissection or formation of thrombus on the damaged endothelium may obstruct any branch of the aorta, and thus stroke, paraplegia (due to spinal artery involvement), renal failure and mesenteric ischaemia may result.

Investigations

- ECG may be normal or show evidence of left ventricular hypertrophy due to long-standing hypertension. Myocardial infarction may occasionally be due to dissection involving the coronary arteries.
- Chest X-ray may show a widened mediastinum: dilated aorta, an enlarged heart due to pericardial effusion and calcification of the aortic intima pushed further than normal within the aortic border.

- The diagnosis is best confirmed with contrast CT or MR angiography. Transthoracic or transoesphageal echocardiography can give valuable information about the aorta and aortic valve, and may also be used to make the diagnosis, particularly in haemodynamically unstable patients.

Management

Dissection of the aorta is a medical (and surgical) emergency. In both types, urgent but careful resuscitation is required, and importantly hypertension should be treated, aiming at a maximal systolic blood pressure of 100–120 mmHg to maintain renal and cerebral perfusion without exacerbating the dissection. Intravenous β-blockers, glyceryl trinitrate and hydralazine may all be needed. Adequate analgesia is required.

- Type A dissections require emergency surgery with cardiopulmonary bypass. The ascending aorta is replaced using a Dacron graft and the aortic valve repaired or replaced as necessary. The aortic arch and its branches may also need repair or replacement.
- Type B dissections should be treated conservatively with antihypertensive therapy. Surgery or endovascular stenting may be indicated if the dissection progresses, or if rupture occurs, but the risk of paraplegia due to spinal artery ischaemia during surgery is high.

Asymptomatic thoracic aortic aneurysms found by screening, e.g. in Marfan's syndrome, are closely monitored with echocardiograms and CT scans for expansion and may be treated electively by surgical repair.

Prognosis

Untreated thoracic aortic dissection results in 50% mortality within 48 hours. In all patients long-term strict blood pressure control is needed.

Acute peripheral arterial occlusion

Definition

Acute loss of the arterial supply to a limb.

Incidence

Commonest vascular emergency.

Age

Increases with age.

Sex

M > F

Aetiology/pathophysiology

The most common causes are emboli and thrombus.

- Ninety per cent of emboli arise from the heart, usually due to mural thrombus (e.g. as a complication of atrial fibrillation or post-infarction) or from abnormal, infected or prosthetic heart valves. Less than 10% arise from the large vessels, e.g. aortic aneurysm or atherosclerotic vessels.
- Thrombosis may cause acute ischaemia usually arising on a pre-existing atherosclerotic plaque or within an aneurysm, causing complete occlusion. Hypovolaemia or hypotension often precipitates complete occlusion. Less commonly thrombosis may arise in non-atherosclerotic vessels as a result of malignancy, polycythaemia or other hypercoagulable states.
- Other causes of acute arterial occlusion include direct trauma and dissection of an aneurysm.

Loss of arterial blood supply causes acute ischaemia and irreversible infarction occurs if the occlusion is not relieved within 6 hours. After the occlusion is relieved there may be secondary damage due to reperfusion injury. This is due to the production of toxic oxygen radicals, which cause further cellular damage.

Clinical features

Patients present with a cold, pale/white and acutely painful limb, which becomes weak and numb with loss of sensation and paraesthesiae, which starts distally (pain becoming painless, pallor, paraesthesia, pulseless and paralysed). Paraesthesiae or reduced muscle power are signs of severe ischaemia. As the condition progresses, the skin becomes mottled with dusky patches. Muscle tenderness is a sign of ischaemic damage. Complete loss of muscle power with tender, firm muscles is a sign of muscle infarction.

Complications

Compartment syndrome may occur (muscle swelling secondary to ischaemia and reperfusion within rigid compartments between the bones and fascial layers causes increased tissue pressure, which rises above capillary perfusion pressures, such that there is further compromise of blood supply to the affected limb). Muscle necrosis leads to the release of high quantities of creatine kinase and myoglobin, which can cause acute renal failure by a direct toxic effect (rhabdomyolysis). Volkmann's ischaemic muscle contracture may also occur.

Investigations

Angiography may be useful but should not delay surgery in critical limb ischaemia. In cases of emboli further postoperative investigation is required to establish the source of the embolus including ECG, echocardiography and abdominal ultrasound scan.

Management

Following assessment and resuscitation treatment involves the following:

- Heparin to minimise propagation of thrombus, in very mild cases this will be sufficient.
- Early cases and distal arteries may be treated medically initially with thrombolytic therapy delivered directly to the vessel under radiographic guidance.
- Acute occlusion with signs of severe ischaemia is treated with emergency surgery. Embolectomy/thrombectomy is usually performed with a Fogarty balloon catheter under local anaesthetic if possible, and complex cases may require arterial reconstruction.
- Compartment syndrome requires urgent fasciotomy.

Prognosis

Acute upper limb ischaemia tends to have a better prognosis, as there is better collateral supply. Unfortunately, acute lower limb arterial occlusion is more common. Amputation is uncommonly necessary, but mortality is as high as 20%, depending on the degree of ischaemia at presentation and overall fitness of the patient.

Deep vein thrombosis

Definition

A thrombus forming in a deep vein most commonly within the lower limb.

Aetiology

Increased risk of thrombosis may result from blood stasis, vascular damage or hypercoagulability (Virkoff's triad).

- Venous stasis: Immobility, obesity, pregnancy, paralysis, operation and trauma.
- Intimal damage: Trauma to a vein, e.g. after a hip operation, can provide a starting point for thrombosis.
- Thrombophilia: Factor V Leiden, antithrombin III deficiency, protein C and protein S deficiency (see page 496), drugs including the combined oral contraceptive pill.

Other risk factors include increasing age, malignant disease, varicose veins and smoking.

Pathophysiology
The starting point for thrombosis is usually a valve sinus in the deep veins of the calf, primary thrombus adheres and grows until flow is occluded. Secondary thrombus forms which then progresses proximally.

Clinical features
The condition is often silent and pulmonary embolism may be the first sign. Calf pain with swelling, tenderness, redness and engorged superficial veins are common. Clinical examination alone is unreliable for diagnosis.

Complications
Pulmonary embolism is a serious complication and may be life-threatening, particularly when the embolus is large, e.g. when it arises from the iliofemoral segment.

Investigations
Ultrasound or Doppler ultrasound scans can be used to confirm the diagnosis; below-knee thromboses cannot be easily seen and may only be diagnosed with venography. Alternatively, in patients with a low clinical risk for deep vein thrombosis may be screened using the D-dimer test. If the D-dimer is normal no further investigation is required.

Management
Bed rest and compression stockings; patients with above-knee thromboses should be initially anti-coagulated with low-molecular-weight heparin and then converted to warfarin for 3 months with the INR maintained between 2 and 3. Thrombolytic therapy is occasionally used for patients with a large iliofemoral thrombosis.

Prophylactic low molecular weight heparin should be given to patients with immobility due to cardiac failure, or surgery to the abdomen, leg or pelvis.

Prognosis
Destruction of deep vein valves occurs in half of patients, with the development of chronic venous insufficiency.

Varicose veins

Definition
Distended and dilated lower limb superficial veins associated with incompetent valves within the perforating veins.

Incidence
Common

Age
Increases with age.

Sex
5F : 1M

Aetiology
Incompetent valves in perforating veins between the superficial and deep venous systems lead to reflux of blood from the deep system. This results in distension and tortuosity of the superficial veins. Familial predisposition, obesity, pregnancy and prolonged standing are established aetiological factors.

Pathophysiology
- Primary varicose veins are common and show a familial tendency, which may either be due to intrinsic valve incompetence or loss of elasticity in the veins.
- Secondary varicose veins develop after valve function has been disrupted by either disease (thrombosis) or occasionally trauma. The valves in the perforating veins are disrupted, so that blood refluxes from the deep veins to the superficial veins.

Impaired venous return 'chronic venous insufficiency', leads to lower limb oedema, fibrosis around the small capillaries and veins, skin changes of eczema and ulceration. These changes are referred to as lipodermatosclerosis.

Clinical features

Patients complain of cosmetically unsightly veins and aching, heavy legs. There may be a family history or history of previous deep vein thrombosis.

Complications

Rupture is uncommon. The superficial veins are prone to thrombus formation due to stasis, causing tender, reddened, painful swollen veins (superficial thrombophlebitis).

Investigations

The site of the incompetent valve can be identified by the Trendelenberg tourniquet test or by Doppler ultrasound.

Management

Elderly patients are managed conservatively with weight reduction, regular exercise and avoidance of constricting garments. Sclerotherapy and laser therapy can be used for small varices, but only surgery is effective if there is deeper valve incompetence. Surgery consists of three parts:
- To interrupt incompetent connections between deep and superficial veins. The sapheno-femoral junction is visualised and the saphenous vein is ligated and divided.
- To strip the main saphenous channels from which pressure is distributed, and the long saphenous vein is stripped out from knee to groin (omitted if a saphenous coronary bypass may be needed at a later date).
- To eradicate varices by dissection or avulsion technique where the varices are winkled out through small incisions.

Superficial thrombophlebitis

Definition

Inflammation of veins combined with clot formation.

Aetiology/pathophysiology
- Thrombophlebitis arising in a previously normal vein may result from trauma, irritation from intravenous infusion or the injection of a noxious agent.
- Spontaneous thrombophlebitis almost invariably arises in a varicose vein due to stasis, with thrombus formation and inflammation.

Clinical features

The pain may be dull or burning, usually superficial and on examination there may be one or more visible cord-like swellings, which are firm and tender with associated erythema.

Complications

If there is a portal of entry, e.g. previous site of cannula, it may become infected, causing a cellulitis. Thrombosis in a superficial vein does not cause pulmonary embolism.

Investigations

No investigations are necessary, except to diagnose underlying deep venous insufficiency.

Management

The condition usually responds to symptomatic treatment with rest, elevation of the limb and non-steroidal anti-inflammatory drugs. Anti-coagulants are not necessary. After the acute attack, treatment of underlying chronic venous insufficiency may be necessary, sclerotherapy or laser therapy may be used as treatment for varicose veins.

Prognosis

Recurrence is common.

Chronic venous ulceration

Definition

Ulceration of the gaiter area (lower leg and ankle) due to venous disease.

Incidence

4% over 60 years of age. It is a major cause of morbidity in the elderly.

Age

Increases with age.

Sex

3F : 1M

Aetiology

Two-thirds are attributable to chronic venous insufficiency. Aggravating factors include old age, obesity, recurrent trauma, immobility and joint problems.

Pathophysiology

Chronic venous ulceration is the last stage of lipodermatosclerosis(the skin changes of oedema, fibrosis around veins and eczema, which occurs in venous stasis).

Clinical features

Distinguishable from arterial ulcers by clinical features and a history of chronic venous insufficiency (see Table 2.11 page 76).

Investigations

Phlebography is performed to assess the underlying state of the veins.

Management

Healing often takes weeks, possibly months. Conservative treatment consists of application of an absorbent nonadherent dressing, preferably under a compression bandage, which reduces venous stasis. Local antibiotics are contraindicated as they do not prevent colonisation and are often irritant and reduce healing rates.

Skin grafts may speed healing, but only if venous pressure is reduced, e.g. by leg elevation. Surgery to remove incompetent veins before ulceration occurs.

Congenital heart disease

Introduction to congenital heart disease

Definition

Developmental abnormalities of the heart.

Prevalence

Up to 1% of live born infants are affected by some form of congenital heart disease.

Age

Congenital.

Sex

M > F

Aetiology

The aetiology of most congenital heart disease is unknown, and associations are as follows:

- Genetic factors: Down, Turner, Marfan syndromes.
- Environmental factors: Teratogenic effects of drugs and alcohol.
- Maternal infections such as rubella, toxoplasmosis.

Pathophysiology

Normally in postnatal life the right ventricle pumps deoxygenated blood to lungs and the left ventricle pumps oxygenated blood at systemic blood pressure to the aorta, with each ventricle morphologically adapted for its task. The pulmonary circulation normally has low resistance.

Congenital heart lesions can be considered according to one or more of

- Abnormal shunting of blood back to the lungs (left to right). Blood from the left side of the heart is returned to the lungs instead of going to the systemic circulation.
- Abnormal shunting of blood from the lungs (right to left) in which de-oxygenated blood bypasses the lungs and enters the systemic circulation.
- Narrowed cardiac outflow channels or valves.
- Abnormal connections or positions of chambers.

Clinically lesions can be divided into two categories:

- Acyanotic heart disease, which include the left to right shunts (atrial septal defects, ventricular septal defects and persistent ductus arteriosus) and obstructive lesions (aortic stenosis, right ventricular outflow tract obstruction, coarctation of the aorta and mitral stenosis).
- Cyanotic heart disease including tetralogy of Fallot and transposition of the great arteries.

Ventricular septal defects

Definition

Abnormal defect in the ventricular septum allowing passage of blood flow between the ventricles.

Incidence

1 in 500 live births, the commonest of all heart defects accounting for around 40%.

Age
Congenital

Sex
M = F

Aetiology
In most cases the aetiology is unknown but may include maternal alcohol abuse. In Down syndrome the combination of atrial and ventricular septal defects may lead to formation of a complete atrioventricular defect with a single AV valve. In other patients ventricular septal defects may also occur in combination with other defects as a part of a complex congenital heart disorder.

Pathophysiology
Most ventricular septal defects occur in the membranous part of the ventricular septum, although muscular defects do occur (see Fig. 2.17).
- Small defects result in little blood crossing to the right side of the heart and no haemodynamic compromise – 'maladie de Roger'. The murmur is loud as there is a small jet of turbulent flow across the defect.
- Large defects with low pulmonary vascular resistance result in a large left to right shunt of blood with volume overload in the left ventricle. The murmur is, however, quieter as there is less turbulent flow.

Initially increased pulmonary blood flow does not cause a rise in pressures within the pulmonary circulation due to the vascular compliance. If, however, there is a

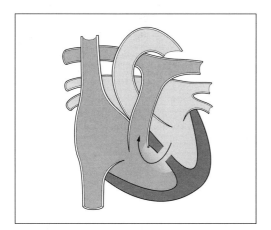

Figure 2.17 Ventricular septal defect.

continued large left to right shunt, the combination of increased pulmonary blood volume and high-pressure shear forces causes hypertrophy and deposition of collagen in the walls of pulmonary arterioles. Eventually these changes become irreversible and pulmonary hypertension develops, usually during childhood. The resultant high pressure in the right side of the heart causes a reduction and eventual reversal of the shunt with associated development of cyanosis termed Eisenmenger syndrome.

Clinical features
VSDs cause a variety of presentations depending on the size of the defect.
- Small defects presents with an asymptomatic loud pansystolic murmur heard loudest at the left sternal edge due to flow across the defect, there may be an associated thrill.
- Large left to right shunts may cause cardiac failure, which may not develop until late childhood. On examination there is usually a pulmonary ejection murmur and there may be tachypnoea and tachycardia if cardiac failure is present.
- Large defects with pulmonary hypertension and hence right to left shunts cause cyanosis. There may be a parasternal heave. The high right heart pressures causes a loud pulmonary component to the second heart sound.

Investigations
- Chest X-ray: Abnormalities are only seen with large defects when cardiomegaly and prominent pulmonary vasculature may be seen.
- ECG is normal in small defects, evidence of left and right ventricular hypertrophy may be seen in larger defects.
- Echocardiography is diagnostic. Measurement of the size of the defect and the blood flow allows prediction of the outcome.

Management
- Prophylaxis against infective endocarditis is advised. If cardiac failure is present it should be treated appropriately.
- Small defects usually close spontaneously, large defects with significant left to right shunts require surgery often before school age to prevent Eisenmenger

syndrome. The defect is closed, often using a Dacron patch, under cardiopulmonary bypass.

- If the pulmonary hypertension has developed and the shunt direction has reversed, surgery is contraindicated. Heart and lung transplant may be considered.

Prognosis

Up to 50% may close spontaneously usually in early childhood, the hole may remain the same size (the heart grows so the defect becomes comparatively smaller).

Atrial septal defects

Definition

Pathological flow of blood between the atria through a septal defect.

Incidence

10% of congenital heart defects.

Sex

F > M

Aetiology

Defects in the ostium primum occur in patients with Down syndrome often as part of an atrioventricular septal defect.

Pathophysiology

The atrial septum is embryologically made up of two parts: the ostium primum and the ostium secundum, which forms a flap over the defect in the ostium primum (see Fig. 2.18). In the foetal circulation right heart pressures are higher than left due to the extensive vasoconstriction within the lungs. This allows blood to flow through the fossa ovalis and hence shunts blood away from the non-functioning lungs. In normal individuals at birth the vasculature within the lungs dilate at birth and hence the right heart pressures fall. Once the left atrial pressure exceeds the right, the ostium secundum flap closes the fossa ovalis.

- Ostium secundum defects (70%) rarely produce symptoms before middle age.
- Ostium primum defects (30%) are situated lower in the septum and are often associated with abnormalities of the atrioventricular valves.

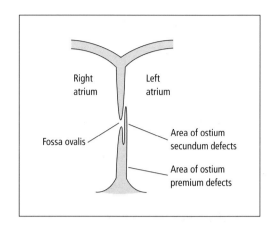

Figure 2.18 Atrial septal defects.

The shunting of blood from left to right increases the volume of blood passing through the right side of the heart leading to right ventricular volume overload and may eventually lead to right heart failure. Prolonged high volume blood flow through lungs can occasionally lead to pulmonary hypertension due to changes in the pulmonary vasculature similar to ventricular septal defects (see page 84).

Clinical features

Atrial septal defects are often asymptomatic in childhood but may cause right heart failure and arrhythmias (especially atrial fibrillation) in later life. On examination there is a fixed widely split second heart sound due to the high volumes flowing through the right side of the heart and the equalisation of right and left pressures during respiration.

Flow through the ASD does not cause a murmur, a systolic murmur is usually heard due to increased flow through the pulmonary valve. A diastolic murmur may also occur due to flow across the tricuspid valve.

Rarely patients may present with paradoxical emboli (where thrombus from a deep vein thrombosis crosses the atrial septal defect and causes stroke or peripheral arterial occlusion).

Investigations

- Chest X-ray may show prominent pulmonary arteries and cardiomegaly.
- ECG often shows some degree of right bundle branch block. Ostium secundum tends to produce right axis

deviation, whereas ostium primum produces left axis deviation.

- Echocardiogram demonstrates abnormal septal motion and can show blood flow between the atria.

Management

In ostium secundum defect repair is safe and advisable. The defect may be closed using an umbrella-shaped occluder placed at cardiac catheterisation. Traditional open surgical repair requires cardiopulmonary bypass and may use a pericardial or Dacron patch to close the defect. Surgical intervention in ostium primum defects is more complex due to involvement of the atrioventricular valves.

Coarctation of the aorta

Definition

Localised narrowing of the descending aorta close to the site of the ductus arteriosus.

Pathophysiology

Coarctation of the aorta tends to occur at the site of the ductus/ligamentus arteriosus, which is usually opposite the origin of the left subclavian artery (see Fig. 2.19). The left ventricle hypertrophies to overcome the obstruction and cardiac failure may occur. Upper body hypertension develops with hypotension in the lower body.

In adult patients longstanding narrowing leads to dilation of the intercostal arteries and may cause systemic hypertension due to poor renal perfusion.

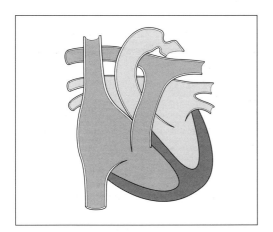

Figure 2.19 Coarctation of the aorta.

Neonatal coarctation is often associated with a patent ductus arteriosus in which the high aortic pressures result in severe left to right shunting and early severe cardiac failure.

Eighty per cent of cases occur in association with a bicuspid aortic valve.

Clinical features

Proximal hypertension may cause headache and dizziness, distal hypotension results in weakness and poor peripheral circulation. On examination the femoral pulses are weak or absent and there is radiofemoral delay. Four-limb blood pressure measurement will demonstrate the difference between upper and lower body. The flow murmur across the coarctation is best heard at the back.

Investigations

- Chest X-ray may show left ventricular hypertrophy and rib notching due to dilated intercostal arteries causing erosion.
- ECG may show left ventricular hypertrophy.

Management

Surgical treatment is used in the majority of cases and is an emergency in coarctation complicated by a patent ductus arteriosus. The chest is opened by left lateral thoracotomy, the stricture is resected and end-to-end anastomosis is performed with a graft inserted in the case of long strictures. The repaired portion of the aorta may not grow and thus a 're-stenosis' may occur, this is often treated by balloon dilatation.

Prognosis

Without treatment 50% of patients die within the first year of life from cardiac failure and complications of hypertension such as intracranial bleeds.

Fallot's tetralogy

Definition

A congenital defect (see Fig. 2.20) of the heart in which there is

- A large membranous ventricular septal defect (VSD).
- Wrongly positioned aorta above the VSD (over riding aorta).

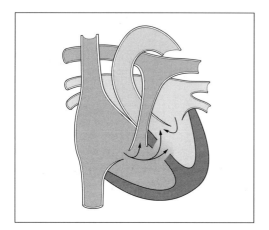

Figure 2.20 Tetralogy of Fallot.

- Right ventricular outflow obstruction (pulmonary stenosis).
- Right ventricular hypertrophy.

Aetiology
Embryological hypoplasia of the conus, which gives rise to the membranous ventricular septum. Occurs in Down syndrome and as part of fetal alcohol syndrome.

Pathophysiology
The pulmonary stenosis results in high right ventricular pressure and hence right ventricular hypertrophy. The large VSD and high right heart pressures cause a right to left shunt. The aorta is over the shunt as the VSD is high and thus there is also flow from the right ventricle directly into the aorta. The degree of pulmonary stenosis is variable (ranging from mild to atresia), thus the clinical picture ranges in severity. The right ventricular outflow tract obstruction is often progressive.

Clinical features
In rare severe cases cyanosis develops within days as the pulmonary circulation is dependent on a patent ductus arteriosus. More commonly presentation is later with progressive cyanosis over a few weeks. Initially it may only be present on exertion, but as the right ventricular outflow obstruction is progressive cyanosis becomes evident at rest, and the characteristic squatting position may be adopted. Squatting traps unsaturated blood in the legs and increases systemic vascular resistance. This reduces the right to left intracardiac shunt and provides some symptomatic relief. On examination cyanosis and clubbing may be present. There is a right ventricular heave. On auscultation there is initially a long systolic murmur across the pulmonary valve, which shortens as cyanosis develops.

Spasm of the infundibular muscle in the right ventricular outflow tract results in further compromises the right cardiac outflow causing worsening cyanosis and often loss of consciousness. These are termed hypercyanotic or tet spells.

Investigations
Chest X-ray often shows a heart of normal size but the left heart border is concave (boot shape) due to the small pulmonary trunk. There is normally pulmonary oligaemia due to low pulmonary blood flow. ECG shows right axis deviation and right ventricular hypertrophy. Echocardiogram is diagnostic.

Management
- Symptomatic infants may require a Blalock–Taussig shunt, using a tube of Gortex to connect the subclavian artery to the pulmonary artery. This provides a left to right shunt replacing the duct as it closes.
- Surgical correction is performed at 4–6 months under cardiopulmonary bypass. It is performed by opening the pulmonary stenosis (by patch enlargement where indicated) and closure of the VSD.

Cardiovascular oncology

Atrial myxoma

Definition
An atrial myxoma is a benign primary tumour of the heart most commonly arising in the left atrium.

Incidence
Primary tumours of the heart are rare, but atrial myxoma is the most common.

Aetiology

The aetiology of atrial myxoma is unknown.

Pathophysiology

The tumour is usually located on a pedicle arising from the atrial septum, and can grow up to about 8 cm across. The pedicle allows the tumour to move within the atrium resulting in various symptom complexes. If the tumour obstructs the mitral valve a picture similar to mitral stenosis will occur. If the tumour passes through the mitral valve, mitral regurgitation will occur. Complete mitral valve obstruction may cause syncope. The tumour may also give rise to thrombosis due to altered flow patterns and resultant systemic embolisation. Local invasion and distant metastasis do not occur.

Clinical features

The clinical picture varies but the diagnosis is suggested by features of mitral stenosis with variable cardiac murmurs and a loud first heart sound especially if coupled to a fever. Many patients have a 'tumour plop' in early diastole. Thromboembolism may result from the abnormal flow pattern through the atrium. It occurs in 40% and is a common presenting feature.

Investigations

ESR is usually raised. Echocardiography demonstrates the mass lesion within the atrium.

Macroscopy

The tumour is usually a polypoid mass on a stalk, its surface covered with thrombus. Histologically the tumour is made up of connective tissue, with a variety of cell types surrounded by extracellular matrix.

Management

The tumour is surgically removed under cardiopulmonary bypass.

Prognosis

Five per cent local recurrence within 5 years. Follow-up with regular echocardiography is therefore indicated even in asymptomatic patients.

Carotid body tumours

Definition

Tumour arising from chemoreceptors at the bifurcation of the carotid artery.

Incidence

Rare

Aetiology

More common in people living at high altitude; it is thought that long-term hypoxia is a predisposing factor.

Pathophysiology

Carotid body tumours are hormonally inactive chemodectomas arising from the chemoreceptor tissue of the common carotid artery at the level of the bifurcation of the artery into internal and external carotid body (anatomically at the level of the hyoid bone). The tumour tends to grow upwards towards the skull base.

Clinical features

Patients present with a pulsatile swelling in the upper neck at the medial border of the sternocleidomastoid muscle. Classically on palpation the lump is mobile from side to side but not up and down, and there may be an associated overlying carotid bruit. It is important to distinguish the rare carotid body tumour from the more common metastatic lymph node from a head and neck tumour, which may have transmitted pulsation. Metastasis of carotid body tumours is very rare.

Microscopy

The tumour has a rich blood supply. It is composed of chief cells with clear cytoplasm and a round nucleus enclosed in a fibrous tissue framework.

Investigations

Angiography shows a splaying of the carotid bifurcation (lyre sign). CT and MRI imaging demonstrate the tumour.

Management

Surgical excision may be performed especially in young healthy patients. In elderly patients surgical removal may not be necessary.

Clinical

Symptoms

Cough and sputum

A cough is one of the most common presentations of respiratory pathology. The timing, onset, precipitating factors and progression of a cough should be noted along with the amount and appearance of sputum produced. The most common patterns are shown in Table 3.1.

Haemoptysis (coughing up of blood from the lungs) may be caused by a number of conditions. It is usually streaky, rusty coloured and mixed with sputum. It should be distinguished from haematemesis (vomiting of blood) which may appear bright red or like coffee grounds.

1 The most common cause is acute infection, particularly with underlying chronic obstructive airways disease.
2 Other important causes are bronchial carcinoma and tuberculosis – these should be looked for, unless in a young, non-smoking patient with an acute infection.
3 Pulmonary oedema in cardiac failure causes pink, frothy sputum and pulmonary infarction such as pulmonary embolism may cause haemoptysis.
4 Other less common causes include Goodpasture's syndrome, vasculitis such as microscopic polyarteritis, cystic fibrosis and clotting abnormalities.

Massive haemoptysis may be caused by bronchiectasis, bronchial carcinoma or tuberculosis.

Dyspnoea

Dyspnoea is an unpleasant sensation of difficulty in breathing. Patients may complain of breathlessness, difficulty in 'catching their breath', a feeling of suffocation, or tightness in the chest. Dyspnoea should be graded by the exertional capability of the patient and the impact on their lifestyle. It is useful to document when breathlessness occurs, e.g. after 200 yards on the flat, up 1 flight of stairs.

In general dyspnoea arises from either the respiratory or cardiovascular system and it is often difficult to distinguish between them. Although the presence of orthopnoea and paroxysmal nocturnal dyspnoea suggests a cardiovascular cause, patients with lung disease may experience orthopnoea due to abdominal contents restricting the movement of the diaphragm.

For diagnosis, respiratory dyspnoea is best considered according to the speed of onset and further differentiated by a detailed history and clinical examination (see Table 3.2).

Wheeze and stridor

Wheeze and stridor are respiratory sounds caused by airflow limitation – when predominantly expiratory these musical sounds are wheezes, inspiratory sounds that do not clear on coughing are only caused by upper airway obstruction and this is called stridor.

A wheeze is described according to where it is best heard and whether it is monophonic (limitation of a

Table 3.1 Patterns of cough

Onset	Timing	Precipitation	Symptoms	Sputum	Most likely diagnosis
Recent (days)			Pyrexia, sinusitis, sore throat	White/clear	Common cold
Recent (days)			Pyrexia, malaise, dyspnoea	Rusty or purulent (yellow/green)	Pneumonia, acute bronchitis
Chronic	Worst mornings		Smoker	White/clear	Chronic bronchitis
Chronic				Large volume purulent	Bronchiectasis
Intermittent, recurrent	Night time/early morning	Exercise, pets, pollen, smoke, etc.	Wheeze	Yellow/white (eosinophils)	Asthma
Recent (weeks)			Smoker, weight loss, occasionally dull chest pain	Haemoptysis	Carcinoma until proved otherwise (often associated pneumonia)

specific size of airway – usually one bronchus) or polyphonic (widespread airway limitation). Asthma is one of the major causes of polyphonic wheeze, but not all asthma attacks are accompanied by wheeze. Other causes include chronic obstructive airways disease and acute bronchitis.

Stridor is due to upper airway obstruction. It occurs because in inspiration, a valve-like effect worsens obstruction in the major airways. On expiration, the in-

creased airway pressure opens the valve, so expiratory wheeze may be minor.

- Acute stridor: Laryngeal trauma or smoke/toxic gas inhalation, acute epiglottitis (drooling, unwell), anaphylaxis, inhaled foreign body.
- Gradual onset: Obstruction by tumours of the upper airway (larynx, pharynx or trachea), extrinsic compression (lymph nodes, retrosternal thyroid), bilateral vocal cord palsy.

Table 3.2 Causes of dyspnoea

Timing	Cause	Accompanying features
Acute	Inhaled foreign body	There is usually a history or suspicion
	Pneumothorax	Pleuritic (sharp, worse on inspiration) chest pain, hyper resonant, no air entry
	Pulmonary embolism	Pleuritic chest pain, haemoptysis, risk factors
Hours	Asthma	Intermittent, previous history of atopy/asthma, precipitating factors, e.g. cold, exercise, allergy
	Pneumonia	Pleuritic chest pain, pyrexia, purulent sputum, lung dull to percussion with bronchial breathing.
	Pulmonary oedema	Cardiac history, intermittent (exertional, orthopnoea, paroxysmal nocturnal dyspnoea) or acute – basal crackles, frothy sputum, cardiac chest pain
	Extrinsic allergic alveolitis	Recurrent, occupational exposure
Days/weeks	Pleural effusions	Dull to percussion, reduced breath sounds
	Carcinoma of the bronchus/ trachea	Obstruction causes collapse and consolidation of lung. Haemoptysis, clubbing, weight loss.
Months/years	Chronic bronchitis/emphysema	Smoking history, cough & sputum
	Idiopathic pulmonary fibrosis	Clubbing and cyanosis, fine crackles
	Occupational fibrotic lung disease	Occupational history

Respiratory chest pain

Chest pain can arise from the cardiovascular system, the respiratory system, the oesophagus or the musculoskeletal system. Respiratory chest pain is usually very different from ischaemic chest pain, as it is characteristically sharp, and worse on inspiration.

On enquiring about chest pain ask about the site, nature (sharp, burning, tearing), radiation, precipitating/relieving factors (deep inspiration, coughing, movement) and any associated symptoms such as dyspnoea. Ask also about the time course, i.e. onset, duration, constant or episodic.

Chest pain made worse by inspiration and coughing is called pleuritic pain. It is sharp and usually localised to one area. It is caused by inflamed pleural surfaces rubbing on one another. Causes include infection (may be associated with pneumonia), pneumothorax, pulmonary embolism and mesothelioma or metastatic tumours to the pleura. Pleurisy may also be caused by connective tissue diseases such as rheumatoid arthritis.

Chest wall pain may be easily confused with pleuritic pain, as it is often sharp, but it can be reproduced by movement of the thoracic spine, chest or shoulders, and by eliciting tenderness with mechanical pressure. Common causes include intercostal nerve entrapment, persistent cough, muscular strains, rib fracture and Tietze's syndrome (costochondritis).

A dull, constant severe chest wall pain may be due to invasion of the thoracic wall by malignancy. Other causes include thoracic herpes zoster – a persistent pain, which may be burning and last several days before the rash appears.

Retrosternal pain may be due to tracheitis or mediastinal disease (lymphoma, mediastinitis) but is more commonly cardiac.

Non-respiratory chest pain

Central chest pain, particularly if radiating to the neck or arms, is more likely to be cardiac. Pericarditis causes a sharp retrosternal/precordial pain which may mimic pleuritic pain as it may be exacerbated by deep inspiration, but is classically relieved by leaning forwards. Pain at the shoulder tip is often referred pain from the diaphragm, and may reflect an abdominal cause such as cholecystitis. Equally, respiratory disease may manifest with abdominal pain, e.g. basal pneumonia causing upper abdominal pain.

Signs

Clubbing

Clubbing is an increased amount of soft tissue in the terminal phalanx of the fingers and toes, concentrated around the nail base. It is seen by inspecting the nails (fingers and toes) from the side. Gross clubbing is usually obvious (drumstick appearance of fingers), but mild clubbing may be difficult to detect (loss of the angle at the base of the nail and sponginess of the nail bed). The pathological mechanism of clubbing is unknown, and causes are shown in Table 3.3.

Breath sounds

Normal breath sounds are caused by the turbulent flow of air through the airways (not the alveoli). They are transmitted to the chest wall through the lungs (see Table 3.4).

Table 3.3 Causes of clubbing

Respiratory	Bronchial carcinoma, more commonly large cell than small cell
	Chronic suppurative lung disease
	Bronchiectasis
	Lung abscess
	Chronic empyema
	Pulmonary fibrosis
	Idiopathic pulmonary fibrosis
	Cystic fibrosis
	Asbestosis
Cardiovascular	Cyanotic congenital heart disease
	Infective endocarditis
Gastrointestinal	Cirrhosis, especially primary biliary cirrhosis
	Inflammatory bowel disease
	Coeliac disease
Idiopathic	Familial usually before puberty
	Idiopathic
Rare	Thyroid acropachy
	Pregnancy
	Unilateral clubbing
	Bronchial arteriovenous aneurysm
	Axillary artery aneurysm

Table 3.4 Breath sounds

Vesicular	This is the normal pattern, a fine rustling or whispering sound. Inspiration and the first part of expiration are heard with no gap in between. Inspiration is slightly louder and longer than expiration.
Reduced	Bilaterally: Chronic obstructive pulmonary disease, severe acute asthma. Asymmetry: Pneumothorax, pleural effusion or lung collapse on the side with reduced sounds.
Bronchial	When the lung is solid it conducts the sounds from the larger airways better, so the whole of inspiration and expiration are heard. Expiration is louder than inspiration. There is often a gap between the two. It occurs over consolidated lung, but may occur in localised pulmonary fibrosis and at the top of a pleural effusion.

Added breath sounds

These are divided into wheezes from the airways, crackles, which come from the large airways, the bronchioles and the alveoli, and friction rubs from the pleura (see Table 3.5)

Wheezes are musical sounds caused by airway obstruction and are usually heard in expiration.

- A low-pitched monophonic wheeze is caused by obstruction of a single large airway (below the trachea). It is caused by bronchial carcinoma or inhaled foreign body, and is frequently inspiratory.

Table 3.5 Summary of added breath sounds

Sound type	Commonest cause
Low-pitched monophonic wheeze	Bronchial carcinoma/foreign body
Polyphonic expiratory wheeze	Asthma COPD
Early inspiratory crackles	
Medium crackles	COPD
Coarse crackles	Bronchiectasis
Late/pan inspiratory crackles	
Fine crackles	Pulmonary fibrosis
Medium crackles	Left ventricular failure
Pleural friction rub	Pleurisy

- A high-pitched expiratory wheeze, often with a mixture of notes 'polyphonic wheeze' is caused by obstruction of many smaller airways as occurs in asthma and chronic obstructive pulmonary disease (COPD). However, these conditions may occur without wheeze, despite severe obstruction.

Crackles/crepitations: Normally the airways do not collapse or obstruct on expiration, but they may due to secretions and oedema or damage by either fibrosis or loss of elasticity. The re-opening of collapsed small airways and alveoli or the presence of secretions in the larger airways cause inspiratory crackles. They are differentiated by their timing and nature:

- Early inspiratory crackles come from the airways, where air reaches them first in inspiration. Late or pan-inspiratory crackles come from the alveoli.
- 'Fine crackles' are usually alveolar (late) and are often described as rubbing hair through fingers. They are typical of pulmonary fibrosis or alveolar oedema.
- Coarse crackles are wet, low-pitched early inspiratory sounds due to airway secretions, often changed in nature by coughing.

Pleural friction rub: A creaking sound in inspiration and expiration, localised over an area of pleural inflammation. Causes include viral or bacterial pneumonia and pulmonary infarct/embolus.

Chest signs in respiratory disease

See Table 3.6.

Respiratory procedures

Lung function testing

The simplest way to assess lung function is from a patient's history, i.e. the exercise capacity, how far the patient can walk before becoming breathless. However, for more repeatable objective assessment various tests are used:

Bedside testing

Peak expiratory flow (PEF): This is quick and simple. It is measured by asking patients (standing where possible) to take a deep breath to full inspiration, then blow

Table 3.6 Chest signs in respiratory disease

Pathological process	Mediastinal displacement	Chest wall movement	Percussion note over affected area	Breath sounds over affected area	Added sounds affected over area	Vocal resonance affected over area
Consolidation (lobar pneumonia)	None	Reduced over affected area/side	Dull	Bronchial	Crackles	Increased
Collapse of lobe or lung: obstruction of major bronchus	Towards lesion	Reduced on affected side	Dull	Absent or reduced	None	Absent or reduced
Pleural effusion	None/away from lesion if very large effusion	Reduced over affected area	Stony dull	Absent over fluid, may be bronchial just above effusion	None or pleural rub above effusion	Absent
Pneumothorax	None, occasionally away from lesion if tension pneumothorax	Reduced over affected area	Hyperresonant	Absent or greatly reduced	None	Absent
Asthma	None	Normal or reduced with prolonged expiration and hyperinflation	Normal	Vesicular (normal) or reduced, prolonged expiration	Polyphonic wheeze	Normal
Chronic obstructive pulmonary disease	None	Normal or reduced with prolonged expiration and hyperinflation	Normal	Prolonged expiration	Polyphonic wheeze and coarse early inspiratory crackles	Normal
Pulmonary fibrosis	None	Slightly reduced bilaterally	Normal	Vesicular (normal)	Fine late inspiratory crackles unchanged by cough	Normal

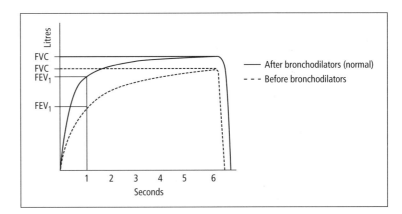

Figure 3.1 Spirometry in reversible obstructive airways disease.

out as hard and fast as they can into a peak flow meter, with a good seal around the tube with their lips. The best of three tries is recorded. This is compared with a predicted value for age, sex and height, although there is considerable individual variation.

It is most useful in monitoring disease patterns, e.g. the day-to-day and diurnal variation in asthma, and for rapid objective assessment and response to treatment. However it is limited in that it only measures the peak expiratory flow, is effort dependent, and can be relatively preserved despite the presence of severe lung disease.

Spirometry: This is now possible with bedside electronic spirometers, which are more portable and convenient than the older Vitalograph models. The patient takes a deep breath to full inspiration, then blows as hard as they can and must continue to blow into the spirometer until the lungs can be emptied no further (≥ 6 seconds in normal people but may require 15–20 seconds in obstructive airways disease). In reversible obstructive airways disease this gives the graph shown in Fig. 3.1.

On this (or calculated by the machine) can be plotted the forced expiratory volume in 1 second (FEV_1) and the forced vital capacity (FVC). Normal values are related to age, sex and height.

1 The FEV_1 falls particularly with airflow limitation, i.e. obstructive airways disease and with reduced lung volumes in restrictive disease.
2 The FVC falls with reduced lung volumes, i.e. restrictive lung disease and more severe obstructive airways disease.
3 The FEV_1/FVC ratio is normally $\sim 75\%$. In restrictive lung disease there is a proportionate reduction in

both values preserving the FEV_1/FVC ratio whereas in obstructive airways disease, although both may be reduced, the FEV_1 falls proportionately more and the FEV_1/FVC ratio is reduced.

Other useful testing which can be done by the bedside includes pulse oximetry to measure oxygen saturations, exercise testing (timed 6 minute walk with PEF, pulse oximetry and even arterial blood gases pre- and post-exertion).

Laboratory testing

More comprehensive tests can be performed in the pulmonary function laboratory, but the equipment requires a specialist technician, is expensive, time-consuming and patients with severe chronic airflow limitation find some of the tests difficult to perform, claustrophobic or exhausting.

These include the assessment of the following:
1 Flow–volume loops: These can localise the site of airflow limitation to extra-thoracic, large airways or smaller airways.
2 Lung volumes: Tidal volume and vital capacity can be measured. A total body plethysmograph can be used to measure total lung capacity (TLC) and residual volume (RV) (see Fig. 3.2). It is characteristic in emphysema for the TLC and RV to be increased due to air trapping, although the FVC is decreased. In restrictive lung disease, the FVC and TLC are decreased together.
3 Transfer factor: This measures the diffusing capacity of the lungs across the alveolar-capillary membrane by indirectly measuring the uptake of carbon monoxide

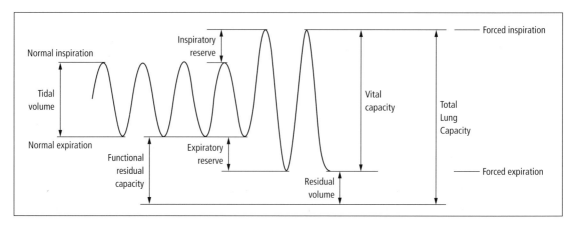

Figure 3.2 Lung volumes.

(CO) by haemoglobin. It depends not only on the thickness of the alveolar-capillary membrane but also on the ventilation/perfusion matching (which is commonly abnormal in lung disease) and on lung volumes. Therefore it is corrected for lung volume to be expressed as the transfer coefficient (K_{CO}).

- The K_{CO} falls in severe emphysema, pulmonary fibrosis, pulmonary oedema, pulmonary embolus.
- It rises in acute pulmonary haemorrhage due to the uptake of CO by blood in the alveoli.

Bronchoscopy

Bronchoscopy allows the visualisation of the bronchial tree and direct access for bronchial and transbronchial biopsies and bronchial and bronchoalveolar washings. It is performed under local anaesthetic and sedation. Flexible fibreoptic bronchoscopy is most commonly used (although rigid bronchoscopy may be required in some instances).

Topical local anaesthetic is applied to the nose and pharynx and supplemental oxygen is given through one nostril. Following sedation the flexible bronchoscope is passed through the nose, the nasopharynx and pharynx. The vocal cords are visualised and sprayed with more topical anaesthetic to minimise coughing. Once in the trachea further topical anaesthesia is administered. Each of the segments and subsegments of both lungs is examined and sampling performed depending on the indication. Radiographic screening can be used for peripheral lesions which cannot be directly visualised.

Investigations

- Biopsy: Central bronchial lesions are easily biopsied, there is a small risk of haemorrhage particularly if it is a vascular lesion or carcinoid tumour. Transbronchial biopsy is used for diagnosis of diffuse parenchymal lung disease. It carries a small but significant risk of pneumothorax. It should be used with caution in ventilated patients for this reason.
- Bronchial brushings: Brushings can be taken for cytology.
- Bronchial/bronchoalveolar lavage: Washings can be taken for cytology (malignancy, differential cell count, e.g. eosinophilia) and microbiology (indicated in particular for *Mycobacterium tuberculosis* and *Pneumocystis jirovecii* (previously called *Pneumocystis carinii*), as well as unresponsive bacterial pneumonia or pneumonia in immunosuppressed patients). Appropriate staining and culture is needed.

Therapies

- Aspiration of mucus plugs.
- Removal of foreign body.
- Laser therapy for obstructing bronchial carcinoma.
- Brachytherapy – application of local radiotherapy sources directly on bronchial carcinomas.
- Transbronchial stenting for obstructing bronchial carcinoma.
- Control of bleeding from vascular tumour.

Complications include hypoxia, airways obstruction, cardiac arrhythmias (usually transient), pneumothorax, haemorrhage and transmission of infection.

Thoracic surgery

Open lung surgery requires intubation and ventilation. Double lumen intubation allows one lung to be collapsed for surgery.

A lobectomy is used for lesions confined to a single lobe. The potential space created by the removal is filled with remaining lung, elevation of the diaphragm and mediastinal shift. Pneumonectomy is the removal of a whole lung usually due to a tumour. The hilar vessels are ligated and the bronchus is divided and closed close to the carina. The space resulting from the operation not occupied by shift of other structures fills with blood and serum which organises and fibroses.

Thoracoscopy is used for diagnosis of pleural disease, mediastinoscopy to sample upper mediastinal lymph nodes and mediastinotomy to sample lower mediastinal lymph nodes. Video-assisted thoracoscopic surgery (VATS) is increasingly used for minimal access surgery. Single lung ventilation is used to allow the collapse of the lung being operated on, e.g. for lung biopsy, overstapling of a broncho-pleural fistula or pleurectomy.

Specific complications following thoracic surgery include pneumonia (related to intubation, ventilation and lung collapse), pneumothorax, haemothorax, empyema, pulmonary oedema and acute respiratory distress syndrome.

Respiratory infections

Acute bronchitis

Definition
An acute infectious condition of the lower respiratory tract.

Incidence
Very common.

Age
Any

Sex
M = F

Aetiology
The primary cause is usually a respiratory virus, e.g. rhinovirus, influenza, parainfluenza and respiratory syncytial virus.

Pathophysiology
The virus enters via the airway by droplet inhalation and causes local inflammation, inducing secretions and impairing ciliary clearance.

Clinical features
Initially there is an irritating non-productive cough. The patient may feel short of breath, wheezy and complain of chest tightness and retrosternal discomfort. There is a low- or high-grade pyrexia. The cough then becomes wet and productive of yellow or green sputum. Discoloured sputum signifies infection, which may be of bacterial or viral origin. Streaky haemoptysis may occur. On auscultation wheezes and medium to coarse late or pan-inspiratory crackles may be heard.

Macroscopy/microscopy
The airway mucosa becomes red and oedematous, there is often an overlying mucopurulent exudate.

Complications
Secondary bacterial infection with *Streptococcus pneumoniae*, *Moraxella catarrhalis* or *Haemophilus influenzae* may occur leading to bronchopneumonia, particularly in the elderly, smokers and individuals with underlying lung disease.

Investigations
These are usually not required, there may be a mild neutrophil leucocytosis even in viral infections.

Management
Antipyretic agents are used. Patients presenting with acute bronchitis during an influenza epidemic may benefit from treatment with a neuraminidase inhibitor if started in the first 48 hours. Only if secondary bacterial infection is suspected should a course of antibiotics be prescribed.

Prognosis
The illness usually lasts up to a week in healthy adults, prolonged symptoms may occur. Changes in the course

of the illness or presence of bronchopneumonia suggest secondary bacterial infection.

Pneumonia

Definition
Pneumonia is an infective, inflammatory disease of the lung parenchyma.

Aetiology
It is useful to classify pneumonia according to the causative organism or the clinical setting, e.g. community-acquired or nosocomial (hospital-acquired), immunosuppressed. This helps to determine the choice of antibiotics for treatment.

Pneumonia most often occurs in children and the elderly, but may also affect young, fit adults. The following risk factors increase the likelihood of pneumonia and also influence the likely organism:
- Cigarette smoking and underlying lung disease.
- Stroke or other neuromuscular disorder (aspiration pneumonia often by anaerobes).
- Immunosuppression and AIDS in particular *P. jirovecii.*
- Intravenous drug abusers.
- Alcoholics and vagrants.
- Hospital patients (more often Gram-negative organisms).

Viral pneumonia is less common, but bacterial pneumonia may be a secondary complication.

Pathophysiology
The infection may be as a result of impairment of one or more normal defence mechanisms (see Table 3.7)

Pulmonary oedema also predisposes to infection by acting as a growth medium. Pathologically pneumonia can be divided into broncho-, lobar or atypical pneumonia depending on the pattern of inflammation.
- Bronchopneumonia is most commonly seen at extremes of age. It is predisposed to by immobility and viral infections which lead to retention of secretions especially in the lower lobes. The infection is centred on the bronchi and bronchioles and spreads to involve adjacent alveoli, which become consolidated with an acute inflammatory exudate. Common causes include *Strep. pneumoniae*, *M. catarrhalis* or *H. influenzae.*
- Lobar pneumonia is seen most commonly in adults who may otherwise be healthy, but particularly va-

Table 3.7 Impaired mechanisms predisposing to pneumonia

Defence mechanism	Conditions impairing defence mechanism
Cough	Coma/anaesthesia Respiratory depression Neuromuscular weakness
Ciliary function	Smoking, influenza, colds Bronchiectasis (including cystic fibrosis and Kartagener's syndrome) Ciliary function can also be impaired mechanically by obstruction, e.g. foreign body, bronchial carcinoma
Phagocytosis	Smoking Alcohol Hypoxia
T-cell response	HIV and AIDS Lymphoma Cytotoxic therapy Immunosuppressive therapy including steroids

grants and alcoholics. Organisms spread rapidly through the alveolar spaces to involve the whole segment, lobe or lung. Ninety per cent of cases in healthy adults are caused by *Strep. pneumoniae*, many of the remaining cases are due to *Klebsiella*. Males are affected more often than females.
- Atypical pneumonias cause predominantly interstitial inflammation in the lung, clinically are less abrupt in onset and slower to resolve. Causes include the atypical bacteria *Chlamydia*, *Coxiella*, *Mycoplasma* and *Legionella*.

Clinical features
Symptoms may include fever, dyspnoea, pleuritic pain and cough often productive of green sputum; however, at extremes of age the presentation may be non-specific. On examination, classically there are signs of consolidation (such as dullness to percussion, increased vocal resonance, bronchial breathing) but even if frank consolidation is not present, most patients have tachypnoea (>20 breaths/minute) and crackles. In atypical pneumonia the signs of consolidation in the lung are often minor or absent, despite severe symptoms. Specific features, investigations and management of different types of pneumonia are summarised in Table 3.8 (see pp. 100–101).

Table 3.9 Histological stages of pneumococcal lobar pneumonia

Stage	Microscopy
Congestion & oedema	Engorgement of the alveolar walls, air spaces filled with oedematous fluid.
Red hepatisation	Organisation of the fluid into a fibrin mesh containing red cells, neutrophils and bacteria.
Grey hepatisation	Clearance of the red blood cells and neutrophils and predomination of macrophages in an attempt to clear the remaining bacteria.
Resolution	The fibrin meshwork is broken down, neutrophil debris is ingested by macrophages which are cleared through the lymphatics.

Macroscopy/microscopy

- Bronchopneumonia: The affected areas of the lung are consolidated. The air spaces are filled with an acute inflammatory exudate causing the lung to be firm and a dark red or grey colour. The bronchi are inflamed and pleural involvement is common.
- Lobar pneumonia: The affected lobe is consolidated with the acute inflammatory exudate being contained in a single segment, lobe or lung. Several identifiable stages are seen in a pneumococcal lobar pneumonia (see Table 3.9):

Complications

Development of lung abscesses and pleural effusion (which may be reactive or infected, i.e. an empyema), pleural infection (pleurisy) and septicaemia.

Investigations

- A chest X-ray will demonstrate areas of consolidation, any abscesses, effusions and masses (such as underlying bronchial carcinoma). X-ray changes generally lag behind clinical features so the X-ray may occasionally be normal at presentation, and may remain abnormal for several weeks after the pneumonia has resolved.
- The white cell count will normally demonstrate a neutrophilia. If patients require admission, sputum and blood cultures should be taken and specific serological tests are available for *Legionella* and other atypical pneumonias.
- Urea and electrolytes are measured for hydration and to detect any co-existing renal disease.
- Blood gases may be required to monitor oxygenation and to assess for respiratory failure.
- In severe cases, immunosuppressed individuals and those unresponsive to standard therapy, broncho-

scopy and bronchial lavage may be considered, as this is more likely to give microbiological results.
- Patients should have a follow-up chest X-ray after 6 weeks to ensure resolution, and to exclude any underlying lesion such as carcinoma causing obstruction.

Management

1 Non-pharmacological: Fluids, physiotherapy to clear secretions, analgesia for pleuritic pain where necessary and oxygen if there is hypoxia (guided by arterial blood gases).
2 Empirical antibiotic treatment should be commenced immediately based on knowledge of the likely organisms, modified where necessary by local microbiology guidelines and on the basis of culture results (see Table 3.10, p. 102).
3 Patients with sickle cell disease, asplenia or severe dysfunction of the spleen, chronic renal disease or nephrotic syndrome, coeliac disease, immunodeficiency or immunosuppression, haematological malignancy, cardiovascular disease, chronic pulmonary disease, chronic liver disease or diabetes mellitus should receive pneumovax prophylaxis.

Prognosis

Outcome depends greatly on the age of the patient and concurrent disease (including diabetes mellitus, chronic renal failure, congestive heart failure and underlying respiratory disease such as chronic obstructive pulmonary disease). Mortality for community-acquired pneumonia is about 14% (about 20% for those requiring hospital admission and up to 35% for those requiring intensive care).

British Thoracic Society guideline for identifying patients with severe community acquired pneumonia:
- Core features (score 1 for each): Confusion, urea $\geq$ 7 mmol/L, respiratory rate $\geq$ 30 breaths per minute,

Table 3.8 Summary of causative organisms and differentiating features in pneumonia

Organism	Epidemiology	Clinical features	Complications	Additional investigations	Specific treatment
Streptococcus pneumoniae	Commonest	Cough productive green/rusty sputum. 90% of cases of lobar pneumonia.		Sputum, blood and urine – pneumococcal antigen	Penicillin (if allergic, erythromycin)
Mycoplasma pneumoniae	4 year epidemic cycle	Atypical pneumonia – cough and sputum absent in 1/3 cases. Preceding flu-like symptoms usually, e.g. headache, myalgia, GI upset before onset of respiratory symptoms	Myocarditis, pericarditis, erythema multiforme, haemolytic anaemia, myalgia, arthralgia, meningo-encephalitis, cold agglutinins	Serology for IgM and IgG antibodies (acute and convalescent titres), cold agglutinins (in 50%)	Erythromycin, azithromycin, clarithromycin or doxycycline
Haemophilus influenzae	Especially seen in the elderly, heavy smokers and COPD patients	No specific features; may be broncho- or lobar pneumonia			Cefuroxime or co-amoxiclav
Moraxella catarrhalis	Common cause of bronchopneumonia especially in the elderly and COPD patients	No specific features; may be broncho- or lobar pneumonia			Cefuroxime or co-amoxiclav
Staphylococcus aureus	More common following influenza pneumonia, intravenous drug abusers, secondary to central line	Severe pneumonia, post-influenza may be rapidly fatal	Abscess formation, pneumothorax, empyema relatively common. Septicaemia: infective emboli causing abscesses in other organs	Nodular consolidation and cavitation on CXR	Flucloxacillin
Chlamydia psittaci 'Psittacosis'	Acquired from avian excreta seen in those exposed to birds.	Malaise, high fever, dry cough, hepatosplenomegaly and rose spots on the abdomen.	Hepatitis, encephalitis, renal failure	Serology for Chlamydia antibodies – complement-fixing antibodies (immuno-fluorescent tests to distinguish types)	Erythromycin, azithromycin, clarithromycin or doxycycline
Chlamydophila pneumoniae	Causes 5–10% of community acquired	Often mild flu-like illness or acute bronchitis recovering spontaneously. Pneumonia also usually mild			Erythromycin, azithromycin, clarithromycin or doxycycline

Organism	Epidemiology	Clinical features	Complications	Investigations	Treatment
Coxiella burnetii (Q fever)	Only 1% of cases overall	Influenza-like illness which causes a pneumonia if it persists, often with multiple CXR lesions	Endocarditis. If untreated chronic infection is fatal	Serology – complement fixing antibody	Erythromycin, azithromycin, clarithromycin or doxycycline
Legionella pneumophilia	• Previously fit people infected from water system. Sporadic cases source unknown • Outbreaks in immuno compromised individuals • Males: Females 2:1	The main diagnostic indications are the presence of 3 of: • A 2–10 day prodromal period • Dry cough, confusion or diarrhoea • Lymphopenia without marked leucocytosis • Hyponatraemia	Hypoalbuminaemia and abnormal LFTs (raised transaminases) are common. Acute renal failure.	Rapid tests: • Urine for specific antigen. • Immunofluorescent tests on sputum or bronchial lavage.	Erythromycin, azithromycin, clarithromycin or ciprofloxacin +/– rifampicin Despite these mortality ~20%
Klebsiella	Elderly with a history of heart or lung disease, diabetes, alcohol excess or malignancy	Sudden onset, severe systemic upset, purulent, mucoid sputum (classically redcurrant jelly). Lobar pneumonia	May cause cavitating lesions – lung abscesses	Extensive lobar consolidation with cavitation	Cefuroxime and gentamicin
Pseudomonas aeruginosa	Nosocomial, cystic fibrosis and neutropenic patients.			Sputum and blood culture, but it does colonise the upper airway as a commensal	Ciprofloxacin or ceftazidime
Anaerobes – *Bacteroides*	Aspiration, e.g. due to stroke. Diabetics				Metronidazole
Pneumocystis jiroveci (PCP) (previously *Pneumocystis carinii*)	The most common opportunistic infection in AIDS (CD4 count <200/mm^3) and immunosuppressed patients	High fever, dry cough, shortness of breath, tachycardia. Marked hypoxia, particularly following exertion. Fine crackles or nothing to find on auscultation.	Mortality now ~10% Long-term prophylaxis is required, e.g. with co-trimoxazole	Typical CXR – perihilar 'butterfly' ground glass shadowing. but may be normal in early disease. CT shows ground-glass shadowing, bronchial lavage or induced sputum for diagnosis by silver staining or by immunofluorescence	Hi-dose i.v. cotrimoxazole or i.v. pentamidine

Viral pneumonia: With the exception of sporadic epidemics due to new viral pathogens such as SARS or H$_5$N$_1$ influenza, most commonly originating in Asia, severe viral pneumonia (e.g. caused by adenovirus) is uncommon in healthy adults. Viral pneumonias are common in the elderly as well as infants and are increasingly recognised with the development of better diagnostics. Any respiratory virus and particularly respiratory synctial virus and those of the *Herpes* family (most commonly *Cytomegalovirus*) may cause pneumonia in the immunosuppressed such as organ transplant and HIV patients. Influenza A may cause a solely viral pneumonia, but is often complicated by secondary bacterial infection, especially *Staph. aureus*.

Table 3.10 Antibiotic therapy for pneumonia

Pneumonia	Therapy
Community acquired	Mild: Amoxycillin and erythromycin p.o.
Streptococcus pneumoniae 40%	Severe: Cefuroxime or amoxycillin i.v. and erythromycin p.o., add flucloxacillin if evidence of *Staphylococcus aureus*
Haemophilus influenzae 10%–30%	
Moraxella catarrhalis 10%–30%	
Atypical bacteria 10%–20%	
Viral 10–20%	
Gram negative organisms <1%	
Nosocomial – hospital acquired	Treatment should include a third generation cephalosporin such as
Gram negative (*Klebsiella, E. Coli,*	ceftazidime. If severe sepsis or in a neutropenic patient combination
Pseudomonas, Proteus) 60%	piperacillin/ tazobactam and gentamicin may be used
Strep. pneumoniae 5%	
Staphylococcus aureus (including MRSA)	

low blood pressure (systolic <90 mmHg or diastolic ≤60 mmHg).

- Additional adverse features include: Age ≥ 50 years, coexisting chronic disease, hypoxia (PaO$_2$ < 8 kPa or oxygen saturation < 92%), bilateral or multilobe involvement on chest X-ray.

A score of 2 or more core features suggest a severe pneumonia with indication for initial combined antibiotic therapy.

Tuberculosis

Definition
Tuberculosis (TB) is a common chronic infectious disease caused by *M. tuberculosis.*

Incidence
Approximately 7000 new cases a year in the United Kingdom and rising throughout Europe and the United States.

Age
Any age

Sex
M = F

Geography
Risk of contracting TB is markedly greater in developing countries, immigrants to the United Kingdom from the Asian sub-continent have a 40 times greater incidence of

TB than non-immigrants. Worldwide the highest rates of tuberculosis are seen in sub-Saharan Africa, India, China and the islands of Southeast Asia. Intermediate rates of tuberculosis occur in Central and South America, Eastern Europe and Northern Africa.

Aetiology
M. tuberculosis is an acid fast aerobic bacillus that grows slowly. It is spread by coughing up of live bacilli after invasion of the disease into a main bronchus (open tuberculosis), which are then inhaled.

The rising prevalence and mortality of tuberculosis is thought to be related to the following:

- Poverty and crowded conditions particularly in urban environments.
- Relaxation of disease control programmes in the mid-twentieth century when TB was declining.
- HIV co-infection.
- The emergence of multiple drug resistance due to non-compliance with medication.

Groups particularly at risk include the elderly, the very young, alcoholics, immunosuppressed, e.g. organ transplant patients, chronic lung disease patients and hospital workers.

Pathophysiology
The cell wall of *Mycobacterium* contains complex lipids and glycolipids which sensitise T-cells to produce abundant cytokines, which recruit macrophages (a Type IV hypersensitivity immune response). The macrophages can phagocytose the organisms, but mycobacterial cell

wall components interfere with the fusion of the lysosomes with the phagocytic vacuole, so that the bacteria can survive intracellularly.

The most common pattern of TB is a primary pulmonary infection:

- The mycobacteria are inhaled into the alveolar spaces of the lung. Conditions for growth are most favourable just below the pleura in the apex of the upper lobe or the apical lobe of the lower lobe. Here the inflammatory process forms the 'Ghon focus' usually just beneath the pleura. Bacteria spread to the draining lymph nodes at the lung hilum, and excite an immune response there also. This pattern forms the primary complex with infection at the periphery of the lung and enlarged peribronchial lymph nodes.
- The outcome of the primary infection depends on the balance between the virulence of the organism and the strength of the host response (see Table 3.11). If the host can mount an active cell mediated immune response the infection may be completely cleared.
- In the vast majority of cases there is an intermediate response and the activated macrophages aggregate and wall off a central area of caseous (cheese-like) necrosis. These are called granulomas or tubercles. Collagen is deposited around these, often becoming calcified. Twenty per cent of these tubercles contain viable mycobacteria, but clinically the infection becomes latent.
- If the immune response is very poor, there is progression of the caesating granulomas in the lymph nodes which erode into a bronchus or blood vessel causing further dissemination. This is called a 'progressive primary infection'. Occasionally the Ghon focus may rupture through the pleura causing a tuberculous pleurisy.

Table 3.11 Predisposing factors towards extension or containment of infection.

Predisposing to extension of infection	Predisposing to containment
Exposure to large numbers of highly virulent organisms	Exposure to a small number of poorly virulent organisms
Poor immune system eg malnutrition, extremes of age, intercurrent disease	Good immune response, e.g. healthy immunised individual
	Use of appropriate antibiotics

Secondary tuberculosis

- Secondary tuberculosis is a reactivation of infection occurring in a previously latently infected individual. It usually occurs due to reactivation of a healed primary lesion due to a weakening of the host defence, e.g. diabetes mellitus, malnutrition, immunosuppression (drugs, HIV). It may occur at any time from weeks up to years after the original infection. Occasionally it may be due to re-infection from an external source. It differs from primary infection in its immunopathology. The lymph nodes are rarely involved, and there is reactivation of the immune response in the tissues.
- In the lung, the bacteria have a preference for the apices (higher pO_2), and form an apical lung lesion known as an Assmann focus. It begins as a small caseating tuberculous granuloma, histologically similar to the Ghon focus, with destruction of lung tissue and cavitation. T cells are re-induced by the secondary infection, with activation of macrophages, and exactly as with primary TB the outcome is a balance between the virulence of the infection and the strength of the host immune system.
  - In patients with a vigorous immune reaction there is healing of the apical region with collagen deposition and eventually calcification by the same process as the healing of the primary infection resulting in a latent apical fibrocaseous tuberculosis lesion.
  - In patients with a poor immune response the lesion enlarges with caseous necrosis destroying lung tissue, thinning of the collagen wall and increasing the risk of erosion of a bronchus or blood vessel.

Patterns of progressive TB infection

See Fig. 3.3.

1 Tuberculous Bronchopneumonia: If an infected lymph node in primary tuberculosis, or an enlarging secondary tuberculous lesion erodes into a bronchus, tuberculous caseous material containing live tubercle bacilli spreads infection throughout that segment of lung. Coughing disperses these bacilli into the atmosphere, transmitting TB to other people. Without treatment, extensive caseating lesions develop rapidly, leading to a high mortality. This disease is sometimes called 'galloping consumption'.

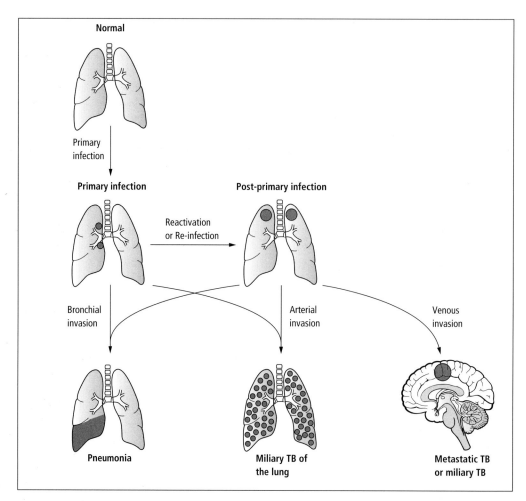

Figure 3.3 Patterns of tuberculosis infection.

2 Miliary Tuberculosis: If an enlarged caseous node erodes into a pulmonary artery the entire lung becomes infected by miliary dissemination with multiple small tubercles. If a lesion erodes a pulmonary vein, there may be systemic miliary dissemination, for example to the meninges, spleen, liver, the choroid and the bone marrow.

3 Metastatic Tuberculosis: If there is systemic dissemination but only a few bacteria are dispersed and the patient mounts a good immune response, organisms may settle in only one or two organs such as adrenal glands, a kidney, bone, joints, brain and meninges or the reproductive tract. There they may remain dor-

mant, reactivating many years later as single organ disease. By that time there may be no evidence of tuberculosis elsewhere.

Clinical features

1 Primary tuberculosis is usually asymptomatic, occasionally there may be a vague pyrexial illness sometimes associated with respiratory symptoms such as a dry cough. The hypersensitivity reaction may produce a transient pleural effusion or erythema nodosum.

2 Secondary pulmonary tuberculosis presents typically with a gradual onset of tiredness, malaise, anorexia and loss of weight over weeks or months. The outstanding

features are fever (drenching night sweats are rare) and cough productive of mucoid, purulent or blood stained sputum. A pleural effusion or pneumonia may be the presenting sign, chest signs are often absent and finger clubbing is only evident in late disease.

3 Miliary tuberculosis may present in a non-specific manner with vague ill health, weight loss and fever. As dissemination progresses there may be tuberculous meningitis, choroidal tubercles seen in the eye and hepatosplenomegaly.

Microscopy

The characteristic lesion, the tubercle (granuloma) consists of a central area of caseous tissue necrosis within which are viable mycobacteria. This central area is surrounded by a layer of activated macrophages and occasional multinucleate macrophages (Langerhans' giant cells). Around the macrophage zone is a collar of lymphocytes and an outer coating of fibroblasts.

Complications

- Fungal infection of cavitated areas of old TB infection forming a mycetoma.
- An enlarged lymph node may compress a bronchus, causing collapse of a segment or lobe of the lung. This usually heals spontaneously but occasionally may persist giving rise to bronchiectasis particularly of the middle lobe (Brock's Syndrome).
- Metastatic TB: Bone marrow invasion may lead to a pancytopenia. Bone involvement may lead to pathological fractures, particularly of the spine together with a paravertebral abscess. Tuberculous meningitis, tuberculous peritonitis or tuberculous pericarditis may occur.

Investigations

- An abnormal chest X-ray is often found incidentally in the absence of symptoms, but it is very rare for a case of pulmonary tuberculosis to be present if the chest X-ray is completely normal. The X-ray shows patchy or nodular shadowing in the upper zone with fibrosis and loss of volume; calcification and cavitation may also be present. There may be calcification in the pericardial sac. In miliary TB the chest X-ray may be normal, as tubercles are not visible until they are 1–2 mm.
- TB can mimic almost any disease, radiographically, so confirmation of the diagnosis must be by staining and culture of material such as sputum, early morning urine samples, cerebrospinal fluid, bronchoscopic washings, pleural, transbronchial, lymph node, or bone marrow solid organ biopsy.
- Microscopy with Ziehl–Nielsen staining or auramine fluorescent stain for acid fast bacilli (AFB). Rapid results can be obtained with polymerase chain reaction (PCR) and DNA probes, which are highly sensitive; however, they may be positive with no active disease. Formal culture of material is the only way of accurately determining virulence and antibiotic sensitivity and should be attempted in every case, results may take 4–6 weeks.
- HIV testing should be performed in all patients diagnosed with TB, even those without known risk factors, as patients with HIV are much more likely to have systemic organ involvement, relapse after treatment and may need lifelong treatment with isoniazid to prevent reactivation. They will also benefit from HIV specific treatment to improve their immune response.
- Tuberculin testing is used for contact tracing and prior to vaccination, it is used to assess exposure and sensitisation to TB. It relies on the hypersensitivity reaction, and is rarely helpful in the diagnosis of tuberculosis:
  i The Tine test and Heaf test are for screening: 4/6 point needles coated with old tuberculin are used to puncture the skin, 72 hours after the test a hypersensitivity reaction is present. If the spots are confluent, the test is positive, indicating exposure. In an immunised adult no TB treatment is required as long as there is no evidence of infection.
  ii The Mantoux test involves injecting a purified protein derivative intra dermally. The reaction is read at 48–72 hours and is said to be positive if the induration is 10 mm or more in diameter, negative if less than 5 mm.

    If the test is positive with a low concentration of purified protein derivative this can indicate active infection requiring treatment. In an immunocompromised host (such as chronic renal failure, lymphoma or HIV) or patients with miliary TB, the tests may be falsely negative.

Management

1 Hospitalisation is required for severely ill patients or where compliance is a particular problem.
2 Standard regimen is with 2 months of rifampicin, isoniazid, ethambutol and pyrazinamide, and a further 4 months of rifampicin and isoniazid alone. These are taken 30 minutes before breakfast to aid absorption.
3 Multi-resistant strains require sensitivity assessment and should be treated with three drugs to which the organism is sensitive for a full 6 months to avoid development of further resistance.

Prevention

In the United Kingdom, vaccination with BCG (Bacille Calmette–Guérin) has been given to Heaf negative 12 year olds since 1954. It is also offered to infants up to 6 weeks after birth (without prior skin testing) in areas with a high incidence of tuberculosis. Contact tracing of cases is essential for screening of all close family members and individuals who share kitchen and bathroom facilities by history, chest X-ray and tuberculin test.

Patients with chest X-ray evidence of previous TB who become immunosuppressed, e.g. renal dialysis, steroid treatment or organ transplant, may have daily isoniazid treatment to prevent reactivation of latent infection.

Prognosis

Five per cent of patients do not respond to therapy, only 1% due to resistance, the remainder due to failed compliance.

Influenza

Definition

Acute infection caused by the influenza viruses type A or B (RNA orthomyxovirus).

Aetiology

Influenza A causes worldwide annual epidemics and is infamous for the much rarer pandemics, the most serious of which occurred in 1918 when ~40 million people died worldwide. Influenza B is also associated with annual outbreaks that are usually milder in nature than those caused by influenza A. Influenza C is of doubtful pathogenicity in humans. Spread is by respiratory droplets.

Pathophysiology

Influenza viruses develop new antigenic variants at regular intervals through random mutations and antigenic drift. Human immunity depends largely on the haemagglutinin (H) antigen and the neuraminidase (N) antigen on the viral surface. Major shifts in these antigenic regions in influenza viruses occur through acquisition of a new H or N from animals such as birds, horses and pigs. These can cause a pandemic, whereas antigenic drift causes the milder annual epidemics. Influenza B only occurs in humans and only undergoes antigenic drift.

Clinical features

Rapid onset of fever usually >38°C, cough, headache, shivering and myalgia start after an incubation period of 1–3 days. Other upper and lower respiratory symptoms may develop. Individuals are infective for 1 day prior to and for around 1 week after symptoms commence.

Complications

- Otitis, sinusitis and viral pneumonia are common. Influenza may exacerbate underlying respiratory disease including asthma and chronic obstructive pulmonary disease.
- Secondary bacterial infection particularly with *Strep. pneumoniae* and *H. influenzae* is common following influenza pneumonia. Less commonly, secondary *Staph. aureus* infection which has a mortality rate of 20%.
- Post-viral syndrome: Debility and depression may develop after the acute illness, and take weeks to months to resolve.
- Post-infectious encephalomyelitis is rare but does occur.

Investigation

Diagnosis is confirmed by detection of virus in nasal or throat swabs by culture, antigen detection or PCR. Retrospective diagnosis can be made by a rise in specific complement-fixing antibody or haemagglutinin antibody measured 2 weeks apart, but this is usually unnecessary.

Management

- Bed rest, antipyretics such as paracetamol for symptoms. Fluids may be needed.

- The neuraminidase inhibitors zanamivir and os-
eltamivir are effective in treating acute influenza occurring during annual influenza epidemics. They
work against Influenza A and B if given within 48
hours of symptoms and especially in the first 24 hours.
They are particularly indicated in the elderly, those
with underlying respiratory disease such as chronic
obstructive pulmonary disease, and those with other
underlying disorders such as cardiovascular disease,
diabetes or renal failure. These drugs are also highly
effective for prophylaxis in family or institutional settings.
- Prophylaxis by vaccination is effective in up to 70%
and in elderly people reduces hospital admission and
mortality by about 50%. Some are manufactured in
chick embryos and these should not be given to anyone
allergic to eggs. Routine vaccination is reserved for
susceptible people with chronic heart, lung or renal
disease, diabetes, immunosuppression and the elderly.
It needs to be given yearly.
- The vaccine needs to be prepared each year based on
predictions of which antigenic variants are present.
These predications depend on global surveillance organised by the World Health Organisation (WHO).
This surveillance depends on viruses being cultured
and therefore on nose/throat swabs being taken and
sent to local labs.

Lung abscess

Definition
Localised infection and destruction of lung tissue leading
to a collection of pus within the lung.

Aetiology
Tuberculosis is the most common cause of lung abscesses
but is considered separately. Organisms which cause cavitation and hence lung abscess include *Staphylococcus*
and *Klebsiella*. It is more common in aspiration pneumonia or bronchial obstruction (by bronchial carcinoma
or a foreign body).

Pathophysiology
The abscess may form during the course of an acute
pneumonia, or chronically in partially treated pneumonia. Multiple lung abscesses may form from septic

emboli, e.g. from right-sided infective endocarditis or
an infected central line. Infarcted lung may cavitate, and
rarely it becomes secondarily infected.

Clinical features
Patients present with worsening features of pneumonia,
usually with a swinging pyrexia, and can be severely ill.
If there is communication between the abscess and the
airways the patient coughs up large amounts of foul sputum. Clubbing may develop.

Investigation
Anaemia, a high neutrophil count and raised inflammatory markers (ESR, CRP) are common. X-ray demonstrates one or more round opacities often with a fluid
level. Sputum and blood cultures may be positive, but
bronchoscopy may be necessary to exclude obstruction,
to look for underlying carcinoma, and to obtain biopsies
and broncho-alveolar lavage for microbiology. Sometimes CT or ultrasound guided aspiration is needed
and can also be therapeutic with insertion of a drain.
Echocardiogram should be considered to look for infective endocarditis.

Complication
Breach of the pleura results in an empyema.

Management
Postural drainage, physiotherapy and a prolonged course
of appropriate antibiotics to cover both aerobic and
anaerobic organisms will resolve most smaller abscesses. Larger abscesses may require repeated aspiration,
drainage and even surgical excision.

Aspergillus fumigatus

Definition
There are essentially three patterns of lung disease caused
by Aspergillus infection: Allergic bronchopulmonary
aspergillosis (ABPA), aspergilloma and invasive aspergillosis.

Aetiology
It is a filamentous fungus, the spores (5 μm in diameter) are ubiquitously present in the atmosphere. It rarely
causes disease. The pattern of disease that arises depends

on the degree of tissue invasiveness, the dose inhaled and the level of the host's defence.

Allergic bronchopulmonary aspergillosis (ABPA)

Pathophysiology

This results from Types I and III hypersensitivity reactions to persistent airway infection with the organism in susceptible (atopic) individuals.

i Initially it causes bronchospasm which commonly presents as asthma.

ii Recurrent episodes of eosinophilic pneumonia occur due to obstruction of the lumen, with the expectoration of firm sputum plugs containing the fungal mycelium.

iii Chronic infection and inflammation leads to irreversible dilatation of the bronchi (classically proximal bronchiectasis).

iv If left untreated progressive pulmonary fibrosis may develop, usually in the upper zones.

Clinical features

ABPA presents as worsening of asthma symptoms with episodic wheeze and cough productive of mucus plugs. There may be intermittent fever and malaise. A large mucus plug may obstruct a bronchus causing lung collapse.

Investigation

The peripheral blood eosinophil count is raised, and sputum may show eosinophilia and mycelia. Eosinophilic pneumonia causes transient lung shadows on chest X-ray. Precipitating antibodies are present in serum. Hypersensitivity is usually confirmed by skin-prick testing. Lung function testing confirms reversible obstruction in all cases, and may show reduced lung volumes in cases where there is chronic fibrosis.

Management

Generally it is not possible to eradicate the fungus. Itraconazole has been shown to modify the immunologic activation and improves clinical outcome, at least over the period of 16 weeks. Oral corticosteroids are used to suppress inflammation until clinically and radiographically returned to normal. Maintenance steroid therapy may be required subsequently. The asthmatic component is treated as per asthma guidelines.

Aspergilloma

This results from Aspergillus growing within an area of previously damaged lung such as an old tuberculous cavity (sometimes called a mycetoma). These are usually asymptomatic but occasionally may cause massive haemoptysis and require resection. Antifungal treatment is rarely effective.

Investigation

Seen on X-ray as a round lesion with an air 'halo' above it. The fungal mycelium may be seen in sputum and the chronic antigenic stimulation gives rise to serum precipitating antibody.

Invasive aspergillosis

In immunosuppressed individuals with a low granulocyte count, the organism may proliferate causing a severe pneumonia, causing necrosis and infarction of the lung. The organisms are present as masses of hyphae invading lung tissue and often involving vessel walls. Invasive aspergillosis presents as a pneumonia or septicaemia in the immunocompromised. Systemic invasive aspergillosis may manifest as meningitis, cerebral abscess or lesions in bone or liver.

Investigation

Invasive aspergillosis can only by diagnosed by lung biopsy.

Management

Invasive aspergillosis is treated with intravenous amphotericin B (often requiring liposomal preparations due to renal toxicity), often combined with flucytosine. Itraconazole and voriconazole have been used more recently but current studies comparing efficacy with amphotericin B have yet to prove definitive.

Obstructive lung disorders

Asthma

Definition

A disease with airways obstruction (which is reversible spontaneously or with treatment), airway inflammation and increased airway responsiveness to a number of stimuli.

Incidence
20% of children, 5–14% of adults, increasing in prevalence.

Age
Can present at any age, predominantly in children.

Sex
M > F under 16 years, F > M over 16 years.

Geography
Varies, e.g. rare in underdeveloped countries.

Aetiology
Asthma can be classified as follows, although the division is not always clear-cut:
1 Extrinsic asthma where there is an external cause
  - It is allergy based and commonly presents in young atopic individuals.
  - Atopy (asthma, eczema, hay fever and other allergies) has a familial component, it describes a disease manifestation related to the development of IgE antibodies against environmental antigens.
  - Common domestic allergens include proteins from house-dust mites, pets and airborne fungi.
2 Intrinsic asthma tends to present later in life. There is no identifiable allergic precipitant.
3 Occupational asthma is a particular type of extrinsic asthma, which may occur in both atopic individuals (who are more at risk) or non-atopic individuals.
  - Some industrial trigger factors are shown in Table 3.12. Patients with occupational asthma from the listed causes are entitled to compensation under industrial injuries legislation in the United Kingdom.
  - For all patients, non-specific irritant trigger factors include viral infections, cold air, exercise, emotion, atmospheric pollution, dust, vapours, fumes and drugs particularly nonsteroidal anti-inflammatories and β-blockers.

Table 3.12 Industrial trigger factors for asthma

Mechanism	Cause
Non IgE related	Isocyanates, colophony fumes (from solder), hardwood dust, complex platinum salts
IgE related	Allergens (from animals, flour, grain and mites), proteolytic enymes

Pathophysiology
The clinical picture of asthma results from mixed acute and chronic inflammation leading to bronchoconstriction, mucosal oedema and secretion of mucus into the lumen of the bronchi. With time this repeated stimulation causes hyperplasia of the smooth muscle and mucus glands within the bronchial wall as well as airway wall fibrosis. The pathophysiology is not yet fully understood. Asthma is a complex mixture of acute and chronic inflammation.
- Acute inflammation is largely mediated by allergen crosslinking of IgE on mast cells, leading to the release of mediators such as histamine, leukotrienes, prostaglandins, proteolytic enzymes and cytokines.
- The chronic inflammation is mediated by T cells producing type 2 cytokines (TH2). IL-5 recruits eosinophils, IL-4 and IL-13 lead to IgE synthesis and mucous secretion.
- Eosinophils are also important, secreting mediators of acute and chronic inflammation including proteolytic enzymes.
- Neutrophils are prominent in severe and virus-induced asthma. They secrete mediators of acute and chronic inflammation including enzymes and oxygen radicals.
- Epithelial cells from the bronchi are activated by allergens, viruses and air pollution and release chemotactic factors that recruit and activate inflammatory cells.
- All of the above cell types release mediators of chronic inflammation recruiting and activating fibroblasts leading to airway fibrosis. They also lead, through mechanisms which are not yet clearly defined, to bronchial hyperresponsiveness – an exaggerated bronchoconstrictor response to non-specific insults to the airways.

The pattern of airway reaction following inhalation of an allergen:
  i An acute reaction occurring within minutes, peaking at ~20 minutes after inhalation (the acute inflammatory response).
  ii A late reaction occurring 4–8 hours after inhalation (the chronic inflammatory response).
  iii A dual phase response incorporating both acute and late phase reactions (the mixed acute and chronic inflammatory response that is characteristic of asthma).

Table 3.13 Assessment of the severity of acute asthma

Mild–moderate attack	Severe attack	Life-threatening attack
• Speech normal	• Unable to complete sentences	• Silent chest
• Pulse <110 bpm	• Pulse ≥110 bpm	• Cyanosis
• Respiratory rate <25	• Respiratory Rate ≥25	• Bradycardia or hypotension
• Peak flow >50% predicted/best	• Peak flow 30–50%	• Peak flow <30% predicted/best

Clinical features

An asthma attack is characterised by rapid inspiration, slow and laboured expiration and polyphonic wheezes in all lung fields heard on expiration. Because of the potential severity of asthma patients require rapid assessment and intervention. An acute asthma attack is classified according to clinical severity (see Table 3.13).

In the long-term management of an asthmatic patient it is important to assess the degree of control that the patient's symptoms are under. Night-time waking, early morning wheeze, acute exacerbations in the preceding year, previous admissions to intensive care and a high requirement for bronchodilator therapy are all markers of poor control.

Complication

Pneumothorax, surgical emphysema due to rupture of alveoli and pneumomediastinum.

Investigations

The PEF (peak expiratory flow) is the most commonly used investigation in asthma. During an attack there is a marked reduction in all expiratory flow indices. In chronic asthma there is a characteristic diurnal variation with PEF >15% lower in early morning as well as day to day variation of >15%. For diagnosis and management patients may therefore be asked to fill in PEF charts with measurements taken AM and PM (prior to any inhaler therapy).

The simplest diagnostic test for asthma is to show a 15% improvement in PEF or forced expiratory volume in 1 second (FEV_1) with an inhaled bronchodilator. However, the test may be falsely negative if the asthma is controlled, in remission, or chronically very severe. If there is diagnostic difficulty in patients with mild symptoms or just cough, exercise tests or peak flow diary card recordings as above. Occasionally, a trial of oral corticosteroids for 2 weeks can be used. Skin tests are used to identify specific allergens and serum can be taken for total and specific IgEs.

Management

Management can be divided into acute and long-term management.

Long-term management
- Asthma is a variable condition which often changes so treatment must be regularly reviewed.
- Allergen avoidance can be advised, e.g. avoid pets, soft toys and dust and employ house dustmite avoidance mechanisms. However these rarely have a major impact on disease.
- Drug therapy includes: short acting β_2 agonists for short term bronchodilation; inhaled steroids for anti-inflammatory activity; long acting β_2 agonists for long term bronchodilation; anti leukotrienes, theophyllines and other agents with additional activities (see Fig. 3.4).
- Except in mild intermittent asthma anti-inflammatory therapy should be started early and must be used regularly. Once disease control is achieved the steroid dose is reduced under regular review to the minimum dose required to maintain disease control.
- Long acting β_2 agonists have been shown to produce better-sustained control. Their introduction is better than increasing inhaled steroids beyond a moderate dose, both in terms of greater effect and reduced side effects.
- Self-management plans in which the patient adjusts medications according to instructions relating to their PEF and/or symptoms have been shown to improve patient education, treatment compliance, disease control and acute exacerbations. They are strongly indicated in moderate to severe asthma.

Consideration should be given to stepping down treatment after a period of stability, but steroids should not be reduced more frequently than every 3 months.

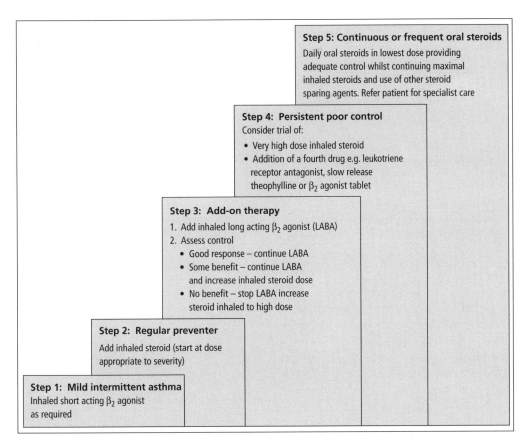

Step 5: Continuous or frequent oral steroids
Daily oral steroids in lowest dose providing adequate control whilst continuing maximal inhaled steroids and use of other steroid sparing agents. Refer patient for specialist care

Step 4: Persistent poor control
Consider trial of:
- Very high dose inhaled steroid
- Addition of a fourth drug e.g. leukotriene receptor antagonist, slow release theophylline or β_2 agonist tablet

Step 3: Add-on therapy
1. Add inhaled long acting β_2 agonist (LABA)
2. Assess control
   - Good response – continue LABA
   - Some benefit – continue LABA and increase inhaled steroid dose
   - No benefit – stop LABA increase steroid inhaled to high dose

Step 2: Regular preventer
Add inhaled steroid (start at dose appropriate to severity)

Step 1: Mild intermittent asthma
Inhaled short acting β_2 agonist as required

Figure 3.4 Stepwise long term management of asthma.

Acute management
This should follow the BTS/SIGN British Guidelines (see Figs. 3.5 and 3.6).

Prognosis
Most children and teenagers with asthma improve as they get older, although asthma may recur in adult life. All patients should be advised not to smoke and to avoid potential work allergens. Mortality is ∼2000 per year in the United Kingdom and is reduced by inhaled steroid therapy.

Chronic bronchitis and emphysema

Definition
Chronic bronchitis has a clinical definition of cough productive of sputum on most days for at least 3 months of the year for more than 1 year. Emphysema is defined as dilation and destruction of the lung tissue distal to terminal bronchioles. The two frequently co-exist to varying degrees as chronic obstructive pulmonary disease (COPD).

Prevalence
COPD has a prevalence of 12% aged 40–64 years. Emphysematous spaces are found in 50% of smokers aged over 60 at autopsy.

Age
Incidence increases with age.

Sex
M > F

Geography
Follows patterns of smoking.

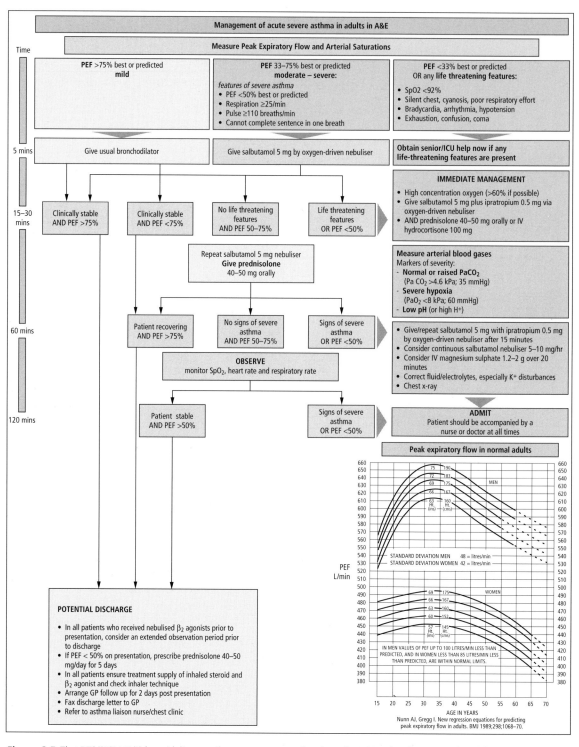

Figure 3.5 The BTS/SIGN British guideline on the management of asthma in A&E. *Thorax* 2003;58(Suppl). Reproduced with permission of the British Thoracic Society.

Management of acute severe asthma in adults in hospital

Features of acute severe asthma
- Peak expiratory flow (PEF) 33–50% of best
  (use % predicted if recent best unknown)
- Can't complete sentences in one breath
- Respirations ≥25 breaths/min
- Pulse ≥10 beats/min

Life threatening features
- PEF <33% of best or predicted
- SpO_2 <92%
- Silent chest, cyanosis, or feeble respiratory effort
- Bradycardia, dysrhythmia, or hypotension
- Exhaustion, confusion, or coma

If a patient has any life threatening feature.
measure arterial blood gases. No other investigations are needed for immediate management.

Blood gas markers of a life threatening attack:
- Normal (4.6–6 kpa, 35–45 mm Hg) $PaCO_2$
- Severe hypoxia; PaO_2 <8 kPa (60mmHg) irrespective of treatment with oxygen
- A low pH (or high H+)

Caution: Patients with severe or life threatening attacks may not be distressed and may not have all these abnormalities. The presence of any should alert the doctor.

Near fatal asthma
- Raised $PaCO_2$
- Requiring IPPV with raised inflation pressures

IMMEDIATE TREATMENT

- Oxygen 40–60%
  (CO_2 retention is not usually aggravated by oxygen therapy in asthma)
- Salbutamol 5 mg or terbutaline 10 mg via an oxygen-driven nebuliser
- Ipratropium bromide 0.5 mg via an oxygen-driven nebuliser
- Prednisolone tablets 40–50 mg or IV hydrocortisone 100 mg or both if very ill
- No sedatives of any kind
- Chest radiograph only if pneumothorax or consolidation are suspected or patient requires IPPV

IF LIFE THREATENING FEATURES ARE PRESENT:
- Discuss with senior clinician and ICU team
- Add IV magnesium sulphate 1.2–2 g infusion over 20 minutes *(unless already given)*
- Give nebulised β_2 agonist more frequently e.g. salbutamol 5 mg up to every 15–30 minutes or 10 mg continuously hourly

SUBSEQUENT MANAGEMENT

IF PATIENT IS IMPROVING continue:
- 40–60% oxygen
- Prednisolone 40–50mg daily or IV hydrocortisone 100 mg 6 hourly
- Nebulised β_2 agonist and ipratropium 4–6 hourly

IF PATIENT NOT IMPROVING AFTER 15–30 MINUTES:
- Continue Oxygen and steroids
- Give nebulised β_2 agonist more frequently e.g. salbutamol 5 mg up to every 15–30 minutes or 10 mg continuously hourly
- Continue ipratropium 0.5 mg 4–6 hourly until patient is improving

IF PATIENT IS STILL NOT IMPROVING:
- Discuss patient with senior clinician and ICU team
- IV magnesium sulphate 1.2–2 g over 20 minutes *(unless already given)*
- Senior clinician may consider use of IV β_2 agonist or IV aminophylline or progression to IPPV

MONITORING

- Repeat measurement of PEF 15–30 minutes after starting treatment
- Oximetry: maintain SpO_2 >92%
- Repeat blood gas measurements within 2 hours of starting treatment if,
  - initial PaO_2 <8 kPa (60 mmHg) unless subsequent SpO_2 >92%
  - $PaCO_2$ normal or raised
  - patient deteriorates
- Chart PEF before and after giving β_2 agonists and at least 4 times daily throughout hospital stay

Transfer to ICU accompanied by a doctor prepared to intubate if:
- Deteriorating PEF, worsening or persisting hypoxia, or hypercapnea
- Exhaustion, feeble respirations, confusion or drowsiness
- Coma or respiratory arrest

DISCHARGE

When discharged from hospital patients should have:
- Been on discharge medication for 24 hours
  and *have had inhaler technique checked and recorded*
- PEF >75% of best or predicted and PEF diurnal variability <25%
  unless discharge is agreed with respiratory physician
- Treatment with oral and inhaled steroids in addition to bronchodilators
- Own PEF meter and written asthma action plan
- GP follow up arranged *within 2 working days*
- Follow up appointment in respiratory clinic *within 4 weeks*

Patients with severe asthma (*indicated by need for admission*) and adverse behavioural or psychosocial features are at risk of further severe or fatal attacks
- Determine reason(s) for exacerbation and admission
- Send details of admission, discharge and potential best PEF to GP

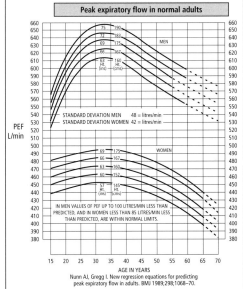

Peak expiratory flow in normal adults

PEF
L/min

STANDARD DEVIATION MEN   48 = litres/min
STANDARD DEVIATION WOMEN 42 = litres/min

MEN

WOMEN

IN MEN VALUES OF PEF UP TO 100 LITRES/MIN LESS THAN
PREDICTED, AND IN WOMEN LESS THAN 85 LITRES/MIN LESS
THAN PREDICTED, ARE WITHIN NORMAL LIMITS.

AGE IN YEARS
Nunn AJ, Gregg I. New regression equations for predicting
peak expiratory flow in adults. BMJ 1989;298;1068–70.

Figure 3.6 The BTS/SIGN British guideline on the management of asthma in hospital. *Thorax* 2003;58(Suppl I). Reproduced with permission of the British Thoracic Society.

Aetiology

Virtually confined to cigarette smokers and related to the number of cigarettes smoked each day. There is a strong genetic element to both components of COPD.

α1-antitrypsin deficiency is a recessive disorder, which causes pan-acinar emphysema and accounts for 5% of patients with emphysema. One in 5000 births have a homozygous deficiency and most these go on to develop the lung disease. Patients tend to be young (below 40 years) especially if smokers, in whom the disease is much worse.

Pathophysiology

There is airway inflammation, dominated by neutrophils and CD8+ T cells. There is also hypertrophy and hyperplasia of the mucus secreting glands causing plugging of airways and luminal narrowing resulting in airway obstruction. This 'chronic bronchitis' co-exists with a greater or lesser degree of emphysema in this patient group.

- In centri-acinar emphysema there is distension of alveoli and damage of lung tissue concentrated around the respiratory bronchioles whilst the more distal alveolar ducts and air spaces tend to be well preserved. The alveolar dilatation results from loss of elastic recoil in the terminal bronchioles, as a result of destruction of lung tissue by neutrophil derived proteases. Smoking also causes glandular hypertrophy (chronic bronchitis) and has an adverse effect on surfactant favouring over distension of the lung.
- In pan-acinar emphysema destruction involves the whole of the acinus.

Clinical features

Chronic bronchitis and emphysema together produce the clinical picture of COPD (also sometimes called chronic obstructive airways disease (COAD), or chronic obstructive lung disease (COLD)). In addition there may be features of asthma as some patients have a degree of reversible airflow obstruction. The clinical features depend on the degrees of chronic bronchitis and of emphysema contributing to the overall picture.

- Symptoms of chronic bronchitis include cough productive of sputum, expiratory wheeze and progressive shortness of breath. Symptoms of emphysema are dominated by progressive breathlessness, initially only on exertion but eventually on mild exertion such

as dressing. Expiratory wheeze and cough are present but the cough is dry.
- Signs in both diseases include expiratory wheeze heard in all lung fields, in chronic bronchitis coarse early inspiratory crackles are also heard. As emphysema becomes more severe other signs become evident including tachypnoea, cachexia, the use of accessory muscles of respiration, intercostal recession, pursed lips on expiration, poor chest expansion (a hyperinflated chest at rest) and loss of cardiac and hepatic dullness due to hyperinflation.
- The two patterns of pink puffer (always breathless, not cyanosed, cachexic) and blue bloater (obese, cyanosed, hypoventilating, often with little respiratory effort) describe the extremes of the spectrum of disease manifest as COPD. The pink puffer is typical of relatively pure emphysema and the blue bloater is typical of relatively pure chronic bronchitis.

Macroscopy

There is secretion of abnormal amounts of mucus causing obstruction and plugging of the airways. Mucus gland hypertrophy and hyperplasia can be quantified by the Reid index which is the ratio of gland to wall thickness within the bronchus.

Microscopy

Both emphysema and chronic bronchitis are inflammatory diseases of the lung. The inflammatory infiltrate is dominated by neutrophils and CD8 +ve T cells. Eosinophils are also seen especially in chronic bronchitis, in which the predominant pathological features are mucus gland enlargement and airway wall inflammation. In emphysema the predominant feature is destruction of the alveolar septae as a result of neutrophil derived proteases. Acute viral or bacterial infections, or chronic bacterial colonisation exacerbates the inflammation. Squamous metaplasia is commonly seen.

Complications

Airway obstruction and alveolar destruction eventually leads to impaired alveolar ventilation and respiratory failure in both conditions. Pulmonary vasculature responds to hypoxia by vasoconstriction which increases the arterial pressure, causing pulmonary artery hypertension, which leads to right heart failure (cor pulmonale). There may be secondary polycythaemia due to hypoxia. In emphysema initially hyperventilation maintains normocapnia. Cyanosis, hypercapnia and cor pulmonale develop only late in the disease after progressive decline in lung function. Amoxycillin resistant *Haemophilus* respiratory infections are common in COPD patients as a result of frequent courses of antibiotic therapy. Acute exacerbations precipitated by viral, bacterial or mixed infections are common resulting in major morbidity and mortality.

Investigations

The diagnosis is frequently made clinically but requires confirmation by demonstration of degree of irreversible airway obstruction manifest by a reduced PEF and FEV_1/FVC after inhaled bronchdilators. In emphysema the K_{CO} (transfer factor) is also reduced. The lung volumes may be normal in chronic bronchitis but are increased in emphysema.

i Chest X-ray: May be normal or there may be bullae, severe over-inflation. There may also be a deficiency of blood vessels in the peripheral half of the lung fields in comparison to the proximal vessels.

ii CT scan is usually performed to assess the degree of alveolar destruction due to emphysema. It frequently shows peribronchial thickening and alveolar coalescence.

iii Haemoglobin and packed cell volume may be elevated.

iv Blood gases are variable as there may be hypoxia and hypercapnia or hypocapnia, depending on the degree of type I or type II respiratory failure and the degrees of respiratory and metabolic compensation.

v ECG for cor pulmonale (right axis deviation, tall R in V_1, peaked P waves) and coexisting cardiac disease.

vi $\alpha 1$-antitrypsin (normal serum range 20–48 mmol/L).

Management

1 Non-pharmacological: By far the most important factor that can affect the prognosis and progression of chronic obstructive pulmonary disease is stopping smoking. Weight loss is vital in the obese. Physiotherapy may help clear sputum, and pulmonary rehabilitation programmes improve exercise capacity and quality of life. Influenza vaccine should be given annually.

2 Pharmacological
- Bronchodilators: Short acting bronchodilators produce significant clinical benefit, helping patients feel less short of breath (although objective improvement in lung function tests may be slight). Salbutamol is usually first line therapy followed by ipratropium bromide. Long acting β_2 agonists and long acting anticholinergics improve lung function, symptoms, reduce exacerbation frequency and are recommended for moderate COPD. Long-term oral theophylline appears to be of some benefit.
- Inhaled corticosteroids have been shown to produce small improvements in lung function, to reduce exacerbation frequency and to slow the decline in FEV_1 over time. The optimum dose and patient group in which they should be used are not yet clearly defined. They are currently recommended for moderate-severe COPD with two or more exacerbations in the last 12 months.
- An oral course of prednisolone, and antibiotics if sputum is purulent, should be given promptly in acute exacerbations in an attempt to minimise lung damage. Amoxycillin resistant *Haemophilus* respiratory infections are treated with erythromycin, co-amoxiclav or cephalosporins.
- Diuretic therapy for oedema in patients with right heart failure.

3 Persistent hypoxia should be treated with long-term domiciliary oxygen therapy to improve prognosis.

4 Non-invasive nasal ventilation is useful in treating acute exacerbations to avoid the need for intubation and formal ventilation. It can also be used for nocturnal hypoxic episodes and to prolong life, e.g. prior to planned transplantation.

5 α_1-antitrypsin infusions are used as replacement for patients with serum levels below 11 mmol/L and abnormal lung function, but it is not known if this improves the prognosis.

6 Surgical management
- Patients of young age who are otherwise fit and well may be considered for lung or heart/lung transplantation. The heart/lung transplant requires cardiopulmonary bypass and is performed through a sternotomy. Bilateral or single lung transplants are performed through a lateral thoracotomy possibly without bypass. Immunosuppression is achieved with triple therapy of cyclosporin, azathioprine

and steroids. The lung is prone to rejection and thus transbronchial biopsies are now used for routine monitoring. Infection is common and may be severe.

- Lung volume reduction surgery has a place in the treatment of some patients with emphysema although its role is still under investigation.

Prognosis
50% of patients with severe breathlessness die within 5 years although even in severe cases stopping smoking improves the prognosis.

Sleep apnoea/Pickwickian syndrome

Definition
Sleep apnoea represents the cessation of airflow at the level of the nostrils and mouth lasting at least 10 seconds, the patient is said to suffer from sleep apnoea if more than 15 such episodes occur in any 1 hour of sleep.

Prevalence
1–2% of the general population.

Age
Middle age.

Sex
Male preponderance.

Aetiology
Risk factors include obesity, smoking, chronic obstructive pulmonary disease and alcohol or other sedatives which exacerbate the problem by causing hypotonia and respiratory depression. Apnoea can be divided into the following:

1 Central apnoea when there is depression of the respiratory drive, e.g. opiate overdose.
2 Obstructive apnoea when air is unable to pass despite a respiratory effort.
3 Mixed central and obstructive apnoea.

Pathophysiology
Snoring arises because of turbulent airflow around the soft palate with partial obstruction. Critical airway obstruction leads to a decrease in arterial oxygen 'hypopnoea' and then occlusion leads to apnoea. There is a reflex increase in respiratory drive, which eventually rouses the patient sufficiently to overcome the obstruction, in the process of which the patients sleep is disturbed, although they do not recall it.

Clinical features
Patients complain of continual tiredness (90%), and may fall asleep during the day. Less than half notice that they have a restless or unrefreshing sleep, and about a third complain of morning headache (due to carbon dioxide retention). Sleeping partners will have noticed loud snoring in 95% and often notice the snore–apnoea–choke–snore cycle. Alcohol and smoking should be enquired about. Classical anatomy is a long soft palate, large neck and excess tissue around the tonsils. Systemic hypertension is common.

Complications
Oxygen saturations may fall very low. The pulmonary vasculature responds to hypoxia by vasoconstriction thus there may be pulmonary hypertension. Hypoxia also increases arrhythmias and there is an increased risk of stroke and myocardial infarction. Twenty per cent experience reduced libido and even impotence.

Investigations
A simple sleep study with overnight pulse oximetry together with a history from sleeping companion may be diagnostic. Many require a full sleep study (polysomnogram), which consists of a pulse oximeter, a tidal volume measurement, oronasal flow and electroencephalography to record sleep and arousal patterns. Polycythaemia (raised haemoglobin and packed cell volume) may occur in advanced cases.

Management
Non-pharmacological treatment includes weight loss, exercise, cessation of smoking and reduced alcohol intake. Mechanical obstruction due to nasal deformities, polyps or adenoids may be correctable.

1 Continuous positive airway pressure (CPAP) via a nasal mask prevents collapse of the upper airway and is the mainstay of treatment.
2 Surgical treatment may be difficult as patients are often a poor anaesthetic risk.
   - Uvulopalatopharyngoplasty (UPPP) trimming of the redundant tissues in the soft palate and lateral pharynx is sometimes performed but its benefit in

true obstructive sleep apnoea is unproven and it may make future CPAP via a nasal mask impossible.

Restrictive lung disorders

Pulmonary fibrosis and honeycomb lung

Definition
Pulmonary fibrosis is the end result of many diseases.

Aetiology
A useful mnemonic for the main causes of pulmonary fibrosis is Breast Ca.

Bleomycin, busulphan (and other cytotoxic drugs)

Radiation

Extrinsic allergic alveolitis

Ankylosing spondylitis and other connective tissue diseases (scleroderma, rheumatoid arthritis, systemic lupus erythematosus)

Sarcoidosis, berylliosis (exposure to this industrial alloy mimics sarcoidosis)

Tuberculosis

Cryptogenic fibrosing alveolitis (idiopathic pulmonary fibrosis)

Asbestosis

The other main groups of causes are the pneumoconioses, which are occupational lung diseases in response to fibrogenic dusts such as coal and silicon, and drug-induced, such as amiodarone.

Pathophysiology
The lung has limited ability to regenerate following a severe noxious insult. Fibrosis may be localised, bilateral or widespread depending on the underlying cause. Honeycomb lung represents late-stage fibrosis. Patients are at an increased risk of secondary infection and even if the original insult is removed may develop progressive fibrosis and subsequent respiratory failure. The alveolar wall fibrosis greatly reduces the pulmonary capillary network, leading to the development of pulmonary hypertension, right ventricular hypertrophy, with eventual right heart failure (cor pulmonale).

Investigations
Chest X-ray shows reticulonodular shadowing in the areas affected, and high-resolution CT shows reticular changes and the cysts seen in honeycomb lung. Lung function testing shows a restrictive defect (reduced lung volumes with relatively preserved peak flows and FEV_1.

Management
Treatment or removal of underlying cause. See also individual conditions.

Idiopathic pulmonary fibrosis – usual interstitial pneumonia

Definition
This condition was previously known as cryptogenic fibrosing alveolitis (CFA) characterised by interstitial infiltrates mainly in the lung bases causing progressive dyspnoea. It has been reclassified as usual interstitial pneumonia, a form of idiopathic interstitial pneumonia.

Prevalence
Uncommon.

Age
Usually late middle age.

Sex
Slightly M > F

Aetiology
Unknown, but an indistinguishable disease is seen in association with a number of other diseases such as asbestosis, rheumatoid arthritis and systemic sclerosis. Antinuclear factor is positive in one third of patients and rheumatoid factor is positive in 50%. Up to 75% of patients are current or former smokers, and smoking appears to be an independent risk factor.

Pathophysiology
There appear to be areas of fibroblast activation, which lay down matrix, and healing of these leads to fibrosis. It is not clear what causes the acute lung injury or the abnormal healing process, but increased levels of cytokines and immune cells are found.

Clinical features
Patients present with dry cough and gradually increasing breathlessness. They may present with secondary

bacterial infection. Classical signs are clubbing, cyanosis and fine end-inspiratory crackles in the mid to lower lungs.

Microscopy

Characteristically chronic fibrotic, scarred zones with collapsed alveoli and honeycombing alternate with areas of relatively unaffected lung. Where there is acute injury, there are foci of activated fibroblasts with little inflammation.

Complications

The disease is progressive and usually unresponsive to treatment, and patients develop respiratory failure, pulmonary hypertension and cor pulmonale. An acute form exists (Hamman–Rich syndrome or acute interstitial pneumonia) with a very high mortality rate.

Investigations

- Chest X-ray shows fine reticular shadows, mainly in the bases and peripheral honeycombing.
- CT scan of the chest show a ground glass appearance in areas of alveolitis with extensive reticular patterns due to fibrosis.
- Respiratory function tests shows a restrictive pattern with reduced lung volumes, FEV_1 and FVC are low but the ratio of the two is normal/high, and gas transfer is reduced. In smokers there may be a superimposed obstructive pattern.
- Blood gases show hypoxaemia with normal or low carbon dioxide levels.
- High erythrocyte sedimentation rate (ESR) in up to one third of patients.
- Broncho-alveolar lavage shows increased cells particularly neutrophils.
- Lung biopsy is indicated if possible, usually transbronchial via bronchoscopy. Because of the patchy nature of the disease, however, surgical lung biopsy of several sites may be needed.

Management

There are no proven effective treatments. A trial of prednisolone 30 mg is indicated if the diagnosis is not well established in case there is a responsive interstitial pneumonitis. Azathioprine and ciclosporin have also been tried. Supportive treatment includes oxygen, long-term oxygen therapy improves the prognosis by delaying the

development of cor pulmonale. Single-lung transplant has been shown to be viable, but most patients have concomitant disease which precludes this.

Prognosis

Median survival of 5 years. Forty per cent die of progressive respiratory failure, most of the others from acute infection or concomitant ischaemic heart disease. Newer anti-fibrotic and immunological therapies are being investigated.

Extrinsic allergic alveolitis

Definition

An immune reaction within the lung to inhaled organic dusts.

Aetiology

See Table 3.14

Pathophysiology

1 After exposure there is formation of antibody–antigen complexes. Normally immune complexes are cleared but if they persist, they activate the complement system resulting in local inflammation, inflammatory cell recruitment and cellular damage (i.e. a type III hypersensitivity reaction).
2 If there is repeated exposure a type IV cell mediated hypersensitivity reaction occurs with the formation of small granulomas. The lung damage is repaired by pulmonary fibrosis.

Table 3.14 Causes of extrinsic allergic alveolitis

Disease	Source	Antigens
Farmer's lung	Mouldy hay/vegetable material	Micropolyspora faeni, thermophilic actinomycetes
Mushroom picker's lung	Mushroom dust	Thermophilic actinomycetes
Bird fancier's lung	Avian excreta and feathers	Various proteins
Malt worker's lung	Germinating barley	Aspergillus clavatus
Humidifier fever	Contaminated humidifiers	Various bacteria and/or amoebae

Clinical features

- Fever, malaise, cough and shortness of breath, sometimes with limb pains, develops several hours after exposure to the antigen and may last up to 2–3 days. On examination there may be tachypnoea and cyanosis, with widespread fine end-inspiratory crackles and mild wheeze.
- Chronic exposure leads to a chronic disease characterised by weight loss, effort dyspnoea, cough and signs similar to idiopathic pulmonary fibrosis (persisting cyanosis, fine crackles and cor pulmonale).

Microscopy

Infiltration with neutrophils, lymphocytes and macrophages. In chronic exposure non-caseating granulomas are seen comprising multinucleated giant cells, within which the antigenic material may be demonstrated.

Complications

Diffuse fibrosis and formation of honeycomb lung in about 5%.

Investigations

- Chest X-ray shows a diffuse haze initially, which develops into micronodular shadowing. The upper lobes are predominantly affected. Advanced cases may show features of honeycomb lung (cystic appearance). CT chest shows ground glass appearance in acute forms due to alveolitis and extensive lung fibrosis with nodule formation in chronic cases.
- There is a raised white count with a neutrophilia following acute exposure. There is no eosinophilia (this would suggest asthma).
- Precipitating antibodies are present in the serum; however, these are markers of exposure and not of the disease.
- Respiratory function tests shows a restrictive pattern with reduced lung volumes, FEV_1 and FVC are low but the ratio of the two is normal/high, and gas transfer is reduced. This is reversible initially, but becomes permanent with chronic disease.
- Bronchoalveolar lavage shows an increase in lymphocytes and macrophages.

Management

1 Avoidance is the most important factor in management, mainly by changing working practice.
2 High-dose prednisolone is used to cause regression of the early stages of the disease, later stages where there is fibrosis are not amenable to treatment.

Prognosis

Recurrent exposure leads to irreversible damage and ultimately respiratory failure, and it is particularly difficult to stop bird fanciers from pursuing their hobby. Farmer's lung is an occupational disease in the United Kingdom with sufferers being entitled to compensation.

Acute respiratory distress syndrome (ARDS)

Definition

An acute form of respiratory failure caused by diffuse pulmonary infiltrates and alveolar damage occurring hours to days after a pulmonary or systemic insult. Previously called adult respiratory distress syndrome it has been renamed as it also occurs in children.

Incidence

Occurs in 20–40% of patients with severe sepsis.

Aetiology

Many conditions are recognised as precipitants, most commonly systemic sepsis.

- Lung-related causes include aspiration and smoke inhalation, pneumonia, near drowning and lung contusion.
- Other systemic causes include shock from any cause, major trauma/burns, disseminated intravascular coagulation (DIC), air, fat or amniotic fluid embolism and heroin overdose. It is also well reported following cardiopulmonary bypass and pancreatitis.

Pathophysiology

1 Acute exudative phase:
- Increased vascular permeability and epithelial damage due to neutrophil-derived toxins, mechanical damage, cytokines and possibly abnormal clotting mechanisms lead to pulmonary oedema

(non-cardiogenic) and exudation of a protein-rich fluid into alveolar spaces.

- Type I pneumocytes, which make up 90% of the alveolar epithelium mostly die, and Type II pneumocytes, which produce surfactant are disrupted in function.

During this phase, there is alveolar collapse, lung compliance falls (i.e. the lungs become stiff) and gas exchange is impaired, and there may also be evidence of airflow obstruction. Increased shunting and deadspace occurs (ventilation–perfusion mismatch) and hypoxaemia results.

2 In some cases the acute phase resolves with complete recovery within a week. In other cases, where damage to lung tissue has been severe the disease progresses to a fibrosing alveolitis phase:

- The mechanism is unclear, but interstitial fibrosis develops with loss of the normal architecture of the lung, obliterating the vasculature and leading to pulmonary hypertension, worsening lung compliance and in the long-term emphysema and honeycomb lung.

Clinical features

The first sign is tachypnoea, followed by hypoxia, worsening dyspnoea and fine bi-basal crackles that become widespread. ARDS is often the first manifestation of multiple organ failure, so the features of other organ failure may develop such as renal and liver failure.

Complications

Often complicated by secondary infection (nosocomial pneumonia).

Investigations

- Chest X-ray and CT scan show bilateral diffuse shadowing with an alveolar pattern. Later the picture may progress to a complete whiteout. With the fibrotic phase, linear opacities become visible.
- Blood gases are used to detect and monitor respiratory failure, other investigations such as U&E and liver function tests may be required, as multiorgan failure is common.
- The pulmonary wedge pressure should be measured by insertion of a Swan–Ganz catheter. In ARDS the pulmonary wedge pressure is normal (although

pulmonary arterial pressure is raised) unlike in cardiogenic pulmonary oedema.

- Other investigations to look for an underlying cause (e.g. blood cultures coagulation screen and d-dimers for DIC, amylase for pancreatitis).

Management

1 Identification and eradication of any underlying cause such as sepsis.
2 Supportive treatment with following:

- Ventilatory support – low volume, pressure-limited cycles reduce further damage.
- Fluid restriction and removal if necessary to minimise pulmonary oedema.
- To attempt to improve ventilation/perfusion mismatch the patient can be alternately nursed prone and supine, or treated with nebulised prostacyclin or nitric oxide.
- High dose steroids are no longer recommended in ARDS for treatment or prophylaxis.

Prognosis

Dependant on the underlying cause, mortality can be very high in patients with septic shock who develop multi-organ failure. Increasing age and pre-existing disease worsen the outcome.

Suppurative lung disorders

Cystic fibrosis

Definition

Autosomal recessive disorder with multisystem involvement including chronic suppurative lung disease, pancreatic insufficiency and liver cirrhosis.

Incidence

1 in 2500 births are homozygous, 1 in 25 carriers (heterozygous) in Caucasians.

Age

90% diagnosed in childhood, and 10% in adolescents and adults.

Sex

M = F

Geography

More common in Caucasians, uncommon in Orientals and Afro Caribbeans.

Aetiology

The condition is caused by mutations of the cystic fibrosis transmembrane conductance regulator (CFTR) gene carried on the long arm of chromosome 7.

Seventy per cent of North European patients have the ΔF508 mutation, which is a specific codon deletion resulting in deletion of a phenylalanine at position 508 within the amino acid sequence of the CFTR protein. Over 1000 other mutations have now been identified. There is poor correlation between the genetics and the clinical disease.

Pathophysiology

In normal mucus secreting epithelium the CFTR acts as an important cAMP-regulated chloride channel to facilitate secretion of sodium chloride and hence water, which results in low viscosity mucus. The mutation results in defective ion transport and nearly all exocrine glands are involved to a varying extent:

1 In the lungs, which appear to be histologically normal at birth, increased production of thick viscous mucus plugs airways, leading to inflammation and secondary infection. Bronchiectasis (thickened, dilated bronchial walls) filled with purulent, thick secretions and areas of atelectasis develop. There may also be immune-mediated damage by an influx of neutrophils releasing proteases.
2 Viscous or solid material also obstructs the lumen of pancreas, small and large intestine, intrahepatic bile ducts and gallbladder.
3 There is increased Na and Cl concentration in the sweat.
4 There is also obstruction or maldevelopment of the vas deferens causing most males to be infertile, and increased viscosity of cervical secretions impairs fertility in some women.

Clinical features

10% of patients escape detection until adolescence or early adulthood.

Presentation:
- 40% with respiratory disease
- 25% with failure to thrive and malabsorption
- 15% at birth with meconium ileus due to viscous meconium
- 10% with liver disease
- 10% with rectal prolapse

With later disease, patients show use of accessory muscles of respiration, a barrel-chest deformity, clubbing and cyanosis. Auscultation of the chest shows widespread coarse crackles.

Investigations

- Diagnosis is by the sweat test which is positive if the Cl is above 60 mmol/L on two sweat tests in at least 75 mg of sweat (preferably 100 mg). Testing involves pilocarpin iontophoresis. Occasionally false positives or negatives occur.
- Pre-natal DNA screening by mutation analysis is possible for those with a previous sibling with CF. Widespread pre-natal screening is not yet recommended.
- Chest X-ray is initially normal, later there is generalised bronchial wall thickening and hyperinflation. Sputum culture for chest infection and lung function testing are useful.

Management

1 Non-pharmacological: Postural drainage, other manoeuvres and exercise, close liaison with a physiotherapist is essential.
2 Pharmacological:
   - Antibiotics used on the basis of regular sputum culture (prophylactic flucloxacillin may be used in first 2 years of life). Respiratory exacerbations should be treated with high-dose antibiotic courses lasting 2 weeks. Oral ciprofloxacin is useful for *Pseudomonas aeruginosa* infections. Regular nebulised gentamicin may be useful.
   - Bronchodilators may prove useful in those with reversible airways obstruction.
   - Agents to reduce the viscosity of the sputum may be used including acetylcysteine, triphosphate nucleotide and inhaled recombinant human deoxyribonuclease (rhDNase).
   - Malabsorption is treated with pancreatic enzyme supplements taken with all meals and snacks. Vitamin A, D and E supplements are used. NG or gastrostomy feeding is possible with either whole or partially digested food.

- Appropriate vaccination against influenza, *H. influenzae Strep pneumoniae*, measles, pertussis and varicella.
- Gene therapy is currently being researched in an attempt to 'infect' individuals with a retrovirus carrying the normal CF gene.

3 Surgical treatment: If the patient has a life expectancy of less than 18 months, lung (or heart–lung) transplantation is used with good result. Liver transplantation has been used in patients with end-stage liver disease.

Prognosis

Median age of survival is 31 years but is expected to rise with improving therapies.

Bronchiectasis

Definition

Bronchiectasis is a condition characterised by purulent sputum production with cystic dilation of the bronchi.

Aetiology

In developed countries, cystic fibrosis is the most common cause, tuberculosis and post-childhood infections are also common.

1 Changes in the normal drainage of bronchial secretions:
  - Airway obstruction such as by a tumour or foreign body.
  - The mucus may not drain if it is excessively thick as in cystic fibrosis.
  - Conditions affecting cilia such as ciliary dyskinesia and Kartagener's syndrome (genetic syndrome associated with dextrocardia and situs inversus).
2 Infections causing damage to the bronchial walls:
  - Childhood respiratory infection in the developing lung, e.g. measles, whooping cough and pneumonia.
  - Persistent infections such as tuberculosis, allergic bronchopulmonary aspergillosis.
  - Immunodeficiency states resulting in recurrent infections.

Pathophysiology

Impairment of the mucociliary transport mechanism leads to recurrent infections, which leads to further accumulation of mucus. Bronchial walls become inflamed, thickened and permanently dilated. The lower lobes of the lungs tend to be most affected because of gravitational pooling of secretions.

Clinical features

In mild cases sputum production only occurs post-infection. More severely affected patients have chronic halitosis, a cough with copious thick sputum, recurrent fevers and episodes of pneumonia. Patients may be dyspnoeic, clubbed and cyanosed. Haemoptysis may occur due to friable granulation tissue and can be massive. Coarse crackles and sometimes wheeze (due to airflow limitation) are heard over affected areas.

Macroscopy

Large dilated air spaces are seen extending out to the lung periphery.

Microscopy

Chronic inflammation in the wall of the abnormal bronchi with replacement of the epithelium with inflammatory granulation tissue, which bleeds. There may be squamous metaplasia of the bronchial mucosa.

Complications

- Pneumonia.
- Pneumothorax, empyema.
- Chronic cases may lead to respiratory failure and cor pulmonale.
- Chronic suppuration causes abscess formation, haematogenous spread of infection (formation of cerebral abscesses) and development of amyloidosis.

Investigations

- Chest X-ray may be normal or may show the dilated thick walled bronchi.
- High resolution CT scans are diagnostic showing the dilated bronchi with thickened walls and adjacent artery forming the typical signet ring appearance.
- Sputum culture is necessary to treat infections. The most common organisms are *Staph. aureus, Pseudomonas aeruginosa, H. influenzae* and anaerobes.
- Serum immunoglobulins, sweat test, cilial motility studies where indicated.

Management

The aim is to prevent chronic sepsis and reduce acute infections.

1 Non-pharmacological: Postural drainage is crucial and requires training by physiotherapists. Patients are taught to tip and hold themselves in the correct positions several times a day.
2 Pharmacological:
   - Antibiotics are given for acute infections and exacerbations.
   - Bronchodilator therapy may be useful if there is airflow obstruction.
3 If hypoxic long term oxygen therapy may delay the onset of cor pulmonale.
4 Surgery may be needed for massive haemoptysis.

Prognosis
Variable depending on cause and severity.

Granulomatous/vasculitic lung disorders

Sarcoidosis

Definition
Multisystem chronic granulomatous disorder of unknown origin.

Incidence
19 per 100,000 in United Kingdom.

Age
Under 40 years; peak 20–30 years.

Sex
F > M

Geography
Affects American Afro Caribbeans more than Caucasians. Uncommon in Japan.

Aetiology
- No HLA association but familial cases seen, suggesting environmental factors.
- Because of the granulomata, atypical mycobacterium, Epstein–Barr virus or other infections have been suggested but never proven.
- Beryllium poisoning can cause an identical clinical picture.

Pathophysiology
Unknown but there is strong evidence for an immunopathological basis:
1 The granulomas consist of macrophages and mainly T lymphocytes, particularly helper (CD4+) cells, and even before granulomas form bronchoalveolar lavages reflect this cell mix.
2 Peripheral blood has decreased T cells and relatively increased B cells (overall lymphopenia).
3 Depressed cell mediated immunity is demonstrated by the depressed responses to tuberculin or other immunological skin testing (this is called 'anergy').

Clinical features
Around half present with respiratory symptoms or are diagnosed following an incidental finding of bilateral hilar lymphadenopathy or lung infiltrates on chest X-ray. Next most common are skin and ocular presentations. Other presentations include arthralgias, nonspecific symptoms of weight loss, fatigue and fever.
   Pulmonary manifestations:
- Bilateral hilar lymphadenopathy with or without pulmonary infiltration.
- Pulmonary infiltration may be progressive leading to fibrosis, increasing effort dyspnoea and eventually cor pulmonale and death.

Extra pulmonary manifestations:
Any organ of the body can be affected, most commonly:
- Skin: Sarcoid is the commonest cause of erythema nodosum (see page 390), when associated with bilateral hilar lymphadenopathy it is diagnostic. Violaceous plaques on the nose, cheeks, ears and fingers known as lupus pernio or skin nodules may occur.
- Eyes: Anterior uveitis is common.
- Enlargement of lacrimal and parotid glands.
- Arthralgia and joint swelling with associated bone cysts.
- Cranial nerve involvement particularly facial nerve palsy occurs but is uncommon.
- Hepatosplenomegaly often present though rarely clinically relevant.
- Cardiac involvement is relatively common: ventricular dysrhythmias, conduction defects and cardiomyopathy with congestive cardiac failure.
- Ten per cent of patients with established sarcoidosis have hypercalcaemia and hypercalciuria which can lead to renal calculi. This is thought to be due to

1α-hydroxylation of vitamin D in sarcoid macrophages, which results in raised levels of 1,25-dihydroxy vitamin D_3.

Microscopy

Non-caseating granulomas consisting of focal accumulation of epithelioid cells, macrophages, (mainly T) lymphocytes and giant cells.

Investigations

- Chest X-ray: Bilateral hilar lymphadenopathy (differential: lymphoma, TB, Ca). Pulmonary infiltration: mottling of mid and lower zones proceeding to bilateral fine nodular shadowing. May be normal even with infiltration.
- Lung function tests show a restrictive pattern with infiltration.
- Full blood count: Mild normochromic, normocytic anaemia with raised ESR and/or CRP.
- Serum angiotensin converting enzyme (ACE): In 75% of patients with untreated sarcoid ACE is >2sd above the mean. Not diagnostic but useful to assess activity of pulmonary infiltrates.
- Transbronchial biopsy: Infiltration of the alveolar walls and interstitial space with lymphocytes. Positive in 90% with or without X-ray evidence.
- Tuberculin test: 80% show anergy, but this is not helpful diagnostically.
- Kveim test: Intradermal injection of sarcoid tissue is not used now due to risk of infection.

Management

1 Acute sarcoidosis, e.g. hilar lymphadenopathy with erythema nodosum usually resolves spontaneously over 2 years and usually does not require treatment if asymptomatic. If symptomatic responds well to steroid therapy.
2 The more chronic form with evidence of infiltration or abnormal lung function is unlikely to improve without treatment and is initially treated with steroids and monitored with lung function tests, ESR, CRP and/or serum ACE levels.

Indications for systemic steroids:

- Progressive deterioration in lung function or symptomatic pulmonary lesions.
- Cardiac, CNS or severe ocular involvement.
- Hypercalcaemia.

- Hepatitis (rare).
- Skin lesions such as erythema nodosum respond rapidly to a short course.
- Constitutional symptoms may also respond.

Prognosis

Once on steroids, many patients require long-term medium dose prednisolone; however, many patients are able to stop steroids after $\sim$2 years. The disease has a high spontaneous remission rate.

- Sarcoidosis is more severe in Black Americans where the death rates are up to 10%.
- In the United Kingdom the death rate is approximately 1 in 20 often due to respiratory problems.
- The chest X-ray provides a guide to prognosis:
  i In patients with only hilar lymphadenopathy two thirds will remit in 2 years.
  ii In patients with lymphadenopathy and infiltration one half will remit in 2 years.
  iii In patients with infiltration alone only one third will remit in 2 years.

Wegener's granulomatosis

Definition

A rare form of necrotising small vessel vasculitis of the upper and lower respiratory tract and the kidneys associated with granuloma formation.

Incidence

Rare

Age

More common over the age of 40 years.

Sex

M > F (2:1)

Pathophysiology

The aetiology is unknown, but it responds to immunosuppression. The small vessel vasculitis in the kidney causes reduced glomerular filtration rate and ischaemia of the glomeruli and hence acute or chronic renal failure.

Clinical features

General malaise is common. In the upper respiratory tract it causes ulceration and granulomas in the nose and sinuses leading to sinusitis, rhinorrhea and epistaxis. It may be very deforming. In the lungs it causes nodular masses, which may cavitate or infiltrations which can lead to cough, dyspnoea, pleuritic pain and haemoptysis. It affects the kidneys in 90% of cases, manifesting as oliguria, haematuria and uraemia.

Macroscopy/microscopy

An inflammatory small vessel arteritis with predominantly mononuclear infiltrates. There are necrotising granulomata of the respiratory tract. Kidney biopsy reveals a focal necrotising glomerulonephritis.

Investigations

1 Full blood count: anaemia of chronic disease, neutrophilia.
2 The ESR is usually very high.
3 U&Es to assess renal function.
4 Urine microscopy shows red cell casts.
5 Lung function testing.
6 The finding of anti neutrophil cytoplasmic antibodies (cANCA) – PR3 (directed against a serine protease termed proteinase C) has a specificity of 90% and a sensitivity of 50% in early disease but closer to 100% in established disease. Finding pANCA (anti-myeloperoxidase) is less specific of Wegener's, i.e. it is found in other inflammatory conditions.
7 Transbronchial or open lung biopsy.
8 Renal biopsy to assess the pattern and severity of glomerulonephritis.

Management

Cyclophosphamide and high-dose steroids to induce remission. Relapse is prevented by long-term low-dose immunosuppression. In pulmonary haemorrhage or severe acute renal failure, plasma exchange may be used. Oral co-trimoxazole is used for nasal involvement.

Prognosis

Once fatal in 1–2 years now much improved due to the use of cyclophosphamide and other immunosuppressive agents.

Goodpasture's syndrome

See page 246.

Polyarteritis nodosa

See page 379.

Churg–Strauss syndrome

See page 380.

Pleural effusion, pneumothorax, pleurisy

Pleural effusion

Definition

A pleural effusion is defined as an accumulation of fluid in the pleural space.

Aetiology

The effusion is classified as transudate or exudate based on the protein content (see Table 3.15).

Table 3.15 Causes of pleural effusion

Type of effusion	Pathogenesis	Cause
Transudate (<30 g/L protein)	Increased hydrostatic pressure	Cardiac failure Constrictive pericarditis
	Decreased oncotic pressure	Hypoalbuminaemia, e.g. nephrotic syndrome, cirrhosis
	Miscellaneous	Hypothyroidism Meigs' syndrome (usually a right-sided effusion and a benign ovarian fibroma)
Exudate (>30 g/L protein)	Infections	Bacterial including TB, empyema, pneumonia
	Neoplasms	Metastatic carcinoma Primary lung carcinoma Mesothelioma
	Pulmonary infarction	Thromboembolic disease
	Connective tissue disease	Rheumatoid disease, SLE
	Abdominal disease	Pancreatitis, subphrenic abscess

Clinical features

Symptoms include shortness of breath and chest pain. Signs of an effusion are only present when >500 mL of fluid is present and include reduced chest expansion on the affected side, stony dull percussion note, reduced or absent breath sounds and vocal resonance.

Investigations

1 Chest X-ray: visible when there is >300 mL, ranges from blunting of the costophrenic angles to dense homogeneous shadow, usually with a meniscus. Mediastinal shift occurs with massive effusion.
2 Diagnostic pleural aspiration with needle and syringe:
   - Biochemistry allows the separation into a transudate and an exudate on the basis of protein content. A pH of less than 7.3 is suggestive of empyema, but may also occur in malignancy, rheumatoid and TB.
   - Microbiology if the aspirate is turbid and to search for an infective course.
   - Blood-staining suggests pulmonary infarction or malignancy.
   - Cytology to detect neoplastic cells, and distinguish acute from chronic inflammation on the basis of the cellular infiltrate.
3 Pleural biopsy if needed: particularly for suspected mesothelioma and TB.

Management

Is aimed at the underlying cause thus identification is of primary importance. Large effusions can be treated by aspiration or chest drainage, but too rapid drainage can cause pain and even pulmonary oedema and hypotension. Recurrent malignant effusions can be treated with chemical or surgical pleuradhesis.

Empyema

Definition

Empyema is pus in the pleural space.

Aetiology

The most common cause of empyema is pneumonia with spread of infection to an associated effusion. A lung abscess can also spread to the pleural space. Exogenous infection may be from a penetrating injury or be iatrogenic, e.g. following chest drain insertion for an effusion. Endogenous infection may be from perforated oesophagus or spread from a subphrenic abscess.

Pathophysiology

Initially the pleural space is filled with a thin watery fluid containing pus cells (purulent effusion). There is then laying down of fibrin between the parietal and visceral pleura, which may become organised to form a thick fibrous wall around the pus filled cavity.

Clinical features

Patients present with similar features to a pleural effusion: dullness to percussion, absence of breath sounds. They often appear generally unwell with tachycardia, tachypnoea and pyrexia.

Investigations

There is a leucocytosis and X-ray shows a pleural opacity classically posteriorly with a D shaped outline. Needle aspiration is used to obtain fluid for microscopy, culture and sensitivities.

Management

The aim of therapy is to drain the fluid and expand the lungs whilst treating the infection with appropriate empirical antibiotics initially. Antibiotics are tailored according to microbiology results from the fluid.
   - In the early stages needle aspiration may be adequate.
   - For thicker pus an intercostal drain may have to be inserted.
   - In some patients, videoscopic assisted thorascopic surgery (VATS) or open thoracotomy and removal of the walls of the empyema is needed for complete resolution, particularly if the effusion is loculated.

Pneumothorax

Definition

Defined as air in the pleural space which may be traumatic or spontaneous.

Aetiology

See Table 3.16.

Clinical features

Sudden onset of unilateral pleuritic pain and/or increasing breathlessness is the usual presenting feature. Large pneumothoraces produce breathlessness, pallor, tachycardia and even hypotension. About one third recur.

Table 3.16 Causes of a pneumothorax

Type	Aetiology
Spontaneous	
Primary	Most commonly thin, tall young men
	Rupture of congenital subpleural bleb
Secondary	Rupture of emphysematous bulla, congenital cyst
	Asthma, COPD
	Pleural malignancy
	Cystic fibrosis
	Pneumonia
	Sarcoidosis
Traumatic	Penetrating chest wounds
	Rib fractures
	Oesophageal rupture
Iatrogenic	Subclavian cannulation
	Positive pressure ventilation
	Pleural aspiration
	Oesophageal perforation during endoscopy
	Lung biopsy

Investigations

Chest X-ray shows the visceral pleura as a thin line with absent lung markings beyond.

Management

- Observation if the pneumothorax is small. The air is reabsorbed gradually over days to weeks.
- If the pneumothorax is >20%, particularly if the patient has underlying lung disease or is significantly dyspnoeic, then simple aspiration is indicated.
- If this fails, i.e. the lung does not re-inflate sufficiently or if the pneumothorax recurs, an intercostal drain with underwater seal is required. If after a few days the drain continues to bubble and the pneumothorax persists this indicates a bronchopleural fistula, i.e. a continued leak of air from the lung to the pleural space. This may require surgical treatment.
- Pleurectomy is indicated in recurrent pneumothoraces or for bronchopleural fistulae that fail to close with conservative management. This is performed by stripping the pleura from the inside of the chest through a limited thoracotomy. Any blebs or bullae are stapled or tied off and the lung re-inflated. The opposition of lung to the raw area on the chest wall causes the surfaces to adhere to one another. Talc or another irritant is often used to improve this adherence.

- Tension pneumothorax (a large pneumothorax causing mediastinal shift) is a medical emergency and requires aspiration immediately.

Pleurisy

Definition

Acute inflammation of the pleura.

Aetiology

The most common cause of pleurisy is infection, related to an underlying bacterial or viral pneumonia. Pleurisy can also be a feature of pulmonary embolism, pulmonary infarction, malignancy and connective tissue diseases such as rheumatoid arthritis.

Clinical features

Sharp, well-localised pain, worse on inspiration or coughing, and a pleural rub heard on auscultation. There may be an associated pleural effusion.

Macroscopy

Fibrinous exudate is seen over the pleural surfaces and there is variable exudation of fluid.

Investigations and treatment

Aimed at identification and treatment of the underlying cause. Nonsteroidal anti-inflammatory drugs and paracetamol are used for analgesia.

Respiratory failure, heart disease and embolism

Respiratory failure

Definition

Respiratory failure is defined as a fall in the arterial oxygen tension below 8 kPa. Carbon dioxide tension defines respiratory failure into type I (normal or low pCO_2) and type II (pCO_2 above 6 kPa).

Aetiology/pathophysiology

- Type I failure, sometimes called 'acute hypoxaemic respiratory failure', is usually due to mismatch between ventilation and perfusion or right to left shunts. It can occur in any respiratory disease most commonly acute exacerbations of asthma or COPD, pulmonary oedema, pneumonia, pulmonary embolus and fibrosing alveolitis. Hyperventilation frequently leads to a low pCO_2.

- Type II failure, sometimes called 'ventilatory failure', is due to alveolar hypoventilation such that the carbon dioxide produced by tissue metabolism cannot be adequately removed and pCO_2 rises. If the failure is chronic the patient with a type II respiratory failure will lose sensitivity to a raised carbon dioxide and therefore rely solely on hypoxic respiratory drive. If aggressive oxygen therapy is initiated the level of oxygen will rise and the respiratory drive is diminished, leading to further decreased ventilation which may be fatal. The most common cause of type II respiratory failure is chronic obstructive airway disease, other causes include any severe respiratory disease, failure of respiratory effort, e.g. central drive depression, chest-wall disease such as deformity and neuromuscular disease such as myasthenia.

Clinical features

In a patient with a normal haemoglobin central cyanosis is visible when the pO_2 falls below 6.7 kPa. Hypercapnia causes a flapping tremor of the outstretched hands, a bounding pulse, vasodilation, increased agitation, then confusion, drowsiness and coma. Other signs include the use of accessory muscles of respiration, tachypnoea, tachycardia, sweating and inability to speak in full sentences.

Complications

- Pulmonary hypertension due to hypoxic pulmonary vasoconstriction. With time the arteries undergo a proliferative change leading to irreversible pulmonary circulation changes. There is increased afterload on the right side of the heart leading to cor pulmonale.
- Polycythaemia results from hypoxia, it causes an increase in blood viscosity and predisposes to thrombosis.

Investigations

Blood gas monitoring is the most important initial investigation to establish the type of failure and will dictate the mode of oxygen therapy.

Management

Acute or acute on chronic respiratory failure

Treat any reversible underlying cause:

- Oversedation or opiate overdose by stopping or reversing sedation (e.g. flumazenil for benzodiazepines, naloxone for opiates).
- Pulmonary oedema with diuretics.
- Asthma by bronchodilators and corticosteroids.
- Pneumonia with appropriate antibiotics.
- Pneumothorax or pleural effusion by aspiration or drainage.
- COPD with bronchodilators, corticosteroids and antibiotics.

Controlled oxygen therapy:

- In patients who have a raised pCO_2 > 6kPa, oxygen therapy can potentially worsen the situation, because of the patient's dependence on hypoxic drive. Controlled 24–28% oxygen is given by Venturi mask and arterial blood gases are repeated to ensure that the pO_2 is rising and the pCO_2 is not rising.
- In patients with acute hypoxaemic failure and a normal or low pCO_2, high-flow oxygen therapy can be used, but they must still be closely monitored with regular arterial blood gases to ensure that they are not tiring and developing type II failure.

If pCO_2 continues to rise or pO_2 cannot be raised adequately with oxygen therapy then assisted ventilation is required, preferably before patients are completely exhausted (see Table 3.17).

Chronic respiratory failure

Long-term oxygen therapy (LTOT) and in some cases non-invasive ventilation, is indicated for chronic respiratory failure. LTOT is indicated in patients with COPD who have a pO_2 < 7.3 kPa when stable or a pO_2 > 7.3 and <8 kPa when stable with polycythaemia, nocturnal hypoxaemia, peripheral oedema or pulmonary hypertension. 19 hours/day of oxygen 1–3 L/minute has been shown to increase survival in patients with chronic bronchitis or emphysema and respiratory failure. Patients must have stopped smoking (for safety reasons), and an oxygen concentrator needs to be installed in their home.

Prognosis

Fifty per cent of patients with severe chronic breathlessness die within 5 years, but in all stopping smoking is the most beneficial therapy.

Table 3.17 Types of assisted ventilation

Type of ventilation	Description	Comments
Non-invasive		
Continuous positive airway pressure (CPAP)	Constant airway pressure via a close-fitting nasal or face mask	Unsuitable for Type II respiratory failure (worsens CO_2 retention). Patients need to be co-operative.
Non invasive positive pressure ventilation (NIPPV), Bilevel positive airway pressure (BiPAP)	Additional supported respiration by mask is provided. In BiPAP inspiratory and expiratory pressures are set separately to increase inspired lung volume, and to maintain some positive end-expiratory pressure to prevent alveoli from collapsing.	Useful for avoiding intubation in exacerbations of COPD, patients need to be co-operative. Administered by tight fitting face or nasal mask.
Invasive		
Intermittent positive pressure ventilation (IPPV)	The inspiratory and expiratory pressures and timing of ventilation can all be altered to give variations.	
Continuous positive pressure ventilation	CPAP can be given via an endotracheal tube.	Used in the weaning of patients from ventilation towards normal breathing.

Pulmonary embolism

Definition
Thrombus within the pulmonary arteries causing lack of lung perfusion. Thrombus within the systemic veins or uncommonly from the heart embolises to the lungs.

Prevalence
Common.

Aetiology
The causes of thrombosis can be considered according to Virkhow's triad:

- Disruption in blood flow particularly stasis: Prolonged bed rest, air travel, pelvic and lower limb fractures, pelvic or abdominal surgery, pregnancy and child-birth. Right sided cardiac thrombosis may occur in atrial fibrillation, septal or right ventricular infarcts.
- Abnormalities of the vessel wall: Following direct trauma to the vein in leg trauma.
- Abnormalities in the blood such as hypercoagulable states – antithrombin III, protein C and S deficiencies and Factor V Leiden (a single point mutation in the Factor V gene, which causes resistance to activated protein C), oral contraceptives, malignant disease and smoking.

Pathophysiology
Following a pulmonary embolus there is a reduction in the perfusion of the lung supplied by the blocked vessel. Ventilation perfusion mismatch occurs, leading to hypoxaemia. Production of surfactant also stops if perfusion is interrupted for a number of hours after which the alveoli collapse. Infarct is rare (only occurring in around 10% of cases) as the lung is also supplied by the bronchial circulation, but there is an increase in pulmonary arterial pressure.

Clinical features
The result of a pulmonary embolism depends on the size and number of the emboli.

- Small emboli may be silent or present with symptoms such as dyspnoea on exertion, haemoptysis, pleuritic pain or rarely cardiac arrhythmias.
- Medium-sized emboli typically present with sudden onset pleuritic pain and dyspnoea. There may be a dry cough or haemoptysis.
- A large embolus may present with syncope, sudden onset of severe central chest pain, shock, loss of consciousness or sudden death. Signs include hypotension, a loud pulmonary component of the second heart sound, tachycardia with third and fourth heart sounds heard as a gallop rhythm. There is a right

ventricular (parasternal) heave due to increased stroke work, a raised JVP with a prominent 'a' wave due to increased right atrial pressure.

- There may be chest signs resulting from alveolar atelectasis or complicating pneumonia. Pleural inflammation results in a pleural friction rub and a low-grade pyrexia.
- Clinical signs of a deep vein thrombosis may also be present.

Macroscopy
Blood enters the pulmonary vasculature and thus there is congestion proximal to the blockage. Affected areas appear haemorrhagic and are frequently wedge shaped. Repair results in the formation of a white scar.

Microscopy
Typical features include haemorrhage (due to extravasation of blood), loss of cell architecture, cellular infiltration and occasionally necrosis.

Complications
Cardiopulmonary arrest and death in the acute stages. Atrial fibrillation and other arrhythmias. Recurrent thromboembolic disease may cause pulmonary hypertension.

Investigations
The chest X-ray may be normal. Atelectasis and areas of hypoperfusion may be seen, and large emboli may cause an elevated hemidiaphragm and enlarged proximal pulmonary arteries. Blood D-dimers (breakdown products of fibrin) are of reasonable sensitivity but high specificity and are therefore useful for exclusion in cases of low clinical suspicion. A ventilation perfusion (V/Q) scan is usually diagnostic, but is less helpful if the chest X-ray is abnormal. Spiral CT pulmonary angiogram normally demonstrates the clot(s) within the pulmonary vasculature. The ECG may be normal or (particularly in larger emboli) reveal:

- Tachycardia.
- A characteristic $S_1 Q_3 T_3$ pattern. This refers to an S wave in lead I, and Q and inverted T wave in lead III.
- Right ventricular 'strain' pattern – T wave inversion in leads V_1–V_4.
- Tall peaked P waves in lead II (p pulmonale).

- Right bundle branch block: RSR' in lead V_1 (may be transient).

Management
1 In massive pulmonary embolism, there is haemodynamic compromise which may require resuscitative therapy. With large emboli, thrombolysis or surgical thrombectomy with cardiac bypass may be life-saving.
2 Prevention of propagation and recurrence: Unfractionated intravenous heparin is started immediately titrated according to the APTT. For small or moderate emboli subcutaneous low molecular weight heparin is as effective and does not require monitoring of APTT. Therapy is converted to warfarin after 48 hours (for 3 months minimum – usually 6 months). Lifelong warfarin may be indicated depending on the underlying cause, or in recurrent embolism.
3 If anti-coagulants are unsuccessful or contraindicated a filter may be inserted into the inferior vena cava to prevent further pulmonary embolism.
4 Standard prophylaxis pre- and postoperatively, and for bed bound patients or those at risk – subcutaneous low molecular weight heparin, graduated compression stockings and early mobilisation if possible.

Prognosis
Ten per cent of symptomatic emboli are fatal.

Pulmonary hypertension

Definition
A pulmonary arterial pressure greater than 30/20 mmHg.

Aetiology
Pulmonary hypertension may be secondary to a variety of diseases, or more rarely a primary idiopathic form. Causes can be divided into
1 Increased blood volume passing through the pulmonary circulation as occurs in left to right shunting (septal defects, persistent ductus arteriosus).
2 Increased left atrial pressure, which causes an increase in pulmonary venous pressure. This in turn raises the pulmonary capillary and arterial pressures (left ventricular failure, mitral valve disease, cardiomyopathy).

3 Increased pulmonary vascular resistance:
- Chronic lung disease such as chronic bronchitis, emphysema and pulmonary fibrosis partly due to the vasoconstriction associated with hypoxia.
- Chronic pulmonary thromboembolic disease due to occlusion of part of the vasculature and hypoxia.

Primary pulmonary hypertension is seen predominantly in young females. A similar syndrome is associated with sytemic lupus erythematosus, scleroderma and Raynaud's disease.

Pathophysiology

Increased pulmonary arterial pressure causes irreversible structural changes in the pulmonary vasculature due to increasing amounts of smooth muscle. The result is a decrease in the lumen of the vessels and hence an increased afterload on the right side of the heart. Progressive failure of the right side of the heart occurs which is called 'cor pulmonale'.

Clinical features

Dyspnoea, syncope and fatigue are common. Symptoms of the underlying cause and of right ventricular failure may also be present.

Signs are a result of the elevated pressures within the pulmonary circulation. There is elevation of the JVP with a prominent 'a' wave, a forceful parasternal heave due to increased right ventricular stroke work, and a loud pulmonary component to the second heart sound. Right heart failure leads to peripheral oedema and hepatomegaly.

A pulmonary mid systolic ejection murmur and an early diastolic murmur of pulmonary regurgitation may be heard (Graham–Steel murmur).

If tricuspid regurgitation develops there will be a pansystolic murmur and a large 'v' wave in the JVP.

Microscopy

If pulmonary hypertension is long-standing, microscopy reveals hypertrophy of the media of the vessels with an increase in the amount of smooth muscle. There is worsening occlusion of the lumen of the vessels.

Investigations

- A chest X-ray may show right ventricular and right atrial enlargement. The central pulmonary arteries are usually prominent and may be 'pruned' peripherally.

- The ECG shows right ventricular hypertrophy with right axis deviation: Prominent R wave in V_1, and inverted T waves in the V_1–V_3. The right atrial enlargement results in tall peaked P waves.
- Underlying causes should be identified wherever possible.

Management

Treatment is aimed at the underlying cause.

- Congenital abnormalities such as septal defects should be corrected wherever possible, mitral valve disease may indicate surgical intervention and left ventricular failure should be treated.
- Pulmonary hypertension secondary to chronic lung disease may benefit from oxygen therapy to reduce the vasoconstrictor effect of hypoxia.
- Long-term intravenous infusion of epoprostenol (prostacyclin) improves the outcome of patients with primary pulmonary hypertension. The administration of bosentan (a nonselective endothelin receptor antagonist) may also be beneficial in patients with primary pulmonary hypertension although long-term follow-up data are not yet available.
- When there are irreversible vascular changes the condition is progressive. Heart–lung transplantation is recommended in younger patients.

Occupational lung disease

Introduction to occupational lung disease

Lung disease resulting from exposure to dusts, vapours and fumes resulting in five basic patterns of disease (see Table 3.18). Most patients with occupational lung disease are entitled to compensation according to their degree of disability.

Definition

Diseases of the lung related to exposure to asbestos.

Incidence

The incidence of asbestos related disease increased dramatically in recent decades but appears to have peaked in the late 1990s, and is expected to gradually decline.

Table 3.18 Patterns of occupational lung disease

Pattern of disease	Causative agents
Pulmonary fibrosis	Mineral dusts such as coal, silicon and asbestos
Occupational asthma	Multiple – may be animal, vegetable, bacterial or chemical precipitants
Extrinsic allergic alveolitis	Organic dusts causing a local allergic response
Acute bronchitis, pulmonary oedema	Irritant gases such as sulphur dioxide, chlorine, ammonia, oxides of nitrogen
Bronchial carcinoma	Asbestos, polycyclic hydrocarbons, radon in mines

Aetiology/pathophysiology

Asbestos is made up of various silicates. It exists naturally as a fibre, and has been widely used for its insulative properties. It was used in sheets in buildings, sprayed on pipes as lagging, in shipbuilding and for boiler insulation. However, it is easily inhaled and the fibres induce a fibrogenic reaction in the lung. The risk of developing pathology from asbestos is dependent on the duration and intensity of exposure, and the type of asbestos (see Table 3.19).

1 Serpentine asbestos (includes white asbestos) is the commonest form. Fibres are long (up to 2 cm) and curly, but only micrometers thick. They are least fibrogenic. It is debatable whether they are carcinogenic, but their use has now been banned in new buildings in the United Kingdom.

2 Amphibole asbestos (including amosite/brown and crocidolite/blue asbestos) fibres are short and straight, this allows them to reach and penetrate the lung parenchyma more easily. They persist in the lung for many years and are very fibrogenic and carcinogenic.

Macroscopy/microscopy

- Asbestos bodies: These are long thin asbestos fibres in the lung parenchyma coated with haemosiderin and protein to form brown filaments with a beaded or drumstick pattern. They are the result of macrophages, which surround and attempt to engulf the fibres, but fail to clear them leading to fibroblast proliferation and fibrosis.
- Pleural plaques are well-circumscribed elevated plaques of white hyaline fibrous tissue arranged symmetrically on the parietal pleura over the ribs and diaphragm. Calcification is common.
- Asbestosis: The lower lobes are usually affected initially, then progressively the mid-upper lobes. There are fibrotic changes in the interstitium, obliteration of

Table 3.19 Patterns of asbestos-related disease

Disease	Exposure	Symptoms	Chest X-ray	Outcome
Asbestos bodies	Light	None	Normal	Normal lung function
Pleural Plaques	Light/moderate	Usually none	Pleural thickening, and calcification	Mild restrictive lung disease at most
Asbestosis	Heavy (5–10 years from exposure)	Progressive dyspnoea	Fine linear shadows initially seen best on CT. Late stage honeycomb lung	Lung fibrosis leads to severe restrictive defect & reduced gas exchange. Poor prognosis
Asbestos-related malignancy: Mesothelioma	Any degree. Peaks 30–35 years from exposure. Not related to smoking	Dyspnoea. Pleuritic or dull chest wall pain	Pleural effusion and knobbly pleural thickenings with reduction in volume in the affected area, possibly with other signs of asbestos exposure	Median survival 2 years after diagnosis
Asbestos-related carcinoma of the bronchus	Risk related to level of exposure and smoking	As for bronchial carcinoma	Evidence of asbestos exposure may be seen together with features of the carcinoma	As for bronchial carcinoma

alveoli and then thickened, cystic spaces (honeycomb lung).

- Malignant mesothelioma: Thoracoscopic or open lung biopsy may be needed to make the diagnosis. Macroscopically the lesion is thick, may be encapsulated, with interlobar fissures. The tumour may be hard and white or glutinous due to the production of hyaluronic acid. Histological pattern is variable, it may be epithelioid, fibrous or mixed. Local invasion is extensive, 50% metastasise.
- Asbestos-related carcinoma of the bronchus: Asbestosis and cigarette smoking act synergistically to cause a fivefold increase in the risk of developing bronchial carcinoma, which is usually adenocarcinoma or squamous cell carcinoma.

Management

- All patients with known asbestos exposure should be advised to stop smoking. Routine surveillance with repeated sputum cytology and chest X-ray does not appear to lead to earlier diagnosis.
- Pleural plaques and asbestos bodies require no treatment. Asbestosis is treated as for respiratory failure when this occurs.
- Mesothelioma treatment is largely palliative, resection may be attempted in early disease. Radiotherapy is ineffective and chemotherapy regimens are under evaluation.
- Patients with bilateral diffuse pleural thickening, asbestosis and (in those with an occupational history or other evidence of asbestos exposure) mesothelioma or carcinoma of the bronchus are entitled to industrial compensation.

Coal worker's pneumoconiosis

Definition

Pathology resulting from inhalation of coal dust and its associated impurities.

Prevalence

Two per 1000 coal workers.

Aetiology

The disease is caused by dust particles approximately 2–5 μm in diameter that are retained in the small airways and alveoli of the lung.

Pathophysiology

Two different syndromes result from inhalation:

- Simple pneumoconiosis in which there is deposition of coal dust within the lung. There are peribronchiolar deposits in the upper parts of the lung, often associated with mild centri-acinar emphysema.
- Progressive massive fibrosis (PMF): The pathogenesis is not understood. Patients develop rheumatoid and antinuclear factor and the damage is thought to be due to immune complexes.

Clinical features

Simple pneumoconiosis is asymptomatic. Patients with progressive massive fibrosis suffer from considerable effort dyspnoea, usually with a cough. The sputum may be black.

Macroscopy/microscopy

- Simple pneumoconiosis is characterised by accumulation of dust in macrophages at the centre of the acinus, with associated emphysema.
- In progressive massive fibrosis there are nodules of >3 cm in the upper lobes. Histologically the nodules can be divided into three types:
  - i Amorphous collection of acellular proteinaceous material, containing little collagen and abundant carbon, which frequently cavitates and liquefies. Seen where silica content is low.
  - ii Dense collagenous tissue and macrophages heavily pigmented by carbon, seen where there is a high silica content in the coal dust.
  - iii Caplan's syndrome seen where there is co-existent rheumatoid disease. Carbon-stained rheumatoid nodules are seen.

Complications

Simple pneumoconiosis is divided into three stages by chest X-ray appearance (see Table 3.20). Stage 1 does not progress, 7% of patients with stage 2 and 30% of patients with stage 3 will go on to develop progressive massive fibrosis. PMF by definition is progressive, and respiratory failure will eventually develop.

Investigations

The diagnosis is made by chest X-ray in those who have been exposed (see Table 3.20).

Table 3.20 Chest X-ray appearance in pneumoconiosis

Pattern	Chest X-ray appearance
Simple pneumoconiosis	
Stage 1	Small round opacities are present but few in number
Stage 2	Small round opacities numerous but normal lung visible
Stage 3	Small round opacities, normal lung totally obscured
Progressive massive fibrosis	Round fibrotic masses, several cm in diameter, in upper lobes

Silicosis

Definition
A rare lung pathology resulting from the inhalation of silica dust (quartz).

Aetiology
This condition is mainly seen in workers in slate mines and granite quarries, metal foundries, stone masonry and tunnelling.

Pathophysiology
The pathogenesis is thought to be a toxic effect on macrophages, which stimulate cytokine generation, precipitating fibrogenesis. Short heavy doses produce acute silicosis with pulmonary oedema and alveolar exudation. Prolonged exposure produces multiple fibrous nodules, which may expand causing extensive destruction of lung tissue and the development of progressive massive fibrosis.

Clinical features
In the early stages there may be no symptoms. The first symptom is usually breathlessness on exertion and a productive cough may follow. Progression leads to respiratory failure.

Microscopy
The nodules in silicosis are made up of collagen and contain silica particles which can be identified using polarised light.

Complications
The development of tuberculosis is a common complication of silicosis (silicotuberculosis). It is thought that this is due to impairment of local defences, as a result of the accumulation of silica in macrophages. Increased risk of lung cancer.

Investigations
Chest X-ray in the early stages shows reticular/nodular shadowing. With progression there are radiological signs of massive fibrosis (destruction and lesions in the upper zones), and thin streaks of calcification around the hilar nodes ('eggshell calcification').

Management
There is no specific treatment, primary prevention through education and exposure prevention remains the only effective strartegy.

Respiratory oncology

Bronchial carcinoma

Definition
A malignant tumour of the bronchial (most common) or rarely alveolar epithelium.

Incidence
Bronchial carcinoma is the most common malignancy of the Western World: 40,000 deaths per year in the United Kingdom, more than 1 million deaths worldwide.

It is the leading cause of death from cancer in men and in women under the age of 65, it has now exceeded breast cancer as the leading cause of death from cancer.

Age
Peak age 40–70 years.

Sex
3M : 1F, but rising in females.

Geography
Follows patterns of smoking, independent of this it is also higher in urban areas.

Aetiology
Around 80–90% of cases occur in smokers (see Table 3.21).

Table 3.21 Risks of cigarette smoking

Cigarettes per day	Never	Ex-	1–14	15–24	>25
Male deaths per 1000 per year	0.1	0.4	0.78	1.27	2.51

- It takes an ex-smoker of ≤20 per day 13 years to return to just above the risk of a non-smoker. Pipe smokers have about 40% the risk of cigarette smokers.
- Occupational and environmental factors include exposure to radioactive material (including radon), asbestos, nickel, chromium, iron oxides and coal gas plants.

Pathophysiology

Lung cancer is characterised by multiple genetic alterations:

1 In >90% of small cell lung cancers the *p53* and *rb* tumour suppressor genes are both mutated, and >50% and 20% respectively in non-small cell lung cancer.
2 Activation of dominant oncogenes – for example, mutations in *ras* genes are associated with 20% of non-small cell lung cancer and confer a poor prognosis, while tumour amplification of c-*myc* is associated with a poor prognosis in small cell lung cancer.
3 Some of these genetic alterations are seen in pre-neoplastic lesions such as hyperplasia, dysplasia and carcinoma-in-situ of the bronchial epithelium, but it appears that as many as 10 of these mutations are needed for the development of lung cancer.

Clinical features

Cough or worsening of a pre-existing cough is the most common early symptom, but may be ignored. Haemoptysis due to ulceration of a tumour is the next most common. Dyspnoea, a dull central chest ache or pleuritic pain, or slowly resolving chest infection are all common. Clubbing and systemic features (weight loss, anorexia and malaise) or complications from metastatic deposits may also be presenting features.

Macroscopy/microscopy

Because of their pathological behaviour malignancies of the lung are divided into 'small cell' and 'non-small cell'. This is useful clinically on deciding treatment. But histologically, lung carcinoma is divided into four cell types:

1 Squamous cell carcinoma, 50%.
2 Small/oat cell carcinoma, 20%.
3 Adenocarcinoma, 20%.
4 Large cell anaplastic carcinoma, 10%.

A few show a mixed pattern: 70% of all tumours arise in relation to the main bronchus (central or hilar) and 30% arise in the peripheral airways or alveoli.

1 Squamous cell carcinoma: Usually located centrally close to the carina and so presents with the sequelae of bronchial obstruction and local invasion. Lesions may cavitate. Histologically squamous cell carcinoma shows a variety of patterns from well-differentiated lesions producing lots of keratin to poorly differentiated lesions containing little keratin.
2 Small cell/oat cell/anaplastic lung cancer is a highly malignant tumour arising from bronchial epithelium, but with properties of neuroendocrine cells containing secretory granules. Tumours are centrally located and are associated with a rapid growth rate with metastases almost invariable at presentation. Often associated with ectopic ADH and ACTH secretion (water/sodium retention and Cushing's syndrome).
3 Adenocarcinoma characteristically develops as a peripheral tumour, but may arise from the main bronchus. A proportion are thought to arise from pre-existing lung scars. It is the most common bronchial carcinoma associated with asbestos and is proportionally more common in non-smokers. Histologically four patterns are seen:
   - Acinar – prominent gland-like spaces.
   - Papillary – fronds of tumour on thin septa.
   - Solid carcinoma – poorly differentiated with mucin production.
   - Alveolar cell carcinoma derived from alveolar or bronchial epithelial cells (Clara cells and type II pneumocytes). These may exist as isolated peripheral nodules, but they characteristically spread through the lung along alveolar septa (seen on chest X-ray as areas of alveolar shadowing). Half are multifocal infiltrative tumours, which replace areas of lung in a manner resembling pneumonic consolidation. Cells are tall, columnar and relatively uniform, have few mitoses and secrete mucin (sometimes copious). The remaining half are single grey masses up to 10 cm in diameter made up of cuboidal cells with hyperchromatic nuclei.

4 Large cell anaplastic carcinomas are poorly differentiated lesions composed of large cells with nuclear pleomorphism and frequent giant cell forms.

Complications

1 Intra-thoracic: Distal pneumonia, lobar collapse and
consolidation, pleural effusions, left recurrent laryngeal nerve palsy (hoarse voice), superior vena cava
obstruction, brachial neuritis (particularly apical tumour (Pancoast tumour)), Horner's syndrome (sympathetic paralysis causing partial ptosis, myosis, anhydrosis, enophthalmos), rib erosion, pericarditis, oesophageal obstruction.
2 Metastases: Haematogenous spread to bone (pain or
fractures), brain, liver, adrenal gland.
3 Endocrine (10%, usually small cell carcinoma): Antidiuretic hormone, ectopic ACTH secretion. Hypercalcaemia seen with squamous cell carcinoma is due
to secretion of a parathyroid hormone related peptide
(PTH-like peptide).
4 Neuromuscular: Neuropathy, myopathy, myositis,
dementia, cerebellar degeneration.
5 Eaton Lambert syndrome: Rare non-metastatic manifestation of small cell carcinoma causing defective
acetylcholine release at the neuromuscular junction
resulting in proximal muscle weakness with absent
reflexes.
6 Systemic: Weight loss, anaemia, clubbing, hypertrophic pulmonary osteoarthropathy (HPOA – this
is clubbing associated with peripheral joint pain and
stiffness in the wrists and ankles caused by a periostitis. It tends to occur more often in squamous cell and
adenocarcinoma).

Investigations

- X-ray evidence only when 1–2 cm (still identifies over
90% of carcinomas). The edge of the lesion appears
typically fluffy or spiked, some may cause cavitation
or collapse. Hilar node enlargement or effusions are
sometimes evident.
- CT is useful for small lesions but not yet proven to
be useful in widespread screening. It is mainly used to
assess the extent and spread, especially lymph nodes
(see Table 3.22).
- Sputum cytology: Examination of expectorated sputum by cytology.
- Cytology of pleural effusion: Examination of pleural
fluid.
- Percutaneous needle aspiration/biopsy under CT
guidance. Open lung biopsy may be needed, particularly for alveolar cell carcinoma.
- Bronchoscopy and biopsy.

Management

1 Identification of histological type is essential.
2 Surgery for all non-small cell carcinomas where possible (see page 95). Surgical resection may be attempted
in limited alveolar cell carcinoma.
3 Chemotherapy and adjuvant radiotherapy is considered in all patients, although chemotherapy is less effective in non-small cell carcinoma.
4 Palliative radiotherapy, laser therapy and tracheo-
bronchial stents.

Surgical treatment: Key elements that offer a reasonable
prospect of success are

- tumour within a lobar bronchus or at least 2 cm distal
to the carina.

Table 3.22 Staging of bronchial carcinoma

Stage	TNM group	Clinical
Stage I	T1 N0 M0	Smaller than 3 cm distal to the carina without spread.
	T1 N1 M0	Smaller than 3 cm distal to the carina with (N1) spread to ipsilateral hilar nodes.
Stage II	T2 N0 M0	Tumour larger than 3 cm, 2 cm distal to the carina invading the visceral pleura (T2), without spread.
	T2 N1 M0	Tumour larger than 3 cm, 2 cm distal to the carina invading the visceral pleura (T2), with spread to ipsilateral hilar nodes.
Stage III	All T3/T4	Tumours involving the carina (T3), involving mediastinal structures (T4), with spread to
	All M1 or N3	contralateral nodes (N3) or metastases (M1).

- no involvement of the heart, great vessels, trachea, oesophagus or vertebrae.
- no malignant pleural effusion.
- no contralateral node involvement.
- no distant metastases (chest CT, serum alkaline phosphatase).
- adequate lung function ($FEV_1 > 1.5$ L, gas transfer >50% normal).

Surgery (only usually possible in 25%) involves the removal of the anatomical unit containing the tumour (segment, lobe or lung) together with the associated lymphatic drainage. 35–40% 5-year survival rate but closer to 90% with peripheral lesions.

Prognosis

- Non-small cell – 20% have successful resection, 10% survive for 5 years. Inoperable non-small cell carcinoma – chemotherapy is effective in ~20% and at best gives a survival benefit of a few months, and it has toxic side-effects. Median survival ~8 months with combination chemotherapy.
- Small cell carcinoma limited to thorax: Median survival 18–24 months with combination chemotherapy and radiotherapy and up to 20% survive 2 years, only 6–12 weeks without treatment. Small cell carcinoma with metastases: Median survival ~8 months with combination chemotherapy, rarely survive to 2 years.
- The rare alveolar carcinoma carries a poor prognosis due to its multifocal nature.

Bronchial carcinoid tumours

Definition

A rare neuroendocrine tumour of the lung.

Pathophysiology

These are highly vascular, low-grade malignant tumours which are locally invasive and can metastasise. They arise from bronchial enterochromaffin (Kulchitsky) cells, and can secrete various amines and peptides, including serotonin (5-hydroxytryptamine (5HT)), histamine and bradykinin. These rarely cause the carcinoid syndrome, as to do so they have to metastasise to the liver first (the peptides are metabolised in the liver).

Clinical features

The tumour can present with obstruction, recurrent haemoptysis or with metastatic disease. There may be weight loss.

Macroscopy/microscopy

They arise from lobar or segmental bronchi into which they protrude as a rounded mass usually covered by intact epithelium. Cells are cuboidal, arranged in a mosaic or trabecular pattern and have a dense core and neurosecretory granules.

Complications

1 Lung collapse and consolidation distal to the obstruction.
2 Local invasion, spread to lymph nodes and distant metastasis.
3 Rarely, the carcinoid syndrome – recurrent episodes of a combination of
   - flushing of the face and neck sometimes leading to telangectasia (due to kinins).
   - abdominal pain, nausea, vomiting and watery diarrhoea (5HT).
   - tricuspid regurgitation or pulmonary stenosis.

Investigations

- Chest X-ray may show a rounded lesion.
- Bronchoscopy usually shows a pedunculated vascular tumour protruding into the lumen.
- 24-hour urinary excretion of the metabolite of 5HT. (5-hydroxyindoleacetic acid (5-HIAA)) on a low serotonin diet (excluding bananas, tomatoes, walnuts, etc.)

Management

Local resection is indicated in all cases.

Prognosis

80% 10-year survival.

Secondary lung tumours

Definition

Metastases to the lung are very common due to haematogenous spread.

Aetiology
The site of primary is usually the kidney, prostate, breast, bone, gastrointestinal tract, cervix or ovary.

Pathophysiology
Secondary tumours nearly always develop in the lung parenchyma where they cause little or no symptoms. Carcinoma, particularly of the stomach, pancreas or breast can spread via the pulmonary lymphatic vessels causing a syndrome of lymphangitis carcinomatosa.

Clinical features
Usually asymptomatic, it is usually found as part of the screening of a patient with known malignancy. Rarely cause chest pain, haemoptysis or breathlessness (the last suggests lymphangitis carcinomatosa).

Investigations
Identification is by chest X-ray usually appearing as round shadow(s) 1.5–3 cm in diameter. CT scan shows up smaller metastases in most cases. Renal tumour metastases may present as a solitary round shadow. In lymphangitis carcinomatosa there is characteristically bilateral lymphadenopathy with dilated intrapulmonary lymphatic vessels appearing as streaky shadowing over both lung fields emanating from the hilar regions.

Management
Truly single metastases can be removed surgically, but this is uncommon.

Prognosis
Lymphangitis carcinomatosa is rapidly fatal.

Gastrointestinal system

Clinical

Symptoms

Abdominal pain

The causes of abdominal pain are diverse, frequently involving inflammation, ischaemia and/or obstruction in different organs.

The characteristics of abdominal pain should be clearly defined when taking a history. A useful mnemonic is SOCRATES (Site, Onset, Character, Radiation, Alleviating factors, Timing, Exacerbating factors and Symptoms associated with the pain).

Site

Well-localised pain suggests involvement of the parietal peritoneum, which has somatic innervation. However, abdominal pain is often 'referred' pain due to the pattern of visceral innervation derived from the embryological development.

- Disease of the embryonic foregut causes pain to be felt in the epigastrium or upper third of the abdomen. This includes the stomach, proximal duodenum (to the opening of the common bile duct), the liver, pancreas and biliary tree. The lower respiratory system and oesophagus are also derived from the foregut, so that occasionally abdominal pain can be due to disease in the chest.
- Pain arising from the midgut, which continues down to two thirds of the way along the transverse colon, is felt in the paraumbilical region.
- Pain arising from the hindgut, which continues to the dentate line, is felt in the suprapubic region.

Pain may begin in one area, then become localised as the peritoneum overlying the organ is involved, e.g. in appendicitis the pain is often initially felt around the umbilicus, then localises to the right iliac fossa.

Radiation

Pain radiating to the back is often due to retroperitoneal structures such as the pancreas, aorta and kidneys. If the disease is sub-diaphragmatic, then pain can be referred to the shoulder-tip because of innervation of the diaphragm by C4.

Onset, character and timing

Acute onset of pain suggests infarction, or an acute obstruction of the biliary tree or urinary tract. The pain may then last for hours. Other gastrointestinal pathology tends to cause a gradual onset of pain. The relationship of pain to posture, meals (including the type of food and timing of onset related to eating) and the pattern of severity should also be noted.

Obstruction of any part of the gut tends to cause 'colicky' pain, i.e. pain that comes in waves caused by contractions (peristalsis). Constant pain may be burning, dull, sharp, mild or severe. It may be recurrent, e.g. the nocturnal pain of peptic ulcer disease.

Alleviating and exacerbating factors

If movement exacerbates the pain, this is suggestive of peritoneal inflammation. Patients with colic tend to roll around in pain, whereas those with appendicitis lie absolutely still. Eating may relieve the pain of peptic ulceration, whereas it may precipitate the pain of ischaemia of the bowel. Vomiting or the passage of stool or flatus may temporarily relieve pain.

Nausea and vomiting

Nausea is the sensation of impending vomiting, whilst retching is the involuntary muscle contractions associated with vomiting, without the expulsion of gastric contents. Vomiting may occur with or without nausea. The causes of nausea and vomiting are diverse, for example alcohol and drugs, motion sickness, pregnancy, many gastrointestinal causes, neurological disorders and myocardial infarction.

Nausea and vomiting can be due to stimulation of the chemoreceptor trigger zones, located in the floor of the fourth ventricle, or by vagal afferents from the gut. These signals stimulate vomiting centres in the medulla.

A history should elucidate the timing, precipitating and relieving factors of the nausea or vomiting and associated symptoms such as abdominal pain. Early morning vomiting is characteristic of pregnancy, but also raised intracranial pressure. Gastrointestinal obstruction may cause vomiting early or late in the condition depending on the site of obstruction. Higher levels of obstruction tend to cause vomiting of less digested food, which occurs more rapidly after eating. Haematemesis is the vomiting of blood, which may appear fresh or partially digested (coffee ground appearance).

A drug history is important as many drugs can precipitate nausea, especially drugs used in chemotherapy. Peptic ulcer disease caused by nonsteroidal anti-inflammatory drugs (NSAIDs) may manifest as nausea and vomiting or even haematemesis, and a typical history of epigastric pain may be elicited.

Dysphagia

Dysphagia or difficulty in swallowing usually indicates organic disease. It differs from odynophagia (pain on swallowing). The history should establish duration, the constant or intermittent nature, and whether it is worse with solids or liquids. If solids are affected more than liquids, the cause is more likely to be obstruction, whereas liquids are affected more in neurological disease. Odynophagia that occurs with liquids suggests upper oesophageal ulceration. Pharyngeal problems are suggested by difficulty in initiating the swallow, or regurgitation into the nose, whereas oesophageal obstruction may manifest with food sticking retrosternally. Causes are as follows:

- Intraluminal blockage from the presence of a foreign body.
- Intramural dysphagia resulting from pharyngitis, tonsillitis, candidiasis, oesophageal web, benign strictures, carcinoma, achalasia or myasthenia gravis.
- Extrinsic compression from thyroid enlargement, pharyngeal pouch, mediastinal lymph node enlargement, aortic aneurysm or paraesophageal hernia.

Investigations that may be useful include videofluoroscopy, contrast swallow, upper gastrointestinal endoscopy and chest imaging. See also under individual conditions.

Diarrhoea

Diarrhoea is the abnormal passage of loose or liquid stools more than three times daily and/or a volume of stool greater than 200 g/day. Patients may use the term diarrhoea in different ways. Diarrhoea lasting for more than 4 weeks is generally considered chronic, likely to be of noninfectious aetiology and warrants further investigation.

Acute diarrhoea occurs with viral gastroenteritis, food poisoning and traveller's diarrhoea. Other symptoms such as pain, fever and vomiting may be present. In most cases specific treatments are unnecessary; however, adequate hydration (preferably using oral rehydration solution) is essential.

Chronic diarrhoea may be caused by organic or functional bowel disorders (e.g. irritable bowel syndrome). Functional bowel disease tends to cause a prolonged history of intermittent diarrhoea, without weight loss. It should be noted however that patients with inflammatory bowel disease might present in this way. Organic disease is suggested by a history of diarrhoea of less than 3 months duration, continuous or nocturnal diarrhoea, or significant weight loss. Malabsorption often causes steatorrhoea (stool that is frothy, foul smelling and floats because of a high fat content).

History taking in chronic diarrhoea should include the following:

- Previous gastrointestinal surgery.
- Any coexistent pancreatic, endocrine or multisystem disease.

- Family history of gastrointestinal neoplasia, inflammatory bowel disease or coeliac disease.
- Medication including previous antibiotics.
- Foreign travel.

Screening tests should include full blood count, ESR, CRP, urea and electrolytes, liver function tests, calcium, vitamin B_{12}, folate, iron studies, thyroid function tests and coeliac serology. Infectious chronic diarrhoea is uncommon in non-immunocompromised patients; however, stool cultures and microscopy should also be sent.

In young patients (under 45 years) with symptoms suggestive of functional bowel disease, a normal examination and negative screening tests, no further investigations are required. If atypical findings are present, a sigmoidoscopy should be performed. In older patients colonoscopy with ileoscopy should be performed with biopsy and histological examination of any suspicious areas.

Rectal bleeding

It is important to determine if the bleeding is fresh bright red or dark, and whether it is on the surface of the stool or mixed in. Bright red blood on the toilet paper after wiping is usually due to haemorrhoids. If the blood is mixed in with the stool, or associated with various abdominal symptoms, other pathology should be sought, in particular gastrointestinal malignancy. Black, tarry, offensive smelling stool is digested blood (melaena) and originates from the more proximal intestine. However, occasionally large upper gastrointestinal bleeds (e.g. varices, peptic ulcers) can cause fresh rectal bleeding, although usually the patient will show signs of volume depletion such as hypotension, postural drop and tachycardia. Rectal blood may occur with infection or inflammation of the bowel (colitis). It is important to consider gastrointestinal malignancy in any case of rectal bleeding.

Constipation

Constipation can be defined as a reduction in the frequency of bowel movements. A normal frequency is considered to be between three times a day and every 3 days, but there is considerable individual variation. Hard, difficult to pass stools are also considered constipation, even if frequent.

Causes include drugs (e.g. opiates), endocrine or metabolic causes (e.g. hypothyroidism, hypercalcaemia,

hypokalaemia) and neurological diseases (spinal cord injury, multiple sclerosis). Constipation may also be the presentation of bowel malignancy, which should be suspected in the older person, particularly if there is a family history, history of rectal bleeding or weight loss. Left-sided colonic malignancies frequently present with a triad of alternating constipation and diarrhoea with weight loss.

Associated symptoms
- Constipation may cause colicky abdominal pains due to peristalsis. This is common and not necessarily due to a serious underlying disease.
- Pain on passage of stool due to anorectal disease may lead to a deliberate suppression of the urge to defecate and therefore the accumulation of large, dry, hard stools and constipation. This is a common cause of constipation in children.
- Occasionally, constipation can present with watery 'overflow' diarrhoea, due to increased gut secretions passing around hard stool in the rectum. Alternating constipation and diarrhoea, often with bloating, passage of mucus, and abdominal pains that are relieved by defecation, is commonly due to a functional bowel disorder, e.g. irritable bowel disease. However, it is important to exclude malignancy if patients are over 45 years or there are any suspicious features.

Weight loss

Loss of appetite (anorexia) and weight loss are important symptoms that may be due to an underlying gastrointestinal cause particularly cancer, but are also associated with other conditions including depression and any malignancy. If there is an increased or unchanged appetite together with weight loss, this suggests either malabsorption or increased metabolic demand/state, e.g. due to hyperthyroidism. The history should establish the duration and severity of weight loss.

GI presentations

The acute abdomen introduction

Patients with an acute abdomen are those with the following clinical presentation:
- Pain that may be local or more generalised.

- Tenderness to palpation with associated guarding (the reflex tensing of their abdominal wall musculature to prevent further pain on palpation).
- Rebound tenderness (pain worse on sudden release of palpation, which is often more severe than on palpation).

The patient is often generally unwell and may be shocked due to dehydration and loss of fluid into extravascular spaces such as the lumen of the bowel and the abdominal cavity. See Table 4.1 for causes.

Investigations

- Full blood count (often normal, but leucocytosis may be present).
- Urea and electrolytes, and liver function tests should be performed.

Table 4.1 Causes of an acute abdomen

Pathological process	Disease
Inflammation	
Appendix	Acute appendicitis
Gallbladder	Acute cholecystitis
Colon	Diverticulitis
Fallopian tube	Pelvic inflammatory disease
Pancreas	Acute pancreatitis
Obstruction	
Intestine	Intestinal obstruction
Biliary system	Biliary colic
Urinary system	Ureteric obstruction/colic. Acute urinary retention
Ischaemia	
Small/large bowel	Strangulated hernia
	Volvulus
	Mesenteric ischaemia
Perforation/rupture	
Duodenum/ stomach	Perforation of peptic ulcer or eroding tumour
Colon	Perforated diverticulum or tumour
Fallopian tube	Ruptured ectopic pregnancy
Abdominal aorta	Ruptured aneurysm
Ruptured spleen	Trauma
Nonsurgical causes	Myocardial infarction, gastroenteritis (inc. typhoid fever, cholera and *E. coli*), diabetes mellitus, Henoch Schönlein purpura, lead colic, basal pneumonia, tuberculosis, porphyria, sickle cell crisis, malaria, phaeochromocytoma

- Serum amylase measurement is useful in diagnosing pancreatitis.
- Urinalysis for sugar, ketones, protein, blood, bilirubin and urobilinogen.
- Imaging: Erect chest X-ray, abdominal X-ray, ultrasound or CT scan may be helpful.

Management

Patients may require resuscitation, and general management includes the following:

- Nil by mouth, nasogastric tube and i.v. fluids if vomiting, obstructed or perforated (drip and suck).
- If shocked, a fluid balance chart should be started and where appropriate urinary catheterisation to monitor output.
- Broad-spectrum antibiotics are often used.
- Subsequent management is directed at the underlying cause.

Dyspepsia

Definition

Dyspepsia is a group of symptoms that suggest disease of the upper gastrointestinal tract.

Prevalence

Dyspepsia has a prevalence of between 23 and 41% in Western populations.

Aetiology/pathophysiology

Diagnoses made at endoscopy include gastritis, duodenitis or hiatus hernia (30%); oesophagitis (10–17%); duodenal ulcers (10–15%); gastric ulcers (5–10%) and oesophageal or gastric cancer (2%); however, in 30% the endoscopy is normal. Functional dyspepsia describes the presence of symptoms in the absence of mucosal abnormality, hiatus hernia, erosive duodenitis or gastritis.

Clinical features

Patients may complain of upper abdominal discomfort, retrosternal burning pain, anorexia, nausea, vomiting, bloating, fullness and heartburn.

Investigations and management

Current UK guidelines suggest

- All patients over the age of 55 years with new onset of uncomplicated dyspepsia and patients of any age with 'alarm symptoms or signs' (see Table 4.2) should

Table 4.2 Alarm symptoms and signs

Unintentional weight loss (≥3 kg)	Unexplained iron deficiency anaemia
Gastrointestinal bleeding	Dysphagia or odynophagia
Previous gastric surgery	Persistent continuous vomiting
Epigastric mass	Suspicious barium meal
Previous gastric ulcer	

undergo an upper gastrointestinal endoscopy. Antisecretory drugs (i.e. H_2 antagonists and proton pump inhibitors) may mask significant diagnoses at endoscopy and should be avoided for 4 weeks before investigation. At endoscopy, biopsy and urease tests should be performed.

- In patients under the age of 55 years with significant symptoms but without any 'alarm symptoms or signs' antisecretory agents may be commenced. It is recommended that such patients should undergo *Helicobacter pylori* testing and where appropriate, eradication therapy (see later in this chapter).

Peritonitis

Definition
Peritonitis is inflammation of the peritoneal lining of the abdomen. Peritonitis may be acute or chronic, primary or secondary.

Aetiology/pathophysiology
Infection can reach the peritoneal cavity from penetrating trauma or surgery, from the abdominal viscera, from the female genital tract or as a result of a septicaemia.

- Primary acute peritonitis is rare: It is most commonly due to *Escherichia coli*: Bacteria are thought to be transferred from the gut or bloodstream. Patients undergoing peritoneal dialysis are at particular risk of recurrent acute peritonitis, which may result in fibrosis and scarring preventing further use of this type of dialysis. Chronic liver disease patients with ascites are at risk of developing a less symptomatic form called spontaneous bacterial peritonitis.
- Chronic infective peritonitis occurs from tuberculous peritoneal infections.

- The most common type of peritonitis is acute suppurative secondary to visceral disease (see section on The Acute Abdomen).
- Postoperative peritonitis may result from persistence of infection present at the time of surgery or from complications such as anastomotic breakdown.

Clinical features
Peritonitis presents with pain, tenderness, rebound tenderness and excessive guarding. Movement exacerbates the pain, so patients often lie very still and have a rigid abdomen on attempted palpation (stiff as a board).

Complications
Infection may spread to the blood stream (septicaemia) form subphrenic or subhepatic abscesses.

Microscopy
An acute inflammatory exudate is seen with cellular infiltration of the peritoneum.

Investigations
The diagnosis is clinical, further investigation depends on the possible underlying cause.

Management
Management in secondary peritonitis is aimed at prompt surgical treatment of the underlying cause (after aggressive resuscitation). Primary or postoperative peritonitis, which is non-surgical in origin, is managed medically.

- Nil by mouth, i.v. fluids and nasogastric tube with aspiration (drip and suck).
- Broad-spectrum antibiotics.
- Drainage of any abscess or collection (either surgically or ultrasound guided aspiration).

Intestinal obstruction

Definition
Intestinal obstruction results from any disease or process that impedes the normal passage of contents. It may be acute, subacute, chronic or acute on chronic.

Aetiology
The common causes vary according to age. Neonatal obstruction may result from a meconium ileus, an atresia of

the small or large bowel, a malrotation or Hirschsprung disease. Children develop intestinal obstruction from external hernia, intussusception or surgical adhesions. In adults external hernia, large bowel cancer, adhesions, diverticular disease and Crohn's disease may all cause obstruction.

Pathophysiology

- The bowel may obstruct from an intraluminal mass, a mural problem or extramural compression. These result in a simple obstruction. The bowel above the lesion becomes progressively distended resulting in painful stretching. There may be compression of blood vessels and a consequent ischaemia.
- In a volvulus, malrotation or hernia there may be strangulation. There is occlusion of the low-pressure veins resulting in congestion and oedema. As the extracellular pressure rises arteries become obstructed causing ischaemia and infarction.

Clinical features

Patients present with pain, vomiting and a failure to pass faeces or flatus. The site of pain is dependent on the embryological gut:

- Foregut (stomach to half way along the second part of duodenum). Pain is felt in the epigastrium.
- Midgut (until two thirds of way along the transverse colon). Pain is felt in the umbilical region.
- Hind gut (down to the dentate line of the rectum). Pain is felt in the suprapubic region.

Physical examination reveals abdominal distension, possibly visible peristalsis. Auscultation reveals exaggerated bowel sounds and high pitched tinkling sounds when bowel becomes distended with fluid or gas.

Complications

- Obstruction may progress to perforation and peritonitis.
- In a volvulus there are two points of obstruction. Similarly in proximal colonic obstruction the ileocaecal valve forms a second point of obstruction. A closed loop obstruction therefore results with rapid compromise of blood supply and high risk of strangulation.

Investigations

Abdominal X-ray reveals the distension and allows assessment of the position within the bowel. Small bowel has markings that cross the whole bowel diameter (valvulae conniventes) whereas large bowel markings (haustra) only partially extend across the diameter. Erect abdominal X-ray may demonstrate fluid levels and any co-existent perforation.

Management

Following resuscitation, prompt diagnosis and operation are essential to avoid strangulation. Nil by mouth, NG suction and i.v. fluids are used in non-surgical causes or patients unable to tolerate procedures.

Small bowel obstruction:

- Hernias are reduced and repaired, adhesions and bands are divided.
- Lesions within the bowel wall such as tumours require resection with end-to-end anastomosis.
- Gallstones or food bolus causing intraluminal obstruction are milked into the colon.
- Strangulated bowel is resected and an end-to-end anastomosis performed.

Right colonic obstruction:

- Obstructive lesions of the right colon are managed by right hemicolectomy and end-to-end ileocolic anastomosis.
- Palliative side-to-side anastomosis between the ileum and transverse colon is performed in cases of inoperable tumours.

Left colonic obstruction: Surgery is often a two-stage procedure to reduce the risk of anastomotic leakage.

- Resection of bowel with both ends exteriorised or a Hartman's procedure (a defunctioning colostomy with closure of the distal stump, which is returned to the abdominal cavity).
- Restoration of continuity at elective surgery some weeks later.

Paralytic ileus

Definition

A cessation of the peristaltic movement of the gastrointestinal tract causing a form of intestinal obstruction.

Aetiology/pathophysiology

Causes of paralytic ileus include abdominal surgery, peritonitis, pancreatitis, metabolic disturbance (including hypokalaemia) or retroperitoneal bleeding. Inflammation of the serosal surface of the small bowel causes paralysis of gut motility leading to dilation. Fluid accumulation within the lumen of the bowel may result in fluid and electrolyte imbalances. This may further exacerbate the paralytic ileus.

Clinical features

There is abdominal distension with little evidence of rebound or guarding. If patients are not nil by mouth they develop copious vomiting. Patients do not pass stool or flatus and bowel sounds are characteristically absent.

Investigations

Abdominal X-ray shows gaseous distension with multiple fluid levels in the lumen of the bowel. This may be optimally seen on an erect film.

Management

It is treated conservatively with i.v. fluids and nasogastric tube (drip and suck). Fluid and electrolyte imbalances should be corrected. Any underlying cause should be identified and treated.

Pseudo-obstruction

Definition

A rare condition in which symptoms suggest obstruction but where no obstruction is present. The condition is seen following major respiratory or renal disease and/or after major trauma.

Clinical features

Symptoms are similar to those of intestinal obstruction, with distension and tinkling bowel sounds.

Investigations and management

Abdominal X-ray reveals gas extending to the rectum, which may be useful to differentiate from true obstruction. It is managed conservatively, any underlying cause should be identified and treated.

Acute upper gastrointestinal bleed

Definition

Acute upper gastrointestinal bleeds arise from the stomach, duodenum and oesophagus.

Incidence

50–150 per 100,000 population per year.

Aetiology

- The most common cause is peptic ulcer disease (35–50%) often exacerbated by the use of nonsteroidal anti-inflammatory drugs.
- Acute gastroduodenal erosions can follow any major illness (8–15%).
- Oesophagitis (5–15%).
- Mallory Weiss tears of the oesophagus resulting from vomiting (15%).
- Oesophageal varices may cause torrential bleeding (5–10%) (see page 199).
- Rarer causes include upper gastrointestinal malignancy and vascular malformations.

Clinical features

Haematemesis is vomiting of blood. It may appear fresh red or as 'coffee ground' altered blood. Melaena is the passage of black tarry stool due to at least 50 mL of digested blood; however, if there is very fast gut transit time or rapid bleeding, bright red blood may be passed rectally. It is essential to identify any coexistent medical conditions especially renal or liver disease and those with widespread malignancy, as these patients (along with the elderly) are at greatest risk of mortality.

Investigations

Urgent full blood count, U & Es, LFTs, coagulation screen and cross match specimens should be sent. The haemoglobin level may not be low despite severe blood loss until fluid redistribution or resuscitation has occurred.

Management

The initial management is to correct fluid loss and hypotension. All patients require large bore cannulae ideally in the anterior antecubital fossae. A central line may also be necessary for measurement of the central venous pressure. If the patient is in a state of shock they should be catheterised for accurate hourly fluid balance. Any coagulopathies should be corrected, e.g. with vitamin K and fresh frozen plasma.

- Young patients with minor bleeds and no comorbidity should be observed and undergo an elective endoscopy.
- Patients with more severe bleeding, particularly older patients or those with comorbidity, require urgent

endoscopic assessment and therapy after adequate resuscitation.

- In non-variceal bleeding failure of endoscopic therapy or further bleeding after a second endoscopic treatment is an indication for surgery.

Prognosis

Ninety per cent of haemorrhages originating from peptic ulcers will stop spontaneously. Indicators of poor prognosis and recurrent bleeds:

- Haematemesis and melaena together.
- Age over 60 years.
- Shock (pulse >100 and systolic BP <100 mmHg).
- Co-morbidity (including obesity).
- Young patient with postural drop >20 mmHg.

Pruritus ani

Pruritus ani is often idiopathic. Causes include the following:

i Lack of hygiene is the most common cause.

ii Skin conditions such as psoriasis or lichen planus. Contact eczema may occur due to cream/lotion application.

iii Infections include candida especially in diabetic and immunosuppressed, lice and anal warts. Thread worms in children.

iv Gastrointestinal disorders causing an anal discharge may result in pruritus.

v Drugs such as quinidine and colchicine may cause pruritus if used long term.

Proctoscopy and sigmoidoscopy may be required to examine for rectal disease. Management where the primary cause cannot be identified or treated includes discontinuation of all local preparations and careful attention to local hygiene. Surgical denervation has been attempted with varying success.

Investigations and procedures

Barium (contrast) studies

Barium is a radiopaque material that is not absorbed, so when swallowed or used as an enema can be used to delineate the internal markings of the gastrointestinal tract and to assess gut motility. Water-soluble contrast should be used if there is significant risk of leakage of contrast outside the lumen (e.g. if assessing for anastomotic leak).

X-rays are taken serially following administration of the contrast. Advantages of contrast studies over endoscopic procedures:

- No requirement for sedation, relatively well-tolerated.
- Motility can be assessed.
- Low risk of perforation, particularly where anatomy is thought to be distorted by previous surgery.

The main disadvantage is lack of ability to biopsy to obtain a tissue diagnosis and to treat, e.g. by removal of polyps or stop gastrointestinal bleeding.

Barium swallow

X-rays of the oesophagus are taken as the patient swallows contrast in the erect and prone positions. If assessing for dysphagia, bread may be given with the contrast to demonstrate how solids move through the oesophagus.

Reflux may be seen in the erect or prone position.

Diagnoses that may be made include candidiasis, oesophageal webs, pouches, stricture and carcinoma, extrinsic compression and achalasia.

Double-contrast barium meal

Barium is given together with effervescent tablets; this raises the diagnostic accuracy to 80–90% for peptic ulcer disease as there is an additional contrast between barium and air. Features of a malignant gastric cancer include a protruding mass into the lumen with a crater (ulcer) on its surface, interrupted nodular or irregular folds around a crater and the stiff 'leather-flask' appearance (linitus plastica) of diffuse gastric carcinoma (which may be missed on endoscopy).

Small bowel follow-through

Barium is swallowed (without effervescent tablets) and X-rays taken as it passes through the small intestine. In both barium meals and follow-through, compression of the abdominal wall may be required to visualise more thoroughly.

Barium enema

Patients are given a low residue diet for 3 days prior to the procedure, with powerful laxatives to cause profuse, watery diarrhoea to clear the large bowel. Barium and air are insufflated into the rectum via a catheter. The patient has to be tipped head-down and rotated to obtain various views of the entire colon, including the terminal ileum in some cases. The procedure can be uncomfortable, unpleasant and requires the patient to be able to stand. Apple-core lesions are classical of colonic carcinoma. Features of colitis can be identified as well as diverticular disease.

In acute illnesses such as possible perforation or diverticulitis, insufflation of air is avoided and a water-soluble contrast is used.

Endoscopy

Endoscopic procedures use flexible fibre-optic tubes, allowing direct vision and usually video imaging. The procedures are done under local anaesthetic and/or sedation, so are usually a day case procedure.

Oesophagogastroduodenal (OGD) or upper gastrointestinal (GI) endoscopy

The patient must be fasted at least 6 hours. Local anaesthetic spray is used on the throat and sedation is sometimes required. The endoscope is passed through the pharynx, into the oesophagus, stomach and duodenum. Diagnoses which may be made include oesophagitis, oesophageal candidiasis, Barrett's oesophagus, carcinoma of the oesophagus or gastric carcinoma, and peptic ulcer disease. Mucosal biopsies can be made for histological diagnosis and testing may be done for the presence of *H. pylori* (see page 162).

In upper GI bleeding, varices or a bleeding ulcer can be treated, e.g. by sclerotherapy, variceal banding, clips, glue, fibrin sealant (e.g. Beriplast) or laser photocoagulation. Upper GI endoscopy should be repeated 4–6 weeks after an endoscopic diagnosis of gastric ulcer has been made to repeat biopsies to exclude malignancy.

Complications of upper GI endoscopy include perforation (of oesophagus or stomach) and bleeding, but these are uncommon.

Colonoscopy

The patient has to have bowel preparation, which commences up to 2 days pre-procedure with a low-residue diet, then clear fluids. Osmotic laxatives or large volumes of electrolyte solutions are then taken to clear the bowel 12 hours before the procedure (essentially causing watery, frequent diarrhoea).

Sedation and analgesia (usually with pethidine) is required. The instrument is passed via the anus and using air insufflation to view the bowel, passed around as far as the caecum and terminal ileum. In 20% of cases, due to insufficient preparation or patient intolerance, it is not possible to obtain good views as far as the terminal ileum.

Polyps can be biopsied or removed. Biopsies can also be taken in suspected inflammatory bowel disease.

Complications: Bowel preparation may cause dehydration, electrolyte or fluid imbalance particularly in the elderly, or those with cardiac or renal disease. Perforation and peritonitis occur approximately 1 in every 2000 examinations and is more likely if biopsy or polyp removal takes place. Polyp removal also carries a 1 in 200 risk of bleeding. Overall colonoscopy has a mortality of 1:100,000.

Flexible sigmoidoscopy

This is a generally well-tolerated procedure that requires only a phosphate enema to clear the lower part of the colon, it is inserted to 70 cm. All patients who have a barium enema, e.g. for possible malignancy, should have a sigmoidoscopy, as barium enemas can miss low lesions.

Proctoscopy

Haemorrhoids are best seen with a proctoscope, which is a shorter, larger diameter tube gently inserted while the patient strains down. It is gently withdrawn whilst the patient continues to strain down. Using a light source haemorrhoids can be directly visualised and can be treated, e.g. with banding or injection of sclerosant.

Gastric surgery

Surgery for uncomplicated peptic ulcer disease is rarely performed since the advent of proton pump inhibitors to reduce acid production and the discovery of *H. pylori*. However in life-threatening upper gastrointestinal bleeding, if gastric outflow obstruction develops or for malignant gastric ulcers surgery is still indicated.

Vagotomy was previously used to reduce acid secretion but caused decreased motility and thus a drainage procedure is required:

- Pyloroplasty in which a longitudinal cut is made in the pylorus, which is then closed transversely, establishing an enlarged outlet from the stomach into the intestine.
- Gastro-enterostomy in which a loop of small bowel is linked to the stomach (the normal pyloric passage remains intact).

The side effects of the procedure are operative mortality, ulcer recurrence, dumping syndrome (see later) and diarrhoea.

Partial gastrectomy is usual (total gastrectomy is uncommon):
- Bilroth I in which the distal part of the stomach is removed and the stomach remnant connected to the duodenum.
- Bilroth II differs in that the stomach remnant is connected to the first loop of the jejunum and the duodenal stump is closed.

Complications following surgery:
- Duodeno-gastric reflux, may lead to chronic gastritis.
- Vomiting due to stoma narrowing.
- Recurrence of the original disease (gastric ulcer, gastric carcinoma).
- Nutritional consequences include weight loss, iron deficiency anaemia, vitamin B_{12} deficiency and malabsorption.
- The dumping syndrome is due to the uncontrolled rapid emptying of hyperosmolar solution into the small bowel characterised by a feeling of epigastric fullness after food associated with flushing, sweating 15–30 minutes after eating. This syndrome may improve with regular small frequent meals. Surgical revision may be indicated.
- Reactive hypoglycaemia is due to rapid absorption of glucose from the upper small bowel, causing a reactive hyperinsulinaemic state and then hypoglycaemia.
- Small increased risk of gastric cancer following partial gastrectomy after a latent period of 20 years possibly due to bacterial overgrowth with the generation of carcinogenic nitrosamines from nitrates in food.

Small bowel surgery

Small bowel resection is normally followed by immediate end-to-end anastomosis as the small bowel has a plentiful blood supply, a stronger wall and a content with a lower bacterial count. Small to medium resections have little functional consequence as there is a relative functional reserve; however, massive resections may result in malabsorption.
- Gastric hypersecretion is common post-resection possibly due to loss of secretary inhibitory factors.
- Nutritional consequences are severe when more than 75% of the bowel is resected.

- Loss of jejunum affects all nutrients, loss of the terminal ileum affects absorption of bile salts and vitamin B_{12}. Iron and folate are absorbed from the upper small bowel.
- Severe diarrhoea causes electrolyte loss, hypertrophy of the mucosa occurs over a period of 2 years after which any residual diarrhoea is likely to be permanent. Following small bowel surgery fluid and electrolytes must be monitored and corrected as required, fat-soluble vitamins should be supplemented.

Large bowel surgery

Resection of the large bowel often requires temporary or permanent stoma to allow healing of the relatively fragile bowel. Patients require counselling wherever possible prior to surgery.

A stoma refers to the exteriorisation of any part of the bowel. These are subdivided into two categories:
1 Colostomy (exteriorisation of the colon), which is flush to the skin. Both ends may be exteriorised as a colostomy and a mucous fistula or the rectal stump can be closed off and left within the pelvis (Hartman's procedure). Both procedures may be reversible.
2 Ileostomy, which requires the creation of a cuff of bowel to prevent skin damage as a result of the digestive enzymes.

In elective procedures such as resection of tumours bowel preparation is performed to clear the bowel of faeces prior to surgery. Prior to emergency surgery aggressive resuscitation is required. Resection of tumours, when of curative intent, involves removal of an adequate region of healthy bowel and as much as possible of the regional lymph drainage.

Complications of intestinal surgery include wound infection (see page 16) and anastomotic failure, the treatment for which is surgical drainage and exteriorisation.

Gastrointestinal infections

Food poisoning

Definition
Bacterial food poisoning is common and can be caused by a number of different organisms.

Aetiology and pathophysiology

- *Bacillus cereus* has an incubation period of 30 minutes to 6 hours. This most commonly causes acute self-limiting vomiting due to pre-formed enterotoxin particularly associated with rice and pulses. Ingested spores (which are resistant to boiling) may cause diarrhoea from production of a different toxin. Recovery occurs within a few hours.
- Staphylococcal food poisoning is caused by ingestion of heat stable enterotoxins A, B, C, D and E. The onset of the clinical disease occurs 2–6 hours after consumption of the toxins. Canned food, processed meats, milk and cheese are the main source. The main characteristic feature is persistent vomiting, sometimes with a mild fever. There may be diarrhoea. Recovery occurs within a few hours.
- *Campylobacter* has an incubation period of 16–48 hours. There is a large animal reservoir (cattle, sheep, rodents, poultry and wild birds). Patients present with fever, headache and malaise, followed by diarrhoea, sometimes with blood and abdominal pain. Recovery occurs within 3–5 days.
- *Clostridium perfringens* Type A produces an enterotoxin which causes watery diarrhoea and cramping abdominal pain as the main symptoms. It has an incubation period of 12–24 hours and recovery occurs within 2–3 days.
- *Salmonella* has an incubation period of 16–48 hours. There are more than 2000 species on the basis of antigens, which can help in tracing an outbreak. *Salmonella enteritidis* (one common serotype is called *Salmonella typhimurium*) is found in both animals and humans. The main reservoir of infection is poultry, though person to person infection may occur. Diarrhoea results from invasion by the bacteria resulting in inflammation. The condition is generally mild with fever, malaise, cramping abdominal pain, bloody diarrhoea and vomiting. Systemic disease may occur in those predisposed individuals, e.g. children, terminally ill patients, sickle cell anaemia patients. The organisms cause septicaemia causing osteomyelitis, pneumonia or meningitis. Recovery may occur within days, but may take up to 2 weeks.

Clinical features

As outlined above the cardinal features of food poisoning are diarrhoea, vomiting and abdominal pain. The severity of each symptom and a careful history of food intake over the past few days may point in the direction of a cause.

Investigations

Microscopy and culture of stool is used to identify cause. All forms of bacterial food poisoning are notifiable to allow contact tracing and investigation of source.

Management

In most cases the important factor is fluid rehydration preferably with oral rehydration solution. Antibiotics are not used in simple food poisoning unless there is evidence of systemic spread. Ciprofloxacin is a common first-line antibiotic, until an organism is identified.

Bacilliary dysentery

Definition

Bacilliary dysentery is a diarrhoeal illness caused by *Shigella* infection.

Aetiology

There are four species of *Shigella* known to cause diarrhoeal illness:

- *Shigella sonnei* (75% of UK infections) cause most of the mild infections.
- *Shigella flexneri* and *Shigella boydii* (travellers) cause intermediate infections.
- *Shigella dysenteriae* is the most serious.

Pathophysiology

Shigella is a human pathogen without an animal reservoir. Spread is by person-to-person contact, faecal–oral route or contaminated food. The incubation period is usually 2 days. The organism attaches to the mucosal epithelium of the distal ileum and colon causing inflammation and ulceration.

Clinical features

Acute watery diarrhoea with systemic symptoms of fever, malaise and abdominal pain develops into bloody diarrhoea. Other features include nausea, vomiting and headaches. Complications include colonic perforation, septicaemia, arthritis and convulsions.

Investigations

Diagnosis is made on stool culture. Sigmoidoscopy if performed reveals an inflamed mucosa with ulceration similar to that seen in inflammatory bowel disease.

Management

Treatment is symptomatic. Severe cases may be treated with trimethoprim or ciprofloxacin. Outbreaks may occur and require notification and source isolation.

Enteric *Escherichia* Coli infections

Definition

The *E. coli* that cause enteric diseases are of different serotypes from those that cause diseases elsewhere. Five main types are recognised.

Aetiology/pathophysiology

1 Enterotoxogenic *E. coli* (ETEC) produces a diarrhoeal illness.
- Pathogenesis: Two toxins are produced, one that is heat stable and one that is heat labile. The toxins are coded for on plasmids and can therefore be transferred between bacteria. The heat labile toxin resembles cholera toxin and acts in a similar way. The heat stable toxin activates guanylate cyclase also resulting in secretory diarrhoea.
- Clinically three syndromes occur with this infection: A cholera-like illness, traveller's diarrhoea and childhood diarrhoea, which may vary in severity.
2 Enteroinvasive *E. coli* (EIEC) produces a very similar illness to bacilliary dysentery (shigellosis).
3 Enteropathogenic *E. coli* (EPEC) causes an infantile gastroenteritis.
- Pathogenesis: Toxins are thought to be involved, the bacteria attaches to and damages intestinal epithelium.
- Clinical: The condition causes a diarrhoeal illness primarily in children below 2 years.
4 Enterohaemorrhagic *E. coli* (EHIC) includes verotoxin producing *E. coli* 0157:H7.
- Pathogenesis: The bacteria produce a shigella-like cytotoxin (Shiga toxin). Infections are associated with contaminated food, particularly hamburgers, only a small bacterial load is required to cause disease.

- Clinical: Patients suffer from bloody diarrhoea and colitis. Haemolytic uraemic syndrome may complicate infections with EHIC.
5 Enteroaggregative *E. coli* (EAEC or EaggEC).
- Pathogenesis: The bacteria produce a cytotoxin and stimulate IL-8 production. It is most common in the developing world but also found in the United Kingdom, especially in immunocompromised hosts.
- Clinical: Traveller's diarrhoea which lasts up to 4 days, or persistent diarrhoea in immunocompromised.

Management

Patients require adequate rehydration, normally orally. Most infections are self-limiting. In severe cases, particularly if there are systemic symptoms, ciprofloxacin is used. It has been suggested from retrospective studies that treatment of *E. coli* 0157 with antibiotics may result in increased rates of haemolytic uraemic syndrome, but the treated patients were also more seriously unwell.

Pseudomembranous colitis

Definition

Pseudomembranous colitis is a form of acute bowel inflammation caused by A and B toxins of *Clostridium difficile*.

Aetiology/pathophysiology

Usually seen in association with the use of broad-spectrum antibiotics particularly clindamycin. Other implicated antibiotics include ampicillin, tetracycline, cephalosporins. Antibiotics reduce the presence of normal protective bowel flora and allows *Clostridium* to multiply, causing inflammation and necrosis of bowel mucosa.

Clinical features

Patients (often already hospitalised) develop diarrhoea with variable fever and abdominal cramps. The stools are green, foul smelling and may contain pseudomembranes, fragments of mucosal slough.

Investigations

- At sigmoidoscopy the mucosa is erythematous, ulcerated and covered by a membrane-like material.

- Identification of the *C. difficile* toxin in the stool by ELISA is specific and is routinely used.
- Culture is possible but usually not required.

Management

The broad-spectrum antibiotics should be stopped and a combination of adequate fluid replacement and oral metronidazole is used. Second-line therapy is with oral vancomycin.

Giardiasis

Definition

Infection of the gastrointestinal tract by *Giardia lamblia* a flagellate protozoa.

Aetiology

Giardia is found worldwide especially in the tropics and is an important cause of traveller's diarrhoea, it is also found in the United Kingdom.

Pathophysiology

The organism is excreted in the faeces of infected patients as cysts. These are ingested, usually in contaminated drinking water. The organism then develops into a trophozoite, which colonises and multiplies in the small intestine. Diarrhoea results from inflammation of the epithelium.

Clinical features

Patients may be asymptomatic carriers or may present 1–2 weeks after ingestion of cysts with diarrhoea, nausea, anorexia, abdominal discomfort and distension. There may be steatorrhoea, and if the condition is prolonged there may be weight loss.

Investigations

- Stool specimen: Identification of trophozoites or cysts.
- Aspirates from the duodenum or jejunal biopsy can be used for identification.
- Serological responses can be measured.

Management

A 3-day course of metronidazole or a single oral dose of tinidazole are highly effective treatments for giardiasis. Prevention is by improved sanitation and precautions with drinking water.

Amoebiasis

Definition

A diarrhoeal illness or dysentery caused by infection with amoebae.

Prevalence

Up to 50% of the population in the tropics.

Geography

Occurs worldwide but most common in the tropics and subtropics.

Aetiology

The condition is caused by *Entamoeba histolytica*, transmission occurs through food and drink contamination or by anal sexual activity.

Pathophysiology

The amoeba can exist as two forms; a cyst and a trophozoite, only the cysts survive outside the body. Following ingestion the trophozoites emerge in the small intestine and then pass to the colon where they may invade the epithelium causing ulceration.

Clinical features

- Asymptomatic carriage and excretion of potentially infective cysts.
- Patients may have a gradual onset of mild intermittent diarrhoea and abdominal discomfort. Subsequently bloody diarrhoea with mucus and systemic upset may occur as a result of colitis, which may be severe. A fulminating colitis with a low-grade fever and dehydration may develop.

Complications

- Severe haemorrhage may result from erosion into a blood vessel. Amoebae may then pass to the liver causing hepatitis and intrahepatic abscesses.
- Amoebic liver abscesses result in tender hepatosplenomegaly, a swinging fever and malaise.
- Progression of fulminant colitis to toxic dilatation risks perforation and peritonitis.
- Chronic infection causes fibrosis and stricture formation.

Investigations

Serodiagnosis is by fluorescent antibody titre, positivity is low in asymptomatic carriers. Stool examination may reveal the trophozoites. Liver disease should be suspected if alkaline phosphatase rises, hepatic ultrasound is used to confirm the diagnosis.

Management

Metronidazole is the drug of choice, large liver abscesses require ultrasound guided percutaneous drainage. Prevention is difficult due to the high prevalence of asymptomatic carriers, boiling water for 10 minutes kills the cysts.

Enteric fever (typhoid and paratyphoid)

Definition

Typhoid (*Salmonella typhi*) and paratyphoid (*Salmonella paratyphi A, B or C*) produce a clinically identical disease.

Aetiology/pathophysiology

Humans are the only reservoir. Transmission is by the faeco–oral route or via contaminated food and water. The incubation period is 10–14 days. Organisms pass via the ileum and the lymphatic system to the systemic circulation causing a bacteraemia. Gut re-invasion leads to the clinical picture. Some secrete salmonella for over a year and measurement of Vi agglutinin is used to detect carrier states.

Clinical features

1 The condition typically runs a course of around 1 month. Week 1 results from the bacteraemia. There is gradual onset of a viral like illness with headache and fever worsening over 3–4 days. There is initially constipation.
2 Week 2 the patient appears toxic with dehydration, constant fever, abdominal pain and diarrhoea. Patients develop an erythematous maculopapular-blanching rash with splenomegaly.
3 During week 3 complications include pneumonia, haemolytic anaemia, meningitis, peripheral neuropathy, acute cholecystitis, osteomyelitis, intestinal perforation and haemorrhage.
4 Over the subsequent week there is a gradual return to normal health.

Investigations

- Blood cultures are positive in 80% in week one and in 30% by week three. Stool cultures are more helpful in the second to fourth weeks.
- Serological testing is by the Widal test measuring serum agglutinins against O and H antigens.

Management

- Ciprofloxacin, chloramphenicol and amoxycillin have all been used.
- Supportive management includes fluid and electrolyte balance and management of complications.
- Carrier state eradication is by 4 weeks of ciprofloxacin and if unsuccessful cholecystectomy can be tried, as the gallbladder is often the site of infection.
- A vaccine is available which gives some protection for up to 3 years.

Botulism

Definition

Botulism is a serious food poisoning caused by the Gram positive bacillus *Clostridium botulinum*.

Aetiology

The bacteria are soil borne, spores are heat resistant to 100°C. The most likely foods contaminated are canned and preserved. Three patterns are recognised:
1 Food borne botulism in which toxin in the food is ingested.
2 Infant botulism in which the organism is ingested and the toxin produced.
3 Wound botulism in which the organism is implanted into a wound.

Pathophysiology

Toxins are transported via the blood stream to the peripheral nerve synapses. Botulinum toxin acts to block neurotransmission.

Clinical features

The illness starts with nausea and vomiting 12–72 hours after ingesting the organism. Neurological features result from neuromuscular blockade: blurred vision, squint due to lateral rectus muscle weakness, the pupil is fixed and unresponsive to light or accommodation. Laryngeal and pharyngeal paralysis heralds the onset of a generalised paralysis and respiratory insufficiency may result.

Investigations
The toxin is demonstrable in the faeces.

Management
Treatment is supportive with respiratory support as indicated. Intravenous antitoxin and guanidine hydrochloride to reverse neuromuscular blockade has been used.

Cholera

Definition
Cholera is an acute infection of the gastrointestinal tract caused by the Gram-negative bacterium *Vibrio cholera*.

Incidence
66 cases in the past 20 years in the United Kingdom, endemic in South East Asia and South America.

Aetiology
V. cholera is found free living in fresh water, it is only pathogenic in humans. It can contaminate shellfish. Transfer from human carriers is via the faeco–oral route.

The serovar 0:1 is the major pathogenic strain and is divided into two biotypes; classical and the more widespread El Tor (named after the quarantine camp in which it was discovered). Phage typing can be used to examine epidemics to try and see if the observed conditions originated from a single source (see Fig. 4.1).

Pathophysiology
1 *V. cholera* is damaged by stomach acid therefore patients on acid suppressing medication are particularly susceptible to infection.
2 Once in the small bowel proliferation occurs and there is production of an exotoxin.

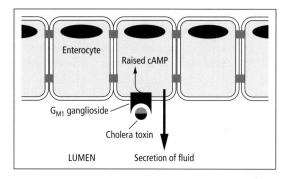

Figure 4.2 Pathophysiology of secretory diarrhoea in cholera.

3 The B subunit of the exotoxin binds to intestinal epithelium expressing the G_{M1} ganglioside and the A unit activates adenylate cyclase (see Fig. 4.2). The result is an increase in cellular levels of cAMP and massive secretion of isotonic fluid into the intestinal lumen.
4 A second toxin termed zonula occludens toxin (ZOT) damages the tight junctions between enterocytes allowing the passage of water and electrolytes.

Clinical features
The incubation period is between a few hours and 1 week. Most patients have a mild self-limiting diarrhoeal illness but in severe cases there may be watery diarrhoea with mucous, termed rice water stool. It is vital to adequately fluid resuscitate patients with such diarrhoea to prevent the onset of hypovolaemic shock.

Investigations
The diagnosis is often made on clinical features alone, pending the results of stool cultures which are diagnostic. However, stool microscopy may reveal the characteristic motile organisms.

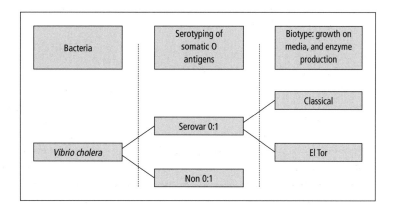

Figure 4.1 Subtypes of cholera.

Management

This depends on disease severity. Assessment of hypovolaemia may be made using clinical indices such as the difference between lying and standing blood pressure, the heart rate, skin turgor, urine output and urea and electrolyte measurement. A postural drop of 15 mmHg or more suggests volume depletion.

- In significant volume depletion intravenous saline should be administered. The fluid input and output should be documented hourly and reviewed with care.
- In mild cases oral rehydration is the treatment of choice using a solution containing sodium, potassium, chloride and citrate. Traditional solutions use glucose to facilitate absorption, rice-based polymers have been used in place of glucose with some evidence of benefit in reducing duration of diarrhoea (see Table 4.3).
- Tetracycline or ciprofloxacin can be used to shorten duration and reduce severity of illness.

Tuberculosis and the GI tract

Definition

Infection of the gastrointestinal tract or the peritoneum by *Mycobacterium tuberculosis* (see also page 102).

Aetiology/pathophysiology

Infections are most common in the immunosuppressed and are more common due to HIV. Sources of gastrointestinal tuberculous infections:

- Reactivation of primary tuberculosis.
- Bovine TB infections from unpasteurised milk.
- Self-infection may occur due to swallowing of infected sputum.

Intestinal tuberculosis occurs at any point of turbulence, e.g. the oesophagus at the indentation of the aorta, the pylorus and the ileocaecal valve, which is most commonly affected. Caseating granulomas and fibrosis may result in stricture formation and obstructions. Tuberculous peritonitis may result from reactivation of TB within an abdominal lymph node.

Clinical features

The presentation depends on the site of infection and often has an insidious onset. Patients may present with diarrhoea, abdominal pain, alteration of bowel habit, blood in stool and systemic features of anorexia and weight loss. Gastric outflow obstruction may result in vomiting and a succussion splash on examination. There may be a palpable abdominal mass. Clinically gastrointestinal tuberculosis may be difficult to distinguish from Crohn's disease.

Investigations

Abdominal ultrasound may demonstrate mesenteric thickening and lymph node enlargement. In patients with vomiting an upper gastrointestinal endoscopy is performed. Diagnosis may be made using histology, culture or PCR of tissue obtained at laparoscopy or colonoscopy (particularly from the ileocaecal valve and terminal ileum). See also Tuberculosis (page 102).

Management

Treatment with a combination of rifampicin, isoniazid, pyrazinamide and ethambutol if resistance is likely. Therapy should continue for 1 year in gut infections and 2 years in peritonitis. Surgical resection of a strictured bowel may be required for obstruction and to exclude a caecal carcinoma.

Disorders of the abdominal wall

Abdominal hernias

Definition

A hernia is the abnormal protrusion of an organ or tissue outside its normal body cavity or constraining sheath (see Fig. 4.3).

Incidence

85% occur in males, with a lifetime risk of 1 in 4 males, but less than 1 in 20 females. They increase with age.

Table 4.3 WHO oral rehydration salts (ORS) formula 2002

	mmol/L
Sodium	75
Chloride	65
Glucose, anhydrous	75
Potassium	20
Citrate	10
Total Osmolarity	**245**

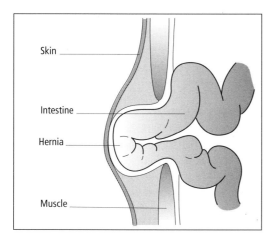

Figure 4.3 Abdominal wall hernia.

Aetiology/pathophysiology

Congenital hernias exploit natural openings and weaknesses. They may not become obvious until later in life and may be predisposed to by coughing straining, lifting, trauma or weak musculature. Examples of hernias include inguinal (direct and indirect), femoral, paraumbilical, umbilical and ventral hernias (see Fig. 4.4).

Of groin hernias, 60% are indirect inguinal, 25% are direct inguinal and 15% are femoral.

- Indirect inguinal hernias are a result of failure of obliteration of the processus vaginalis, a tube of peri-toneum dragged down into the testes during the embryonic descent of the testes from the posterior abdominal wall. It is usually obliterated leaving the tunica vaginalis as a covering of the testes.
- Direct inguinal hernias occur as a result of weakness in the floor of the inguinal canal (through Hesselbach's triangle which is formed inferiorly by the inguinal ligament, the inferior epigastric vessels laterally and the internal oblique muscle superiorly).
- Femoral hernias are due to a weakness of the femoral sheath, the top of which is the femoral ring bounded by the inguinal ligament anteriorly, the femoral vein laterally, the lacunar ligament medially and the superior ramus of the pubis posteriorly. Femoral hernias are particularly prone to incarceration or strangulation, as the angle of the canal makes the hernia difficult to reduce. Females have femoral hernias more often than males, but inguinal hernias are still the most common hernia in females (by 4 to 1).
- Incisional hernias occur at weakened areas caused by surgical incisions and muscle splitting. They occur in approximately 5% of postoperative patients, risk factors include infection, poor wound healing, coughing and surgical techniques.

Clinical features

Hernias may be completely asymptomatic, or present with a painless swelling, sudden pain at the moment of herniation and thereafter a dragging discomfort made worse by coughing, lifting, straining and defecation (which increase intra-abdominal pressure). Persistent or severe pain may be a sign of one of the complications of hernias, i.e. incarceration or strangulation. In most cases the hernia is not visible when the patient is lying supine. They are best examined standing and when the patient is coughing or straining. A bulge may be visible and a cough impulse is normally palpable. It can be difficult to distinguish the groin hernias.

- Indirect hernias once reduced can be controlled by pressure applied to the internal ring. This distinguishes indirect from direct hernias, which cannot be controlled, and where on reduction the edges of the defect may be palpable.
- An inguinal hernia passes above and medial to the pubic tubercle whereas a femoral hernia passes below and lateral.

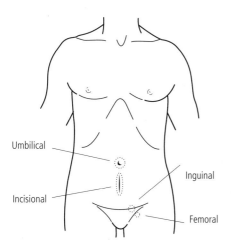

Figure 4.4 Sites of abdominal wall hernias.

Complications

- Hernias are irreducible when the contents cannot be manipulated back into the abdomen. Irreducibility (incarceration) is more likely if the neck of the sac is narrow (e.g. femoral and paraumbilical hernias) or if the contents become distended. Obstruction of the intestine may occur causing abdominal pain, vomiting and distension.
- Strangulation denotes compromise of the blood supply of the contents and significantly increases morbidity and mortality. The low-pressure venous system obstructs first, the resultant back pressure results in arterial insufficiency, ischaemia and ultimately infarction.

Investigations

These are rarely necessary to make the diagnosis, although imaging such as ultrasound is sometimes used.

Management

Surgical treatment is usually advised electively to reduce the risk of complications. However, longstanding, large hernias which are relatively asymptomatic may be treated conservatively, as they have a low risk of incarceration and strangulation. Treatment can be by open or laparoscopic repair. Direct hernias are reduced and the defect closed by suture or synthetic mesh. Indirect hernias are repaired by surgical removal of the herniation sac from the spermatic cord. If the internal ring is enlarged it is reduced surgically. For other hernias, the principle is to excise the sac and obliterate the opening either by suturing or mesh.

Prognosis

The recurrence rate of direct inguinal hernias is approximately 10%, but less with mesh techniques.

Disorders of the oesophagus

Gastrooesophageal reflux disease

Definition

Reflux of acidic gastric contents into the oesophagus via the lower oesophageal sphincter.

Aetiology

Factors include hiatus hernia, pregnancy, obesity, excessive alcohol ingestion, cigarette smoking, coffee, red wine, anticholinergic drug, oesophageal dysmotility and systemic sclerosis.

Pathophysiology

The lower oesophageal sphincter is formed of the distal few centimeters of the oesophageal smooth muscle. Normally after the passage of a food bolus the muscle rapidly contracts preventing reflux. Sphincter tone can increase in response to a rise in intra-abdominal or intra-gastric pressure.

Reflux results from low resting tone of the lower oesophageal sphincter and failure of increase in tone to rises in pressure further down the GI tract.

The normal squamous epithelium of the oesophagus is sensitive to the effects of acid and thus acute inflammation may be caused, called reflux oesophagitis. Continuing inflammation may manifest as ulceration, scaring, fibrosis and stricture formation.

Continuing inflammation may result in glandular epithelial metaplasia (a change from the normal squamous epithelium to glandular epithelium) termed Barrett's oesophagus, which predisposes to neoplasia.

Clinical features

Patients complain of symptoms of dyspepsia (see earlier in this chapter) particularly heartburn, a retrosternal burning pain aggravated by bending or lying down. Effortless regurgitation of food and acid (waterbrash) into the mouth may occur.

Investigations

Patients should be investigated as for dyspepsia including upper GI endoscopy where appropriate (see page 147).

- Barium swallow may show a hiatus hernia, true reflux of barium must be demonstrated to be diagnostic. A negative test however does not exclude reflux.
- 24-hour intraluminal pH monitoring is a gold standard test for acid reflux.

Management

Patients are managed as for dyspepsia, i.e. patients under the age of 55 years without 'alarm symptoms and signs' (see page 143) are treated without endoscopy.

Older patients and those with suspicious features should undergo endoscopy prior to commencing treatment. Although *H. pylori* infection is no more likely to be present in patients with gastrooesophageal reflux disease compared to the normal population, patients are tested as part of the investigation of dyspepsia and treated if found to be positive. See also Dyspepsia and *H. pylori* (pages 142–162).

- Patients should be advised to lose weight if obese, and avoid precipitating factors such as alcohol and coffee. Raising the head of the bed may be of benefit.
- The most effective relief is provided by proton pump inhibitors; however, many patients have adequate symptom control from antacids, alginates, H$_2$ antagonists or prokinetic agents such as domperidone or metoclopramide. An initial course of 4 weeks of treatment is used.
- Indications for anti-reflux surgery include continued symptoms despite high dose proton pump inhibitor therapy for at least 6 months, complications or high grade oesophagitis in young/fit patients and reflux after previous upper gastrointestinal tract surgery. A fundoplication (open or laparoscopic) is performed in which the mobilised gastric fundus is wrapped completely or partially around the lower end of the oesophagus. Endoscopic techniques are now available. Oesophageal strictures may require endoscopic dilatation to stretch the stricture to achieve a luminal diameter of 10–15 mm. Complications include haemorrhage, perforation and bacteraemia.

Hiatus hernia

Definition
Hiatus herniation is the abnormal passage of part or all of stomach through the diaphragm. It may be axial/sliding, paraesophageal/rolling or mixed.

Prevalence
Increases with age, very common in elderly patients (up to 70%).

Aetiology/pathophysiology
See Fig. 4.5.

- In a sliding hernia the stomach passes up through its own opening. Sliding hernias are initially intermittent. Incompetence of the lower oesophageal sphincter results in reflux, which may cause chronic inflammation and fibrosis. This can eventually shorten the oesophagus, fixing the stomach in the thorax.
- In a para-oesophageal hernia there is a defect in the diaphragm allowing the greater curve to roll upwards into the mediastinum. As the gastro-oesophageal sphincter remains in place patients do not develop reflux. Symptoms may result from pressure on the heart or lungs. These are most commonly seen in the elderly.

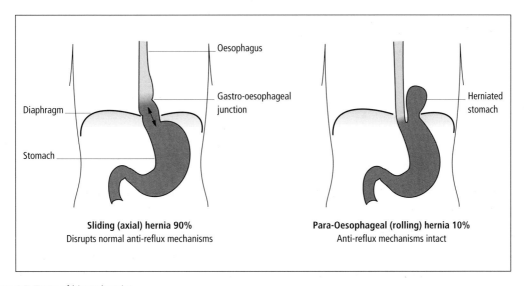

Figure 4.5 Types of hiatus hernias.

Clinical features

Most patients are asymptomatic. Patients with a sliding hernia may present with symptoms of dyspepsia due to gastro-oesophageal reflux. Para-oesophageal hernias may cause dyspnoea or palpitations. However 20% of patients with para-oesophageal/mixed hernias present acutely with acute upper gastrointestinal haemorrhage, strangulation, infarction or perforation of the intrathoracic stomach.

Investigations

Chest X-ray may reveal a gas bubble above the diaphragm, diagnosis is confirmed on barium swallow which may require a head down position or pressure applied to the abdomen. Endoscopy can establish the extent and severity of inflammation and exclude oesophageal carcinoma.

Management

- In sliding hernias management of symptoms is achieved either with medical anti-secretory agents (see section on Gastro-oesophageal Reflux page 156) or fundoplication. In fundoplication (open or laparoscopic) the gastric fundus is mobilised and wrapped around the lower end of the oesophagus. Increase in intra-gastric pressure therefore results in the closing off of the lower oesophagus. Endoscopic techniques may also be used.
- In para-oesophageal hernias surgery is indicated (in fit patients) to reduce the risk of strangulation and other life-threatening complications. Surgery consists of excision of the peritoneal sac, reduction of the hernia and closure of the defect. A fundoplication is usually then performed.

Pharyngeal pouch

Definition

A false diverticulum arising at the junction of the oesophagus and the pharynx.

Aetiology/pathophysiology

In co-ordination between the contraction of the pharynx and relaxation of the upper oesophageal sphincter causes the pharyngeal mucosa to herniate posteriorly between the upper and lower fibres of the inferior constrictor muscle (Killian's dehiscence).

Clinical features

Patients may present with a lump in the throat and dysphagia with regurgitation of undigested food some hours after eating. Complications include aspiration pneumonia, loss of weight and loss of appetite.

Management

A barium swallow will demonstrate the pouch. Diverticulectomy in which the pouch is excised and the defect repaired. Endoscopic techniques may be used in elderly patients, with a large dependent pouch, who are unfit for surgery.

Plummer–Vinson syndrome

Definition

Plummer–Vinson syndrome or Paterson–Brown–Kelly syndrome is an unusual combination of iron deficiency anaemia and dysphagia.

Aetiology/pathophysiology

There is atrophic, inflamed mucosa in the pharynx and the upper oesophagus with the formation of a post-cricoid web. The dysphagia is thought to be due to oesophageal spasm.

Clinical features

Patients present with dysphagia, glossitis, koilonychia and iron deficiency anaemia. There is a high risk of upper oesophageal or pharyngeal malignancy.

Management

Webs are dilated endoscopically to relieve obstruction, iron deficiency anaemia is treated. If malignancy occurs the prognosis is poor.

Achalasia

Definition

Achalasia is a disordered contraction of the oesophagus of neuromuscular origin.

Aetiology

Degeneration is seen in the vagus nerve associated with a decrease in ganglionic cells in the Auerbach's nerve plexus within the oesophageal wall. Chagas' disease in

South America is very similar where infection by *Trypanosoma cruzi* causes destruction of the myenteric plexus.

Pathophysiology
The neuromuscular damage causes disordered motility along the whole length of the oesophagus. On manometry there is aperistalsis and incomplete relaxation of the lower oesophageal sphincter in response to swallowing. The gastrooesophageal sphincter classically remains tightly closed and there is dilation of the oesophagus.

Clinical features
Patients present with progressive dysphagia, regurgitation and nocturnal aspiration. Retrosternal burning pain occurs in around a quarter of patients. Patients are often underweight.

Complications
Patients may aspirate and develop respiratory symptoms. Achalasia may predispose to oesophageal carcinoma even after successful treatment (incidence of 5–10%).

Investigations
- A chest X-ray may reveal a fluid level behind the heart.
- Diagnosis is made by barium swallow, which reveals a markedly dilated 'megaoesophagus'. There may be superficial mucosal erosions with a very narrow passage of barium (rat's tail) into the stomach through the contracted lower oesophageal sphincter.
- 24-hour pH and manometry studies can differentiate achalasia from other oesophageal motility disorders.
- Upper gastrointestinal endoscopy is performed to exclude a tumour. Classically there is a dilated oesophagus containing food debris. The gastrooesophageal junction may or may not be tight. A normal upper gastrointestinal endoscopy does not exclude the diagnosis of achalasia. Biopsy reveals inflammation and mucosal ulceration in the oesophagus secondary to bacterial overgrowth.

Management
Patients require long-term treatment with a proton pump inhibitor. Treatment is by repeated dilatation of the lower oesophageal sphincter with a hydrostatic balloon and/or injection of botulinum toxin into the lower oesophageal sphincter. Surgical intervention is indicated in those who fail to respond; a 10–12 cm incision is made into the anterior wall of the oesophagus without breaching the mucosa (Heller's cardiomyotomy). Laparoscopic techniques are also used. Gastro-oesophageal reflux is a complication with both procedures.

Diffuse oesophageal spasm

Definition
A severe form of abnormal oesophageal mobility.

Aetiology/pathophysiology
There is a generalised abnormality of the oesophagus with resultant hypermotility leading to painful oesophageal spasms. The resting pressure and relaxation of the lower oesophageal sphincter is normal.

Clinical features
Pain is retrosternal and ranges from mild to severe colicky spasms that occur spontaneously or on swallowing.

Investigations
Barium swallow may show a corkscrew appearance due to contracted muscle (nutcracker oesophagus). Manometry can be used to identify the diseased segment and is required prior to surgery.

Management
Calcium channel blockers can reduce the amplitude of the contractions. Nitrates have also been used with some success. Surgical intervention with open or thoracoscopic myotomy is considered in refractory cases. The myotomy should extend the entire length of the involved segment of oesophagus and through the lower oesophageal sphincter. To prevent gastrooesophageal reflux a fundoplication should also be performed (see page 158).

Mallory-Weiss tear

Definition
A tear in the mucosa normally at or just above the oesophageal gastric junction.

Aetiology/pathophysiology
The tear in the mucosa is a result of a sudden increase in intra abdominal pressure associated with vomiting,

particularly on a full stomach or after large amounts of alcohol.

Clinical features

Patients present with haematemesis which is usually small. The bleeding typically occurs after a number of retches, i.e. not on the first vomit.

Investigations

Young patients with a typical history do not require investigation. Other patients with an upper gastrointestinal bleed require endoscopy to confirm the diagnosis and exclude oesophageal varices (see page 199).

Management

Almost all stop spontaneously. Continuing bleeding suggests other causes.

Oesophageal perforation

Definition

Perforation of the oesophagus resulting in leakage of the contents.

Aetiology

A rare complication of endoscopy, foreign bodies and trauma. Occasionally a rupture following forceful vomiting may occur (Boerhaave's syndrome).

Pathophysiology

Perforation usually occurs at the pharyngeo-oesophageal junction. It results in release of secretions into the mediastinum.

Clinical features

Presentations include surgical emphysema of the neck; intense retrosternal pain, tachycardia and fever in mediastinitis; subdiaphragmatic perforation causes peritonitis.

Investigations

CXR may reveal air in the mediastinum or soft tissues (surgical emphysema).

Management

Small perforations occurring in the neck are managed with broad-spectrum antibiotics and nasogastric tube. Large thoracic perforations are repaired with a gastric fundus patch. Oesophageal perforation secondary to malignancy at or above the lower oesophageal sphincter can be treated with a covered metal stent placed endoscopically.

Disorders of the stomach

Gastritis

Gastritis is inflammation of the gastric mucosa, which can be considered as acute or chronic and by the underlying pathology (see Fig. 4.6).

There is little correlation between the degree of inflammation and symptomatology. Patients may complain of epigastric burning pain and occasionally vomiting. Endoscopy can be performed to confirm the diagnosis but is rarely indicated in acute gastritis.

Acute erosive gastritis

Definition

Superficial ulcers and erosions of the gastric mucosa develop after major surgery, trauma or severe illness.

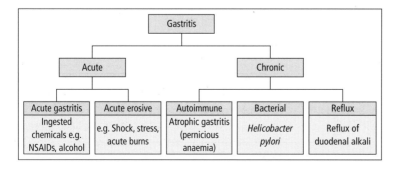

Figure 4.6 Causes of gastritis.

Aetiology

This pattern of gastritis is seen in patients with shock, severe illness. It may also be seen with the use of nonsteroidal anti-inflammatory drugs, steroids and heavy alcohol ingestion. *H. pylori* can cause an acute gastritis, which typically starts in the antrum and may extend to involve the entire gastric mucosa.

- Curling's ulcers are a form of stress ulcers occurring in patients following burns.
- Cushing's ulcers occur in patients with neurosurgical illness possibly due to the increased intracranial pressure causing an increased in vagal secretormotor stimulus.

Clinical features

Patients develop epigastric pain, burning in nature associated with vomiting and occasionally haematemesis and perforation.

Macroscopy/microscopy

The gastric mucosa appears hyperaemic with focal loss of superficial gastric epithelium (ulceration) and small erosions.

Investigations

Diagnosis may be confirmed by endoscopy with a urease (CLO) test for *H. pylori*.

Management

Identification and management of the underlying cause is required, specific interventions include the use of H_2 antagonists and proton pump inhibitors.

Peptic ulcer disease

Definition

A peptic ulcer is a break in the integrity of the stomach or duodenal mucosa.

Incidence

15% of the population will suffer from a duodenal ulcer and 5% a gastric ulcer at some time during their life.

Age

More common with increasing age.

Sex

Duodenal ulcers 4M : 1F.

Geography

In the United Kingdom duodenal ulcers are more common in North England and Scotland.

Aetiology

Factors involved include presence of *H. pylori* within the stomach, the use of nonsteroidal anti-inflammatory drugs (NSAIDs) and aspirin. Rarely pathological hypersecretion of gastrin (Zollinger–Ellinson syndrome) may be the cause of multiple ulcers. Most duodenal ulcers occur in the proximal duodenum, most gastric ulcers occur on the lesser curve. Rare sites include the following:

- The oesophagus following columnar metaplasia due to gastrooesophageal reflux.
- The jejunum in Zollinger–Ellinson syndrome.
- A Meckel's diverticulum containing ectopic gastric mucosa.

Pathophysiology

Ulceration results from an imbalance between the gastric secretion of acid and the ability of the mucosa to withstand such secretion. Normal protective mechanisms include mucous, bicarbonate and prostaglandins. Patients with *H. pylori* infection have elevated basal and stimulated concentrations of serum gastrin and a decreased concentration of somatostatin resulting in increased acid production. *H. pylori* also releases proteases which degrade mucous glycoproteins which normally protect the gastric mucosa.

Clinical features

Clinically patients present with dyspepsia, which they often describe as indigestion, nausea and occasionally vomiting. Gastric ulcers tend to cause pain that is worse during the day and after meals. Duodenal ulcers tend to cause well-localised epigastric pain that may radiate to the back. It occurs a few hours after meals or on an empty stomach and is often worse at night or in the early hours of the morning when circadian acid secretion is maximal.

Macroscopy/microscopy

Chronic ulcers have sharply defined borders, without any heaping up of the edges (which would be suggestive of a malignant ulcer). There is a break in the integrity of the epithelium extending down to the muscularis mucosa. Active inflammation is seen with granulation tissue and fibrosis.

Complications

- Perforation occurs much more commonly with duodenal ulcers. It results in peritonitis and an acute abdomen, free air is seen under the diaphragm on plain erect chest X-ray. Patients require resuscitation and emergency surgery to locate and close the duodenal perforations, a partial gastrectomy may be required in gastric ulcers.
- Haemorrhage may be slow and chronic presenting as anaemia. More rapid loss may cause melaena and haematemesis. Peptic ulcer disease is the most common cause of acute upper gastrointestinal haemorrhage and may cause hypovolaemia and shock. Acute bleeds require resuscitation to stabilise the patient and may require urgent endoscopic treatment (see page 147). Early endoscopy can reduce the risk of rebleeding by injection or argon plasma coagulation of bleeding ulcers. Surgery may be needed if bleeding is uncontrollable or endoscopy is unsuccessful.
- Scarring of the pyloric region results in gradual development of outflow obstruction (pyloric stenosis). The patient presents with upper abdominal distension after meals and projectile vomiting. X-ray reveals a distended stomach, barium meal is diagnostic. Fibrotic stenosis requires surgical intervention following treatment of any electrolyte imbalances resulting from copious vomiting.

Investigations

Patients are investigated and managed as for dyspepsia, i.e. patients under the age of 55 years without 'alarm symptoms and signs' (see under section Dyspepsia) are treated without endoscopy. Older patients and those with suspicious features should undergo endoscopy to exclude malignancy prior to commencing treatment.

Management

Duodenal ulcer:

- *H. pylori* positive (90%): Patients should receive eradication therapy (see below). If asymptomatic following this treatment a further endoscopy is not necessary. If symptoms persist or recur (or in all patients initially presenting with complications) a urea breath test should be performed at 4 weeks and further eradication therapy used if positive. If negative clinical re-evaluation is necessary.

- *H. pylori* negative (10%): Antisecretory therapy such as H_2 receptor antagonists (first line) or proton pump inhibitors are used. If the patient is taking NSAIDs these should be stopped if possible.

Gastric ulcer:

- *H. pylori* positive (70%): Eradication therapy is used (see below) followed by antisecretory therapy for 2 months.
- *H. pylori* negative (30%): The majority of these are NSAID or aspirin induced. Standard antisecretory therapy should be given for 2 months and NSAIDs should be stopped if possible.

Repeat endoscopy with biopsies is essential in all gastric ulcers until completely healed, as there may be an underlying malignancy. If the ulcer does not heal within 6 months then surgery should be considered.

In all patients with peptic ulcer disease who continue to require NSAIDs, long-term treatment with a proton pump inhibitor (or misoprostol in gastric ulcers) should be considered. In patients with rheumatoid arthritis or osteoarthritis a COX2 specific antagonist may be considered in place of the NSAID.

Helicobacter pylori

Definition

H. pylori is a spiral bacterium which is implicated in the causation of chronic gastritis, peptic ulcer disease, gastric carcinoma and mucosal associated lymphoid tissue (MALT) lymphoma.

Aetiology

The transmission of *H. pylori* is not fully understood; however, intrafamilial clustering suggests person-to-person spread and there is an association with lower socio-economic class.

Pathophysiology

H. pylori binds to the gastric epithelium beneath the protective mucus layer. It produces an enzyme that breaks down the glycoproteins within the mucus. There are also changes in the secretory patterns within the stomach along with toxin-mediated tissue damage. Initial infection causes an acute gastritis which rapidly proceeds to chronic inflammation. Prolonged inflammation results in metaplasia and predisposes to dysplasia and neoplasia.

Clinical features
Most people become colonised by *H. pylori* during their lifetime; however, only a minority develop symptoms of dyspepsia.

Microscopy
H. pylori causes a mixed acute and chronic inflammatory reaction within the lamina propria and superficial epithelium.

Investigations
Invasive tests are performed at time of endoscopy and biopsy.
- Rapid urease (CLO) test is performed by mixing the biopsy specimen with a urea solution. The presence of *H. pylori* is detected as ammonia formation causes a rise in pH changing the colour of indicator solution.
- Biopsy specimens can be cultured on selective media and the sensitivities determined.
- Histological identification can also be performed.

Noninvasive tests can be performed if an endoscopy is not indicated.
- The urea breath test uses ingestion of ^{13}C or ^{14}C labelled urea, if the bacteria is present the urea is broken down releasing labelled carbon dioxide which is detected in the breath. This test can be used to confirm successful eradication, but patients must not be taking proton pump inhibitors or bismuth and must not have had antibiotics in the preceding 4 weeks.
- Serological testing is simple, non-invasive and widely available, but remains positive after clearance or successful eradication.

Management
First line eradication (triple) therapy consists of a proton pump inhibitor, amoxycillin or metronidazole, and clarithromycin for 1 week. Second line (quadruple) therapy is with a proton pump inhibitor, bismuth subcitrate, metronidazole and tetracycline. Compliance with treatment is very important for successful treatment. If symptoms persist or recur a repeat urea breath test should be performed.

Zollinger–Ellinson syndrome

Definition
Pathological secretion of gastrin resulting in hypersecretion of acid.

Aetiology/pathophysiology
The condition is usually caused by a gastrinoma in the G cells of the pancreatic islets it occurs most commonly in males between 20–50 years of age. 60–90% of gastrinomas are malignant often with metastases at diagnosis.

Clinical features
Patients present with epigastric burning pain and with complications of peptic ulcer disease. The excess acid causes inactivation of duodenal/jejunal lipases and hence steatorrhoea also occurs.

Investigations
A fasting serum gastrin level is taken (>150 ng/L is suggestive, >500 ng/L strongly suggestive). The patient should not be taking a proton pump inhibitor as these increase gastrin levels. Tumour location is attempted with isotope scanning and CT of the abdomen.

Management
Resection of the gastrinoma should be attempted but problems with locating the tumour, which is often multifocal, makes surgery difficult. High-dose proton pump inhibitors are also used. Other treatment options include octreotide, interferon α, chemotherapy and hepatic artery embolisation.

Prognosis
In inoperable tumours 60% of patients survive 5 years and 40% survive 10 years.

Disorders of the small bowel and appendix

Acute appendicitis

Definition
Inflammatory disease of the appendix, which may result in perforation.

Incidence
Commonest cause of emergency surgery of childhood (3–4 per 1000).

Age
Any age but usually over 5 years.

Sex

No sex predisposition.

Geography

Disease of Western civilisations.

Aetiology/pathophysiology

Acute appendicitis typically commences with colicky pain suggesting that obstruction of the lumen may be a factor, e.g. by lymphoid hyperplasia, faecoliths, adhesions, fibrosis or neoplasia. The pain is initially felt in the periumbilical region due to the pattern of visceral innervation, but becomes localised to the right iliac fossa as the parietal peritoneum becomes inflamed. Accumulation of secretions result in distension, mucosal necrosis and invasion of the wall by commensal bacteria. Inflammation and impairment of blood supply lead to gangrene and perforation. Once perforation has occurred there is migration of the bacteria into the peritoneum (peritonitis). The outcome depends on the ability of the omentum and surrounding organs to contain the infection.

Clinical features

This is a classic cause of an acute abdomen. Pain is initially periumbilical, then migrates to the right iliac fossa. There is mild to moderate fever, nausea and anorexia. Vomiting is uncommon. The presentation may be less specific in the young, pregnant and elderly. Development of the disease may be over hours to days partly depending on host resistance.

Once there is peritonitis, the patient will have severe pain, exacerbated by movement and has a rigid abdomen with tenderness and guarding over the right iliac fossa. A mass may be felt through the abdominal wall or rectally particularly if the omentum is wrapped around the appendix, or an abscess has formed.

Macroscopy

The appendix appears swollen and the surface vasculature is yellow. There is a rough, yellow, fibrinous exudate on the surface.

Microscopy

Initially there is acute inflammation of the mucosa, which undergoes ulceration. There may be pus in the lumen. As the condition progresses the inflammation spreads through the wall until it reaches the serosal surface. There is then necrosis within the wall and a site of perforation may be seen.

Investigations

There are no diagnostic tests. FBC may show a raised white cell count, CRP may be raised. Ultrasound is increasingly being used but does not exclude the diagnosis. CT of the abdomen or laparoscopy may be indicated if another diagnosis is suspected. In women of childbearing age a pregnancy test should be performed to exclude an ectopic pregnancy.

Management

Conservative treatment has little place, except in patients unfit for surgery. Fluid resuscitation may be required prior to surgery and intravenous antibiotics are commenced.

- Under general anaesthetic the abdomen is opened by an incision along the skin crease passing through McBurney's point (one third of the distance from a line drawn from the anterior superior iliac spine to the umbilicus). The muscle fibres in each muscle layer are then split in the line of their fibres (grid iron incision). The mesoappendix is divided with ligation of the appendicular artery. The appendix is ligated at its base and removed. The stump is invaginated with a purse string suture. Peritoneal washout is performed if there is pus in the abdomen. The wound is then closed in layers.
- If there is an appendix abscess this should be surgically drained.

Discovery of a normal appendix means other pathology must be excluded (i.e. convert the operation to a diagnostic laparotomy). In most cases, the appendix is removed to avoid confusion if patients ever re-present with an acute abdomen.

Prognosis

Uncomplicated appendicitis has an overall mortality of 0.1%. Mortality rates may be as high as 5% following perforation.

Meckel's diverticulum

Definition

An ileal diverticulum occurring as a result of persistence of part of the vitellointestinal duct.

Incidence
2% of the population, the most common congenital abnormality of the GI tract.

Age
Congenital

Sex
2M > 1F

Aetiology
The vitellointestinal duct runs from the umbilicus to the ileum. By birth the duct has either disappeared or is normally only a small fibrous cord. Persistence of the duct may result in a Meckel's diverticulum (persistence of the ileal end of the duct), an umbilical sinus (persistence of the umbilical end of the duct) or an umbilical ileal fistula (see Fig. 4.7).

Pathophysiology
The diverticulum arises from the antimesenteric border of the ileum 2 ft from the ileocaecal valve and is on average 2 inches long. Ten per cent of diverticula are joined to the umbilicus by a fibrous cord. Acid secreting gastric mucosa is found in 50% of cases which may result in ulceration of the surrounding mucosa.

Clinical features
Ninety-five per cent of cases are asymptomatic, symptomatic patients present most commonly with bleeding due to ulceration of the adjacent ileum. Intestinal obstruction may result from intussusception of the diverticulum or from a volvulus.

Investigations
Presence of gastric mucosa can be detected by scintiscanning with ^{99m}Tc labelled sodium pertechnetate, which is taken up by parietal cells (the Meckel's scan).

Management
Symptomatic Meckel's diverticula are excised by wedge resection.

Malabsorption syndromes

Absorption of food occurs within the small bowel. The process involves breakdown of macromolecules by enzymes and transport across the specialised small bowel mucosa. Disorders of any of the elements potentially leads to malabsorption. The most common causes of malabsorption are pancreatic insufficiency, coeliac disease, resection of the ileum, Crohn's disease and liver disease (see Fig. 4.8).

Coeliac disease

Definition
Coeliac disease is a permanent inability to tolerate gluten.

Incidence
1 in 2000.

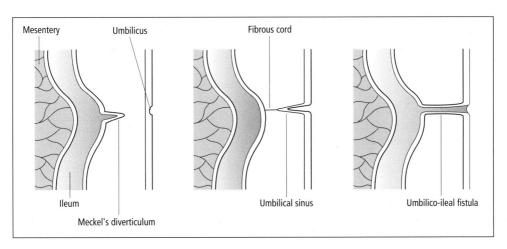

Figure 4.7 Persistence of the vitellointestinal duct.

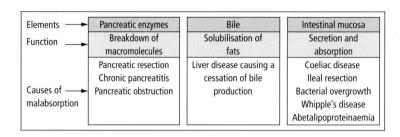

Figure 4.8 Malabsorption syndromes.

Age
Can present at any age.

Sex
F > M in adult diagnosed disease.

Geography
Common in Europe, (1 in 300 in Ireland) rare in Black Africans.

Aetiology
Thought to be an autoimmune disease with genetic and environmental components.
- Genetic: 90% of patients have the HLA A1,B8,DR3, DR7,DQW2 haplotype. 70% concordance of monozygotic twins.
- Environmental: There is amino acid sequence homology between gliadin and adenovirus 12, increased childhood incidence in those exposed to gluten containing foods from a young age.

Pathophysiology
Gluten ingestion results in mucosal damage causing a flattening of villi (subtotal villous atrophy) which in turn leads to a more generalised malabsorption.

Clinical features
Patients may present with irritability and failure to thrive in childhood, delayed puberty, short stature, or vomiting, diarrhoea, anorexia or abdominal distension at any age.

Complications
There is an association with development of small bowel lymphoma and a small increased risk in the development of small bowel adenocarcinoma. There is also an association with dermatitis herpetiformis (HLA B8 linkage is shared) and other organ specific autoimmune conditions, e.g. primary biliary cirrhosis.

Microscopy
There is lymphocytic infiltration of the lamina propria, and an increase in intra-epithelial lymphocytes (which bear the $\gamma\delta$ eceptor). Loss of normal villous architecture ranges from blunting (partial villous atrophy) to complete loss (total villous atrophy) with crypt hyperplasia in an attempt to compensate.

Investigations
- Serology: Screening by IgG gliadin and IgG anti-reticulin antibodies is sensitive but not specific. Screening by IgA gliadin and IgA anti-reticulin antibodies is specific but not sensitive. Antiendomysial antibodies (IgA) are found in the serum of most patients (sensitivity 98% specificity 93–99%), but total IgA must also be measured as coexistent IgA deficiency is not uncommon. ELISA for transglutaminase antibody has been shown to be sensitive and specific.
- Small bowel biopsy is diagnostic when taken at diagnosis, later when on a gluten free diet showing recovery of architecture and after gluten challenge showing villous loss again.

Management
A gluten free diet leads to a restoration of normal villous structure and resolution of dermatitis herpetiformis (see page 394). Haemoglobin and antiendomysial antibodies may be checked at routine follow-up to look for inadvertent gluten intake.

Whipple's disease

Definition
Rare multisystem disorder with malabsorption, lymphadenopathy and arthritis.

Aetiology

Caused by an infection by *Tropheryma whippelii*, an actinomycete. The route of infection is unknown. The organism is found in intestinal macrophages.

Clinical features

Patients present with steatorrhoea, abdominal pain and systemic symptoms of fever, weight loss, lymphadenopathy and arthritis. Heart, lung and CNS involvement may occur.

Investigations and management

Electron microscopy can demonstrate the organism. PCR is now available for diagnosis. Various antibiotics are used often in combination and for prolonged courses (up to 1 year).

Tropical sprue

Definition

A severe malabsorption syndrome endemic in Asia, some Caribbean islands and parts of South America.

Aetiology/pathophysiology

The condition occurs in epidemics and improves on antibiotics thus it is likely that it has an infective cause.

Clinical features

Patients present with diarrhoea, anorexia, abdominal distension and weight loss. The onset may be acute or insidious.

Investigations

The diagnosis can be made on jejunal biopsy, there is colonisation of the gut lumen by toxin producing enterobacteria associated with partial villous atrophy.

Management

Severely ill patients require resuscitation for dehydration and electrolyte imbalance. Nutritional deficiencies should be corrected and antibiotics given, but patients often improve when they leave endemic areas.

Disorders of the large bowel and inflammatory bowel disease

Diverticular disease

Definition

A diverticulum is a mucosal out-pouching, diverticular disease is a general term that encompasses diverticulosis (the presence of diverticula) and diverticulitis (inflammation of a diverticulum).

Incidence

Rare before the age of 35, but by 65 years one third of the population is affected.

Geography

Primarily a Western condition (due to diet). Immigrants to the West are also at risk.

Aetiology

Diverticulae are associated with high intraluminal pressure, muscle hypertrophy can be seen before diverticulae develop. There is a relationship with a low fibre diet and chronic constipation.

Pathophysiology

They occur most commonly in the sigmoid colon and may become obstructed with a faecolith. Repeated inflammation and scarring may result in an ulcer difficult to distinguish from carcinoma. Diverticulitis is caused by obstruction of the neck of the diverticulum resulting in mucosal inflammation.

Clinical features

- Diverticulosis is frequently asymptomatic. Patients may however report intermittent lower abdominal and left iliac fossa pain, altered bowel habit or occasional minor rectal bleeding.
- Diverticulitis presents as pyrexia, nausea, vomiting, with pain and tenderness, a mass may be palpable.

Macroscopy/micropscopy

On the surface of an opened section the slit like openings of diverticula can be seen.

Complications

- Perforation presents as an acute abdomen with peritonitis.
- Bleeding which may be significant.
- Obstruction due to oedema, fibrosis or adherence of small bowel loops.
- Stricture formation in long-standing disease difficult to differentiate from malignant strictures.
- Fistulae may occur to skin or viscera. A colovesical fistula presents with painful passage of pneumaturia.

Investigations

Barium enema can be used to demonstrate the presence of diverticulae. They may be seen on colonoscopy (contraindicated in acute diverticulitis).

Management

Most patients improve on a high-fibre diet and bulk-forming laxatives such as Fybogel.

- Acute diverticulitis is treated with bowel rest, intravenous fluids and broad-spectrum antibiotics.
- Surgery may be indicated for refractory symptomatic diverticulosis. A sigmoid colectomy and end-to-end anastomosis is performed.
- Perforation is treated with resuscitation and surgical resection. If there is peritonitis a Hartman's procedure (distal segment is oversewn and returned to the abdomen, proximal segment brought to surface as a colostomy) or exteriorisation of both ends of the bowel is performed, with secondary anastomosis 6–8 weeks later.
- Strictures or obstructions are treated by surgical resection followed by primary or secondary anastomosis.
- Severe bleeding may require embolisation or surgery.

Irritable bowel syndrome

Definition

A condition of disordered lower gastrointestinal function in the absence of known pathology of structure.

Prevalence

Common, affecting ∼10% of the population.

Age

Any

Sex

1M : 2F

Aetiology/pathophysiology

- 50% of patients seen in gastroenterology clinics attribute the onset of their symptoms to a stressful event including physical or sexual abuse as child or adult. Patients have a higher incidence of psychological symptoms, psychiatric disease and other somatic complaints.
- 10–20% of patients relate the onset of their symptoms to an acute gastrointestinal illness. Food allergy is rare but many patients believe that certain foods exacerbate symptoms. There is no consistent evidence of abnormal motility.
- Some patients with irritable bowel syndrome exhibit evidence of altered CNS processing of visceral pain.

Clinical features

Patients complain of recurrent abdominal pain, most often in the left iliac fossa, associated with disturbed bowel habit (including the passage of mucous). There is often a sensation of bloating and the frequent passage of small volume stool, which may relieve discomfort. Non-gastrointestinal symptoms include lethargy, poor sleep, generalised aches and pains. Examination is unremarkable.

Investigations

Investigation is required if there is weight loss, rectal bleeding, nocturnal symptoms, anaemia or an atypical history particularly in older patients. Investigation may include flexible sigmoidoscopy, with colonoscopy/barium enema in patients with onset of symptoms over the age of 45 years.

Management

- Psychological support and reassurance is essential. Coexistent psychological disorders should be identified and treated; relaxation therapy, biofeedback training and cognitive behavioural therapy may be of benefit.
- A sensible balanced diet avoiding food fads and excessive caffeine.
- Antispasmodics may help, e.g. hyoscine butylbromide, mebeverine. Alternatively a tricyclic antidepressant

can be tried. Urgency and diarrhoea can be treated with loperamide or codeine, whereas constipation can be helped by increased soluble fibre intake.

Ulcerative colitis

Definition
Chronic inflammatory bowel disease affecting only the large bowel, characterised by the formation of crypt abscesses (see Table 4.4).

Incidence
5 per 100,000 per year.

Age
Peak in young adult life.

Sex
F > M

Aetiology
Multifactorial aetiology including
1 Familial: Familial tendency, some concordance between monozygotic twins.
2 Genetic: HLA B27 is more common in patients.
3 Smoking: Patients presenting with ulcerative colitis are more likely to be non-smokers or recent ex-smokers.
4 Immunological: pANCA may be found in ulcerative colitis.

Pathophysiology
Ulcerative colitis is characterised by continuous inflammation starting in the rectum (proctitis) and extending variably to the descending colon or there may be a total colitis (pancolitis). In a few patients inflammation of the distal terminal ileum occurs termed backwash ileitis.

Clinical features
The condition is characterised by acute exacerbations interspersed by clinical remission. In acute episodes, patients present with diarrhoea containing blood and mucous which may be copious and associated with urgency. There may be extra-gastrointestinal features including erythema nodosum and pyoderma gangrenosum in the skin, iritis, arthropathy of large joints, sacroiliitis and ankylosing spondylitis (HLA B27) and chronic liver disease.

Table 4.4 Inflammatory bowel disease

Criterion	Ulcerative colitis	Crohn's disease
Extent	Large bowel only	May involve entire gastrointestinal tract
Rectal involvement	Almost invariable	Variable
Disease continuity	Continuous	Discontinuous
Depth of inflammation	Mucosal	Transmural
Mucosal appearance	Multiple small ulcers Pseudopolyps	Cobblestone, discrete deep ulcers and fissures
Histological features	Crypt abscesses No granulomas	Transmural inflammation Granulomas (50%)
Presence of anal lesions	25% of cases	75% of cases with large bowel disease 25% of cases with small bowel disease
Frequency of fistula	Uncommon	10–20% of cases
Risk of developing cancer	Significant	Rare
Medical management	Topical agents, then oral or systemic treatment. 5-ASA drugs +/− steroids used to induce remission. Steroids not used in maintenance.	5-ASA drugs +/− steroids to induce remission and for maintenance. Oral agents often required due to multifocal disease.
Surgical management	Pan proctocolectomy is performed in patients with complications, failure to thrive, or as prophylaxis against carcinoma.	90% of patients require surgery at some time. Surgery is non curative and thus only symptomatic bowel is resected with the aim of maintaining continuity

Macroscopy/microscopy

1 During acute exacerbation there is superficial mucosal haemorrhagic ulceration, interspersed with more normal mucosa appearing as an inflammatory polyp (pseudopolyps). On microscopy there is oedema and lymphocytic infiltration of the lamina propria. Neutrophils migrate through the wall of mucosal glands to form crypt abscesses.
2 During remission there is little ulceration, the mucosa appears hyperaemic and thin. Microscopy reveals chronic inflammatory cell infiltration.
3 Confluent inflammation and ulceration extending into the muscle layer is seen in fulminant disease.

Complications

Severe fulminant disease may manifest as toxic colonic dilation, septicaemia, obstruction and perforation. Chronic bowel inflammation is associated with increased risk of cellular dysplasia and a significant risk of carcinoma.

Investigations

- Anaemia due to blood loss, iron deficiency or chronic disease, acute inflammation may also cause a rise in platelet count. Inflammatory markers such as ESR are often raised in acute exacerbations.
- Barium enema may cause perforation in acute disease and is therefore contraindicated. In mild disease a diffusely reticulated pattern is seen with punctate collections of barium in small ulcers. In chronic disease a featureless colon with complete loss of folds is seen. Repeated plain abdominal X-ray is of value in acute flares to diagnose acute colonic dilation.
- Colonoscopy with biopsy is diagnostic but may induce megacolon or perforation in severe, extensive disease. Flexible sigmoidoscopy is safer and usually adequate.
- Stool culture and microscopy is used to exclude additional infection.

Management

1 Mild attacks of proctitis or proctosigmoiditis can be treated topically with 5-aminosalicylic acid (5-ASA) suppositories or enemas or steroid enemas. If these are not tolerated, or if there is involvement of more of the colon, oral 5-ASA or steroids may also be used.

2 Severe attacks or fulminant colitis should be treated with high dose steroids (oral or intravenous). Fluid and antibiotic management is often required. Ciclosporin may induce remissions in refractory attacks.
3 Maintenance therapy is with low dose 5-aminosalicylic acid. Steroids can maintain remission but due to long term side effects steroid sparing agents such as azathioprine are often used. Azathioprine requires careful monitoring as it may cause abnormal liver function tests or bone marrow suppression. Azathioprine should be avoided in patients who are TPMT (thiopurine-S-methyltransferase) deficient as they are at particular risk of bone marrow suppression.
4 Alternative treatments: Intravenous heparin and nicotine patches have been shown in some studies to help induction of remission in refractory UC, but are not recommended as maintenance therapy.
  - Surgical treatment: Pan-proctocolectomy with permanent ileostomy involves removal of all the colonic mucosa and is curative.
  - Colectomy and ileorectal anastomosis does not require ileostomy but proctitis may persist causing diarrhoea and cancer surveillance is still necessary.
  - Pan colectomy with retention of the anal sphincters allows anastomosis via an ileal pouch. This removes all diseased mucosa.
  - Emergency surgery for perforation, toxic dilation, massive bleeding and refractory severe exacerbations may be necessary but carries a significant mortality.

Prognosis

Relapses and remissions with overall prognosis related to the extent of the disease. 3–5% of patients with UC develop colonic carcinoma, the risk is much greater in those with active disease for more than 10 years.

Crohn's disease

Definition

A chronic granulomatous inflammatory bowel disease (IBD), which may affect the whole bowel (see Table 4.4).

Incidence
5–6 per 100,000 per year.

Age
Peak incidence 20–50 years.

Sex
M = F

Geography
Incidence varies from country to country, most common in the West.

Aetiology
1 Familial: There is significant concordance between monozygotic twins. Crohn's disease is more common in relatives of patients.
2 Genetic: HLA B27 is more common in patients with IBD. A specific susceptibility gene for Crohn's disease has been found on chromosome 16, IBD1. This encodes a protein, NOD2, which regulates macrophage activation in response to intracellular lipopolysaccharide.
3 Smoking: Patients with Crohn's disease are more likely to be tobacco smokers.
4 Some suggestion of infective trigger, but no clear evidence.

Pathophysiology
Crohn's disease is a chronic relapsing and remitting inflammatory disease that can affect any part of the gastrointestinal tract. The site most commonly affected is the terminal ileum. The disease may affect a small area of the bowel or may be extensive affecting the whole bowel. Multiple areas may be affected with normal bowel inbetween termed 'skip lesions'.

Clinical features
The clinical picture is dependent on the area affected. Colonic disease presents with passage of blood and mucus, terminal ileal disease often presents with diarrhoea, abdominal pain and weight loss. Abdominal pain is variable from chronic to acute, and may occur in any part of the abdomen. It may mimic other pathologies such as intestinal obstruction or acute appendicitis. Specific features to be elucidated include oral or perianal ulceration, joint pain and swelling, rashes such as erythema nodosum, and signs of iritis.

Macroscopy
In early disease there is oedema of the mucosa and submucosa resulting in a loss of transverse folds. Later in the course there is a cobblestone effect due to submucosal oedema and deep fissured ulcers. Bowel wall thickening and strictures result from oedema and fibrosis. These areas are interspersed by normal areas of bowel.

Microscopy
Transmural (full thickness) inflammatory cell infiltrates are seen. Ulcers extend deep within the bowel wall, fissures and fibrous scars are also seen. Non-caesating granulomas in the presence of mucosal changes of inflammatory bowel disease are characteristic and diagnostic of Crohn's disease.

Complications
Fibrosis and scarring leads to stricture formation and intestinal obstruction. Inflammation of the serosal surface may cause adhesions and intestinal obstruction. Transmural inflammation may lead to fisulae, perforation and abscess formation. In long-standing disease there is an increased incidence of carcinoma of the bowel.

Investigations
- Anaemia may be due to chronic disease, iron deficiency or vitamin B_{12} or folate deficiency. The platelet count may be raised in active disease.
- Inflammatory markers such as C reactive protein and ESR may be raised.
- A small bowel contrast follow through may reveal deep ulceration and areas of narrowing (sting sign). Strictures are also demonstrated.
- Colonosocopy with biopsy is diagnostic. Capsular endoscopy can be used to visualise the small bowel.
- Other investigations include a white cell scan to identify areas of active inflammation and MRI scanning for perianal disease.

Management

Symptomatic treatment includes anti-diarrhoeal agents such as loperamide or codeine phosphate. Anaemia is supported with ferrous sulphate.

Acute exacerbations:

- Induction of remission. Mild cases may be treated initially with 5-aminosalicylic acid (5-ASA) drugs such as mesalazine. The next step is often antibiotics in ileitis or colitis (usually ciprofloxacin and metronidazole) – these may work by reducing inflammation due to infection, or transmigration of bacteria through the gut wall. Moderate or severe cases require corticosteroids which may be given as enemas in colonic disease or orally/parenterally, often in combination with 5-ASA drugs and antibiotics. Steroids are withdrawn following induction of remission, but relapse may occur.
- Maintenance of remission – apart from 5-ASA drugs, steroid-sparing agents such as azathioprine and 6-mercaptopurine may be used to allow the reduction and withdrawal of steroid dose. Azathioprine requires careful monitoring as it may cause bone marrow suppression particularly in TPMT deficient patients (see above) or abnormal liver function tests.
- Infliximab (a monoclonal antibody directed against tumour necrosis factor alpha –TNFα) is used in moderate to severe Crohn's disease, particularly for fistulising Crohn's.
- Elemental and polymeric diets may be used, particularly in children.

Surgical: 80–90% of patients will require some form of surgical intervention during their lifetime. Surgery may be required for complications or if there is failure of medical treatment and severe symptoms. The procedure involves resection of affected bowel; however, poor wound healing may lead to fistulas, so surgery is avoided if possible.

Prognosis

The condition runs a course of relapses and remissions. Virtually all patients will have a significant relapse within 20 years. Mortality is twice that of the general population, operative mortality of 5%. The risk of malignancy is 2–3% (slightly higher than the general population).

Disorders of the rectum and anus

Haemorrhoids (piles)

Definition
Enlarged and engorged veins in or around the anus.

Aetiology
Associated with constipation and straining to pass stool or during labour. Suggested that low fibre Western diet accounts for increased incidence.

Pathophysiology
It is thought that increased abdominal pressure causes dilatation of the internal haemorrhoidal plexus of blood vessels. These drain to the portal system and contain no valves.

- First degree piles bulge into the lumen without prolapsing through the anus.
- Second degree piles prolapse on defecation but return spontaneously.
- Third degree piles remain prolapsed but can be actively returned.
- Fourth degree piles are those that can not be returned to the anal canal. The anal sphincter contracts around a prolapsed haemorrhoid causing venous congestion and a risk of thrombosis.

Clinical features
Patients normally present with rectal bleeding which is typically a bright red streak on the toilet paper. Severe bleeding may cause blood in the toilet. Prolapse may be noted and cause a mucus discharge. Pain occurs with strangulated or thrombosed piles.

Investigations
Proctoscopy visualises the piles, prolapse is demonstrated on straining. Flexible sigmoidoscopy is essential in cases of rectal bleeding to exclude other pathology and a barium enema or colonoscopy may be indicated depending on the index of suspicion of inflammatory bowel disease or malignancy.

Management

Small asymptomatic piles are managed conservatively, a high-fibre diet may reduce constipation. First-degree piles can be treated by sclerosing injection into the pedicle. More severe haemorrhoids may be treated by following:

- Ligation: The pile is pulled down through a proctoscope and a rubber band is applied to the pedicle. One pile is treated at a time with intervals of 3 weeks between treatments.
- Infrared photocoagulation causes necrosis within the haemorrhoid and hence shrinkage.
- Haemorrhoidectomy requires ligation and excision. Post-operative pain is common especially on defecation. Complications include haemorrhage and rarely anal stenosis, abscesses, fissures or fistulas.

Rectal prolapse

Definition

Prolapse of the rectum through the anal canal. Rectal prolapses may be incompletely through the anus (Type I), complete prolapse by intussusception of the rectum (Type II) or complete prolapse due to a sliding hernia of the pouch of Douglas (Type III).

Incidence

Type I is more common in children, type II and III in adults, 85% female.

Aetiology

Partial prolapse is more likely when there is a shallow sacral curve such that the rectum is directly above the anus. Complete prolapse results from poor pelvic floor muscle tone, which may follow gynaecological surgery. 10% of children with cystic fibrosis present with rectal prolapse.

Pathophysiology

Initially prolapse only occurs on defecation with spontaneous return; however, with time the prolapse becomes more permanent.

Clinical features

There is often discomfort on passing stool possibly with bleeding and mucus due to inflammation of the prolapsed segment. Weakness in the surrounding musculature may cause irregular bowel motions, faecal incontinence may occur. The prolapse may only be demonstrated on straining.

Management

- Children are often managed conservatively, it is rare for the prolapse to persist beyond the age of 5. Constipation should be avoided by dietary intervention.
- Partial prolapsing mucosa is excised by dissection and ligation. If the sphincter control is poor, surgery will not affect bowel habit which may improve with sphincter exercises.
- Complete prolapse requires a pelvic repair procedure including mobilisation of the rectum, fixation to the sacrum and suture of the levator ani muscles to the front of the rectum. If incontinence persists suturing of the sphincters may help. Colostomy may be considered in frail elderly patients.

Fissure-in-ano

Definition

An anal fissure is a tear in the skin lining the lower anal canal.

Aetiology

1 Primary fissure-in-ano are idiopathic, they are generally posterior. Patients often report the onset of symptoms when passing hard, constipated stool.
2 Secondary fissure-in-ano are seen in inflammatory bowel disease when they are often multiple and may occur anywhere around the anal circumference.

Pathophysiology

Fissures are longitudinal tears, which develop into canoe shaped ulcers involving the lower third of the internal sphincter. Swelling and inflammation at the anal verge may form a sentinel pile (haemorrhoid).

Clinical features

Severe burning pain on defecation that may last for hours so that defecation is avoided. The sentinel pile may be visible on examination, rectal examination is very painful and often impossible. Examination under anaesthesia (proctoscopy/sigmoidoscopy) allows diagnosis.

Complications
Infections may form a perianal abscess.

Management
Primary anal fissures may heal spontaneously. Refractory fissures may require surgical management. An incision is made into the perianal skin on one side of the anal canal and the internal sphincter is divided without entering the lumen.

Fistula-in-ano

Definition
A fistula is an abnormal communication between one epithelial surface and another. A fistula-in-ano connects the anal canal to the perianal skin.

Aetiology
Most anal fistulae have no obvious cause. Associations include inflammatory bowel disease, tuberculosis and carcinoma of the rectum.
1 Low anal fistula is the commonest form with a communication from the anal canal below the level of the anal crypts to the perianal skin.
2 High anal fistulas have a track which extends above the pectinate line below the anorectal ring. The muscle fibres of the internal and external anal sphincter surround the rectum. In both low and high fistulas the track of the fistula may pass through the fibres of both sphincters or descend in the intersphincteric space.
3 Anorectal fistula
   • Pelvirectal fistula is a direct communication between the rectum and the skin bypassing the anal canal and passing through the levator ani muscle.
   • Ischiorectal fistula is similar to a low fistula, but with additional extension upwards towards the rectum without penetrating the levator ani muscle.

Pathophysiology
Goodsall's rule states that if the fistula lies in the anterior half of the anal area then it opens directly into the anal canal, while if a fistula lies in the posterior half of the canal then it tracks around the anus laterally and opens into the midline posteriorly.

Clinical features
Patients often present with an abscess, the incision of which completes the fistula. Patients with a completed fistula present with a discharging sinus that causes localised pruritus and excoriation.

Investigations
Proctoscopy may reveal the internal opening with a flexible probe used to demonstrate the track. Sigmoidoscopy is required to exclude associated rectal diseases.

Management
Primary fistulas are laid open to granulate and epithelialise. In pelvirectal fistulas such an incision would divide the anorectal ring causing incontinence. These and secondary fistulae are treated conservatively.

Pilonidal sinus

Definition
A sinus of the natal cleft containing hair that often becomes infected.

Aetiology/pathophysiology
It is thought that sinuses arise from penetration of hairs subcutaneously with secondary infection. A post anal pilonidal sinus typically occurs around 2 cm posterior to the anus and extends superiorly and subcutaneously for about 2–5 cm.

Clinical features
The sinus only becomes symptomatic when infection causes an abscess with swelling, tenderness and discharge.

Management
Abscesses are drained, de-roofed and cleaned under general anaesthetic. The cavity is left open to granulate. Pilonidal sinuses tend to recur.

Anorectal abscess

Definition
Anorectal abscesses may occur as perianal, ischiorectal or high muscular abscess.

Age
Most common 20–40 years.

Sex
2M : 1F

Aetiology
In the majority of patients there is no apparent cause for abscess formation. Recurrent abscesses occur in inflammatory bowel disease, HIV and rectal carcinoma.

Pathophysiology
Infection of an anal gland may cause a tracking down to form a perianal abscess, or tracking out to form a ischiorectal abscess, or upwards to produce a high intermuscular abscess.

Clinical features
- Perianal abscess is common and presents in well patients with an acute tender swelling at the anal verge.
- Ischiorectal abscess present with a diffuse hard painful swelling lateral to the anus, which may extend behind the anal canal to form a horseshoe abscess. Patients have significant systemic upset.

- High intermuscular abscesses cause pain exacerbated on defecation, a boggy tender swelling is felt on rectal examination.

Management
Perianal and ischiorectal abscesses are drained under general anaesthetic and de-roofed by making a cruciate incision and excising the resultant 4 triangles of skin. 25% of abscesses recur.

Vascular disease of the bowel

Intestinal ischaemia
Intestinal ischaemia results from a failure of the blood supply to the bowel. Certain areas of bowel are more susceptible to ischaemia (e.g. the splenic flexure) due to the pattern of blood supply. Three underlying pathologies are in operation resulting in a number of clinical entities all with three possible outcomes (see Fig. 4.9).

Focal ischaemia of the bowel

Definition
Localised bowel pathology may result in focal area of ischaemia.

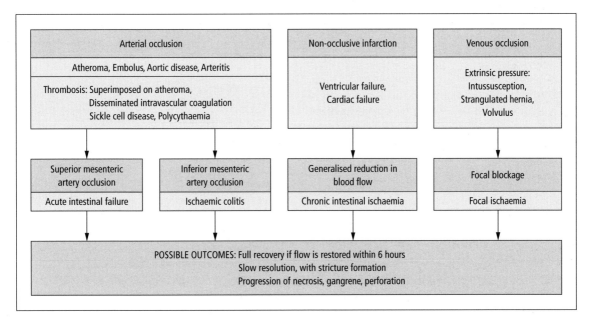

Figure 4.9 Intestinal ischaemia.

Aetiology
Underlying causes include strangulation of a hernia, intussusception, or a volvulus in which a loop of bowel twists on itself usually around a fibrous peritoneal band or adhesion.

Pathophysiology
The ischaemia results from venous infarction due to strangulation. The thin draining veins are occluded by external pressure resulting in venous congestion and hence a failure of arterial supply to the segment of bowel.

Clinical features/management
The underlying cause requires identification and treatment. If blood flow is not restored, a progression to infarction and necrosis necessitates bowel resection.

Ischaemic colitis

Definition
Ischaemia of the colon due to interruption of its blood supply.

Aetiology
In most cases the underlying cause is thrombosis of the inferior mesenteric artery, embolisation of mural thrombus in atrial fibrillation, or non-occlusive infarction.

Pathophysiology
In around half the ischaemia is transient with damage confined to the mucosa and submucosa. The splenic flexure is most often affected due to the territories of the arteries supplying the bowel. If the blood supply is not restored, ischaemia progresses to gangrenous ischaemic colitis. The presentation and treatment is as for acute intestinal failure (see page 177).

Clinical features
The patient presents with lower abdominal pain, nausea, vomiting and bloody diarrhoea. There is lower abdominal tenderness and guarding in the lower abdomen.

Microscopy
There is ischaemic loss of mucosa, ulceration and later healing with oedema and inflammatory infiltrate.

Complications
Ischaemic strictures may result from scarring at the splenic flexure or sigmoid colon. These are confirmed on barium studies and require resection.

Investigations
A barium enema can be used to show oedema or mucosal sloughing. Bleeding into the bowel wall produces a thumb print appearance. Mesenteric angiography will demonstrate the stenosis or occlusion.

Management
The condition generally is self-limiting within a few days with uncomplicated cases managed conservatively.

Chronic intestinal ischaemia

Definition
Slow progressive ischaemia of the gut due to atheroma generally occurring in the elderly.

Aetiology
Atheroma within the mesenteric vessels causes reduced blood flow and ischaemia. Risk factors:
- Fixed: Age, sex, positive family history, familial hyperlipidaemia.
- Modifiable: Smoking (direct relationship to the number of cigarettes smoked), hypertension, diabetes mellitus, LDL and total cholesterol levels (HDL are protective).

Pathophysiology
Progressive atheroma occludes the lumen of the vessels causing reduced blood flow. The clinical presentation depends on the position and degree of occlusion and the presence of collateral blood supply.

Clinical features
Patients describe pain occurring after food, weight loss, malabsorption and signs of vascular disease.

Investigations
The diagnosis is made on angiography.

Management
Surgical revascularisation depends on the results of angiography. A variant of this condition is coeliac axis

compression due to the median arcuate ligament of the diaphragm. This may be amenable to surgery.

Acute intestinal failure

Definition
Complete necrosis and gangrene of the midgut resulting from cessation of blood flow in the superior mesenteric artery. It is predominantly a disease of the elderly.

Clinical features
There may be a preceding history of non-specific symptoms (variable abdominal pain, diarrhoea, vomiting and weight loss). Signs of acute intestinal failure include abdominal tenderness, guarding, loss of bowel sounds and rigidity, due to perforation.

Investigations
Calcification within the abdominal aorta may be evident on abdominal X-ray. Gas filled, thickened, dilated bowel loops and free gas within the peritoneal cavity due to perforation may also be seen. Angiography or spiral CT can identify the vascular occlusion.

Management
Following adequate resuscitation laparotomy and resection (which may be massive) are required. Removal of the vascular occlusion may be possible (e.g. embolectomy). A second look laparotomy can be performed 24 hours later to re-examine any segment of bowel the viability of which was questionable.

Prognosis
The overall prognosis is poor with 70–90% mortality. If the patient survives they have considerable malabsorption problems.

Gastrointestinal oncology

Oesophageal carcinoma

Definition
Primary malignant cancer arising in the oesophagus.

Age
Rare below the age of 40 years.

Sex
M > F

Geography
Particularly common in Japan and China.

Aetiology
- Squamous carcinoma accounts for more than 90% of cases. These usually occur in the middle third of the oesophagus although the lower third may also be affected. Aetiological factors include high alcohol consumption, smoking and chewing betel nuts.
- Adenocarcinoma makes up the remaining 10% and affects the lower third of the oesophagus particularly the gastrooesophageal junction possibly following epithelial metaplasia from squamous to columnar cells as a result of gastro oesophageal reflux (Barrett's oesophagus).
- Familial forms have been noted.

Pathophysiology
Carcinomas spread along the mucosa and submucosa, invading adjacent structures and lymph nodes, distant metastases are rare. Adenocarcinoma tends to metastasise earlier.

Clinical features
Patients may present with progressive dysphagia, but often present late with weight loss, anaemia and malaise. On examination there may be cervical lymphadenopathy, cervical mass and hepatomegaly.

Investigations
Barium swallow demonstrates an apple core defect or stricture without proximal dilatation. Endoscopy allows visualisation and biopsy of oedematous friable mucosa proximal to the obstruction. Initial staging (TMN) should include spiral CT of the chest and abdomen to look for metastases. In the absence of metastases endoscopic ultrasound is useful to assess operability. Other techniques include abdominal ultrasound scanning, MRI scanning, bronchoscopy and laparoscopy.

Management
- Wherever possible surgical resection is the primary treatment with those occurring in the lower third being the most amenable to surgery. Anatomical

reconstruction requires either a gastric pull up, or a section of colon on a pedicle flap. Neoadjuvant chemotherapy with cisplatin and 5-fluorouracil (5-FU) improves short term survival over surgery alone.

- Squamous cell carcinoma may be sensitive to radiotherapy in inoperable cases, this is usually used in conjunction with combination chemotherapy (chemoradiation). Chemoradiation is the treatment of choice for localised squamous cell carcinoma of the proximal oesophagus.
- Palliative treatments include stricture dilation, or endoscopic insertion of covered/uncovered metal stent, argon plasma coagulation (APC) and laser.

Prognosis

Surgical resection carries an operative mortality of up to 20%. Prognosis remains poor with only 5% 5-year survival.

Benign gastric tumours

Definition

Benign tumours and polyps of the stomach. These can be divided into epithelial and mesenchymal derived tumours:

Epithelial derived, polypoid structures:

- Hyperplastic polyps are common overgrowths of gastric mucosa often resulting from the healing of an ulcer.
- Adenomatous polyps are rare benign tumours of the surface epithelium which may be single or multiple. They have a significant risk of malignant change most likely in large polyps.
- Hamartomas are seen in Peutz–Jeghers syndrome.

Mesenchymal derived benign tumours:

- Leiomyomas appear as mucosal or intramural nodules.

Clinical features

Most benign tumours are asymptomatic and found on endoscopy or barium meal. Rarely bleeding or obstruction with vomiting may occur.

Management

All suspicious polyps require examination by endoscopic excision biopsy, multiple polyps may require gastric resection. Leiomyomas are treated by surgical excision.

Gastric adenocarcinoma

Definition

Malignant tumour of the stomach.

Incidence

10 per 10,000 per year, accounts for 10% of cancer deaths due to late presentation.

Age

More than 30 years. Incidence rises above age 50 years.

Sex

2M > 1F

Geography

Highest in Japan and Chile.

Aetiology

Pre-malignant conditions include chronic atrophic gastritis with intestinal metaplasia and adenomatous polyps of the stomach.

- *H. pylori* causes atrophic gastritis resulting in dysplasia and neoplasia.
- Dietary carcinogens possibly including nitrates and alcohol. Salt may be involved.

Pathophysiology

Gastric adenocarcinomas are derived from mucus secreting epithelial cells most occurring in the antrum. Tumours may be of three types:

- Ulcerating (most common) with appearance similar to benign ulcers but with raised edges and no normal mucosa.
- Polypoidal which often bleed leading to earlier presentation.
- Infiltrating when fibrous tissue causes a firm non-distendable or linitis plastica (leather bottle) stomach.

It tends to present late with non-specific symptoms.

Spread may be direct invasion to the liver and pancreas, transcoelomic spread resulting in a malignant ascites and ovarian Krukenberg tumour, lymphatic spread to regional and distant lymph nodes (Virkow's node) and via the portal circulation to the liver.

Clinical features

Patients tend to present late with non-specific weight loss, anorexia and anaemia. There may be dyspepsia or haematemesis. In early stages there may be occult blood in faeces. Examination reveals epigastric tenderness and often a mass. Dermatomyositis and acanthosis nigricans may be manifestations of an underlying gastric malignancy.

Microscopy

Histologically gastric adenocarcinomas may have an intestinal pattern with gland like spaces or they may be diffuse infiltrative carcinoma with sheets of anaplastic cells which have a mucin containing vacuole.

Investigations

Diagnostic testing usually involves an endoscopy and biopsy, which may be preceded by a barium meal. If there is an associated ascites diagnostic tapping and cytological examination may be useful. Anaemia is a non-specific finding and liver metastases may cause a rise in liver function tests. A CT scan is used for staging and surgical planning.

Management

Treatment of choice is surgical resection wherever possible. At laparotomy if there is no evidence of local invasion or spread beyond local nodes, a partial gastrectomy is performed for distal carcinoma (Bilroth II with anastomosis to the jejunum and closure of the duodenal stump) or in proximal carcinomas a total gastrectomy is performed. Lymph node clearance is performed of regional nodes. Palliative resections may be performed for blood loss or obstruction. Combination chemotherapy may be used in disease not amenable to surgery.

Prognosis

In Japan early disease cure rates are up to 90%. Overall 5-year survival in the United Kingdom is around 10% due to late presentation.

Gastric lymphoma

Definition

A primary lymphoma of the stomach which accounts for 3% of malignant gastric tumours.

Aetiology/pathophysiology

Gastric lymphoma is a non-Hodgkin B cell lymphoma. Tumours arising in the mucosa associated lymphoid tissue (MALT) result from *H. pylori* infection in over 90% of cases.

Clinical features

Patients present similarly to gastric adenocarcinoma with non-specific weight loss, anaemia and malaise and associated epigastric tenderness. Symptoms may be mild despite a large tumour mass.

Microscopy

Lymphoma cells range from small cells to large immunoblastic cells.

Investigations

Endoscopy and biopsy is diagnostic.

Management

Lymphoma often responds to *H. pylori* eradication therapy. As there is potential for recurrence frequent upper gastrointestinal endoscopy and multiple biopsies are recommended for all patients following eradication therapy. Patients who do not respond to, or who relapse following eradication therapy are treated with single agent chemotherapy (e.g. cyclophosphamide or chlorambucil) or radiation therapy. Patients with advanced or aggressive disease and those who fail to respond or recur after single agent chemotherapy are treated with multiagent chemotherapy, such as CHOP (cyclophosphamide, doxorubicin, vincristine and prednisone). Surgery is now rarely indicated.

Prognosis

Postoperative 5-year survival of 80–90%.

Small intestine lymphoma

Definition

A non-Hodgkin lymphoma which occurs within the small bowel particularly in the ileum.

Aetiology/pathophysiology

- Non-Hodgkin B cell lymphoma arises in the mucosal associated lymphoid tissue (MALT) and occurs within the distal ileum.

- T cell lymphomas form ulcerated plaques or strictures in the proximal small bowel. Coeliac disease predisposes to a T cell lymphoma, treatment with gluten free diets may reduce the risk.
- A Burkitt lymphoma like tumour occurs in children from North Africa and the Middle East.
- Immunoproliferative small intestine disease (IPSID) is a condition characterised by plasma cell proliferation in the lamina propria of the small bowel. IPSID occurs mainly in the Mediterranean and presents with malabsorption. Transformation into lymphoma may occur.
- Perforation, bleeding and obstruction may occur with any form of lymphoma.

Management

Resection is performed where possible, radiotherapy and chemotherapy are often used postoperatively, although their efficacy is uncertain. Inoperable disease is treated by combination chemotherapy; radiotherapy is used for palliation. IPSID not complicated by lymphoma is treated with antibiotics.

Carcinoid tumours of the intestine

Definition

Tumours originating from neuroendocrine or APUD (amine precursor uptake and decarboxylation) cells of the intestine.

Aetiology/pathophysiology

Carcinoid tumours most commonly occur in the appendix, terminal ileum and rectum. Small bowel, colonic and stomach lesions grow slowly and metastasise to the liver. Rectal and appendix carcinoids almost never metastasise.

Clinical features

Most lesions are asymptomatic although appendix carcinoids may present with acute appendicitis. Carcinoid syndrome occurs in 5% with liver metastases, the features of which (see Table 4.5) depend on the hormones produced.

Table 4.5 Features of carcinoid syndrome

System	Symptom	Frequency (%)
Skin	Flushing	85
	Telangectasia	25
	Cyanosis	18
Gastrointestinal	Diarrhoea and pain	80
Cardiac	Valvular lesions	50
Respiratory	Bronchospasm	19

Macroscopy/microscopy

Carcinoid tumours appear as a yellow–white mural nodule composed of cords and nests of cells with secretory granules.

Investigations

Plasma chromogranin A is raised in carcinoid tumours. Urinary 5-hydroxyindoleacetic acid (a 5 HT metabolite) is useful for carcinoid tumours of the midgut. Staging investigations include octreotide scanning, liver ultrasound, spiral CT scanning, MRI scanning and endoscopic ultrasound.

Management

Resection of the primary tumour (e.g. by appendicectomy) is performed where possible. Octreotide (somatostatin analogue) relieves diarrhoea and flushing and may reduce tumour growth. Other treatments include chemotherapy, embolisation and thermal ablation.

Large bowel neoplastic polyps

Definition

A polyp is defined as a tumour attached by a stalk to the surface from which they arise. Neoplastic polyps of the colon are also known as adenomas.

Incidence

Affects 5–10% of the population in the Western world.

Age

Sporadic cases increase with age.

Aetiology/pathophysiology

Polyps may be solitary (sporadic) or multiple, e.g. familial adenomatous polyposis. Neoplastic polyps may be tubular, villous or tubular-villous dependent on histological features.

- Tubular polyps account for 90% and consist of glandular tubules with a fibrovascular core covered by a mucous membrane.
- Villous adenomas are composed of finger like epithelial projections, spread over a large area within the mucosa.
- Tubular villous adenomata are composed of both patterns.

Clinical features

Most are asymptomatic but they may cause bleeding and diarrhoea.

Complications

All neoplastic polyps are pre-malignant, low lesions may prolapse through the anus.

Management

Tubular polyps are resected endoscopically, villous lesions require transmural excision or formal resection.

Prognosis

There is a 30–50% risk of recurrence therefore surveillance with 3–5 yearly colonoscopy in patients under 75 years is suggested.

Large bowel carcinoma

Definition

Large bowel malignant adenocarcinoma.

Incidence

Lifetime incidence of 1 in 25. Second most common cause of cancer death.

Age

Average 60–65 years.

Sex

Rectal cancer M > F; colonic cancer F > M.

Geography

Rare in Africa and Asia (thought to be environmental).

Aetiology

Most colorectal cancers arise from adenomatous polyps with a median transition of 20 years. Ulcerative colitis is associated with an increased incidence.

- Genetic predisposing conditions include familial adenomatous polyposis, hereditary non-polyposis colon cancer. There is an overall increased incidence in first-degree relatives.
- Dietary factors such as a high animal fat and low fibre intake.

Pathophysiology

Colonic cancer occurs in the sigmoid colon and rectum (50%), caecum and ascending colon (30%) and transverse and descedending colon (20%). Carcinomas may be polypoidal, ulcerating or stenosing. The tumour spreads by direct infiltration into the bowel wall and circumferential spread. Subsequent invasion of the blood and lymphatics results in distant metastasis most frequently to the liver.

Clinical features

Presentation is dependant on the site of the lesion, but in general a combination of altered bowel habit and bleeding with or without pain is reported. Up to a third of patients present with obstruction, or perforation. Caecal or ascending colonic cancers often present later with iron deficiency anaemia. Examination may reveal a mass (on abdominal palpation or rectal examination), ascites and hepatomegaly.

Macroscopy/microscopy

Raised red lesions with a rolled edge and central ulceration. Adenocarcinomas are composed of glandular tissue made up of pleomorphic neoplastic epithelial cells.

Investigations

- Endoscopic examination of the large bowel with biopsy is diagnostic.
- Barium enema or CT pneumocolon may also detect tumours.
- LFTs, liver ultrasound scan and chest X-rays are used to look for metastatic spread.
- Pre-symptomatic disease may be identified by surveillance colonoscopy in at risk patients.

Table 4.6 Dukes classification of colorectal carcinoma

Dukes stage	Tumour spread	5-year survival (%)
A	Not extending through the muscularis propria	>90
B	Extending through the muscularis propria but no node involvement	70
C	Any nodal involvement	30
D	Distant metastases	5

- In a recent study the use of faecal occult blood testing as screening has a positive predictive value was 11% for cancer and 35% for adenoma. 48% of all detected cancers were Dukes stage A (see Table 4.6).

Management
Primary resection is the treatment of choice in fit patients (see also page 148).
- Tumours of the right and transverse colon require right hemicolectomy and ileocolic anastomosis.
- Tumours of the descending colon are treated with left hemicolectomy.
- Tumours of the sigmoid colon are treated with a sigmoid colectomy.

In all the procedures the associated mesentery and regional lymph nodes are removed en bloc.

Most rectal tumours are treated by anterior resection. In very low rectal lesions an abdominoperineal (AP) resection with formation of a permanent colostomy in the left iliac fossa may be required.

Resections may be curative or palliative, if resection is not possible a bypass procedure may be carried out. Adjuvant chemotherapy based on 5-fluorouracil (5-FU) is performed in patients with Dukes stage C (see below) but has not been shown to be beneficial in Stage A or B disease, or in elderly patients who have a higher incidence of complications. Patients with limited hepatic metastases may benefit from resection of the metastases.

Rectal carcinomas are just as likely to recur locally as metastasise distantly, so treatment is best with local radiotherapy and adjuvant chemotherapy.

Prognosis
The overall 5-year survival rate is 40% but this depends on Dukes staging (see Table 4.6).

Anal squamous cell carcinoma

Definition
The anal canal is lined with stratified squamous epithelium and thus is prone to development of epithelial derived tumours.

Incidence
Much less common than rectal carcinoma.

Sex
M > F

Clinical features
Patients present with a localised ulcer or a wart like growth, there is often associated bleeding and discharge. Inguinal lymph nodes may be stony hard if spread has occurred. In female patients an ano-vaginal fistula may result in offensive vaginal discharge.

Investigations
Suspect lesions require biopsy.

Management
Treatment is by combined local radiotherapy and chemotherapy rather than abdominoperineal resection. Early metastases are frequent.

Familial adenomatous polyposis

Definition
Familial adenomatous polyposis is a rare genetic condition in which patients develop multiple polyps.

Aetiology/pathophysiology
This is an autosomal dominant condition in which there is a defect in the adenomatous polyposis (apc) gene on the long arm of chromosome 5. Multiple polyps develop during childhood throughout the large bowel.

Clinical features
Patients may be identified through screening of known relatives. The presence of multiple polyps may lead to bleeding, diarrhoea and mucus discharge.

Complications

Malignant change is inevitable as each polyp carries a risk of transformation. Adenocarcinoma is unlikely before the age of 20.

Investigations

Colonoscopy is used to screen relatives above 12 years.

Management

Definitive treatment involves a total colectomy and ileo-rectal anastomosis with ileal pouch formation. The rectal stump requires continuing surveillance.

Peutz–Jegher syndrome

Definition

Syndrome characterised by intestinal polyposis and freckling of the lips.

Aetiology

Autosomal dominant inheritance pattern, most cases involve mutations in the PJ gene on chromosome 19.

Clinical features

Patients are found to have mucocutaneous pigmentation characteristically around the mouth, hands and feet. Gastrointestinal hamartomatous polyps are found in the small bowel, colon and stomach.

Complications

Polyps may bleed or cause intussusception, but are not pre-malignant.

Management

Multiple polypectomies may be required, but bowel resection should be avoided.

Clinical

Symptoms

Pain from the liver, biliary and pancreatic systems

Pain originating from the liver, biliary tree or pancreas is usually felt in the upper third of the abdomen. The features of the pain that should be elicited in the history are the same as those for abdominal pain (see page 139).

Pain from the liver

This is usually felt in the right upper quadrant of the abdomen, right loin or epigastrium. It may radiate through to the back. The pain is due to stretching of the liver capsule following recent swelling of the liver, as caused by right heart failure and acute viral or alcohol-induced hepatitis. It is typically a dull, constant, aching pain. Liver metastases may also cause pain as a presenting feature, especially in later stages. Associated symptoms may include nausea and jaundice.

Pain from the gallbladder and biliary tree

- Biliary colic is the term used to describe the pain due to obstruction of the biliary system, for example by a stone. The patient complains of very severe constant pain with excruciating colicky spasms felt in the upper abdomen, which may radiate to the back or right subscapular region. The onset is sudden, often after a meal

(postprandial) or at night and the pain usually lasts up to 2 or 3 hours without relief except with strong analgesia. Associated features commonly include nausea, vomiting and sweating. Jaundice occurs in about a fifth of patients.

- Acute cholecystitis, when the gallbladder becomes inflamed due to infection, causes more well-localised, constant pain as the parietal peritoneum becomes involved. The patient complains of pain in the right hypochondrium, which often radiates to the right shoulder tip. The pain is exacerbated by movement and breathing and persists until analgesia is given, and the underlying cause is treated. Unlike biliary colic, the pain lasts more than 3 hours. Associated symptoms include fever, nausea, vomiting and anorexia.

- Gallstones may also cause postprandial indigestion or pain, usually with an onset up to half an hour after eating, lasting 30 minutes to 1.5 hours. It is often worse after fatty foods, and symptoms may recur over several months to years (see also page 215).

Pain from the pancreas

Inflammation of the pancreas, as occurs in acute pancreatitis (see page 218), causes epigastric pain which is often sudden in onset, constant and increasing in severity. The pain may radiate through to the back and towards the left shoulder. Movement and lying down exacerbate the pain and characteristically patients prefer to sit up and lean forwards. Commonly there is persistent nausea, with retching and vomiting. Strong analgesia is required.

Jaundice

Definition

Yellow pigmentation to the sclera and skin, it is clinically evident when the plasma bilirubin level is above 50 mcmol/L (2.5 mg/dL).

Aetiology/pathophysiology

Jaundice is due to an abnormality in the metabolism or excretion of bilirubin, which is derived from haem containing proteins such as haemoglobin.

Unconjugated (water insoluble) bilirubin is transported to the liver bound to albumin. It is taken up by hepatocytes and conjugated in a two-stage process to a water soluble form. Bile containing conjugated bilirubin, bile salts, cholesterol, phospholipids and electrolytes is secreted into the intrahepatic bile ducts and passes to the gallbladder via the common hepatic duct where it is stored. Gallbladder contraction (e.g. following a meal) causes bile to pass via the cystic duct into the common bile duct and hence into the duodenum through the ampulla of Vater (see Fig. 5.1).

Prehepatic jaundice results from excess bilirubin production (e.g. haemolytic anaemia) or abnormalities in bilirubin conjugation such as occur in some forms of congenital hyperbilirubinaemia (Gilbert's syndrome and Crigler–Najjar syndrome). The mildly raised serum bilirubin is unconjugated and other liver function tests are normal.

Hepatic jaundice results from hepatocyte damage with or without intrahepatic cholestasis. Causes include hepatitis of any cause, cirrhosis, drugs, liver metastases, sepsis, other liver diseases and some forms of congenital hyperbilirubinaemia (Dubin–Johnson syndrome and Rotor syndrome). There is raised conjugated and unconjugated bilirubin, and often liver function tests are abnormal due to hepatocyte damage (see page 189).

Posthepatic jaundice results from obstruction of the biliary tree distal to the bile canaliculi of the liver. Causes include gallstones in the common bile duct, pancreatic cancer, cholangiocarcinoma, primary biliary cirrhosis and primary sclerosing cholangitis. There is a conjugated hyperbilirubinaemia with increased urinary excretion of water-soluble conjugated bilirubin. If there is complete

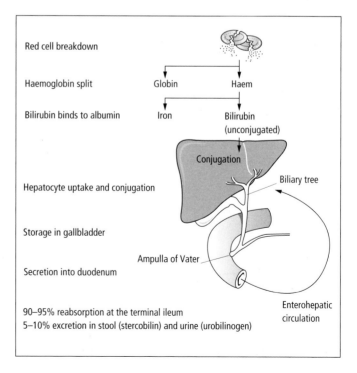

Red cell breakdown

Haemoglobin split — Globin — Haem

Bilirubin binds to albumin — Iron — Bilirubin (unconjugated)

Conjugation

Hepatocyte uptake and conjugation

Biliary tree

Storage in gallbladder

Ampulla of Vater

Secretion into duodenum

Enterohepatic circulation

90–95% reabsorption at the terminal ileum
5–10% excretion in stool (stercobilin) and urine (urobilinogen)

Figure 5.1 Bilirubin metabolism.

obstruction no bile reaches the bowel. This results in dark urine and pale stools. Liver function tests are usually abnormal. Obstruction of the bile system causes alkaline phosphatase to rise first and proportionally more than the aminotransferases.

Clinical features

A careful history should be taken including the following:

- Prodromal 'flu-like' illness up to 2 weeks before onset of jaundice suggests viral hepatitis.
- Other risk factors for infectious causes include previous blood transfusions, intravenous drug use, body piercing, tattoos and high-risk sexual practice.
- Patients should also be asked about jaundiced contacts.
- Previous or present biliary colic/gallstones suggest obstructive jaundice.
- A drug history including prescribed and non-prescribed medication, herbal remedies, alcohol and recreational drugs.

Examination may reveal hepatomegaly and/or splenomegaly, signs of chronic liver disease and portal hypertension.

Investigations

Routine tests:

- U&Es, LFTs (see page 189), FBC, blood film and reticulocytes, clotting profile.
- Viral serology: EBV, CMV, hepatitis A, B and C.
- An ultrasound should be performed to look for dilated bile ducts, gallstones or other causes of biliary obstruction. Further imaging including ERCP and CT scan of the abdomen may be required.
- Other investigations should be considered for specific causes such as autoimmune hepatitis, haemochromatosis, primary biliary cirrhosis and Wilson's disease.

Signs

Hepatomegaly

Hepatomegaly is the term used to describe an enlarged liver. Normally, the liver edge may be just palpable below the right costal margin on deep inspiration, particularly in thin people. It may also be palpable without being enlarged due to downward displacement, e.g. by hyper-

expansion of the thorax in chronic obstructive airways disease, a subdiaphragmatic collection or a Riedel's lobe (an enlarged tongue-like growth of the right lobe of the liver which is a normal variant). To define the size of the liver its span should be percussed. A diseased liver may not always be enlarged, and in late cirrhosis it is more common for it to become small and scarred.

If the liver is palpable, other features should be elicited such as whether it feels soft or hard, regular and smooth or irregular, tender or non-tender, and pulsatile or non-pulsatile. The liver should be auscultated for a bruit. Associated features, depending on the underlying cause, may include splenomegaly, signs of chronic liver disease, lymphadenopathy and/or a raised jugular venous pressure.

The most common causes of a palpable liver in the developed world:

- Cardiac failure – right heart failure leads to a smooth, firm, tender liver due to congestion.
- Cirrhosis – particularly in early alcoholic cirrhosis. The liver is non-tender and firm.
- Cancer – metastases in the liver cause a hard, craggy, irregular or nodular surface.

Less common causes:

- Haematological malignancies (chronic leukaemia, lymphoma) and myeloproliferative disease can cause massive hepatomegaly.
- Infections such as acute hepatitis (smooth, tender), liver abscess or hydatid cysts.
- Primary hepatocellular carcinoma (may be tender and may have an arterial bruit).
- Fatty liver.
- Haemochromatosis.
- Sarcoid, amyloid.

A tender liver indicates recent stretching of the liver capsule by enlargement, such as caused by cardiac failure or acute hepatitis. A pulsatile liver is most commonly caused by tricuspid regurgitation.

Signs of chronic liver disease

There are many signs of chronic liver disease, but in some cases examination can be entirely normal, despite advanced disease (see Fig. 5.2).

The hands:

- Clubbing of the fingers (see page 92).

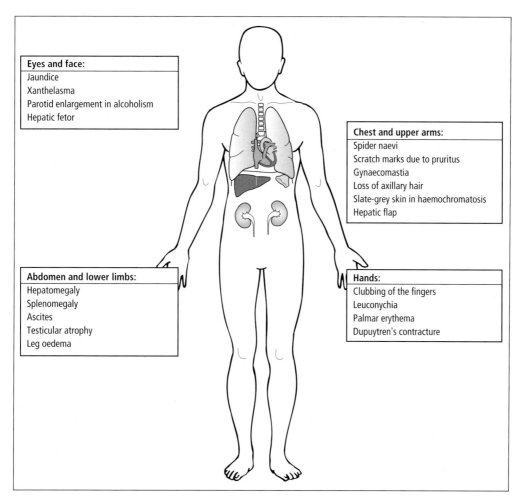

Eyes and face:
Jaundice
Xanthelasma
Parotid enlargement in alcoholism
Hepatic fetor

Chest and upper arms:
Spider naevi
Scratch marks due to pruritus
Gynaecomastia
Loss of axillary hair
Slate-grey skin in haemochromatosis
Hepatic flap

Abdomen and lower limbs:
Hepatomegaly
Splenomegaly
Ascites
Testicular atrophy
Leg oedema

Hands:
Clubbing of the fingers
Leuconychia
Palmar erythema
Dupuytren's contracture

Figure 5.2 Signs of chronic liver disease.

- Leuconychia – the nail appears white and opaque, but the distal end is often spared, it is thought to be due to hypoalbuminaemia.
- Palmar erythema although commonly seen in liver disease, it is also associated with pregnancy, thyrotoxicosis, other diseases and may occur in healthy people. It has been attributed to increased levels of circulating oestrogens, due to altered metabolism.
- Dupuytren's contracture is a thickening of the palmar fascia which may be palpable as thickening or cords and as it progresses flexes the fingers (most commonly the ring and little fingers). It has many causes, including an inherited tendency, but is associated with alcoholic cirrhosis.

The eyes and face:
- Jaundice should be looked for (see page 185).
- Xanthelasma (cholesterol deposits on the eyelids) are seen in primary biliary cirrhosis.
- Parotid enlargement occurs in alcoholism.
- Hepatic fetor is a sweet smell of the breath, which occurs in advanced liver failure.

The chest and upper arms:
- Spider naevi are telangiectases that consist of a central arteriole with radiating small vessels. They blanch if pressure is applied to the centre, then refill outwards. Up to five spider naevi are said to be normal.
- Scratch marks due to pruritus, particularly in primary biliary cirrhosis.

- Gynaecomastia, which may be due to increased oestrogen levels or drugs such as spironalactone. Loss of axillary hair is another sign.
- Tattoos may indicate a possible source of previous hepatitis infection.
- Slate-grey pigmentation of the skin occurs in haemochromatosis.
- There may be a hepatic flap, which is a flapping tremor of the outstretched hands.

The abdomen and lower limbs:

- Hepatomegaly and/or splenomegaly (see page 463).
- Ascites (see page below).
- Caput medusa (see below).
- Testicular atrophy in males.
- Ankle oedema (due to right heart failure or hypoalbuminaemia).

In early cirrhosis liver function is adequate, so that patients are asymptomatic and do not have complications. In more severe disease portal hypertension, low serum albumin and other complications occur. This is called decompensated cirrhosis. Patients may fluctuate back and forth, depending on intercurrent events such as infections.

Signs of decompensated cirrhosis:

- Deep jaundice.
- Ascites, with or without peripheral oedema.
- Hepatic encephalopathy, i.e. any drowsiness, confusion, hepatic flap and hepatic fetor.
- Development of dilated collateral veins, i.e. veins around the umbilicus (caput medusa, which are very rare) or oesophageal varices, which can lead to upper gastrointestinal haemorrhage.

Ascites

Definition
Ascites is the accumulation of fluid within the peritoneal cavity.

Aetiology/pathophysiology
Ascites may be a transudate or an exudate dependent on the protein content (see Table 5.1).

Clinical features
Ascites presents as abdominal distension with shifting dullness and a fluid thrill on examination. Discomfort

Table 5.1 Causes of ascites

Transudate	Exudate
Hypoalbuminaemia (e.g. nephrotic syndrome)	Malignancy
	Chylous ascites
Raised central venous pressure	Hepatic vein obstruction (Budd–Chiari syndrome)
Chronic liver disease	Pancreatitis
Portal vein obstruction	Inflammatory bowel disease
Congestive cardiac failure	

is common but severe pain is more likely to result from the underlying cause.

Investigations
The diagnosis can be confirmed by ultrasonography. A diagnostic aspiration of the fluid should be obtained. A transudate is suggested by a protein of ≥ 11 g/L below the serum albumin level.

- Clear fluid is seen in liver disease and hypoalbuminaemia. Bloodstained fluid suggests malignancy. Milky fluid suggests chylous ascites.
- Very high protein counts are found in tuberculous ascites, pancreatic ascites and Budd–Chiari syndrome.
- Ascitic fluid amylase is raised in pancreatic ascites.
- Fluid is sent for microscopy, Gram stain and culture (in blood culture bottles). More than 250 white blood cells per millilitre indicates infection (subacute bacterial peritonitis).
- Fluid should also be sent for cytology.

Management
Treatment depends on the underlying cause. The progress of ascites can be monitored using repeated weight and girth measurements. Sodium intake should be restricted but protein and calorie intake should be maintained. Water restriction is only necessary if the serum sodium concentration drops below 128 mmol/L. The combination of spironolactone and furosemide is effective in the majority of patients. Patients who not respond to this treatment may require

- therapeutic paracentesis, the removal of fluid over a number of hours. If more than 1 L of fluid is removed then intravenous albumin or plasma expander is required to prevent hypovolaemia.
- refractory ascites may be treated by TIPPS (see page 199).

Investigations and procedures

Liver function testing

Liver function testing includes blood tests to look for evidence of hepatocyte necrosis, as well as assessing the actual functions of the liver, i.e. its synthesis of proteins including albumin and clotting factors and bile metabolism and excretion. In most laboratories, if liver function tests (LFTs) are requested, this means measurement of the serum levels of bilirubin, aminotransferases, alkaline phosphatase (ALP) and total protein. γ-glutamyl transpeptidase (γ-GT) may be included amongst the standard tests, but often needs to be requested separately. For assessing the synthetic function of the liver, two other blood tests are needed, the prothrombin time and serum albumin.

Hepatocyte necrosis/damage

- Aminotransferases: Two are measured, aspartate aminotransferase (AST) and alanine aminotransferase (ALT). These are raised by most causes of liver disease, but paradoxically, in severe necrosis or in late cirrhosis levels may fall to normal indicating a lack of viable hepatocytes. ALT is more specific than AST, the latter being found in many other organs (see Table 5.2).

Table 5.2 Non-hepatic causes of abnormal liver function tests

Blood test	Non-hepatic causes
AST	Myocardial infarction
	Congestive cardiac failure
	Muscle injury (e.g. polymyositis, rhabdomyolysis)
	Haemolysis
Bilirubin	Haemolysis
	Sepsis
ALP	Pregnancy (normal)
	Bone disease (e.g. Paget's disease, osteomalacia, metastases, hyperparathyroidism)
γ-GT	Alcohol
	Enzyme-inducing drugs
Albumin	Malnutrition
	Nephrotic syndrome
	Congestive cardiac failure
PT	Anti-coagulant use
	Dietary deficiency or gastrointestinal loss of vitamin K
	Disseminated intravascular coagulation

Obstruction

- Bilirubin: Raised bilirubin levels indicate abnormalities in its synthesis, metabolism or excretion. It often rises in causes of obstructive (cholestatic) jaundice, but it is not specific for obstruction or even for liver disease (see Table 5.2 and page 185).
- ALP: This enzyme is found in the liver, where it is produced by the cells lining the small bile ducts. It is also found in bone, placenta and intestine. If the liver disease is primarily due to obstruction of the intrahepatic or extrahepatic bile ducts (cholestatic), the ALP rises first and proportionally more than the aminotransferases.

If the ALP is raised due to liver disease, γ-GT measurement is also raised as it shares a similar pathway of excretion. If γ-GT levels are normal with a raised ALP then a non-hepatic cause should be suspected such as bone disease. Alternatively, it is possible to differentiate the bone and liver isoenzymes.

- γ-GT: Alcohol and drugs such as phenytoin induce this enzyme even when there is no liver damage. It may be used to detect if patients continue to drink alcohol, but it does have a long half-life. In cholestasis it rises in parallel with the ALP.

Synthetic function

- Serum proteins:
  - The liver synthesises many proteins. Total protein itself is not that useful, without measuring the serum albumin level and immunoglobulin levels.
  - Albumin constitutes about 65% of the total protein and as it has a short half-life of about 3 weeks, it is a good marker of synthetic function. It falls in both acute and chronic liver disease, although levels may be normal early in the disease. Low albumin levels (hypoalbuminaemia) may lead to the development of ascites and oedema. Other causes of hypoalbuminaemia include gastrointestinal losses or heavy proteinuria.
  - Serum immunoglobulins are often non-specifically raised in liver disease. IgM is particularly raised in primary biliary cirrhosis, whereas IgG is raised in autoimmune hepatitis.
- Prothrombin time (PT): Most clotting factors are synthesised by the liver. They have a much shorter half-life than albumin, and a prolonged PT may occur in both acute and chronic liver disease.

Vitamin K deficiency including that caused by obstructive jaundice (due to reduced absorption from the intestine) causes a prolonged PT (see page 465). Parenteral replacement of vitamin K should lead to improvement of the prolonged PT within a few days if hepatic synthetic function is intact.

Pancreatic function tests

Exocrine function

- Serum amylase is a marker for pancreatic damage. A rise of more than 4 times normal with suggestive clinical features is diagnostic of acute pancreatitis, although lesser rises may occur due to other causes, e.g. mesenteric infarction and acute cholecystitis. A normal amylase level does not exclude acute pancreatitis. Serum lipase is also a marker for pancreatic damage.
- Steatorrhea which is thought to be caused by chronic pancreatitis may be investigated using faecal fat estimation and/or a breath test to compare the absorption of a radiolabelled fatty acid versus a radiolabelled triglyceride. If the fatty acid is absorbed normally but the more complex triglyceride is not, then the steatorrhea is caused by pancreatic disease.
- Other tests to assess the exocrine function, such as measuring the levels of enzymes in the duodenum after a food challenge, are available but not commonly performed.

Endocrine function

- Chronic pancreatitis may lead to secondary diabetes mellitus. Tests for endocrine function in this context are not required.
- Endocrine tests may be needed in the diagnosis of islet cell tumours. Pancreatic polypeptide is raised in all of these types of tumour and see page 222 for specific tests.

Imaging of the liver, biliary system and pancreas

Plain abdominal X-ray

This is usually unhelpful, but occasionally abnormalities may be detected. Up to 10% of gallstones are radio-opaque and visible on X-ray. Pancreatic calcification may be seen in chronic pancreatitis. The finding of air in the biliary tree suggests infection with gas-producing organisms, trauma, a fistula between the intestine and gallbladder, or may be seen after endoscopic or surgical instrumentation.

Abdominal ultrasound scan (USS)

This is a safe, non-invasive test, which can be used to visualise the liver, biliary tree and pancreas. It is particularly useful in patients who have

- jaundice or abnormal liver function tests where it is useful to look for gallstones, dilated intra- or extra-hepatic bile ducts, and to assess the size and appearance of the liver.
- signs of chronic liver disease.
- hepatomegaly or splenomegaly.
- suspected gallstone disease, including cholecystitis.
- acute pancreatitis, particularly to look for gallstones, pseudocysts and abscesses.
- suspected intra-abdominal abscess, e.g. liver abscess including amoebic abscess.

Other abnormal findings include ascites, abdominal masses and lymphadenopathy. Ultrasound may also be used for liver biopsy, and doppler ultrasound is used to look for hepatic blood flow, particularly portal vein flow direction and venous patency.

Computed tomography (CT)

This can visualise the liver, biliary tree, lymph nodes and the pancreas in more detail. Preferably a spiral CT is performed after intravenous contrast, as this allows imaging in the arterial and portal venous phases, which characterises liver lesions more precisely. Precautions should be taken in case of allergy or risk of contrast nephrotoxicity. This includes stopping metformin and ensuring patients are well-hydrated prior to the tests. CT is particularly useful for assessing focal lesions of the liver, staging of malignancy, and it is more sensitive for pancreatic lesions, such as assessing the severity of acute pancreatitis and to look for complications such as pseudocysts.

Magnetic resonance imaging (MRI) and magnetic resonance cholangiopancreatography (MRCP)

This is sometimes used for more sensitive imaging of the liver, particularly for focal lesions. MRCP is sometimes used as a non-invasive alternative to endoscopic retrograde cholangiopancreatography (ERCP) to visualise the pancreatic and biliary ducts, particularly in patients suspected of having biliary obstruction, stone or post-liver transplant.

Endoscopic retrograde cholangiopancreatography (ERCP)

ERCP is used in the diagnosis and treatment of conditions of the biliary tract and pancreas, such as in obstructive jaundice or if obstruction of the pancreatic ducts is suspected. It provides more detailed information than an ultrasound scan. A side-viewing endoscope is passed into the duodenum and a radio-opaque dye injected into the biliary and pancreatic systems by means of a cannula inserted into the papilla of Vater. This is followed by real-time radiography.

Further diagnostic and therapeutic manoeuvres:
- Biopsy of periampullary tumours.
- Sphincterotomy or balloon dilatation to allow gallstone removal.
- Dilatation of benign biliary strictures.
- Insertion of stents to relieve obstructive jaundice.

The rate of complications with a diagnostic ERCP is approximately 1%, but this rises with any therapeutic procedure. The most common complication is acute pancreatitis. Haemorrhage and perforation occur less commonly. Ascending cholangitis may be prevented by antibiotics, which are given prophylactically to all patients with possible biliary obstruction.

Percutaneous transhepatic cholangiography (PTC)

Percutaneous transhepatic cholangiography is used to image the biliary tree, particularly the upper part, which is not well outlined by endoscopic retrograde cholangiopancreatography (ERCP). For example in obstructive jaundice with obstruction of the upper biliary tree and when malignancy of the biliary tract is suspected or being evaluated. Prior to the procedure the clotting profile is checked and the patient is given prophylactic broad-spectrum antibiotics.

A slim flexible needle is passed into the liver percutaneously and a radio-opaque dye injected. The image can be followed by real-time radiography and still pictures obtained. Complications include haemorrhage, bile leakage, bacteraemia and septicaemia. Emergency surgery may be required.

Liver biopsy

Liver biopsy is used to diagnose the cause of liver disease. In jaundiced patients, imaging such as an ultrasound (US) scan and endoscopic retrograde cholangiography should initially be used to exclude an obstructing lesion. It is also used for diagnosis of a space-occupying lesion such as a tumour or abscess. Biopsy may be preceded by a CT scan to determine if metastatic disease is present and may be guided by CT or ultrasound.

Prior to the biopsy coagulation studies should be checked and a sample sent to transfusion for group and save serum. Hepatitis B and C surface antigen status should be known. Patients with abnormal clotting should have their liver biopsy postponed until this is corrected. If uncorrectable, biopsy may be undertaken through the hepatic veins, using a transjugular approach.

A biopsy needle is passed percutaneously, and the biopsy taken whilst the patient holds their breath in expiration. Percutaneous aspiration of an abscess is occasionally performed. Complications include haemorrhage, bile leakage and pneumothorax. After the procedure the patient should rest on their right side for 2 hours in bed and should gently mobilise after bed rest for a further 4 hours.

Liver resection

Liver resection may be indicated in abdominal trauma, and in tumours of the liver. However, in many cases of malignant tumours only complete removal of the liver and liver transplantation is curative. Localised metastases may also be resected.

The liver is composed of several segments, as defined by the blood supply and drainage, this is important in liver resection. The hepatic artery and portal vein each have a left and right branch and these supply the left and right hemi-livers respectively. The left hemi-liver comprises of the left lobe and the caudate and quadrate lobes; together these form four segments. The right hemi-liver comprises of the remainder of the right lobe and is also further divided into four segments (see Fig. 5.3).

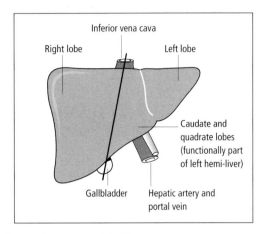

Figure 5.3 Anatomy of the liver.

This means that right hepatectomy, left hepatectomy and extended right hepatectomy (right lobe plus caudate and quadrate lobes) or individual segments may be resected. The liver is first mobilised from its peritoneal attachments. The appropriate vessels for the segment(s) are ligated and divided before the segment(s) are dissected away from the remainder of the liver. Careful identification and ligation of biliary ducts and smaller vessels is required to reduce blood loss and therefore morbidity and mortality. Drainage is required postoperatively, to prevent bile from pooling intra-abdominally.

Cholecystectomy

Surgical removal of the gallbladder and associated stones in the biliary tract may be by open surgery or laparoscopic surgery.

Cholecystectomy may be indicated for symptomatic gallstones. Cholecystectomy is also considered in younger patients with asymptomatic gallstones in order to prevent complications such as acute pancreatitis. Carcinoma of the gallbladder is treated by wider resection, including neighbouring segments of the liver and regional lymph nodes.

Open cholecystectomy is usually performed through a right subcostal (Kocher) incision or by a paramedian or midline incision. Cholangiography may be used to visualise the duct system. The gallbladder is removed with ligation and division of the cystic duct and artery. If stones have been found, the common bile duct may be opened longitudinally and the stones removed. A

T-tube is sited into the opening, which is brought out to the abdominal wall. The T-tube allows drainage of bile and also allows a cholangiogram later. Alternatively, common bile duct stones are removed at endoscopic retrograde cholangiopancreatography (ERCP).

Laparoscopic cholecystectomy requires three or four cannulae inserted through the anterior abdominal wall, for visualisation and access with operative instruments. The cystic duct and artery are clipped and dissected, while the gallbladder is held retracted.

Open cholecystecomy often requires quite a long stay in hospital, possibly a week or more, whereas laparoscopic cholecystectomy may be conducted as a day case.

Complications include haemorrhage, respiratory problems and wound infection. Bile leakage and haemorrhage may require further surgery. Laparoscopic technique reduces the incidence of respiratory problems and surgical site infection.

Disorders of the liver

Introduction to the liver and liver disease

Introduction to the liver

The liver is divided into two lobes, left and right (which includes the caudate). It has two blood supplies: 25% of its blood originates from the hepatic artery (oxygenated) and 75% originates from the portal vein that drains the gastrointestinal tract and spleen. This blood is therefore relatively low in oxygen, but rich in glucose, lipids and amino acids.

The functions of the liver are carried out by the hepatocytes, which have a special architectural arrangement. Blood enters the liver through the portal tracts, which contain the triad of hepatic artery, portal vein and bile duct. It then filters from the edges of the lobule to the central (efferent) vein. The lobule is classically used to describe the histology of the liver (see Fig. 5.4a) but the acinus forms the functional unit (see Fig. 5.4b).

The hepatocytes in zone 1 of the acinus receive well-oxygenated blood from the portal triads, whereas the hepatocytes in zone 3 receive poorly-oxygenated blood and are therefore more vulnerable to damage when the blood supply is compromised.

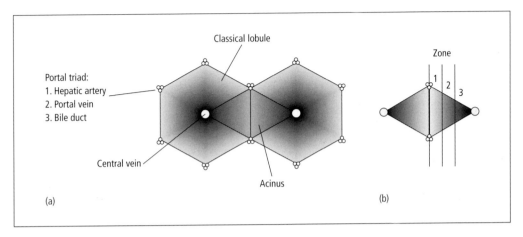

Figure 5.4 (a) Lobule and (b) acinus.

The liver has multiple functions, which may be impaired or disrupted by liver disease:

- Carbohydrate metabolism: The liver is one of the major organs in glucose homeostasis under the control of pancreatic insulin. Excess glucose following a meal is converted to glycogen and stored within the liver. In early starvation states this glycogen is mobilised, and once this store is exhausted glucose is synthesised via the gluconeogenesis pathway within the liver.
- Protein: The liver is involved in the synthesis of all circulating proteins apart from immunoglobulin. This includes carrier proteins, albumin and coagulation factors. The liver is also involved in the breakdown of amino acids producing ammonia, which is converted to urea and excreted by the kidneys.
- Fat: The liver is involved in synthesis of lipoproteins (lipid protein complexes), triglycerides and cholesterol.
- Bile synthesis and metabolism.
- Drug and hormone inactivation and excretion.

Liver disease can be considered according to the aetiology, the pathology (such as acute hepatitis) or the clinical picture of presentation.

Patterns of liver disease

Acute hepatitis

Definition
Acute inflammation of the liver parenchyma.

Aetiology
The causes of acute hepatitis:

- Acute viral hepatitis may be caused by the hepatotrophic viruses (A, B and E) or other viruses such as Epstein–Barr virus, cytomegalovirus and yellow fever virus.
- Alcohol-induced hepatitis.
- Nonalcoholic steatohepatitis.
- Drug-induced hepatocellular damage which may be histologically indistinguishable from viral hepatitis, e.g. paracetamol.
- Wilson's disease.

Pathophysiology
Cellular damage results in impairment of normal liver function: bilirubin is not excreted properly resulting in jaundice and conjugated bilirubin in the urine, which appears dark. Less bile reaches the gut, so that the stool contains less stercobilinogen and appears pale. There is reduced protein synthesis, e.g. albumin and clotting factors.

Dying hepatocytes release enzymes, mainly transaminases.

Swelling of the liver results in stretching of the liver capsule which may result in pain.

Clinical features
The features of acute liver damage are malaise, jaundice, anorexia, nausea, right upper quadrant pain and in severe cases, evidence of liver failure. In cases of acute viral hepatitis, there is often a history of a 'flu-like' illness

preceding the onset of jaundice. On examination there may be an enlarged, tender liver, pale stools and dark urine. Stigmata of chronic liver disease should be looked for to exclude acute on chronic liver disease.

Microscopy

Acute viral hepatitis has a histological appearance which can be mimicked by drug reactions. Hepatocytes undergo ballooning degeneration appearing swollen and vacuolated. There is a lymphocytic infiltration. Cell death is by apoptosis and results in the formation of Councilman bodies. As regeneration occurs the normal architecture is disrupted. In severe cases, necrosis spreads from one portal tract to the central vein or from central vein to central vein, so that confluent areas of necrosis form termed bridging necrosis.

Complications

Fulminant liver failure, chronic hepatitis, and cirrhosis.

Investigations

- Serum bilirubin and transaminases (aspartate transaminase (AST) and alanine aminotransferase (ALT)) are raised in acute liver injury.
- Prothrombin time and albumin should be measured.
- Ultrasound may be needed to exclude obstructive jaundice, if applicable.
- Serological testing will identify viral infections.
- Specific tests depend on suspected causes, e.g. paracetamol levels. A liver biopsy may be required if the cause is not identified.

Management

In most cases supportive management is the only available treatment. This includes careful fluid balance, adequate nutrition and anti-emetics. Where possible removal of the causative agent, e.g. alcohol or specific therapies should be given (see Wilson's Disease page 211 and Paracetamol poisoning page 527). Patients require serial liver function tests (including clotting) to follow the course of the hepatitis.

Chronic hepatitis

Definition

Chronic hepatitis is a clinical and pathological syndrome characterised by a variable degree of hepatocellular necrosis and inflammation, without improvement for at least 6 months. However, it is sometimes diagnosed earlier than this.

Aetiology

The main causes of chronic hepatitis:
- Viral hepatitis: Hepatitis B virus ($+/-$ hepatitis D), hepatitis C virus.
- Autoimmune: Autoimmune chronic hepatitis, primary biliary cirrhosis (PBC).
- Toxic: Alcohol-induced hepatitis (rare), drug-induced hepatitis (methyldopa, isoniazid, ketoconazole, antiretroviral drugs).
- Nonalcoholic hepatosteatosis (NASH).
- Inherited: Wilson's disease, α_1 antitrypsin deficiency, haemochromatosis.

Clinical features

Patients may present with non-specific symptoms (malaise, anorexia and weight loss) or with the complications of cirrhosis such as portal hypertension (bleeding oesophageal varices, ascites, encephalopathy). Following acute viral hepatitis persistently raised serum transaminases (aspartate transaminase, alanine aminotransferase) may be detected during follow-up. Asymptomatic patients with chronic viral hepatitis may be detected during screening at blood donation.

Microscopy

Features include lymphocyte infiltration, fibrosis and fat deposition. Histologically three patterns of chronic hepatitis are seen.

- Chronic active hepatitis (CAH). A severe pattern which is likely to progress rapidly to cirrhosis with chronic inflammatory cells infiltrating the portal tracts and extending into the lobule with 'piecemeal necrosis'. Fibrous tissue formation links portal tracts to central veins or central veins to each other (bridging necrosis).
- Chronic persistent hepatitis (CPH) has a more favourable prognosis unless caused by hepatitis C virus. CPH may also develop into CAH in some e-antigen positive hepatitis B infected patients. Inflammation is confined to the portal tracts.
- Chronic lobular hepatitis (CLH) is most commonly associated with viral hepatitis. Hepatitis B patients who are e-antigen positive may develop CAH.

Inflammation of the portal tracts with spotty inflammation in the parenchyma of the lobules, but there is no liver cell necrosis.

Complications

Cirrhosis is the most common complication. There is increased risk of hepatocellular carcinoma in patients with chronic viral hepatitis especially in hepatitis B.

Investigations

Chronic hepatitis is diagnosed by a combination of persistently abnormal liver function tests and the findings on liver biopsy. Other investigations are aimed at diagnosing the underlying cause and providing a prediction of prognosis including serum viral markers and autoantibodies (e.g. antimitochondrial antibodies suggest primary biliary cirrhosis).

Management

- Symptomatic management includes adequate nutrition and hydration.
- Specific treatments depend on the underlying cause, e.g. anti-viral treatment.
- Liver transplantation may be indicated.

Cirrhosis

Definition

Cirrhosis is an irreversible change of the liver architecture, characterised by nodules of regenerated liver cells separated by bands of fibrous scar tissue.

Aetiology

Cirrhosis results from continued hepatocellular necrosis and chronic inflammation. Fibrous scarring causes disruption of the normal architecture, although regeneration of hepatocytes occurs between the fibrous tracts, their function, which depends on intact architecture, is impaired.

- Alcohol accounts for more than 80% of cirrhosis in the United Kingdom.
- Viral hepatitis due to hepatitis B and C is the most common cause worldwide.
- Other conditions include primary biliary cirrhosis (PBC), autoimmune hepatitis, nonalcoholic steatohepatitis (NASH), haemachromatosis, α_1 antitrypsin

disease, galactosaemia, cystic fibrosis, Wilson's disease and drugs.

Pathophysiology

All the liver functions are impaired (bilirubin metabolism, bile salt synthesis, specialised protein synthesis, detoxification of hormones, drugs and toxins). Impaired blood flow through sinusoids leads to an exacerbation of the functional deficit and portal hypertension. Feminisation in males and amenorrhea in females are common in alcoholic liver disease and haemochromatosis due to alterations in the hypothalamic–pituitary–gonadal axis. Reduced immune competence and increased susceptibility to infection also occur.

Clinical features

Patients may present with complications such as bleeding from oesophageal varices or encephalopathy. Patients with active chronic hepatitis may present with features of chronic liver disease before cirrhosis is established. Signs of chronic liver disease:

1 General appearance: Jaundice, pigmented (haemochromatosis), pallor (anaemia), bruises (clotting abnormalities), petechiae (thrombocytopenia), scratch marks (pruritus), spider naevi on trunk, muscle wasting (malnutrition).

2 Hands: Leuconychia (if hypoalbuminaemic), clubbing, palmar erythema, Dupuytren's contracture, hepatic flap (asterixis, sign of hepatic encephalopathy), tremor may occur in alcoholism and Wilson's disease.

3 Abdomen: Dilated veins around the umbilicus, striae may result from abdominal distension. The liver is usually enlarged, firm and irregular, but is shrunken in late disease. The spleen may be enlarged due to portal hypertension. Ascites may be present.

Macroscopy

The liver is often enlarged and nodular, with a bosselated surface. The cut surface shows nodules of liver tissue, separated by fine or coarse fibrous strands. Micronodular cirrhosis consists of nodules less than 3 mm, if larger nodules are seen it is termed macronodular cirrhosis.

Complications

Bleeding oesophageal varices secondary to portal hypertension, hepatocellular carcinoma.

Table 5.3 Child–Pugh grading

Grading system	1	2	3
Encephalopathy	None	Grade I–II	Grade III–IV
Ascites	Absent	Mild–moderate	Severe
Bilirubin (micromol/L)	<35	35–50	>50
Albumin (g/L)	>35	28–35	<28
Prothrombin time (seconds over control)	1–3	4–6	>6

Child–Pugh grade A = score of 5–6; Child–Pugh grade B = score of 7–9; Child–Pugh grade C = score of 10–15

Investigations

Aimed at diagnosis of underlying cause and assessment of severity/degree of reversible liver injury. The severity of liver disease may be graded A–C by means of a modified Child–Pugh grading system (see Table 5.3). Liver biopsy is often required for assessment.

Management

Treatment is largely supportive. Withdrawal from alcohol is essential in all patients. Malnutrition is common and may require nutritional support. Liver transplantation may be required when end stage liver failure occurs.

Prognosis

Cirrhosis is an irreversible, progressive condition which often continues to end-stage liver failure despite the withdrawal of precipitating factors. The higher the Child–Pugh grade, the worse the prognosis, particularly for death from bleeding varices or following surgery.

Fulminant hepatic failure

Definition

The rapid development of severe hepatic failure causing encephalopathy and impaired synthetic function in a person who previously had a normal liver or had well-compensated liver disease.

Incidence

Rare

Aetiology

Any cause of an acute hepatitis may progress to fulminant hepatic failure. Over 50% of cases in the United Kingdom have a viral cause, most of the remainder being due to paracetamol poisoning. Other rare but important drug-induced causes are halothane, isoniazid and rifampicin.

Pathophysiology

Widespread multiacinar necrosis with or without fatty change causes a severe loss of liver function. Hepatic encephalopathy is thought to be due to failure of the liver to metabolise toxins. Serum amino acid levels rise affecting the balance of cerebral neurotransmitters. Hepatic dysfunction also results in renal failure (hepatorenal syndrome).

Clinical features

Patients may have altered behaviour, euphoria or sedation and confusion (see Table 5.4). Fever, vomiting abdominal pain and bleeding may also occur.

On examination patients are jaundiced, there may be fetor hepaticus (sickly sweet odour on breath), flapping tremor, slurred speech, difficulty in writing and copying simple diagrams (constructional apraxia) and generalised hypertonia.

Complications

- Central nervous system: Cerebral oedema in 80% causing raised intracranial pressure.
- Cardiovascular system: Hypotension, arrhythmias due to hypokalaemia including cardiac arrest.
- Respiratory system: Respiratory arrest.
- Gastrointestinal system: Haemorrhage, pancreatitis.
- Genitourinary system: Acute renal failure due to hepatorenal failure or acute tubular necrosis.
- Metabolic: Hypoglycaemia, hypokalaemia.
- Haematology: Coagulopathy.
- Infections.

Table 5.4 Grading of hepatic encephalopathy

Grade I	Altered mood or behaviour
Grade II	Increasing drowsiness, confusion, slurred speech
Grade III	Stupor, incoherence, restlessness, marked confusion
Grade IV	Coma

Investigations

Liver function tests show hyperbilirubinaemia, high serum transaminases, abnormal coagulation profile. Liver ultrasound may be of value to show underlying chronic liver disease. Specific tests depend on the suspected underlying cause, e.g. viral serology, paracetamol levels. Other tests include full blood count, urea and electrolytes, glucose, calcium, phosphate and magnesium levels.

Management

Treatment is supportive as the liver failure may resolve:

- Specialist hepatology input is essential, ideally patients should be managed in a specialist liver unit. Positioning at a 20° head up tilt can help ameliorate the effects of cerebral oedema. Monitoring of intracranial pressure may be necessary in severe encephalopathy. Whilst adequate nutrition is essential the protein intake should be restricted to 0.5 g/kg/day or less. Lactulose and phosphate enemas may be used to empty the bowel and minimise the absorption of nitrogenous substances. Oral neomycin can decrease enteric bacteria. Sedatives should be avoided.
- Any treatable cause, e.g. paracetamol overdose should be managed appropriately.
- Complications should be anticipated and avoided wherever possible. Regular monitoring of blood glucose and 10% dextrose infusions are used to avoid hypoglycaemia. Other electrolyte imbalances should be corrected. Coagulopathy should be treated with intravenous vitamin K (although this may not be effective due to poor synthetic liver function), fresh frozen plasma should be avoided unless active bleeding is present or prior to invasive procedures as it can precipitate fluid overload. Antisecretory agents, e.g. H_2 antagonists or proton pump inhibitors may reduce the risk of gastrointestinal haemorrhage. Renal support may be necessary.
- Systemic antibiotics and antifungals may be used to prevent sepsis.
- Liver support using cellular and non-cellular systems are under development; however, liver transplantation remains the treatment of choice if the patient fails to improve.

Prognosis

Outcome is dependent on the degree of encephalopathy. There is over 80% mortality for those with grade IV encephalopathy. However, long-term sequelae, e.g. cirrhosis or chronic hepatitis is rare in survivors.

Complications of chronic liver disease

Portal hypertension

Definition

Raised portal venous pressure is usually caused by increased resistance to portal venous blood flow and is a common sequel of cirrhosis. When the portal venous pressure is consistently above 25 cm H_2O, serious complications may develop.

Aetiology

By far the most common cause in the United Kingdom is cirrhosis of the liver. Causes may be divided into those due to obstruction of blood flow, and rare cases due to increased blood flow (see Fig. 5.5).

Pathophysiology

Venous blood from the gastrointestinal tract, spleen and pancreas (and a small amount from the skin via the paraumbilical veins) enters the liver via the portal vein. As the portal vein becomes congested, the pressure within it rises and the veins that drain into the portal vein become engorged. If the portal pressure continues to rise the flow in these vessels reverses and blood bypasses the liver through the porto-systemic anastamoses (paraumbilical, oesophageal, rectal). This portosystemic shunting eventually results in encephalopathy.

Clinical features

The presenting symptoms and signs may be those of the underlying disease, (most commonly cirrhosis), of reduced liver function or features of portal hypertension. Portal hypertension causes oesophageal varices, splenomegaly, distended paraumbilical veins (caput medusa), ascites and encephalopathy.

Complications

Oesophageal varices can cause acute, massive gastrointestinal bleeding in approximately 40% of patients with cirrhosis. Anorectal varices are common, but rarely cause

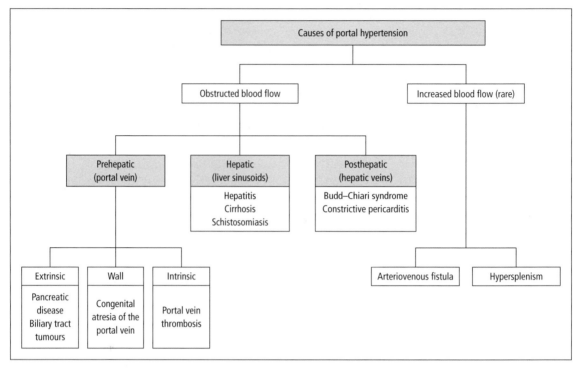

Figure 5.5 Causes of portal hypertension.

acute bleeding. Surgical shunting may exacerbate portosystemic encephalopathy.

Investigations

These are aimed at discovering the cause of the portal hypertension and assessing the degree of portal hypertension, when considering surgical intervention. The severity of liver disease may be graded A–C by means of a modified Child–Pugh grading system (see page 196). Ultrasound of the liver and spleen is performed to assess size and appearance. Additional Doppler studies can assess the direction and flow of blood within the portal and hepatic veins. Liver biopsy may be required. The hepatic wedge pressure may be directly measured.

Management

- Portal hypertension is significantly improved by abstinence from alcohol in cases of alcohol-induced disease.
- Primary prophylaxis against variceal haemorrhage:

1 β-blockers, in particular propranolol, cause splanchnic vasoconstriction and reduce cardiac output. This reduces the portal pressure gradient, the azygos blood flow and variceal pressure, which reduces the likelihood of variceal bleeding.
2 Endoscopic variceal band ligation may be performed in patients with significant varices who are unable to tolerate β-blockers.
3 If both β-blockers and endoscopic banding are contraindicated isosorbide mononitrate has been shown to be effective.

- Specific complications requiring intervention include ascites (see page 188), bleeding varices (see page 199) and encephalopathy (see Table 5.4).
- Portosystemic shunting is used in patients with reasonably good liver function and who are not being considered for a liver transplant. There are various techniques, for example connecting the:
1 Portal vein to inferior vena cava.
2 Splenic vein to left renal vein (Warren shunt): useful for portal vein obstruction and maintains liver

blood flow, so that there is a lower risk of encephalopathy afterwards.

3 Insertion of a transjugular intrahepatic portosystemic shunt (TIPSS) can be performed without general anaesthesia and laparotomy. A transjugular approach is used to pass a guidewire through the hepatic vein piercing the wall to the intrahepatic branches of the portal vein, a stent is then passed over the guidewire. The risk of encephalopathy is the same as for other shunts, but operative morbidity and mortality is improved.

- Liver transplantation offers the only hope of cure.

Bleeding oesophageal varices

Definition
Oesophageal varices are dilated vessels at the junction between the oesophagus and the stomach and occur in portal hypertension. They may rupture and cause an acute and severe upper gastrointestinal bleed.

Incidence/prevalence
30–50% of patients with portal hypertension will bleed from varices.

Aetiology
Varices result from portal hypertension, the most common cause of which is cirrhosis. Factors predicting bleeding in varices include pressure within the varix, variceal size and severity of the underlying liver disease.

Clinical features
Patients with acute upper gastrointestinal bleeding present with haematemesis, which is usually a large volume of fresh blood. Melaena may also be present. Severe blood loss results in hypovolaemic shock. Signs of chronic liver disease may be present (jaundice, pallor spider naevi, liver palms, opaque nails, clubbing). Other features of portal hypertension may be seen.

Investigations
The diagnostic investigation is endoscopy, which may also be therapeutic during an acute bleed. The varices must be confirmed to be the source of bleeding, because up to 20% of patients with varices also have peptic ulcers and/or gastritis. The varices are seen as tortuous columns in the lower third of the oesophagus. They usually bleed from the lowest point of the oesophagus. Urgent blood samples should be sent for full blood count, group and cross-match for at least 6 units, U&Es, glucose, liver function tests and clotting profile.

Management
Resuscitation:
- At least two large bore peripheral cannulae should be sited for fluid resuscitation. Packed red blood cells should be given as soon as possible, O −ve blood may be required before cross-matched blood is available.
- Any abnormalities in prothrombin time or platelet count should be corrected.
- Careful fluid balance assessment is essential and may require urinary catheterisation and central venous pressure measurements.
- Elective intubation may be required in severe uncontrolled variceal bleeding, severe encephalopathy, in patients unable to maintain oxygen saturation above 90%, or in patients with evidence of an aspiration pneumonia.

Further management:
- An upper gastrointestinal endoscopy should be performed as soon as the patient is haemodynamically stable. Variceal band ligation is the treatment of choice. If banding is not possible, the varices should be injected with a sclerosant.
- If endoscopy is unavailable, vasoconstrictors, such as octreotide or glypressin, or a Sengstaken tube may be used while more definitive therapy is arranged.
- In case of bleeding that is difficult to control, a Sengstaken tube should be inserted until further endoscopic treatment, transjugular intrahepatic portosystemic shunting (TIPSS) or surgical treatment is performed.
- Infection may occur following a variceal haemorrhage in cirrhotic patients resulting in significant morbidity and mortality. All patients should receive a course of broad-spectrum antibiotics as prophylaxis.

Secondary prophylaxis following a variceal bleed in cirrhosis:
- Following control of active bleeding the varices should be eradicated using endoscopic band ligation (sclerotherapy if banding unavailable). Following successful eradication of the varices repeated upper gastrointestinal endoscopy is required to screen for recurrence.

Table 5.5 Hepatotrophic viruses

Virus	Type	Transmission	Incubation period
Hepatitis A virus (HAV)	ssRNA	faecal/oral	~1 month
Hepatitis E virus (HEV)	ssRNA	faecal/oral	~1–2 months
Hepatitis B virus (HBV)	dsDNA	blood/sexual	~2–3 months
Hepatitis D virus (HDV)	Defective RNA	blood/sexual	Needs HBV for replication
Hepatitis C virus (HCV)	ssRNA	blood/sexual	~2–3 months

- β-blockers may be used as secondary prophylaxis either in combination with endoscopic therapies or alone. If they are used alone, it is recommended that hepatic venous pressure gradient is measured to confirm the success of treatment.
- TIPSS is more effective than endoscopic treatment in reducing variceal rebleeding but does not improve survival and is associated with more encephalopathy.

Prognosis

There is a 50% mortality in patients presenting for the first time with bleeding oesophageal varices. Prognosis is worse in patients with high Child–Pugh grading (see page 196). Without treatment to prevent recurrence two thirds of patients re-bleed whilst in hospital and 90% re-bleed within a year.

Viral hepatitis

Definition

The term viral hepatitis usually refers specifically to the diseases of the liver caused by the hepatotropic viruses, which include hepatitis A, B, C, D, E (see Table 5.5). Other viruses such as the Epstein–Barr virus and cytomegalovirus may cause acute hepatitis.

Pathophysiology

The hepatotrophic viruses can cause a range of pathologically and clinically evident liver disease (see Fig. 5.6).

Hepatitis A

Definition

Hepatitis A virus (HAV) is one of the hepatotrophic viruses, which cause viral hepatitis.

Geography

Endemic in developing countries, with exposure in early childhood being common and adults universally immune. In developed countries, most cases are sporadic and the numbers are declining.

Aetiology/pathophysiology

ssRNA enterovirus of the picorna group. HAV is transmitted by the faecal–oral route (especially in seafood) and has an incubation period of 2–6 weeks. It is infectious from 2 weeks before clinical symptoms until a few days after the onset of jaundice. The mechanism of hepatocyte necrosis is unclear; the virus is not cytopathic in tissue culture.

Clinical features

Exposure and infection in early childhood is usually asymptomatic. Symptoms and severity increase with age. A history of contact/travel abroad may be found, although many asymptomatic cases occur. Patients present with a prodromal phase (malaise, anorexia, nausea, aversion to fatty foods and cigarettes) lasting about a week. Jaundice appears after the prodromal phase and lasts about 2 weeks. The liver may be palpably enlarged and tender.

Complications

Intrahepatic cholestasis resulting in dark urine and pale stools. Rarely, aplastic anaemia in children, which has a high mortality. Very occasionally fulminant hepatic failure occurs.

Investigations

Diagnosed by the finding of HAV-specific IgM. IgG anti-HAV appears as IgM, disappears over the following months and persists for years, giving immunity.

Management

Treatment is supportive. Prevention by HAV vaccination, a killed whole virus vaccine.

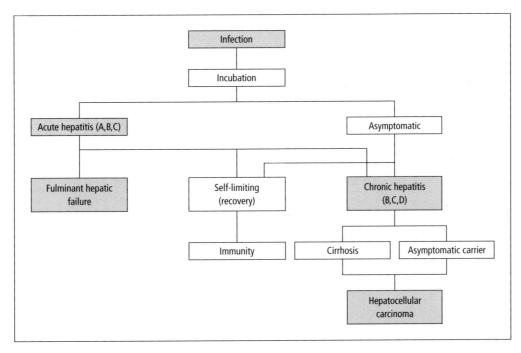

Figure 5.6 Patterns of disease in viral hepatitis.

Prognosis
Case fatality rate less than 1 per 1000. No long-term carrier state.

Hepatitis B

Definition
Hepatitis B (HBV) is a predominantly sexually or vertically transmitted virus, which causes hepatitis.

Prevalence
Worldwide 300 million people carry the hepatitis B virus, 1 million die annually from HBV-related disease. In the United Kingdom it is uncommon: 0.1–2%.

Geography
More common in the developing world with highest levels in Africa and SE Asia.

Aetiology
HBV is a dsDNA virus of the hepadna group.
- Vertical transmission is the most common route in high endemic areas. It occurs at or after birth and is most common in babies of e-antigen positive mothers.

Post exposure prophylaxis has reduced this transmission in the developed world.
- Horizontally transmission occurs between young children in the developing world possibly through a minor skin break or close bodily contact with affected children.
- Sexual intercourse: The virus is most readily transmitted by rectal intercourse. At risk individuals include those with multiple sexual partners. Barrier contraceptive methods prevent transmission.
- Blood-borne transmission may occur with transfusions, other blood products or at organ transplantation. All blood and transplant donors are screened in the United Kingdom. Nosocomial infections may occur due to needle stick injuries or contaminated instruments.

Pathophysiology
The incubation period is approximately 2–3 months. The virus is not cytopathic, the liver damage is immune-mediated by the cytotoxic T lymphocytes response to viral antigen expressed on the surface of liver cells during the period of viral replication. The mechanisms of

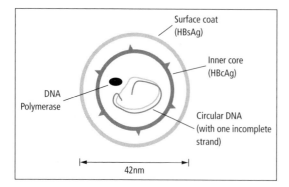

Figure 5.7 The Dane particle.

cell death include bystander damage from T cell derived cytokines and antibody-dependent cell-mediated cytotoxicity. The complete virion or Dane particle is spherical, 42 nm in diameter (see Fig. 5.7).

The Dane particle is found in the serum of HBV-infected patients, its presence denoted by HBsAg. This denotes when there is first a viraemia.

The viral particle is seen in body fluids, saliva, semen, vaginal secretions, faeces, breast milk as well as serum.

- HBcAg is found in the nuclei of liver cells, where HBV replicates.
- The e-antigen or HBeAg is related to the core proteins. The presence of the e-antigen denotes active viral replication. It is detectable in acute hepatitis, chronic active hepatitis or in high infectivity carriers (super-carriers). Conversely, anti-HBe antibodies indicate a better prognosis.
- Carrier status is defined as presence of HbsAg for more than 6 months. Carrier status is associated with chronic hepatitis in people with lowered immunity and with neonatal or childhood infection. It has also been noted that patients who present with jaundice during the acute infection rarely convert to a carrier status, compared to those who have an anicteric acute hepatitis.

Clinical features

Hepatitis B can cause a range of clinical disease, from asymptomatic to fulminating hepatic failure or chronic hepatitis. The likelihood of these conditions depends on the age of the patient:

- Neonatal infections are normally asymptomatic (98%), but often become chronic with a 40% risk of developing cirrhosis.
- Infections in adulthood generally cause an acute symptomatic hepatitis (70%) which may rarely result in fulminant hepatic failure (0.1–0.5% of infections). Only 1–2% of infections during adulthood result in cirrhosis.

Complications

Increased risk of cirrhosis and hepatocellular carcinoma. Carriers may develop extra-hepatic disease, such as glomerulonephritis in children and polyarteritis nodosa following chronic hepatitis. These may be due to immune complex formation.

Investigations

Hepatitis B is diagnosed and followed using serological markers (see Fig. 5.8).

In carrier states the HBsAg remains high with an absence of anti-HBs indicating continued presence of virus. If the e-antigen (HBeAg) remains present and there is no anti-HBe, there is active viral replication indicating a super-carrier or high-infectivity state. Presence of anti-HBs alone (without other antibodies) indicates a previous successful vaccination.

Management

Acute hepatitis is managed supportively.

In patients with chronic high infectivity (HBeAg positive) and the evidence of active hepatitis (elevated ALT) interferon α can be used. If there is no response or relapse following treatment, nucleoside analogues and other antiviral drugs can be tried.

Vaccines are available which are effective:

- Active immunisation by recombinant protein (HBsAg made in yeast cells) is given to at risk individuals including health-care workers and in areas of high prevalence. The WHO recommends that hepatitis B vaccine should be included in routine childhood immunisation schedules for all children in all countries.
- Active immunisation should be given to all infants born to HBsAg-positive mothers, passive immunisation with hepatitis B immunoglobulin is given, in addition, to infants born to HBeAg positive mothers. Combined active and passive immunisation is also used as post-exposure prophylaxis for needlestick injuries.

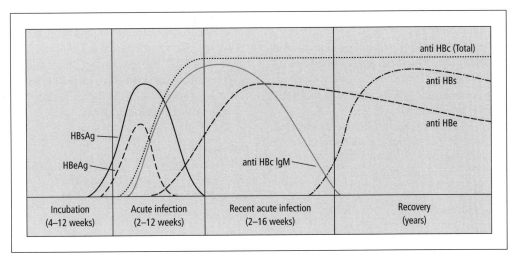

Figure 5.8 Serological changes following acute infection with hepatitis.

Prognosis
Up to 40% eventually die from liver disease.

Hepatitis C

Definition
Hepatitis C is one of the hepatotrophic viruses, which predominantly causes a chronic hepatitis.

Incidence/prevalence
Common worldwide. Carrier rate of 0.2% in northern Europe.

Geography
Five per cent carrier rate in Far East; 1–2% in Mediterranean.

Aetiology/pathophysiology
ssRNA virus of the flavivirus group. It was discovered in 1988 as being the most common cause of non-A, non-B hepatitis, particularly in blood transfusion recipients. The main route of HCV transmission is parenteral, most patients will give a history of either intravenous drug abuse or a blood/blood product transfusion prior to testing. There is some evidence of sexual transmission, which may be facilitated by co-infection with HIV. Vertical transmission may occur especially if the mother is HIV positive or has a high viral load.

Clinical features
Less than 10% of patients have an acute flu-like illness with jaundice, the remainder are asymptomatic at the time of infection. Very rarely hepatitis C can cause fulminant hepatic failure. Following infection most patients develop chronic hepatitis C, which predisposes to cirrhosis and hepatocellular carcinoma. Chronic hepatitis C is often asymptomatic but may cause fatigue, myalgia, nausea, anorexia and right upper quadrant pain. Symptoms and signs of chronic liver disease occur years after initial infection.

Microscopy
Lymphocytic infiltration within the vascular sinusoids. Fatty change is seen in the hepatocytes, with little active hepatocellular necrosis.

Complications
Chronic active hepatitis may be associated with autoimmune hepatitis, Sjogren's syndrome, lichen planus, thyroiditis, membranous glomerulonephritis, polyarteritis nodosa and mixed essential cryoglobulinemia.

Investigations
- Seroconversion occurs several months after infection, but anti-HCV is found in chronic sufferers of hepatitis, carriers (using ELISA) and those who have recovered from infection.

- Acute infection is diagnosed by the presence of HCV RNA in the serum, using PCR. A positive PCR indicates current viraemia whereas a negative test with positive anti-HCV antibodies suggests non-viraemic infection, transient absence of viraemia or recovered infection. Quantification of the viral load may be of use in tailoring treatment.
- Liver biopsy is used for assessing liver inflammation, potential progression of fibrosis and the presence or absence of cirrhosis.

Management

Counselling regarding transmission is essential. In acute infection supportive treatment may be necessary. Combination therapy with pegylated interferon α and ribavirin is recommended for the treatment of people aged 18 years and over with moderate to severe chronic hepatitis C (histological evidence of significant scarring and/or significant necrotic inflammation). If ribavirin is contraindicated or not tolerated, pegylated interferon α monotherapy should be used. Patients with severe cirrhosis may require liver transplantation. There is no available vaccine.

Hepatitis D

Definition

Hepatitis D virus (HDV) or delta agent is a virus that only causes hepatitis in conjunction with hepatitis B.

Aetiology/pathophysiology

Hepatitis D, a single stranded RNA virus, has a genome which does not encode for its own protein coat. It therefore has to use proteins made by the HBV. It is therefore not pathogenic in the absence of HBV replication. Unlike HBV, it has a direct cytopathic effect, which may contribute to the clinical features. Any patient at risk of hepatitis B is at risk of hepatitis D, particularly intravenous drug users.

Clinical features

Two patterns of disease are seen:
- When hepatitis B and D simultaneously infect the host a co-infection occurs. The resulting hepatitis is of variable severity, but is more likely to cause fulminant hepatic failure. The chronic carrier state is rare.

- If hepatitis D occurs in patients carrying hepatitis B, i.e. a super-infection, it may precipitate an acute hepatitis or convert a mild chronic disease to fulminant hepatitis. HDV super-infection has a strong tendency (10–40%) towards chronic progressive disease, leading to an increased risk of rapidly developing cirrhosis and hepatocellular carcinoma.

Investigations

Finding antibodies to HDV (IgM or IgG) is diagnostic. Alternatively, a cDNA probe can be used to detect HDV in the blood, and HDAg can be detected in liver cells using immunofluoresence.

Management

There is no vaccine for hepatitis D; however, vaccination against hepatitis B will prevent hepatitis D infection. Interferon α can be used to treat patients with chronic hepatitis B who also have hepatitis D infection.

Prognosis

Recovery from hepatitis B leads to clearance of hepatitis D also. However, chronic hepatitis D infection has a poor prognosis.

Hepatitis E

Definition

Hepatitis E virus (HEV) is a member of the group of hepatotrophic viruses, which cause hepatitis.

Incidence/prevalence

Epidemics of tens of thousands of cases in developing world.

Geography

Cause of water-borne epidemics in the Indian subcontinent and North Africa.

Aetiology/pathophysiology

HEV is an ssRNA virus of the calicivirus group. Hepatitis E, like hepatitis A, is transmitted via the faecal–oral route and has an incubation period of 2–9 weeks. It causes a self-limiting acute hepatitis, with no chronic or carrier state.

Clinical features
HEV causes acute hepatitis, with a prodromal phase of a 'flu-like' illness, followed by jaundice. Generally there is a 1% risk of fulminant liver failure, except in women in the last trimester of pregnancy where there is a 25% risk.

Management
Supportive care may be required.

Other liver diseases

Alcohol-induced liver disease

Definition
Liver disease caused by alcohol range from a fatty liver to hepatitis and cirrhosis.

Incidence/prevalence
Alcohol is the most common cause of liver disease in the West.

Geography
Increasing importance in developing countries.

Aetiology
The risk of developing chronic disease is related to quantity, types of beverage, drinking pattern (see page 521), nutrition and genetic susceptibility.

Pathophysiology
- Any alcohol ingestion causes changes in liver cells, which can be seen by electron microscopy. Alcoholic hepatitis refers to alcohol-induced liver injury visible by light microscopy. Alcohol may alter and/or enhance the effects of other chemicals on the liver, including other hepatotoxins and carcinogens.
- Alcohol increases lactate and fatty acid accumulation resulting in fatty liver.
- Chronic alcohol use activates the microsomal oxidising system, which increases metabolism of alcohol and other drugs (see Fig. 5.9). Cirrhosis may result from fibroblast proliferation and collagen synthesis. Liver cell membranes may become immunogenic resulting in a lymphocyte-mediated cytotoxic response against the liver cells.

Clinical features
Differing patterns are seen:
- Acute alcoholic hepatitis resembles acute viral hepatitis, (malaise, anorexia, jaundice, abdominal pain and fever).
- Fatty liver is asymptomatic, it may be detected with abnormal liver function tests.
- Chronic alcohol-induced liver damage may present with signs of chronic liver damage or with complications of cirrhosis.

Microscopy
There are three main patterns of liver damage:
- Alcoholic hepatitis is focal necrosis of hepatocytes, with neutrophil infiltration. Fibrosis around the central veins is present in later cases. Characteristically Mallory's bodies composed of cytoskeletal fragments and ubiquitin, a heat shock protein that labels proteins as being damaged and targets them for breakdown. It appears as bright eosinophilic amorphous globules within hepatocytes.

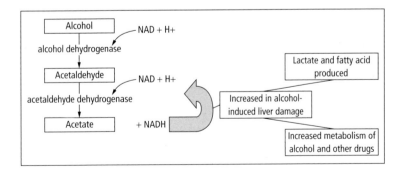

Figure 5.9 Alcohol metabolism.

- Fatty change is reversible sublethal cell injury. Cells are swollen pale and vacuolated. This form of change is seen in those ingesting more than 80 g alcohol per day (6 units, 1 bottle of wine or 3 pints of beer).
- Cirrhosis: Repeated damage has led to fibrosis, with damage to the normal architecture upon which function is dependent.

Complications
Acute hepatitis may rarely lead to fulminant hepatic failure. Up to 10% of patients with cirrhosis, secondary to alcohol use, develop hepatocellular carcinoma.

Investigations
Patients have deranged liver function tests especially γGT, the MCV is also raised. Assessment of severity requires a liver biopsy, as significant liver damage can be present with a few symptoms or enzyme changes. Ultrasound may show significant cholestasis and be mistaken for extra-hepatic obstructive jaundice.

Management
Abstinence is the best treatment. In late stages patients may be considered for liver transplant if they have proved abstinence.

Prognosis
Abstinence results in an improved prognosis, but alcohol-induced liver damage is a progressive disorder continuing to cirrhosis in many patients despite abstinence.
- Fatty liver is reversible, with complete recovery.
- Asymptomatic patients with biopsy-proven alcoholic hepatitis who continue to drink progress to cirrhosis in 90%. However, if they abstain from drinking 90% have a full recovery.
- Patients with established cirrhosis who present with an acute episode of hepatitis have the poorest prognosis ($\sim$60–70% 5-year survival rate).

Nonalcoholic fatty liver disease

Definition
Nonalcoholic fatty liver disease (NAFLD) is a condition with histological features resembling alcohol-induced

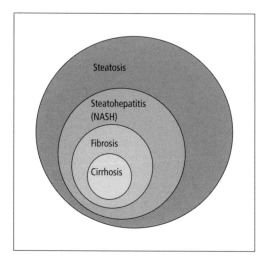

Figure 5.10 Non-alcoholic fatty liver disease (NAFLD).

liver injury, occurring in patients with little or no history of alcohol consumption. The exact significance of NAFLD is currently unknown.

NAFLD encompasses a histological spectrum that ranges from fat accumulation in hepatocytes (hepatic steatosis) to hepatic steatosis with hepatic inflammation (nonalcoholic steatohepatitis or NASH) that may or may not have associated fibrosis, (see Fig. 5.10). NASH may progress to cirrhosis in up to 20% of patients.

Aetiology/pathophysiology
The pathogenesis of nonalcoholic fatty liver disease is not fully understood.
- Hepatic steatosis results from excessive triglyceride accumulation in the liver as a result of increased free fatty acid entering the liver, decreased free fatty acid leaving the liver or impaired beta-oxidation of free fatty acid. Insulin resistance appears to be important in the development of hepatic steatosis and steatohepatitis. Obesity, type II diabetes and insulin resistance are frequently seen in patients with NAFLD.
- Oxidative injury may be required for the development of hepatic inflammation and necrosis. Suggested mechanisms include increased hepatic iron, anti-oxidant deficiencies and intestinal bacterial overgrowth.

Clinical features
Most patients are asymptomatic, fatigue, malaise and right upper abdominal discomfort may occur in some patients with NASH. Hepatomegaly is a frequent finding. Most cases are found on incidental abnormal liver function tests.

Complications
Histologic progression occurs in a small proportion of patients (up to 20%), a few of which progress to end-stage liver disease. Patients who develop cirrhosis may be at increased risk for hepatocellular carcinoma.

Investigations
Serum AST and ALT are raised (>90% of patients) and alkaline phosphatase is often normal as are serum bilirubin levels; however, patients with severely abnormal liver histology may have normal liver function tests. Ultrasound scan may indicate fatty infiltration. Liver biopsy is the only definitive method to diagnose or exclude NAFLD, although its exact role in the management of patients without definitive evidence of liver damage is undecided.

Management
- Obesity, hyperlipidemia and diabetes should be managed; however, weight loss should be gradual as rapid weight loss may exacerbate the condition.
- Potential treatments under investigation include vitamin E and C supplementation, oral hypoglycemic agents and ursodeoxycholic acid.
- In the few patients who progress to end stage, liver failure transplantation may be required; however, recurrence in the transplanted liver has been reported.

Drug-induced liver disease
Hepatic injury caused by drugs accounts for 2–5% of hospital admissions for jaundice. Drugs that cause hepatotoxicity may be subdivided into predictable (dose-dependent) and idiosyncratic, although more than one mechanism may occur with a single drug (see Fig. 5.11).
- Direct hepatotoxins have a direct physico-chemical effect on the cells, e.g. membrane disruption which leads to metabolic defects.
- Cytotoxic indirect hepatotoxins interfere with the hepatocytes' integrity, most commonly this manifests as fatty change and necrosis due to decreased removal of lipid from the cell.
- Cholestatic drugs interfere with the uptake or excretion of bile by hepatocytes, which manifests as cholestasis in the upper biliary tree.
- Idiosyncratic hepatotoxins appear to cause a chronic active hepatitis similar to autoimmune chronic hepatitis and there may be antinuclear and anti smooth muscle antibodies present in serum. Though rare, they are important because the disease is reversible on withdrawal.

The pathophysiology of drug hepatotoxicity may also be divided into the liver pathology caused (see Table 5.6).

Autoimmune chronic hepatitis

Definition
A chronic hepatitis of unknown aetiology characterised by circulating autoantibodies and inflammatory changes on liver histology.

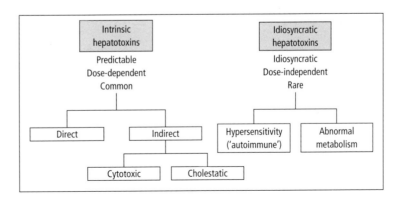

Figure 5.11 Mechanisms of drug-induced liver disease.

Table 5.6 Examples of drugs causing hepatotoxicity

Acute hepatitis	Isoniazid, rifampicin, methyldopa, enalapril, ketoconazole, cytotoxic drugs
Acute hepatocyte necrosis	Paracetamol, salicylates, ferrous sulphate
Fatty liver	Methotrexate, tetracycline, sodium valproate, amiodarone
Granulomatous change	Hydralazine, allopurinol, carbamazepine
Cholestatic	Sex hormones, chlorpromazine, haloperidol, erythromycin, flucloxacillin, cimetidine, ranitidine. Sclerosing cholangitis can be caused by intra-arterial injection of 5-fluorodeoxyuridine.
Chronic active hepatitis	Methyldopa, fenofibrate, isoniazid
Chronic fibrosis and necrosis	Methotrexate, hypervitaminosis A, retinoids
Vascular change	Oral contraceptive steroids, anabolic steroids, azathioprine, cytotoxic drugs, alternative medicine such as Bush Tea
Liver tumours	Oral contraceptive steroids, androgens, (haemangioma, hepatic adenomas, rarely hepatocellular carcinoma)

Prevalence

Most common cause of chronic active hepatitis in developed countries.

Age

10–30 and 40–60 years.

Sex

F > M (6:1)

Aetiology/pathophysiology

No autoimmune mechanism has yet been proven, although high titres of autoantibodies are characteristic. Patients may have features that overlap with primary biliary cirrhosis and primary sclerosing cholangitis. Autoimmune chronic hepatitis is also commonly associated with other autoimmune disorders e.g. haemolytic anaemia, idiopathic thrombocytopenic purpura, type I diabetes mellitus, thyroiditis and ulcerative colitis (more often associated with primary sclerosing cholangitis).

Clinical features

The illness may be asymptomatic with elevated liver enzymes. Patients may have an acute hepatitis or complications of cirrhosis such as portal hypertension (e.g. bleeding oesophageal varices or hepatic encephalopathy).

Investigations

Diagnosis of chronic active hepatitis is made by liver biopsy, there is often a normochromic anaemia, raised bilirubin, moderately raised transaminases, alkaline phosphatase and γ globulin levels. Autoantibodies that may be detected include anti-smooth muscle antibodies, anti-nuclear antibodies, anti-mitochondrial antibodies, anti-microsomal antibodies or anti-liver cystosol antibodies.

Management

The condition may respond to immunosuppressant drugs, such as corticosteroids and azathioprine. In patients who develop end stage liver disease despite medical treatment liver transplantation may be considered although hepatitis may recur in the transplanted organ.

Prognosis

Drug treatment may be withdrawn after 2 years of remission, but relapse is common (60–80%). The risk of hepatocellular carcinoma is low, in contrast to chronic active hepatitis due to viral causes.

Primary biliary cirrhosis (PBC)

Definition

Ongoing autoimmune damage to the intralobular bile ducts causing liver failure.

Incidence

5 per 100 000 population per annum.

Age

20–80 years, mean age 50 years.

Sex

>90% female

Aetiology

Associated with other autoimmune disorders and also HLA-DR8 haplotype. Antibodies to mitochondria are present; however, their exact role in pathogenesis is unclear as titres do not correlate with disease.

Environmental triggers suggested include enterobacteria such as *E. coli.*

Pathophysiology

Chronic inflammation of the small intrahepatic bile ducts leads to cholestasis and destruction of bile ducts. This leads on to portal tract fibrosis and cirrhosis. Duct epithelium in the pancreas, salivary and lacrimal glands are also affected.

Clinical features

Up to half of patients are asymptomatic at diagnosis. Patients may complain of fatigue and pruritus, followed some months later by jaundice. Any sign of liver disease may be present, such as clubbing, hepatomegaly, spider naevi, xanthomata. Asymptomatic patients are discovered through abnormal biochemical findings or during investigation of another autoimmune disorder such as thyroiditis.

Macroscopy/microscopy

Throughout the disease, copper accumulates due to the chronic cholestasis.

- Stage I: Lymphocytic infiltration of small bile ducts and portal tracts with occasional granuloma formation.
- Stage II: More widespread inflammation in the periportal parenchyma, leading to loss of bile ducts.
- Stage III: Fibrous septa extend between triads and form fibrous bridges (bridging necrosis).
- Stage IV: Cirrhosis with absent bile ducts, scarring, distorted architecture and nodular regeneration.

Complications

- Oesophageal varices, osteoporosis, osteomalacia, pancreatic hyposecretion, renal tubular acidosis (possibly copper induced).
- Increased risk of hepatocellular carcinoma and breast cancer.
- Associated with many other disorders, such as Sjögren's, hypothyroidism, systemic lupus erythematosus, scleroderma, dermatomyositis.

Investigations

Definitive diagnosis is made on liver biopsy. Antimitochondrial antibodies (AMA) are present in >99%. Raised alkaline phosphatase suggests damage to bile ducts. Raised cholesterol and raised total IgM are also found.

Management

Supportive treatment involves ursodeoxycholic acid (which helps the pruritus), calcium and vitamin supplementation, management of complications such as varices, hyperlipidaemia. The disease may recur after liver transplantation.

Prognosis

Asymptomatic patients may have a normal life expectancy. In symptomatic patients advancing age, hepatomegaly, high bilirubin, low albumin and cirrhosis correlate with shortened survival (5–7 years in severe disease).

Primary sclerosing cholangitis (PSC)

Definition

A disease of unknown aetiology in which chronic inflammation of the bile ducts leads to stricture formation and progressive obstructive jaundice.

Age

Peak 25–40 years.

Sex

M > F

Aetiology

The cause is unknown but there is a strong association with HLA haplotype (HLA-B8, DR-3, DR-2 and DR-52a). There is also a strong association with inflammatory bowel disease, which is present in 60–75%, but may be asymptomatic. Also associated with HIV infection.

Pathophysiology

Chronic inflammation of the intra- and extra-hepatic bile ducts leads to fibrosis and short strictures form which obstruct the passage of bile. Chronic obstruction leads to jaundice and cirrhosis develops over about 10 years.

Clinical features

Patients usually present with progressive jaundice and pruritus or ascending cholangitis.

Investigations

Endoscopic retrograde cholangiopancreatography (ERCP) shows a beaded appearance of the large bile ducts. Liver biopsy is diagnostic demonstrating concentric, (onion-skin) fibrosis around medium-sized bile ducts, including those in portal tracts. Small bile ducts scar and vanish.

Management

Corticosteroids, azathiporine and methotrexate have been tried, but have no proven benefit. Drainage is usually ineffective. Liver transplantation is used in advanced cases.

Prognosis

Slowly progresses to chronic liver disease with risk of fulminant hepatic failure, cholangiocarcinoma and hepatocellular carcinoma. There is an increased risk of colon cancer.

α_1 Antitrypsin deficiency

Definition

Inherited cause of chronic liver disease and panacinar emphysema.

Aetiology

The gene for α_1 antitrypsin (Pi, for Protease Inhibitor) is found on chromosome 14. It has more than 30 different alleles which are defined according to their motility on electrophoretic gel. The normal phenotype is designated PiMM. Z is the most abnormal allele, it encodes for a defective protein which cannot be excreted from hepatocytes.

Pathophysiology

α_1 antitrypsin is an extracellular inhibitor of neutrophil elastase. In its absence, damage to cells is not controlled. Individuals who have a PiMZ phenotype have an increased risk of developing emphysema. Cigarette smoke probably contributes to this by inhibiting any functioning antitrypsin which is present. Those with a ZZ phenotype develop emphysema and cirrhosis.

Clinical features

ZZ homozygotes usually present in the first year of life, with symptoms of neonatal hepatitis, i.e. pale stools, dark

urine and an enlarged liver. Occasionally, the individual is asymptomatic until adulthood, when they present with cirrhosis.

Investigations

Liver function tests are abnormal. Liver biopsy shows variable histology including hepatocellular necrosis, inflammation, fibrosis and cirrhosis. α_1 antitrypsin levels can be measured and are low.

Management

Supportive, patients must not smoke, end-stage liver failure may require liver transplantation.

Hereditary haemochromatosis

Definition

Inherited disorder resulting in abnormal accumulation of iron in the body.

Incidence/prevalence

Homozygous mutation 1 in 350, clinical disease rare.

Age

Clinical disease; most common in middle age.

Sex

Clinical disease, M > F.

Aetiology

Hereditary haemochromatosis is inherited in an autosomal recessive manner. The carrier frequency is 1 in 10. The gene (HFE) is located on the short arm of chromosome 6, closely linked to HLA A3. The commonest mutation is a cysteine-to-tyrosine substitution at amino acid 282 (C282Y). Although 80–90% of patients with hereditary haemochromatosis are homozygous for the C282Y mutation, 75–99% of homozygotes are clinically disease free.

Pathophysiology

The mechanism by which HFE mutation causes disease is unclear. It is thought that there is a gradual accumulation of iron over decades. Women accumulate less iron due to menstrual losses and therefore present later. Iron accumulates in the tissues as haemosiderin particularly within the liver, pancreas, pituitary, heart and skin.

- Hepatocyte necrosis leading to cirrhosis.
- Islet cell death, leading to diabetes mellitus.
- Cardiomyopathy and heart failure.
- Pituitary and gonadal abnormalities.

Clinical features

Pigmentation of the skin (due to increased melanin), diabetes and hepatomegaly is the classical description of the disease. Arthritis due to calcium pyrophosphate deposition may occur, usually affecting the knees and metacarpophalangeal joints. Other presenting features include pituitary dysfunction, cardiac enlargement and/or failure.

Macroscopy/microscopy

The tissues appear rusty brown. The iron is mainly around the portal tracts. Portal fibrosis is seen, prior to cirrhosis.

Complications

There is a high risk of hepatocellular carcinoma if cirrhosis develops.

Investigations

Diagnosed on liver biopsy.

1 Liver function tests may be normal.
2 Serum iron is high, with >90% saturation of total iron binding capacity.
3 Serum ferritin is a measure of the total body iron content and is useful for follow-up.

Management

Regular venesection reduces the iron load and the risk of cirrhosis and hepatocellular carcinoma. Other manifestations are treated symptomatically, e.g. insulin for diabetes, testosterone for gonadal failure. First degree relatives should undergo screening with serum ferritin levels.

Prognosis

The earlier the diagnosis and treatment, the better the prognosis. With treatment, symptoms tend to improve, including diabetes. However, cirrhosis is not reversible.

Wilson's disease

Definition

Inherited disorder causing copper accumulation in the liver, brain, kidney, cornea and bone.

Prevalence

Rare; 1 in 50,000 of the population.

Age

May present at any age. Unusual before 5 years.

Sex

M = F

Aetiology

Inherited in an autosomal recessive manner. The mutation is in a copper-transport ATPase gene on chromosome 13.

Pathophysiology

In Wilson's disease the mutation is thought to affect the excretion of copper from hepatic lysosomes into the bile. Excess copper in the hepatocytes causes lipid to collect in the cytoplasm. There is increasing inflammation and fibrosis and untreated, it progresses to cirrhosis.

Clinical features

Heterozygous individuals are asymptomatic and usually have a completely normal copper balance. In homozygotes, the condition may present with acute hepatitis or may remain clinically silent until cirrhosis is established or neurological symptoms develop including reduced performance at school, clumsiness or slurred speech. Kayser–Fleischer rings (green/brown rings around the edge of the cornea) are a late diagnostic sign, but are variably present.

Microscopy

Excess copper can be seen in the liver using special staining. It is ~2–20 × normal, but this also occurs in chronic cholestatic disorders, such as primary biliary cirrhosis.

Investigations

Reduced serum copper and ceruloplasmin levels (not specific and 25% of patients will have normal levels). Urinary copper is high and increases markedly following a test dose of D-penicillamine. A slit-lamp examination of the eyes should be performed.

Management

D-penicillamine (a copper-chelating agent) depletes copper stores. Patients should avoid foods high in copper (chocolate, nuts and dried fruits). Siblings and children of affected individuals should be screened. If diagnosed and treated sufficiently early, there is some improvement in liver function and further deterioration is arrested.

Pyogenic liver abscess

Definition

The development of liver abscesses is thought to follow bacterial infection elsewhere in the body.

Aetiology/pathophysiology

Enteric Gram negative and anaerobic organisms, e.g. *Strep. milleri*. Infection may reach the liver by the portal vein from a focus of infection drained by the portal vein, e.g. diverticulitis, appendicitis, infected haemorrhoids. Infection may also result from a generalised septicaemia or direct spread from the biliary tree.

Clinical features

Symptoms and signs range from mild to severe, often the symptoms are less marked in elderly patients, with a mild fever with or without pain and hepatomegaly. In severe cases patients present with upper abdominal pain, swinging fever, anorexia, malaise and weight loss.

Macroscopy/microscopy

May be single or multiple lesions ranging from a few millimetres to several centimetres in size.

Investigations

Ultrasound scan is useful for screening, and pus may be aspirated for culture under its guidance. Further imaging may include CT or MRI of the abdomen. Blood cultures, liver function tests and inflammatory markers should be sent. A raised alkaline phosphatase may be the only marker.

Management

Repeated ultrasound guided aspirations may be required. Extensive, difficult to approach abscesses are drained by open surgery, with soft pliable drains.

Intravenous broad-spectrum antibiotics until bacterial culture and sensitivities are available.

Prognosis

Poor prognostic factors are co-existent biliary tract disease, old age and multiple abscesses.

Amoebic liver abscess

Definition

Infection of the liver by *Entamoeba histolytica*.

Aetiology/pathophysiology

E. histolytica is a protozoan that infects the large intestine. The infection water is food borne and is most common in parts of the world with poor sanitation, e.g. Far East and Africa. Ingestion of the cysts results in the release of trophozoites in the intestine, which are thought to invade through the mucosa gaining entry to the portal blood system and then spread to the liver.

Clinical features

The onset of symptoms may be sudden or insidious. Symptoms include right upper quadrant pain, anorexia, nausea, weight loss and night sweats. Tender hepatic enlargement without jaundice is usual. Basal pulmonary collapse and pleural effusion may occur.

Complications

Rupture, secondary infection and septicaemia. Metastatic brain abscesses have been reported.

Investigations

Ultrasound or CT of the abdomen can show the abscess. Blood tests include blood culture and serological tests. Guided aspiration and stool ova, cyst and parasite examination may demonstrate the organism.

Management

Treated with metronidazole. Percutaneous aspiration is used in resistant cases.

Hydatid disease

Definition

A tapeworm infection of the liver common in sheep rearing areas such as Greece, Australasia and Wales.

Aetiology/pathophysiology

In man hydatid disease is caused by one of two tapeworms *Echinococcus granulosus* and *Echinococcus multilocularis*. *Echin. granulosus* infections occur following ingestion of food contaminated with infected dog faeces. *Echin. multilocularis* is carried by foxes and small rodents. Sheep and cattle perpetuate the life cycle. In humans the embryos hatch in the duodenum and enter the liver via the portal system. Once in the liver the embryos form a hydatid cyst and may be disseminated to the lung, kidney or brain.

Clinical features

The disease may be symptomless but chronic right upper quadrant pain with enlargement of the liver is the common presentation. The cyst may rupture into the biliary tree or peritoneal cavity and may cause an acute anaphylactic reaction.

Investigations

Eosinophilia is common and serological tests are available. Small, calcified cysts may be seen on plain abdominal X-ray. Ultrasound or CT scanning can demonstrate cysts.

Management

Mebendazole or albendazole is commenced prior to any intervention. Percutaneous ultrasound guided fine needle aspiration with injection of scolicidal agents and re-aspiration may be used. Large symptomatic cysts may be surgically excised intact taking great care to avoid contamination of the peritoneal cavity.

Tumours of the liver

Benign tumours of the liver

Benign tumours of the liver must be differentiated from malignant tumours such as metastases or primary hepatocellular tumour and cysts or abscesses. There are four main types:

- Cavernous haemangiomas are the most common benign tumours of the liver. Usually asymptomatic, they rarely become large and produce pain, enlarged liver or haemorrhage. They may be detected at ultrasound or at laparotomy. Biopsy may cause haemorrhage.
- Hepatic adenomas are oestrogen dependent tumours generally only seen in women. They are strongly associated with the oral contraceptive pill. Usually asymptomatic, they may rupture causing intraabdominal bleeding and pain. Removal is advised because of difficulty differentiating them from a well-differentiated hepatoma.
- Focal nodular hyperplasia is also seen more commonly in women and oestrogen plays a role.
- Solitary simple liver cysts are rare but multiple liver cysts may be seen in patients with inherited polycystic kidney disease.

Primary hepatocellular carcinoma

Definition

Also called hepatoma, this is a tumour of the liver parenchyma.

Incidence/prevalence

Relatively uncommon in the Western world (2–3%), but by far the most common primary tumour of the liver worldwide.

Age

Usually in middle-aged and elderly.

Sex

M > F (3–4:1)

Geography

High incidence (40% of all cancers) in countries where predisposing factors such as hepatitis B are common, e.g. in Africa and the Far East.

Aetiology

Tumours arise in a chronically damaged liver especially in cirrhosis independent of the cause. Hepatitis B virus carrier states and chronic active hepatitis predisposes to primary hepatocellular carcinoma, especially when hepatitis B infection occurs in early life. Hepatotoxins such as mycotoxins present in food, increase the incidence of primary cancer. Aflatoxin, produced by *Aspergillus flavus*, is frequently found in stored nuts and grains in tropical countries. Other risk factors include drugs such as oral contraceptives following long-term use and androgens.

Pathophysiology

Tumour growth causes further impairment of liver function in already cirrhotic patients. Sometimes rare syndromes occur such as hypercalcaemia, hypoglycaemia and porphyria cutanea tarda (bullae on the skin following sun exposure or minor trauma due to a defect in a hepatic enzyme).

The tumour marker alpha-fetoprotein (αFP) is normally synthesised by the fetal liver, but in adults is present at very low levels (<10 ng/mL). When the tumour secretes αFP, as it does in most cases, it can reach very high levels. It is also raised in germ cell tumours (testicular and ovarian carcinoma).

Clinical features

Insidious onset with anorexia, weight loss and poorly localised upper right quadrant abdominal pain. On examination, the liver is usually enlarged and there may be an arterial bruit.

Macroscopy/microscopy

The right lobe is more frequently affected than the left. There is usually one large, haemorrhagic, soft mass or multifocal nodules. Sometimes the tumour is diffusely infiltrating with invasion of veins. Histologically cells range from well differentiated to anaplastic, with atypical nuclear cytology and abnormal architecture.

Complications

Metastases most commonly occur via the bloodstream to the lungs. Direct spread may also occur to abdominal lymph nodes and to other abdominal organs.

Investigations

- Persistently high levels of serum α feto-protein is very suspicious of carcinoma.
- Ultrasound and CT abdomen are used to image tumours.
- Definitive diagnosis is by liver biopsy.

Management

- Curative treatment by partial liver resection is feasible in patients with tumour in only one lobe and with sufficient liver functional reserve, i.e. no cirrhosis.
- Palliative treatment: Analgesia, arterial embolisation or percutaneous injection of alcohol may also cause tumour reduction and pain relief.

Prognosis

Primary hepatocellular tumour is a rapidly growing tumour, which usually presents late in patients who already have a serious underlying pathology, cirrhosis. The prognosis is very poor. Median survival is <6 months from diagnosis.

Metastatic liver tumours

Definition

Secondary tumours in the liver are very common.

Aetiology

The most common sites of the primary tumour are bronchus, breast, bowel (stomach, colon) and pancreas. The liver is also an important site of growth for lymphomas and leukaemias.

Pathophysiology

Haematogenous spread via the portal vein or the hepatic artery. One or more tumours may develop. Large or multifocal tumours cause loss of liver parenchyma and liver impairment. Liver metastasis may be the first sign that there is a primary tumour present, or it may occur in a patient with known past or present malignant disease.

Clinical features

Insidious onset of fatigue, anorexia and weight loss occurs. Jaundice is a late sign. Pain and tenderness may be felt over the liver, which may be irregular, firm and enlarged.

Investigations

Liver function tests may be abnormal. Ultrasound or CT abdomen may demonstrate the tumours, guided biopsy may be required if the diagnosis is unclear or if the primary tumour is unknown.

Management

Treatment depends on the natural history of the primary tumour.

- Chemotherapy may be effective in certain tumour types such as small cell lung carcinoma, lymphoma and breast cancer. Drugs can be infused through a catheter into the hepatic artery.

- Rarely curative excision of a liver metastasis is performed, particularly for slow-growing tumours.
- In most cases liver metastases indicate a poor prognosis and treatment of the liver tumour will not be curative. Patients should receive palliative care.

Prognosis

Depends on the primary tumour type. Obstructive jaundice is a poor prognostic factor.

Disorders of the gallbladder

Gallstone disease (cholelithiasis)

Definition

Gallstones form from bile constituents in the gallbladder and bile ducts.

Incidence/prevalence

The most common disease affecting the biliary tract and is increasing in frequency. It affects more than 20% of women and 8% of men in the United Kingdom, although >70% remain asymptomatic.

Age

Increases with age, most patients >40 years.

Sex

F > M (2:1)

Geography

More common in developed world.

Aetiology

Gallstones may be cholesterol stones (more common in the developed world), pigment stones (more common in the Far East) or mixed stones.

Cholesterol stones are predisposed to by supersaturation of bile with cholesterol. Normally bile salts and lecithin keep the cholesterol soluble, forming micelles.

- Increased cholesterol: Obesity and rich, fatty diets can cause cholesterol-rich bile to be secreted. Conversely, sudden weight reduction and cholesterol-reducing diets may precipitate gallstones by mobilising cholesterol stores from the liver. However,

hypercholesterolaemia has not been associated with gallstones.
- Increased concentration: Stone formation is more likely when the bile is concentrated, due to stasis, reduced gallbladder contractility or a reduced bile salt pool.
- Precipitants: Gallstone formation may be around a focus or 'nucleus' such as bacteria, cells or other particulate matter.
- Reduced bile salt pool: Bile salts are normally recycled by reabsorption at the terminal ileum through the enterohepatic circulation. Malabsorption (e.g. in cystic fibrosis, Crohn's disease or resection of the terminal ileum) can lead to reduced amounts of bile and predispose to nucleation.
- Hormonal influences have been implicated: Pregnancy, the oral contraceptive pill and hormone replacement therapy all increase the incidence of stone formation.

Pigment stones mainly consist of calcium bilirubinate. Predisposing factors:

- Increased production of bilirubin: Chronic haemolysis such as in congenital spherocytosis, haemoglobinopathies and malaria leads to increased production of conjugated bilirubin.
- Cirrhosis, biliary stasis and chronic biliary infections also predispose, although the mechanism is unknown. Bacterial action on bilirubin has been postulated.

Mixed stones are associated with anatomical abnormalities, stasis and previous surgery.

Pathophysiology

Several different patterns of disease may result from gallstones depending on where the gallstones are located (see Fig. 5.12).

Clinical features

- Gallstones in the gallbladder are asymptomatic in 90% of cases.
- Impaction of a gallstone in the outlet of the gallbladder or in the cystic duct produces biliary colic, a severe colicky pain in the epigastrium and right hypochondrium, radiating to the back. Onset is often after a meal or in the evening, the pain is variable in intensity over several hours. Associated features are nausea, vomiting and retching. Jaundice may occur.

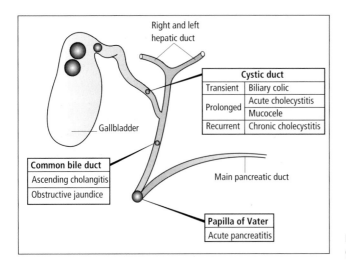

Figure 5.12 Disease resulting from gallstones.

- Acute cholecystitis may result from gallstone obstruction. Inflammation is initially caused by concentrated bile. Secondary infection is common usually due to *Escherichia coli, Klebsiella aerogenes* and *Streptococcus faecalis*. Patients develop acute onset of severe griping pain in the right upper quadrant radiating to the right subscapular region and occasionally to the right shoulder. Associated features include fever, tachycardia, nausea, vomiting and occasionally jaundice. On examination there is abdominal tenderness and guarding in the right upper quadrant, which may become generalised due to peritonitis, a gallbladder mass may be felt due to wrapped omentum. Murphy's sign is usually present (inspiration during right hypochondrial palpation causes pain and arrest of inspiration as the inflamed gallbladder moves downwards and impinges on the fingers).
- Chronic cholecystitis probably results from a combination of gallstones, chemical inflammation due to bile and repeated attacks of acute cholecystitis. Patients complain of a vague intermittent right upper quadrant discomfort, with feelings of distension flatulence and an aversion to fatty foods.
- Patients may also present with ascending cholangitis (abdominal pain, high fever and obstructive jaundice) or acute pancreatitis.

Macroscopy

Cholesterol stones are yellow to green in colour with a rough surface, typically rounded, faceted and large (usually up to 3 cm in size). Pigment stones are often multiple, small and irregular in shape. They are usually <1 cm across.

Complications

A mucocele occurs when long-standing obstruction occurs without infection, the bile is resorbed and instead the epithelium secretes clear mucus. Acute cholecystitis may lead to empyema (pus-filled gallbladder), perforation with abscess formation and biliary peritonitis (chemical and bacterial).

Investigations

- Full blood count (and investigation for haemolytic anaemia in pigment gallstones). Liver function tests, blood cultures, inflammatory markers and amylase should be sent.
- ERCP (endoscopic retrograde cholangiopancreatography) is used for the detection and removal of stones from the common bile duct or papilla of Vater.
- Ultrasound can demonstrate the presence of gallstones and detect dilatation of ducts.
- Plain abdominal X-ray demonstrates radio-opaque stones (15%).

Management

- Patients with asymptomatic gallstones are usually managed conservatively.
- Patients with impacted stones or acute cholecystitis require adequate analgesia and antibiotics to prevent

or treat cholangitis. Stones impacted at the papilla of Vater may need to be removed at ERCP.

- Patients with empyema or acute ascending cholangitis may require drainage procedures.
- Cholecystectomy may be performed as an open or laparoscopic procedure. It may be performed as an emergency (severe or complicated acute cholangitis), early elective (during initial admission for acute cholangitis) or delayed elective (following biliary colic, acute pancreatitis, acute cholangitis or chronic cholangitis)

Prognosis
In acute cholecystitis 90% of patients settle with conservative management within 4–5 days. Ascending cholangitis has a mortality of up to 20% in severe cases requiring emergency decompression.

Carcinoma of the gallbladder

Definition
Carcinoma of the gallbladder is rare, but almost always associated with gallstones.

Age
Usually >70 years.

Sex
F > M (4:1)

Aetiology/pathophysiology
Unknown, but associated with gallstones and chronic cholecystitis. Histologically 90% of tumours are adenocarcinomas and 10% are squamous carcinomas.

Clinical features
Patients may have a history of gallstone disease. Invasion of the bile duct or porta hepatis leads to unremitting jaundice. A mass is often palpable in the right upper quadrant. Many tumours are detected following cholecystectomy for symptomatic gallstones. Direct invasion of local structures, especially the liver, is almost invariable at presentation. Spread via the lymphatics and blood occurs early.

Investigations
Ultrasound, percutaneous transhepatic cholangiography (PTC), CT scan.

Management
Surgical resection is often not feasible due to local spread and metastases. Sometimes aggressive segmental resection of the liver and regional lymph nodes is carried out. Once jaundice occurs, resection is not curative and palliation by stenting or surgical bypass is needed.

Prognosis
Five-year survival rate is <5%.

Carcinoma of the bile ducts

Definition
Carcinomas of the bile ducts are called cholangiocarcinomas. They may be intrahepatic or extrahepatic.

Incidence/prevalence
Uncommon. Increasing in frequency in the West.

Age
Elderly

Aetiology/pathophysiology
Predisposed by chronic inflammation (e.g. primary sclerosing cholangitis associated with ulcerative colitis) and chronic infection with the parasites *Clonorchis* and *Opisthorchis*. Specific risk in patients with choledocal cysts. The tumour can arise anywhere in the biliary system and may be multifocal. It causes obstruction and hence dilatation of the proximal ducts.

Clinical features
The usual presentation is progressive obstructive jaundice. Other symptoms include vague epigastric or right upper quadrant pain, pruritus, anorexia and weight loss. Obstruction of the gallbladder may cause a mucocele or empyema presenting with biliary colic and a non-tender swelling in the right hypochondrium.

Macroscopy/microscopy
The carcinoma commonly appears as a sclerotic stricture anywhere along the biliary tree from the intrahepatic

ducts down to the common bile duct. Histologically it is an adenocarcinoma.

Investigations
- Ultrasound may show dilated intrahepatic ducts and a collapsed gallbladder.
- Percutaneous transhepatic cholangiogram shows a stricture, may show multifocal disease.
- CT scan may show hepatic metastases and nodal involvement.

Management
Curative treatment is only attempted if the tumour is localised and the patient is fit for radical resection.
- Carcinoma of the common bile duct is treated by the Whipple's operation (see page 221).
- Carcinoma of the upper biliary tract is only resectable in 10% of patients. Hepatic resection is often advised. The remaining biliary tree is anastomosed to a Roux loop of jejunum.

Palliative treatments include insertion of a stent or anastomosis of a Roux loop of jejunum to a biliary duct in the left lobe of the liver.

Prognosis
The majority of patients die within 1 year of diagnosis. The prognosis is better for patients with carcinoma of the common bile duct who are suitable for a Whipple's operation.

Disorders of the pancreas

Introduction to the pancreas

The pancreas has two important functions: the production of pancreatic juice, which contains enzymes vital for normal digestion and absorption of food, and the production of the hormones insulin and glucagon in the islets of Langerhans, which are released into the blood and have numerous effects on cell metabolism. Inflammation of the pancreas, which may be due to many causes, including pancreatic duct obstruction, alcohol and viruses causes an initial insult to pancreas, but further damage results from the release of intracellular enzymes and their abnormal activation, so that the pancreas autolyses itself.

The endocrine pancreas
The islets of Langerhans are islands of endocrine cells scattered throughout the pancreas. They are clustered around a capillary network into which they secrete their hormones. The islets contain three main cell types, which cannot be distinguished histologically but secrete different hormones:
- α cells secrete glucagon.
- β cells secrete insulin.
- δ cells secrete stomatostatin.

Acute pancreatitis

Definition
Acute inflammation of the pancreas with variable involvement of local tissue and other organs.

Incidence
Almost 5–25 per 100,000 per year and rising.

Age
More common >40 years.

Sex
M > F

Aetiology
Biliary tract disease (80%), especially cholelithiasis, gallstones are present in up to half of all cases although often in the gallbladder rather than impacted. Alcoholism is the second most common cause (20% in the United Kingdom). Causes are as follows:
- Obstruction: Gallstones, biliary sludge, carcinoma of the pancreas.
- Drugs/toxins: Alcohol, azathioprine, steroids, diuretics.
- Metabolic: Hypercalcaemia, hyperlipidaemia.
- Infections: Coxsackie, mumps, *Mycoplasma*.
- Trauma: Blunt or penetrating injury, post-surgery, post-ERCP.
- Autoimmune: Polyarteritis nodosa, systemic lupus erythematosus.

Pathophysiology
The pancreatic acini and ducts become damaged, this leads to release and activation of the digestive enzymes of the pancreas which autolyse the tissues. Proteolysis

due to proteases, fat necrosis due to lipases and phospholipases and haemorrhage occur. Translocation of gut bacteria can result in local infection and septicaemia. Shock may result from the release of bradykinin and prostaglandins, or secondary to sepsis.

Clinical features

Patients present with severe abdominal pain, which is continuous epigastric pain radiating to the upper back, often associated with vomiting. On examination there is epigastric guarding. Less commonly, the patient may be jaundiced and shocked. Haemorrhage may cause Grey–Turner's sign, which is bruising around the left loin and/or Cullen's sign, bruising around the umbilicus.

Macroscopy/microscopy

The pancreas appears oedematous with grey-white necrotic patches. Bacterial infection leads to inflammation and pus formation. Healing results in fibrosis with calcification.

Complications

In the most severe cases there is systemic organ failure:

- Cardiovascular system: Shock (hypotension, tachycardia, arrhythmias).
- Respiratory system: Adult respiratory distress syndrome, respiratory failure.
- Kidney: Acute renal failure.
- Metabolic: Hypocalcaemia, hypoglycaemia.
- Haematology: Altered haematocrit (raised or lowered), clotting abnormalities (thrombosis, disseminated intravascular coagulation).
- Central nervous system: Neurological symptoms include confusion and irritability.
- Local complications include pancreatic haemorrhage, pseudocyst (a collection of fluid and pancreatic enzymes walled off by compressed tissue), pancreatic abscesses (which may contain gas indicating infection with gas-forming bacteria) and duodenal obstruction.

Investigations

When supportive clinical features are present the diagnosis can be made with a serum amylase more than four times normal, or by a lipase activity greater than twice normal. Patients with acute on chronic pancreatitis may have a smaller rise in serum amylase, in such cases a urinary amylase may be useful to confirm the diagnosis.

Table 5.7 Glasgow system to predict severity of pancreatitis

Within 48 hours of admission
Age >55 years
Glucose >10 mmol/L (not diabetic patient)
White blood cell count >15 $\times$ 10^9/L
LDH >600 i.u./L
Transaminases >100 i.u./L
Hypocalcaemia (serum Ca <2.0 mmol/L)
Blood urea >16 mmol/L despite adequate fluid therapy
Low arterial PaO$_2$ (<8kPa)
Serum albumin <32g/L

Ultrasound (to look for gallstones) of the gallbladder and biliary tract should be performed, but CT scanning is the most useful imaging modality for the pancreas.

Other investigations are required to assess the severity and to monitor for complications: full blood count, clotting screen, urea and electrolytes, liver function tests, lactate dehydrogenase, calcium levels, blood glucose, C reactive protein and arterial blood gas (see Table 5.7).

Management

The early management depends on the severity of the disease, and later management depends on the aetiology and any complications.

- Mild attacks can be admitted to a general ward. Initial treatment is supportive with correction of hypovolaemia and electrolyte imbalances, insertion of a nasogastric tube and analgesia (opiates are often required). Antibiotics should only be given if there are focal signs of infection, e.g. biliary sepsis or pneumonia.
- Severe cases should be managed on a high dependency unit (or intensive care unit if they require respiratory support). Patients require careful fluid balance using central venous pressure monitoring and urinary catheterisation to allow accurate urine output measurement. Regular arterial blood gases are needed to detect early respiratory compromise. Prophylactic broad-spectrum antibiotics are given to reduce the risk of infective complications.
- Gallstone-associated pancreatitis: in mild cases which settle with supportive therapy, early (within 2–4 weeks) cholecystectomy should be performed, with operative cholangiography if ERCP is not performed perioperatively. In cases which do not settle,

particularly those with biliary obstruction or sepsis, urgent ERCP and papillotomy is indicated.

- Laparotomy may be required to drain retroperitoneal collections of pus, resect any necrotic pancreatic and peripancreatic tissue, and perform peritoneal irrigation. Pancreatic pseudocysts which do not resolve with conservative management require laparoscopic drainage into the stomach.

Prognosis

Pancreatitis is a serious condition: overall mortality is 10%. The prognostic factors are listed in Table 5.7. If less than three criteria are met then the pancreatitis is considered mild and has <3% mortality. If more than three criteria are met the pancreatitis is considered severe and has >60% mortality.

Chronic pancreatitis

Definition

Chronic pancreatitis is an inflammatory condition that results in irreversible morphological change and impairment of exocrine and endocrine function.

Age

Usually >40 years.

Sex

M > F

Aetiology/pathophysiology

Two patterns of chronic pancreatitis are seen, a chronic relapsing course with recurring acute pancreatitis and stepwise deterioration, or a truly chronic gradual deterioration leading to pancreatic insufficiency. Risk factors include alcohol abuse, hereditary pancreatitis, ductal obstruction (e.g. trauma, pseudocysts, stones, tumours), systemic lupus erythematosus and cystic fibrosis. Hypercalcaemia, hyperlipidaemia and congenital pancreatic malformations are recognised associations.

Clinical features

Patients may present with an acute episode of pancreatitis or an insidious onset with persistent or recurrent episodes of abdominal pain and weight loss. Late complications include impaired glucose tolerance, diabetes mellitus and malabsorption (steatorrhoea) associated with profound weight loss and oedema due to hypoalbuminaemia.

Complications

Predisposes to pancreatic cysts, pseudocysts and pancreatic cancer. Ascites and persistent obstructive jaundice may occur.

Investigations

Serum amylase fluctuates, but may be moderately raised on testing.

Plain abdominal X-ray may show calcification.

Ultrasound and CT scanning demonstrates cysts, calcification and enlarged ducts.

Endoscopic retrograde cholangiopancreatography may show scarring of the ductal system and even stones in the pancreatic duct. Magnetic resonance cholangiopancreatography is increasingly being used.

Management

Precipitating factors especially alcohol need to be removed. Adequate analgesia is required, thoracoscopic splanchnicectomy may be required in refractory pain not associated with main pancreatic duct dilatation. Steatorrhoea is managed with pancreatic enzyme supplementation and diabetes may need oral hypoglycaemics or insulin. Surgery is indicated for obstruction. Surgical techniques include sphincteromy or sphincteroplasty, partial pancreatectomy or opening the pancreatic duct along its length and anastomosing it with the duodenum or jejunum. Total pancreatectomy can be carried out, with replacement oral pancreatic enzymes and insulin.

Tumours of the pancreas
Carcinoma of the pancreas

Definition

Malignant tumours of the exocrine pancreas.

Incidence

10 per 100,000 per annum and rising.

Age

Mainly >60 years.

Sex

2M : 1F

Geography

In many Western countries it is the fourth commonest cause of cancer death in males and in females, the sixth.

Aetiology

There appears to be some familial clustering and hence it is suggested that genetic susceptibility may play an important role. Specific inherited risks include familial pancreatitis and familial cancer syndromes such as Peutz–Jegher syndrome and Von Hippel Lindau syndrome. Smoking is the only environmental factor firmly associated although high-fat diets and exposure to chemical carcinogens are thought to be contributory.

Pathophysiology

The majority of carcinomas of the pancreas are ductal adenocarcinomas. Acinar cell carcinomas, cystadenocarcinomas and sarcomas are all rare. Most tumours develop in the head of the pancreas and these tend to present early with obstructive jaundice.

Clinical features

Pancreatic cancer is associated with several clinical syndromes:

- One third of patients present with painless obstructive jaundice, i.e. dark urine and pale stool, with palpable dilatation of the gallbladder (Courvoisier's sign).
- Weight loss, anorexia are common. Chronic epigastric pain radiating to the back similar to chronic pancreatitis develops in most patients at some stage.
- Migratory thrombophlebitis and deep vein thrombosis of the legs (Trousseau's syndrome).
- Pancreatic insufficiency: One third of patients have impaired glucose tolerance or diabetes mellitus. Steatorrhoea is common and failure to absorb the fat-soluble vitamin K may cause coagulopathy.

Macroscopy/microscopy

The tumour is hard yellow-white in appearance. 60% of tumours arise in the head of the pancreas, 10% in the body, 10% in the tail and 20% diffusely involve the whole pancreas. Most tumours are moderately differentiated adenocarcinoma with a prominent fibrous stroma.

Complications

The main routes of spread are local causing obstructive jaundice or invasion of the duodenum, lymphatic to adjacent lymph nodes which drain into the coeliac and superior mesenteric lymph nodes and haematogenous mainly to the liver. Seventy-five per cent of patients have metastases at the time of presentation.

Investigations

There are no useful tumour markers or pancreatic function tests for diagnosis, which must be histological.

- Ultrasound scan shows a dilated biliary tree, excludes gallstones and may show the mass lesion in the pancreas or metastases in the liver. Endoscopic ultrasound is increasingly used.
- CT scanning has sensitivity of greater than 95% for the detection of pancreatic tumours.
- Percutaneous fine-needle aspiration or Tru-cut needle biopsy under ultasound or CT guidance can be carried out.
- ERCP allows assessment of both pancreatic and biliary ducts and may also be used for intervention. Biopsies along with aspiration of pancreatic juice and bile can be sampled for cytology.

Management

Surgical resection offers the only chance of cure, but only about 10–15% of patients are suitable for radical surgery depending on tumour size, invasion of blood vessels and the presence of ascites or metastases.

- Whipple's procedure is a radical pancreaticoduodenectomy with block resection of the head of pancreas, distal half of the stomach, duodenum, gallbladder and common bile duct. Reconstruction involves anastomoses of the jejunum and the pancreatic remnant, the common hepatic duct and gastric remnant are anastomosed to the jejunum. There is significant perioperative morbidity and mortality.
- Palliative treatment aims are to relieve jaundice, pruritus, pain and duodenal obstruction. Stents of the bile duct and/or duodenum tend to become blocked and have to be replaced.

Prognosis

The prognosis is extremely poor with an overall 5-year survival of <5% (most in the first 6 months). The 5-year survival of patients who undergo curative resection is 30%.

Islet cell tumours

Insulinoma: A usually benign islet-cell tumour that may occur in the pancreas or at ectopic sites causing the hypersecretion of insulin. There may be gradual intellectual and motor impairment with insidious personality changes. Severe attacks of hypoglycaemia can produce sweating, palpitations, tremulousness and a range of bizarre psychoneurological behaviours. Patients may present with a hypoglycaemic coma. Histology shows encapsulated yellow/brown nodules containing cords and nests of well-differentiated β-cells.

Investigations/management

- Fasting hypoglycaemia with inappropriately high insulin secretion (exogenous insulin can be excluded by measuring C-peptide levels).
- The tumour is found by conventional imaging in less than 50% of cases. Selective venous sampling of concentrations of insulin may be helpful, endoscopic ultrasound is increasingly being used.

- Many pancreatic endocrine tumours express somatostatin receptors. Radiolabelled octreotide (a somatostatin analogue) can be used for localisation of the primary tumour and detection of any metastases.
- Surgery is the treatment of choice.
- Several options are available for the treatment of metastatic neuroendocrine tumors including octreotide, interferon α, chemotherapy and hepatic artery embolisation.

Glucagonoma: This is a very rare tumour of the islet cells of the pancreas which is often asymptomatic. Patients may present with necrolytic migratory erythema, painful glossitis, stomatitis, gastrointestinal upset, weight loss, diabetes mellitus and anaemia. Plasma glucagon levels are raised. Imaging and systemic treatment are as for insulinoma. Resection of the tumour is usually curative.

Other islet cell tumours: Very rarely islet-cell tumours secrete VIP or gastrin. VIPomas cause a profuse watery diarrhoea, hypokalaemia and achlorhydria. The patient may present as an acute abdomen, with ileus and abdominal distension suggestive of intestinal obstruction. Treatment is by resection where possible, or systemic treatment as for insulinoma. Gastrinomas cause the Zollinger–Ellison syndrome (see page 161).

Genitourinary system

6

Clinical

Symptoms

Loin pain

Definition

Loin pain or flank pain is pain felt unilaterally or bilaterally in the back, below the twelfth rib. It has two main causes: obstruction and inflammation. Most kidney diseases do not cause loin pain.

On taking the history of any pain consider the Site, Onset, Character, Radiation, Alleviating factors, Timing, Exacerbating factors and Symptoms associated with the pain (SOCRATES).

The classic form of loin pain is from obstruction to the outflow of urine, usually caused by a renal stone (often called renal colic, although the pain may not always be colicky).

- Site: The pain is usually unilateral, as bilateral renal obstruction is uncommon without there being bladder obstruction as well.
- Onset tends to be sudden.
- Character: The pain can be dull, but is usually severe and constant if the stone has obstructed the kidney, or may come in spasms (colicky) if the stone is in the ureter, and the patient will often walk around, or roll around, trying to get comfortable.
- Radiation occurs down towards the symphysis pubis, groin or into the testis.

- Alleviating factors: Nothing relieves the pain until either the stone is passed (which may be felt as 'gravelly' urine), or strong analgesia is given.
- Associated symptoms include nausea, vomiting, frank haematuria (blood in the urine).

Loin pain is associated with fever, and loin tenderness is strongly suggestive of infection of the kidney (pyelonephritis). There may be nausea and vomiting, but lower urinary tract symptoms (such as stinging, burning on passing urine or urinary frequency may be minimal or absent). Pain felt in the loin may also result from other abdominal organs (see under Gastrointestinal System and Liver Biliary Pancreas), and musculoskeletal pain. Rarer causes include psoas haematoma and abscess.

Dysuria

Definition

Dysuria is the sensation of burning or stinging on passing urine.

This is usually caused by a urinary tract infection and is frequently accompanied by increased urinary frequency and increased urgency (a sudden urge to pass urine). There may be accompanying fever, and systemic upset such as nausea and vomiting, although these are less common with simple cystitis, compared to cystitis complicated by prostatitis, pyelonephritis or obstruction.

It can also be caused after instrumentation of the urinary tract, e.g. by a catheter or cystoscopy, and by urethritis (sexually transmitted diseases causing an inflamed urethra).

Change in urinary frequency, flow and volume

Urinary frequency is recorded as by day and by night so D×6, N×3 means urine is passed six times by day, with three episodes of nocturia. It is difficult to say what is normal, as individuals vary considerably, but it is important to look for changes and also to assess the degree of disruption to the individual. Nocturia more than once is probably abnormal.

- Pregnancy is an important physiological cause of increased urinary frequency, including nocturia.
- Associated symptoms of urgency and dysuria, usually with low volumes passed each time suggest a urinary tract infection.
- Urgency and frequency, without dysuria, suggests urge incontinence (see page 264).
- Increased urinary volume with frequency is caused by polyuria (see below).

Urinary flow: Most individuals will empty their bladder within 30 seconds. The beginning of flow after initiation should be prompt – if delayed, this is called *hesitancy*, and dribbling more than a few drops after the end of micturition is called *terminal dribbling*. Poor flow, hesitancy and terminal dribbling are characteristic of bladder outflow obstruction, usually caused by prostatic enlargement.

Volume: The volume of urine passed is usually about 1000 to 2500 mL/day in healthy individuals. It should be approximately 500 mL less than the intake. However, in many young, active individuals who exercise (and therefore sweat) and those 'too busy' to drink enough fluid, this volume can often drop to ~700–800 mL. Less than this is seen in low body mass, low salt diets, dehydration and also in acute renal failure, although often patients do not notice this. *Oliguria* is reduced urine excretion, often used as a term when <20 or 30 mL/hour is passed. Oliguria occurs in prerenal and renal failure. *Anuria* (no urine) suggests that the urinary tract is obstructed, either bladder outflow, or both kidneys, or a single functioning kidney (which will, if not rapidly treated, go on to cause postrenal failure). *Polyuria* is the passage of increased volumes of urine, as much as 6–8 L can be passed. Polyuria has many causes, including diabetes mellitus,

diabetes insipidus, increased fluid intake and loss of urinary concentrating ability by the kidneys (which may occur in some forms of renal failure, often in the recovery phase).

Haematuria and discoloured urine

Haematuria is blood in the urine, which may be macroscopic or microscopic. Macroscopic haematuria is suggested by a reddish or pink discoloration of the urine, or may range to the passage of bright red, dark or even clotted blood. Microscopic haematuria can only be diagnosed by use of a 'dipstick' test, or on microscopy, as it cannot be seen by the naked eye.

Blood can come from anywhere within the urinary tract, from the glomeruli, down to the urethra. Pink tinged urine at the start of micturition, which then clears, suggests urethral inflammation/trauma or prostatic disease. Haematuria that only occurs at the end of micturition suggests disease of the trigone of the bladder.

When the urine appears pink, but does not contain red blood cells on urine microscopy, this is 'spurious haematuria'. If the dipstick test is positive, then this means that there is either haemoglobin or myoglobin in the urine, such as occurs in rhabdomyolysis. Certain drugs (such as rifampicin) and beetroot ingestion can make the urine appear orange, pink or red, but the dipstick test will be negative (see Table 6.1).

Dark urine should not be interpreted as 'concentrated', as this is an unreliable sign. Dark urine does occur in conjunction with pale stools in obstructive jaundice. Urine turns dark after standing for some time in porphyria. Cloudy urine has many causes, including pus (pyuria), blood ('smoky' urine) and phosphate crystals. A high concentration of phosphate in the urine is quite common, usually completely benign, and can be reduced by drinking plenty of fluids (not milk), but occasionally can signify a tendency to develop urinary stones.

Clinical features

It is important to take a history, which may suggest a cause:

- Dysuria suggests cystitis. This should be treated, then urine re-tested to ensure the haematuria has cleared.
- Renal colic, or a previous history of urinary stones.
- Recent upper respiratory tract infection suggests IgA nephropathy or post-infectious glomerulonephritis.

Table 6.1 Causes of positive dipstick test for blood in the urine

Haematuria	Cause
Renal	Glomerular Disease
	Polycystic Kidney Disease
	Pyelonephritis
	Trauma
	Carcinoma (renal cell, transitional cell)
	Vascular malformations, emboli
Extra-renal	Cystitis, Prostatitis, Urethritis
	Urinary stones
	Trauma
	Neoplasm (papilloma, bladder cancer)
	Drugs, e.g. cyclophosphamide (haemorrhagic cystitis)
Systemic	Coagulation disorders/anti-coagulant therapy
	Sickle cell trait/disease (causes papillary necrosis)
Spurious (no rbc's on microscopy)	Haemoglobinuria, myoglobinuria

- If the patient is a female of childbearing age ensure she is not menstruating (repeat the test mid-cycle).
- A drug history, including anti-coagulants such as warfarin.
- Occupational history (for exposure to carcinogens – see page 277).
- A history or family history of polycystic kidneys, or other kidney disease.

Perform an examination including blood pressure. Urine dipstick is vital and considered part of the clinical examination.

Investigations

Transient microscopic haematuria (without proteinuria) without any other symptoms or signs is generally benign, and may be followed up clinically in young individuals.

Separate samples of urine can be collected on commencing micturition, midway through micturition and at the end of micturition (the three-glass test).

- If haematuria is greatest in the first sample the source of bleeding is likely to be the anterior urethra.
- Haematuria greatest in the third glass suggests a source in posterior urethra, bladder neck or trigone (base of the bladder).
- Haematuria that occurs equally in all glasses indicates bleeding in the bladder or upper urinary tract.

It is useful to try to differentiate between urological and nephrological causes, after initial tests such as a midstream urine for culture, urine microscopy looking for casts, FBC and U&Es, to determine which further investigations are needed and which specialist should see the patient. A raised urea and creatinine may be caused by nephrological or urological cause, such as glomerular disease or urinary obstruction (see Fig. 6.1).

- If there is proteinuria or red cell casts, glomerular disease should be suspected, and patients should be referred to a nephrologist (see page 240).

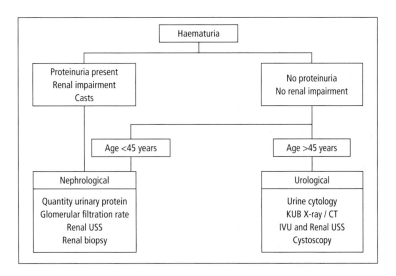

Figure 6.1 Investigation of haematuria.

- In the absence of proteinuria, it is important to exclude cancer of the urinary tract and patients should be referred to a urologist.

Investigations and procedures

Urine tests

Dipstick testing

The basic test includes blood, protein, glucose, specific gravity and urinary pH. More complex dipstick tests are available which test for ketones (raised in starvation and diabetic ketoacidosis), leucocyte esterase, which signifies white cells, and nitrites, which signifies the presence of certain bacteria that convert nitrates (found in normal urine) to nitrites.

- Blood: Dipstick testing for blood is much more sensitive than the naked eye. False positives occur with myoglobinuria and haemoglobinuria. Cross-contamination may occur if females are menstruating. If truly positive, it should be investigated as for haematuria (see page 224).
- Protein: Normal protein excretion is <150mg/day, of which albumin normally forms about 35 mg. Dipstick for protein will be negative unless protein excretion is >300–500 mg/day. It mainly detects urinary albumin, and is insensitive for other proteins such as immunoglobulin light chains (Bence Jones protein) which require specific tests. Very dilute urine will underestimate the degree of proteinuria, and concentrated normal urine may show a trace of protein. If 1+ or more of protein is detected, further quantification of protein should be done (see below). False positives can occur with radiocontrast agents.
- Glucose: Presence of glucose is almost always due to diabetes mellitus. Glucose is not normally found in the urine until the plasma glucose concentration is ≥10 mmol/L. If found with lower levels, this suggests an inability of the kidney to reabsorb filtered glucose due to dysfunction in the proximal tubule, such as occurs in multiple myeloma, renal tubular acidosis (RTA) and pregnancy.
- Specific gravity (SG): This gives an estimation of urine concentration, it is useful in acute renal failure, investigation of polyuria or syndrome of inappropriate anti-diuretic hormone (SIADH). If there are high levels of glucose or myeloma chains in the urine, SG is high even when the patient is not dehydrated.
- Urinary pH: In metabolic acidosis, urine pH falls to below 5.3, unless the cause of metabolic acidosis is RTA. Urinary tract infections with bacteria such as Proteus, which produce urease, cause the urine pH to rise to neutral or even alkaline levels.

Quantification of proteinuria

This is done on patients who have persistent proteinuria. There are two main methods.

1 24-hour urine collection: Unfortunately this method is inaccurate and often inconvenient for the patient. They must empty their bladder when they get up in the morning, then begin collecting in a container every single drop of urine passed for the next 24 hours, up to and including the first emptying of the bladder the next morning. This is then sent to the laboratory for total protein quantification.

2 Protein-to-creatinine ratio: This is performed on a random urine specimen and is accurate, straightforward and convenient. This test is simpler using conventional units as used in the USA, because urinary protein concentration and serum creatinine concentration are both expressed in mg/dL, so a ratio of 3.8 represents a 24-hour protein excretion of 3.8 g/1.73 m^2. In the United Kinddom, urinary creatinine is expressed in mmol/L so the result needs to be multiplied by 0.088:

$$\text{Protein excretion } (g/1.73m^2)$$
$$= \frac{\text{Urinary protein } (mg/dL) \times 0.088}{\text{Urine creatinine } (mmol/L)}$$

Microalbuminuria

Patients with proteinuria, which is greater than normal but less than detectable on dipstick, have 'microalbuminuria'. This is defined as albumin excretion of between 35 and 200 mg/24 hour. It is an early indicator of diabetic kidney disease, and is also found in other conditions such as cardiovascular disease even without renal impairment. There are now bedside testing kits for detecting microalbuminuria (extra sensitive forms of dipsticks), but laboratory testing is more accurate, using a random urine sample to compare urinary albumin-to-creatinine concentration (>3 is abnormal).

Urine microscopy

This is performed on fresh mid-stream urine.

- White blood cells: >10 WBCs per high power field (HPF) on uncentrifuged urine is abnormal. Causes include cystitis, tubulointerstitial nephritis and calculi.
- Red blood cells: >1 RBC per high power field is abnormal. Red cells from the lower urinary tract look like normal, round RBCs seen on a blood film. If they are of variable size and shape, with blebs, budding or as though a 'bite' has been taken out of an edge, they are dysmorphic RBCs, which are a sign of glomerular disease.
- Bacteria: Visible bacteria may be due to contamination of the specimen, or a urinary tract infection. Whether treatment is needed depends on the number of WBCs per HPF present.
- Crystals: Uric acid crystals and calcium oxalate or calcium phosphate crystals are commonly seen in normal urine. Other types may signify an underlying disease.
- Casts: These are cylinders formed in the renal tubules from Tamm–Horsfall protein, which is normally secreted by tubular epithelium. In glomerular or tubular disease, cells in the urine become incorporated into the casts. Red cell casts are diagnostic of glomerular disease. White cell casts occur in tubulointerstitial disease and pyelonephritis. Other sorts of casts such as granular or epithelial cell casts exist.

Urinary electrolytes

Comparing urinary and serum sodium concentration is useful in the assessment of fluid balance. In hyponatraemia, a low urinary sodium is physiological, whereas a high urinary sodium suggests renal failure. In a patient with a normal serum sodium, a low urinary sodium indicates salt-and-water depletion (dehydration). Urinary sodium is also useful in differentiating types of acute renal failure. Following abdominal or pelvic surgery, it can be useful to measure urea and creatinine concentrations in fluid from drains or aspirated from a collection. If these are similar to the urine urea and creatinine concentrations, this indicates a urinary leak.

Proteinuria

Definition

A greater than normal amount of protein in the urine.

Table 6.2 Causes of proteinuria

Cause	Examples
Physiological (up to 300mg/24h)	Fever
	Exercise
	Orthostatic proteinuria
Renal	Glomerular disease
	Amyloidosis
	Pyelonephritis
	Acute tubular necrosis
Lower urinary tract	Cystitis
	Obstructive uropathy
Extra-renal causes (most of these cause some degree of intra-renal damage)	Diabetes mellitus
	Pre-eclampsia
	Hypertension
	Congestive cardiac failure
	Myeloma (or other cause of increased plasma protein)

Aetiology

Causes of proteinuria include those shown in Table 6.2.

Pathophysiology

The glomeruli normally filter 7–10 g of protein per 24 hours, but less than 2% of this is actually excreted because protein is actively reabsorbed in the proximal tubules. Normal urinary protein excretion is <150 mg/24 h, of which less than 35 mg is albumin. Proteinuria may occur by various mechanisms.

1. Overflow: Increased plasma protein exceeding tubular resorptive capacity, such as occurs in multiple myeloma.
2. Glomerular proteinuria is due to increased permeability of the glomerular basement membrane. Glomerular proteinuria may range from mild to heavy. Heavy proteinuria (>3 g/day) is termed nephrotic range proteinuria which indicates glomerular pathology. Nephrotic range proteinuria with hypoalbuminaemia and oedema is termed nephrotic syndrome.
3. Tubular disease causes impaired reabsorption of protein. Urinary β_2-microglobulin can be used as a measure of tubular function, because this small peptide is completely filtered by the glomeruli and completely reabsorbed by normal tubules. The proteinuria is usually mild in tubular disease, such as in acute tubular necrosis or pyelonephritis.
4. Increased secretion of protein (Tamm–Horsfall protein) by the kidneys or uroepithelium, which normally

accounts for half of the total protein excretion, occurs in orthostatic proteinuria, fever and exercise.

Clinical features

Proteinuria is usually asymptomatic, although heavy proteinuria may be noticed as frothy urine, or if nephrotic syndrome develops. Protein excretion increases in the upright position, and proteinuria, which disappears on early morning collection before ambulation is called orthostatic proteinuria, a benign condition affecting 2–5% of adolescents, but uncommon over the age of 30 years. If significant proteinuria is found, a careful history and examination should be made to look for an underlying cause, together with appropriate investigations.

Investigations

All positive urine dipstick measurement of protein should be confirmed by laboratory testing. Dipstick detects albumin most sensitively, but false positives are caused by alkaline urine, antibiotics and X-ray contrast media. False negatives occur when there is proteinuria without much albuminuria, e.g. Bence Jones protein.

24-hour urinary protein should be quantified with a formal 24-hour urine collection, although this is being superseded by spot urinary protein:creatinine ratios ($\leq$0.1 g = normal; 0.1–0.2 g = trace, 0.2–1.0 g = low-grade proteinuria, 1.0–3.0 g = moderate proteinuria, $\geq$3.0 g = nephrotic range proteinuria).

Initial investigations include:
- Urinalysis and microscopy to look for haematuria and evidence of urinary tract infection.
- U&E's, glucose to look for diabetes. Serum immunoglobulins and plasma protein electrophoresis.
- Renal ultrasound.
- Urine electrophoresis for Bence Jones protein or differentiating glomerular (mainly albumin) from tubular loss (lighter chain proteins).
- Renal biopsy may be necessary to make a diagnosis.

Management

Depends on underlying cause and severity. Often mild isolated proteinuria is treated expectantly after baseline investigations (BP, U&Es, plasma creatinine) have been done.

Prognosis

Microalbuminuria (30–200 mcg albumin/24 h or an early morning urine albumin:creatinine ratio >3) predicts mortality and renal failure in diabetes mellitus and cardiovascular deaths in the elderly. It also occurs in hypertension, myocardial infarction and as part of the acute phase response.

Imaging of the urinary tract

Plain X-ray of the kidneys, ureters and bladder (KUB)

On a plain X-ray radiopaque (calcium-containing, struvite and cystine) stones and renal tissue calcification, calcification of vessels (e.g. an atheromatous aorta) and calcification in tumours will show up. The outlines of the kidneys are unreliably seen because of overlying bowel gas.

Renal ultrasound scan (USS)

This is a useful imaging method of the kidneys. It avoids the use of contrast dyes, which have to be given intravenously, are nephrotoxic, and to which patients occasionally develop an allergic reaction. USS is particularly useful for the following:
- Renal obstruction, an important reversible cause of renal failure. The pelvicalyceal systems and ureter(s) look dilated except in early obstruction, or if the patient is oligoanuric. Occasionally a cause is seen such as a stone.
- To assess the size of the kidneys. In renal failure, small kidneys mean chronic renal failure, normal size kidneys usually mean acute renal failure which is potentially reversible. The exceptions are diabetes mellitus, amyloid and multiple myeloma.
- Assessment of cysts and mass lesions.
- In refractory pyelonephritis to look for a renal abscess, obstruction or an underlying anatomical abnormality such as a stone.
- For USS-guided kidney biopsy.
- Doppler USS - to look for renal blood flow, renal vein thrombosis and renal artery stenosis.

Bladder and prostate USS

Bladder USS can assess residual volumes after bladder emptying. Prostate USS is best done transrectally, and can demonstrate its size, any asymmetry, or suspicious areas. USS-guided prostatic biopsy may be performed.

Intravenous urogram/pyelogram (IVU/IVP)

This is commonly used in the investigation of renal colic, although it is also a useful tool in assessing the anatomy of the urinary tract.

A plain film is taken first as the comparison film, then a slow intravenous injection of an iodine-containing contrast dye is given (prophylaxis with high-dose steroids are given to asthmatics and those with a known allergy to iodine, to prevent an allergic reaction). Serial X-rays are then taken, which show the passage of the dye through the renal parenchyma, outlining the kidneys clearly. The dye then normally passes rapidly into the ureters. If there is obstruction, dye will be 'held-up' on one or both sides. The exact site of obstruction can often be seen with dilatation above. A filling defect within the ureter suggests a radiolucent stone or tumour. Pre and post-voiding films are taken to look for any filling defects in the bladder (stone or tumour), and to assess bladder emptying.

IVU/IVP should be avoided in significant renal impairment because of nephrotoxicity and poor dye excretion makes the test difficult to interpret. All patients should be well hydrated. Diabetics are particularly at risk of nephrotoxicity, metformin should be stopped prior to giving contrast.

Other urographic studies

These two methods are more invasive than IVU/IVP, but as the dye is given directly into the urinary tract, avoids the risk of nephrotoxicity and allergy. Therapeutic stents may be placed as part of the procedure to relieve obstruction.

1 Nephrostomy and antegrade pyelography – for upper tract obstruction, a fine-bore catheter is introduced into the dilated renal pelvis percutaneously under local anaesthetic. This relieves the obstruction and allows urine to drain out. Contrast is then injected through the catheter, to demonstrate the cause and site of obstruction.

2 Retrograde pyelography – following cystoscopy, a catheter is passed into the ureteric orifice normally under general anaesthetic. Contrast is injected and images are obtained. This is useful for defining lower ureteric lesions such as stones, and to look for transitional cell carcinoma of the ureter.

Computed tomography (CT)

In most cases, the diagnostic ability of CT is improved by giving intravenous contrast, but as noted above, certain precautions should be taken.

- Renal cysts and masses – CT can help differentiate benign cysts from malignancy.
- It can be used for staging in all types of genitourinary malignancy, including renal cell carcinoma, bladder cancer and testicular tumours.
- It is able to detect radiolucent stones missed on plain X-ray.
- In polycystic kidney disease it can be useful if one cyst is thought to be infected or malignant.

Nuclear medicine scans

A non-nephrotoxic radioisotope is given intravenously, which is taken up and excreted by the kidneys. Imaging may be 'static' (for anatomical detail), or 'dynamic' (for function).

- Static DMSA scans are more sensitive than IVU to look for scarring and ischaemia.
- Dynamic DTPA and MAG3 are used to look for renal parenchymal disease and obstruction. To look for obstruction, furosemide is given – the radioisotope will flush out promptly if there is no obstruction.

Magnetic resonance imaging/angiography (MRI/MRA)

MRI is sometimes used to further assess renal cysts and solid lesions. It is also used with gadolinium contrast to perform angiography (MRA) as a non-invasive alternative to renal angiography. Gadolinium is non-nephrotoxic.

Renal angiography

This is mainly performed for suspected renal artery stenosis. A sheath is placed in the femoral artery, and an arterial catheter passed to the aorta. Each renal artery is selectively catheterised and contrast injected. Conventional or digital subtraction angiography (DSA) may be used. DSA uses less contrast, which reduces the risk of contrast nephropathy (acute renal failure secondary to the nephrotoxic contrast). Other complications include cholesterol emboli and arterial dissection. Percutaneous renal angioplasty (PRA) and renal artery stenting can also be performed.

Cystoscopy

A rigid or flexible fibreoptic cystoscope is introduced through the urethra in order to visualise the interior of the bladder. Flexible cystoscopy can be done under local anaesthetic, as a daycase procedure, but rigid cystoscopy is performed under an epidural or general anaesthetic. The bladder is distended with distilled water or saline, and forceps or diathermy loops can be inserted through the instrument to take biopsies, and treat superficial bladder cancer (transurethral removal of bladder tumour – TURBT). The ureteric orifices can be inspected, and fibreoptic ureteroscopes can be passed up, to look for ureteric lesions such as stones or carcinoma. In addition, the ureteric orifice can be cannulated using a fine-bore catheter, so that retrograde pyelography can be performed. Prophylactic antibiotics are needed, to reduce the risk of a urinary tract infection.

Measuring renal function

Renal function testing involves measuring urea and creatinine and glomerular filtration rate (GFR). Urea and creatinine may remain normal until more than half of renal function is lost.

Normal kidneys receive 25% of the cardiac output. The volume that is ultrafiltrated per minute is the GFR, and it is the sum of the filtration that occurs in all the functioning nephrons. When nephrons are lost or are not functioning properly, there is compensation by the remaining nephrons by hyperfiltration, and improved solute clearance. If there is poor blood supply to the kidneys, due for example to hypotension or cardiac failure, the GFR will fall – even though the nephrons are intact.

Serum urea: Urea is freely filtered at the glomeruli, but variably reabsorbed by the tubules, and its production fluctuates considerably, even within an individual. It is higher following protein intake, in a catabolic state, after steroids or gastrointestinal (GI) haemorrhage, and lower when patients are not eating, and in liver disease. In dehydration, urea rises proportionally more than creatinine because it is avidly reabsorbed at the proximal tubules in a fluid-depleted state.

A urea above normal therefore suggests renal failure, GI bleeding or dehydration. If the creatinine is also proportionally raised (creatinine is normally ~20× urea) above normal, this indicates intrinsic renal failure.

Serum creatinine: Creatinine is produced as a waste product when creatine phosphate is broken down in muscle. The amount produced is lower in those with low muscle bulk, in women, children and the elderly. It is freely filtered, a small amount is also secreted at the tubules. Plasma creatinine is increased by strenuous exercise, ingestion of meat, certain drugs (trimethoprim and cimetidine) impair tubular secretion. It is decreased in malnutrition, wasting diseases, immediately after surgery and by corticosteroids. For these reasons there is wide variation in normal creatinine levels between individuals. In most patients, serial or previous measurements of creatinine are useful to monitor the progress of renal function.

Glomerular filtration rate (GFR): To assess the GFR the rate at which a substance is cleared from the plasma is measured. The normal GFR = 80–130 mL/min/1.73 m^2 body surface area. Clearance is defined as the 'virtual' volume of blood cleared (by the kidney) of solute per unit time. If a substance is completely filtered by the glomeruli and not secreted, absorbed or metabolised by the renal tubules then its urinary clearance equals GFR. Creatinine almost fulfils these criteria, and is used in clinical practice to measure GFR using a 24-hour urine collection:

$$\text{Urinary clearance} = \frac{UV}{P} \text{ (usually expressed in mL/min)}$$

where U = urinary concentration, V = urine flow rate and P = plasma creatinine.

Blood creatinine levels are inversely related to clearance. This means that with normal renal function a small rise in creatinine means a large fall in GFR. Conversely in patients with moderate to severe renal failure, i.e. a low GFR, even a small further fall in GFR will result in a large increase in creatinine (see Fig. 6.2).

24-hour urinary collections are inconvenient and inaccurate. The creatinine clearance can be calculated from a patient's serum creatinine using formulae correcting for factors like the patient's age, sex and weight (which adjust for muscle mass). The best known of these is the Cockcroft and Gault formula:

$$\text{CrCl (mL/min)} = \frac{1.23 \times (140 - \text{age}) \times \text{weight (kg)}}{\text{Cr (μmol/L)}}$$

For women multiply by 1.04 rather than 1.23. When accurate GFR measurement is needed the rate of clearance of a radioisotope is used. This is indicated in severe

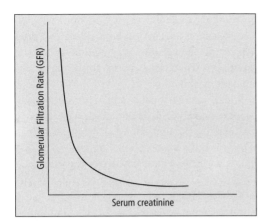

Figure 6.2 Relationship of GFR to creatinine.

renal failure (creatinine clearance becomes inaccurate), for kidney donors and patients receiving chemotherapy.

Anion gap

Anion gap calculation is useful in metabolic acidosis, to differentiate causes. It is a measure of the unestimated anions (phosphate, ketones, lactate) and cations. The formula used to calculate the anion gap varies from source to source, and the normal range depends on the methods by which the laboratory measures each electrolyte. For example:

$$\text{Anion gap} = K^+ + Na^+ - Cl^- - HCO_3^-$$
$$\text{Normal range} = 8 - 16 \text{mmol/L}$$

In metabolic acidosis, an increased anion gap occurs due to raised acid levels:
- Lactic acidosis (exercise, shock, hypoxia, liver failure).
- Acid ingestion (aspirin, ethylene glycol).
- Ketoacidosis.
- Uraemia.

In metabolic acidosis, a normal anion gap indicates that there is failure to excrete acid or loss of base:
- Failure to excrete acid occurs in renal tubular disease and Addison's disease.
- Loss of base (bicarbonate) occurs in diarrhoea, proximal renal tubular acidosis, or iatrogenically, due to carbonic anhydrase inhibitor or ureterosigmoidostomy.

Renal biopsy

Renal biopsy is indicated when glomerular disease is suspected, and in unexplained acute renal failure. It may also

be performed in cases of deterioration of renal function in patients with known kidney disease, to help guide treatment, for example in systemic lupus erythematosus, and relatively frequently in renal transplant patients particularly to look for rejection.

The biopsy can be performed percutaneously, or at open surgery (unusual unless the other method is not possible, or contraindicated, e.g. single kidney). Ultrasound guidance is used, and usually two cores are obtained using a spring-loaded biopsy needle. These are examined under light microscopy, electron microscopy and immunofluoresence or immunoperoxidase staining.

Complications include haematuria, bleeding under the renal capsule and bleeding out into the retroperitoneal space, arteriovenous aneurysm formation (if very large may need treatment) and discomfort. In up to 3% of individuals, blood transfusion is required for bleeding, and in 0.1–0.4% surgery or interventional radiology (artery embolisation using coils) is needed to stop the bleeding. Nephrectomy or death occur rarely.

Contraindications to percutaneous renal biopsy:
- Clotting abnormality or low platelets (unless corrected).
- Small kidneys (<9 cm), as this indicates chronic irreversible kidney damage.
- Uncontrolled hypertension.
- Multiple bilateral cysts or tumour.
- Active urinary tract infection.
- If there is hydronephrosis, then obstruction should be corrected, and renal biopsy re-considered and performed if there is still an indication.

Relative contraindications include obesity (technically difficult), single kidney (except of a transplanted kidney) and pregnancy, as this carries special risks, but biopsy may be necessary if urgent diagnosis and treatment are needed.

Dialysis

When the kidneys fail to a degree that causes symptoms and complications of renal failure, renal replacement therapy (RRT) is needed to remove waste products and fluid, and to restore electrolytes and fluid balance to as normal as possible. There are several types of RRT, including haemodialysis, haemofiltration and peritoneal dialysis. Despite advances in technology, these are still unable to completely mimic renal function, and none are able to replace the endocrine functions of the kidney.

Renal transplantation is a special form of RRT which most closely restores a physiological state, including the endocrine functions. Patients may switch modality many times whilst on RRT.

Haemodialysis

Blood has to be pumped from the patient, and passed through a 'dialyser', sometimes called an artificial kidney. The dialyser consists of an array of semi-permeable membranes. The blood flows past the membrane on one side, whilst on the other side, a solution of purified water, sodium, potassium, calcium, magnesium, chloride, dextrose and bicarbonate or acetate is kept flowing in the other direction (counter-current – see Fig. 6.3).

Solutes diffuse across the semi-permeable membrane down a concentration gradient. Small solutes with a large concentration gradient diffuse rapidly, e.g. urea and creatinine, whereas diffusion is slower with larger molecules or if the concentration gradient is low.

The diffusion gradient is kept high by keeping blood and dialysate flows high, and also by using counter-current flow. Proteins are too large to cross the membrane. fluid is removed by generating a transmembrane pressure, so that fluid is pushed out from the blood compartment into the dialysate compartment. Water drags small and medium molecular weight solutes with it. This is called ultrafiltration. Several hours of dialysis, usually three times a week, are needed to achieve satisfactory urea and creatinine clearance. Underdialysis (lack of adequate dialysis) is associated with an increase in cardiovascular and other morbidity and mortality. To remove and return blood, the patient must have vascular access such as an arteriovenous fistula or a double-lumen central venous line. The blood needs to be anticoagulated (usually with heparin) to stop it clotting in the dialysis machine.

Although many patients cope very well with dialysis, common symptoms include headache, joint pains and fatigue during and after a dialysis session. Complications include hypotension, line infections, dialysis amyloid and increased cardiovascular mortality.

Haemofiltration

Continuous renal replacement therapy, as takes place on intensive care units, uses ultrafiltration as the main method rather than dialysis. Convection carries water and solutes across a highly permeable membrane and this is removed. Before the blood is returned to the body, fluid is replaced using a lactate or bicarbonate-based solution containing solutes in the desired concentrations (see Fig. 6.4).

The advantage of continuous therapy is that removal of fluid and changes in electrolyte concentration take place more gradually, reducing this risk of hypotension. It is expensive in both materials and staffing and therefore only takes place on intensive care units.

Peritoneal dialysis

In peritoneal dialysis (PD), fluid and solutes are exchanged across the peritoneal membrane by putting dialysis solution into the abdominal cavity. Peritoneal access is obtained by putting a tube through the anterior abdominal wall. Dialysate is run under gravity into the peritoneal cavity and the fluid is left there for several hours. Small solutes diffuse down their concentration gradients between capillary blood vessels in the peritoneal lining and the dialysate. Fluid removal takes place by osmosis. The osmotically active agent in PD fluid is usually dextrose.

Dialysate exchanges are usually performed by the patient, four or five times a day (CAPD – continuous ambulatory peritoneal dialysis), or some or all of the exchanges can by performed by an automated cycling device to which the patient is attached at night (APD – automated peritoneal dialysis). Patients often develop some constipation which can limit the flow of dialysate, they are treated with laxatives. Hernias should be repaired before starting PD.

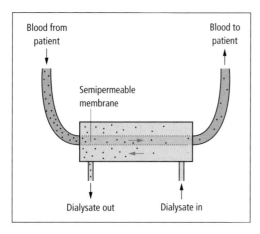

Figure 6.3 Principles of haemodialysis.

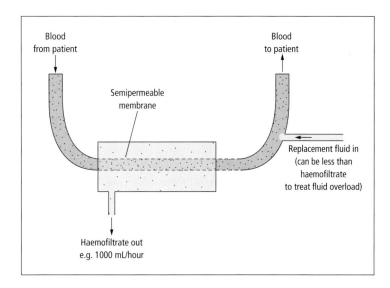

Figure 6.4 Principles of haemofiltration.

Bacterial infection of the tunnelled catheter and bacterial peritonitis are the most common serious complications. Patients with PD peritonitis present with abdominal pain (80%), 'cloudy bags', fever and nausea, vomiting and diarrhoea without classical signs of peritonitis. This can be treated by adding antibiotics to the peritoneal dialysate. In the longer term, PD may become unable to adequately dialyse a patient, as the peritoneal membrane fails.

Disorders of the kidney

Renal failure

Definition
Renal failure is defined as a reduction in the glomerular filtration rate (GFR), which leads to a loss of the ability of the kidney to perform its functions properly.

The kidneys have three important functions:
1 Fluid and electrolyte balance, including acid–base balance.
2 Excretion of waste products and many drugs and toxins.
3 Hormone synthesis (such as erythropoietin, vitamin D and renin).

A normal kidney has 1 million nephrons. The nephron is the basic unit of the kidney. It consists of the glomerulus and its associated vascular supply and the tubules, loop of Henle and collecting ducts. There is a large degree of redundancy in the kidney, so many nephrons may be lost before there is a noticeable change in fluid and electrolyte balance, and even more before there are symptoms of renal failure.

It is useful when considering the causes of renal failure to divide the kidney into three parts (see Fig. 6.5).
• Blood supply (aorta, renal arteries etc.) – prerenal.
• Parenchyma (the 'meat' of the kidney, consisting of nephrons and interstitium) – renal.

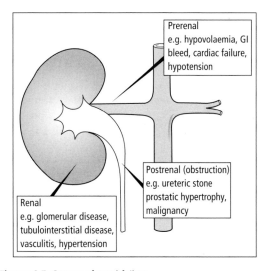

Figure 6.5 Causes of renal failure.

- Draining system (the renal pelvis, ureters and bladder outflow) – postrenal.

More than one type may co-exist, as prerenal or postrenal failure can lead to parenchymal involvement.

- In prerenal failure, the kidney is not damaged but functionally compromised due to ischaemia, so reversal of the cause leads to prompt recovery of renal function, although in some cases correction can be difficult.
- In renal failure, there is evidence of parenchymal disease. There may be a pre-existing prerenal factor, which led to renal damage. Recovery may be possible, though if the disease is severe and scarring results, full functional recovery is unlikely.
- With postrenal failure as with prerenal failure, early treatment can avert irreversible damage to the kidneys. If left undetected for some time, for example one kidney is first affected without causing symptoms, then the other precipitates renal failure, there may be permanent loss of function.

Renal failure causes

1 A rise in serum concentrations of urea, creatinine, hydrogen ions (causing a metabolic acidosis) and potassium (hyperkalaemia). The rate at which these rise depends on a number of factors, including how catabolic the patient is, i.e. the rate of tissue breakdown, in particular muscle breakdown causes a marked rise in potassium. Uraemia (a term used to describe raised urea and creatinine) is associated with anorexia, nausea, vomiting and increased bleeding tendency (due to a reduction in platelet function). Neurological effects include confusion, myoclonus and lowered seizure threshold. It is thought that urea and creatinine are not directly responsible for the observed clinical features but that there are other uraemic toxins which rise in parallel with urea and creatinine.

2 Loss of the kidneys' ability to manage salt and water. Oliguria (urine output <15 mL/hour or <400 mL/24hour) is common, but does not occur with all causes of renal failure. This can cause fluid overload, i.e. peripheral oedema and pulmonary oedema, particularly in those with impaired cardiac function, the elderly, and those given excessive amounts of intravenous fluids in order to try and reverse a preceding hypovolaemic state. Water retention can lead to hyponatraemia.

3 Reduced production of 1, 25-dihydroxycholecalciferol, which can lead to low calcium, and reduced excretion of phosphate causes hyperphosphataemia. High phosphates cause pruritus (itching), chronic renal failure leads to renal osteodystrophy.

4 Anaemia (normocytic, normochromic) can occur reduced erythropoietin production.

The presentation of renal failure may be asymptomatic (diagnosed on blood tests), with symptoms and signs of acute renal failure or the more insidious symptoms of chronic renal failure.

Acute renal failure

Definition

A deterioration of renal function (loss of GFR) over a period of days to weeks.

Aetiology/pathophysiology

The causes may be divided into prerenal, renal and postrenal, whilst they all have different mechanisms, the result is loss of the three functions of the kidney: fluid and electrolyte balance, excretion of waste products and toxins, and hormone synthesis (see Table 6.3).

Clinical features

The main clinical features are usually those of the underlying cause together with symptoms and signs caused by the renal failure. Acute renal failure (ARF) may be difficult to differentiate from chronic renal failure (CRF) without a recent onset in symptoms of an underlying cause, e.g. loin pain, a previous serum creatinine measurement or further investigations.

- In asymptomatic patients, ARF may be detected by a rise in plasma creatinine or abnormality on urine dipstick.
- Reduced urine output or a change in urine appearance. Complete anuria is only seen with bladder outflow obstruction, bilateral (or unilateral in a single functioning kidney) ureteric obstruction.
- Loin pain – this is suggestive of a renal stone (or other cause of obstruction), pyelonephritis or renal infarction.
- Anorexia, vomiting, fever, malaise, hiccoughs, confusion, seizures.
- Hyperventilation may be due to hypoxia or respiratory compensation for metabolic acidosis.

Table 6.3 Causes of acute renal failure

Cause	Examples
Prerenal	
Hypovolaemia and/or hypotension	Bleeding, dehydration, diuretics
	Sepsis, cardiac failure, drugs
Renal ischaemia or congestion	Renal artery stenosis (acutely exacerbated by an ACE-inhibitor), aortic dissection, renal vein thrombosis
Severe liver disease	Hepatorenal syndrome*
Renal	
Acute tubular necrosis (ATN)	Any cause of pre-renal failure, drugs and toxins
Acute glomerulonephritis	Primary and secondary causes of glomerular disease
Acute interstitial nephritis	Pyelonephritis, drugs
Cast nephropathy	Myeloma
Diseases of glomerular capillaries or small/medium sized blood vessels	Haemolytic uraemic syndrome, vasculitis, systemic sclerosis, accelerated phase hypertension, pre-eclampsia
Postrenal	
Obstruction of the bladder outflow or bilateral upper tracts	Stones (bilateral), pelvic malignancy, bladder outflow obstruction, retroperitoneal disease (lymphoma, aortic dissection, retroperitoneal fibrosis)

*Mechanism unclear, resolves with hepatic recovery.

It is important to assess the volume status by assessing blood pressure, jugular venous pressure, skin turgor, ankle or sacral oedema and pulmonary oedema. Hypertension may be a feature.

Complications

Hyperkalaemia may cause cardiac arrhythmias and sudden death. Fluid overload may cause cardiac failure, pulmonary oedema. Gastric erosions and GI bleeding are quite common. Uraemic pericarditis can rarely lead to tamponade. During recovery of ATN, there may be polyuria in which it is often difficult to maintain sufficient water and electrolyte input.

Investigations

The aims are to try to distinguish acute and chronic renal failure, between prerenal, renal or postrenal causes, as well as the underlying cause.

- Urgent urinalysis, followed by microscopy (to look for cells and casts) and culture.
- Urine sodium concentration. In prerenal failure, or in renal failure without tubular dysfunction the kidney will reabsorb sodium so that urinary sodium is less than 20 mmol/L (exceptions to this are in the presence of diuretics, in pre-existing chronic renal failure). If there is tubular damage, then the ability of the kidney to concentrate sodium falls, so that urinary sodium rises to >40 mmol/L.
- Bloods
  1 Anaemia (normochromic, normocytic if underlying disease or in chronic renal failure).
  2 Raised urea, creatinine, K^+, urate.
  3 Reduced Ca^{2+} with increased PO_4.
  4 Na^+ may be high, normal or low.
  5 Arterial/venous blood gas shows a metabolic acidosis usually with increased anion gap.
  6 LFTs.
  7 Creatine kinase (CK) – raised in myocardial infarction but also very high in rhabdomyolysis (muscle breakdown).
- ECG, chest X-ray.
- Renal imaging to exclude obstruction – a renal ultrasound should be obtained as soon as possible to look for hydronephrosis (dilated renal pelvis, calyces and ureters) and for renal size.
- Consider further tests for causes of ARF if diagnosis still unclear. These include autoantibody profile, complement levels, blood and urine tests for myeloma and possibly a renal biopsy.

Management

Acute renal failure is an emergency, with possible life-threatening complications.

Reversible causes should be treated as soon as possible; withdraw any potentially nephrotoxic drugs, treat sepsis, malignant hypertension, and relieve any obstruction.

Fluid management

- If volume depletion is causing renal failure then appropriate fluid replacement (usually colloid, crystalloid or blood) should be given. Fluid challenges may be required with regular review to ensure that the patient does not become fluid overloaded. Central venous pressure measurement may be helpful, but should not be relied upon over clinical assessment especially in the presence of cardiac or pulmonary disease. Urinary catheterisation is not always required, and carries a risk of introducing infection. Urine output should increase in response to filling. If it does not, and the patient is well filled, then there is likely to be concomitant renal ARF. If blood pressure remains low despite filling (such as due to cardiac insufficiency, sepsis), then additional treatment, usually inotropic support is needed with specialist help.

- Once the patient is normovolaemic intravenous fluids should be reduced to maintenance levels to avoid precipitating fluid overload.
- In fluid overload, or in oliguric renal failure high doses of furosemide may be effective in causing a diuresis. However, there is no good evidence that furosemide speeds the recovery from renal failure, and it should be avoided in those thought to have pre-renal failure.
- Pulmonary oedema which does not respond to diuretics may have to be treated initially with vasodilators (intravenous GTN, diamorphine) and ventilatory support including non-invasive ventilation, but the only definitive treatment is haemodialysis or haemofiltration.

Hyperkalaemia

- Treat severe hyperkalaemia (K > 6.0 mmol/L) urgently to avoid cardiac arrhythmias (see page 7).
- Stop any drugs that cause high potassium (ACE-inhibitors, spironalactone).

General measures

- A multidisciplinary approach is required, involving physiotherapists, nurses and nutritionists.
- Monitor fluid in/out, daily weight (this is a useful, accurate way of monitoring fluid balance).
- Low salt and potassium diet. Ensure adequate nutrition.
- Review all medication for dosages in renal failure.
- Consider prophylaxis against gastrointestinal bleeding.
- Referral to a renal physician should be considered if there are red cell casts or heavy proteinuria, if the diagnosis is unclear or if there is acute-on-chronic renal failure.

Indications for urgent dialysis

- Persistent hyperkalaemia >6 mmol/L despite medical therapy
- Severe acidosis
- Refractory pulmonary oedema
- Pericarditis, cardiac tamponade, encephalopathy (flap)
- Rapidly progressive renal failure

Prognosis

Depends on underlying cause and concomitant medical conditions. Oliguric ARF has a higher mortality.

Acute tubular necrosis (ATN)

Definition

Necrosis of renal tubular epithelium as caused by hypoperfusion of the kidneys and certain toxins.

Aetiology

The main causes are hypoperfusion, i.e. the causes of pre-renal failure (more common) and toxins (see Tables 6.3 and 6.4).

Pathophysiology

The renal medulla is particularly susceptible to ischaemia, because of high metabolic activity. In addition, in shock renal blood flow is particularly likely to suffer because of constriction of renal vessels due to

Table 6.4 Causes of acute tubular necrosis

Causes of ATN	Examples
Hypoperfusion	
Hypovolaemia	Severe burns, haemorrhage, diarrhoea
	Intravascular hypovolaemia, e.g. nephrotic syndrome
	Diuretics
Impaired cardiac output	Cardiac failure
Septic shock	
Toxin induced	
Endogenous	Haemoglobinuria, myoglobinuria, hepatic toxins, uric acid, Bence–Jones protein
Exogenous	Drugs, e.g. antibiotics, NSAIDs, cytotoxics
	X-ray contrast
	Organic solvents: chloroform, carbon tetrachloride

sympathetic activity and the release of vasoconstrictive substances. The glomerular filtration rate (GFR) falls in response to hypoperfusion, and ischaemia causes the tubules to lose function.

Toxins may have a variety of mechanisms such as causing vasoconstriction, a direct toxic effect on tubular cells causing their dysfunction, and they may also cause the death of tubular epithelial cells which block the tubules. The glomeruli (which are well perfused) may continue to filter urine in large volumes, and if the tubules are not reabsorbing the filtrate, urine output may be maintained (non-oliguric renal failure) or even increased (polyuric renal failure).

Ischaemia or toxins can cause tubular epithelial cells to die and slough away from the basement membrane, blocking the tubules. Blockage of the renal tubules causes a secondary reduction in glomerular blood flow.

If the basement membrane is intact, tubular epithelium regrows within 10–20 days, restoring function to the nephrons. Dead material is phagocytosed. The epithelial cells take time to differentiate and develop their concentrating function.

Clinical features

ATN presents as with acute renal failure. It typically passes through three phases:

- Oliguric phase (reduced GFR): Acute renal failure with complications of hyperkalaemia, metabolic acidosis and fluid overload (pulmonary oedema). This phase may last many weeks, depending on the initial severity of insult.
- Polyuric phase: This is during early recovery, patients may pass 5 L or more of urine a day and are at risk of developing secondary problems with water and electrolyte (Na^+, K^+, Ca^{++}) depletion. Initially uraemia may persist, but this usually gradually improves.
- Recovery to baseline renal function, or with some residual deficit.

Management

The management is similar to that of acute renal failure.

Prognosis

In acute tubular necrosis the mortality is high but if the patient survives the prognosis for renal recovery is good.

Table 6.5 Causes of chronic renal failure

Uncertain	19%
Diabetes mellitus	17%
Glomerulonephritis	12%
Pyelonephritis/reflux nephropathy	10%
Renovascular disease	7%
Hypertension	6%
Adult polycystic kidney disease	6%
Other (inc. not sent)	23%

Chronic renal failure

Definition

Chronic renal failure (CRF) is a loss of renal function occurring over months to years because of the destruction of nephrons. End-stage renal failure (ESRF) is loss of renal function requiring any form of chronic renal replacement therapy, i.e. long-term dialysis or transplanbreaktation.

Incidence

The exact number of people with chronic renal failure is difficult to estimate, as many are undetected. The number who progress to end-stage renal failure and commence renal replacement therapy is ~100 per million population per year in the U.K.

Aetiology

The main causes in England and Wales (2002) are listed in Table 6.5. Certain systemic diseases commonly cause renal disease such as amyloid, myeloma, systemic lupus erythematosus and gout.

In a significant proportion of patients no underlying cause is found. These patients are often labelled as ESRF secondary to hypertension, but this may be a result of the renal failure rather than the cause.

Pathophysiology

Progressive destruction of nephrons leads to gradual reduction in renal function, with loss of the three functions of the kidney:

1 Electrolyte and water homeostatic disturbance may cause fluid overload, hypertension, hyperkalaemia and metabolic acidosis as well as rises in serum urea and creatinine. Initially there may be a phase of large volumes of dilute urine production due to reduction in tubular reabsorption. As the glomerular filtration rate (GFR) falls further urine volumes fall to less than normal.

2 Excretion of waste products, drugs and toxins is reduced leading to complications of toxicity.

3 The hormone functions of the kidney are also affected: reduction of vitamin D activation causes hypocalcaemia and hyperparathyroidism; reduced erythropoietin production causes anaemia.

As renal function declines to about 10–20% of normal, i.e. a GFR of ~15 mL/min, symptoms develop. Acute renal failure (ARF) may also lead to these symptoms, although they are more commonly seen in CRF. This is called uraemia – which literally means 'urine in the blood'. The onset of uraemia is insidious, but by the time serum urea is >40 mmol/L, creatinine >1000 μmol/L, most patients have symptoms. No single toxin has been identified, and in fact urea itself is not thought to be very toxic, but it acts as a convenient marker for other products.

Clinical features

The onset of symptoms is variable. Early symptoms are mostly due to anaemia (malaise, fatigue and shortness of breath on exertion). Late symptoms include pruritis, anorexia, nausea and vomiting – very late symptoms are pericarditis, encephalopathy (confusion, coma, seizures) and tachypnoea due to metabolic acidosis.

There are few signs of ESRF, although there may be signs of the underlying cause such as diabetic retinopathy, renal or femoral bruits, an enlarged prostate or polycystic kidneys. It is important to assess the fluid status by looking at the jugular venous pressure, skin turgor, lying and standing blood pressure, and for evidence of pulmonary or peripheral oedema (see Fig. 6.6).

Complications

CRF patients are much more prone to ARF (acute-on-chronic renal failure), for example due to drugs, radiographic contrast and dehydration. Patients with CRF are affected by accelerated atherosclerosis which occurs due to long-term hypertension, hyperlipidaemia, disordered calcium and phosphate metabolism (calcified vessels) and uraemia. They also develop left ventricular hypertrophy due to hypertension. Cardiovascular morbidity and mortality are much higher than in patients with normal renal function.

Macroscopy/microscopy

The kidneys are usually small and shrivelled, with scarring of glomeruli, interstitial fibrosis and tubular atrophy.

Investigations

The aim of investigations is to make a diagnosis of the cause, and in addition, to consider if there is any acute condition precipitating the renal failure, e.g. prerenal failure, sepsis, obstruction or a nephrotoxin. Any previous historical urea and creatinine measurements are very useful.

The investigations for ARF on CRF or undiagnosed CRF are similar to those for ARF (see page 235), including the blood tests, imaging and possibly renal biopsy.

Chronic renal failure is now classified as stages 1–5 of chronic kidney disease, according to GFR and other features (see Table 6.6).

In the routine follow-up of CRF, the usual investigations include the following:

- FBC to look for anaemia.
- U&E to assess progress of the renal failure, ensure Na^+ and K^+ are normal.
- Bicarbonate to look for acidosis.
- Calcium, phosphate, ALP, PTH (X-ray hands to assess for renal osteodystrophy).
- CRP (ESR is normally raised in CRF, but a raised CRP suggests infection).
- Hyperlipidaemia should be looked for.
- Urinalysis is performed to look for proteinuria and haematuria (if new or increasing these may need further investigation) and urinary tract infections.
- Underlying causes may need to be monitored, e.g. HbA_1C for diabetes mellitus and urate for gout.

Table 6.6 Staging of chronic kidney disease (CKD)

Stage 1 CKD	Kidney damage but normal GFR (>90 mL/min)
Stage 2 CKD	Mild kidney damage (GFR 60–89 mL/min)
Stage 3 CKD	Moderate kidney damage (GFR 30–59 mL/min)
Stage 4 CKD	Severe kidney damage (GFR 15–29 mL/min)
Stage 5 CKD	Kidney failure (GFR <15 mL/min or ESRF on renal replacement therapy)

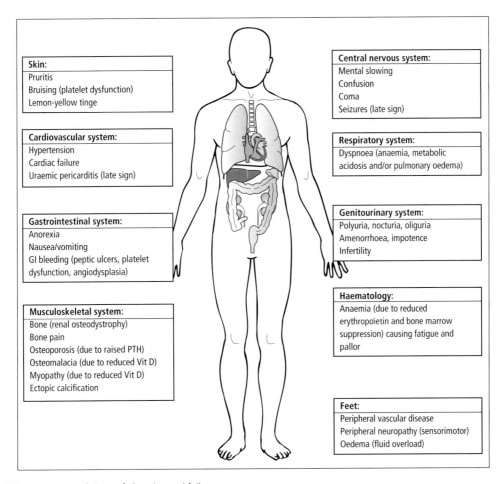

Skin:
Pruritis
Bruising (platelet dysfunction)
Lemon-yellow tinge

Cardiovascular system:
Hypertension
Cardiac failure
Uraemic pericarditis (late sign)

Gastrointestinal system:
Anorexia
Nausea/vomiting
GI bleeding (peptic ulcers, platelet
dysfunction, angiodysplasia)

Musculoskeletal system:
Bone (renal osteodystrophy)
Bone pain
Osteoporosis (due to raised PTH)
Osteomalacia (due to reduced Vit D)
Myopathy (due to reduced Vit D)
Ectopic calcification

Central nervous system:
Mental slowing
Confusion
Coma
Seizures (late sign)

Respiratory system:
Dyspnoea (anaemia, metabolic
acidosis and/or pulmonary oedema)

Genitourinary system:
Polyuria, nocturia, oliguria
Amenorrhoea, impotence
Infertility

Haematology:
Anaemia (due to reduced
erythropoíetin and bone marrow
suppression) causing fatigue and
pallor

Feet:
Peripheral vascular disease
Peripheral neuropathy (sensorimotor)
Oedema (fluid overload)

Figure 6.6 Symptoms and signs of chronic renal failure.

Management

The aim is to delay the onset of end-stage renal failure (ESRF) and uraemia as long as possible. Refer early to a renal specialist (certainly if the serum creatinine is ≥ 150 μmol/L).

- Identify and treat any underlying causes appropriately such as glomerulonephritis, diabetes, hypertension, obstruction, recurrent urinary tract infections. Proteinuria may be reduced by ACE inhibitors and/or angiotensin II receptor antagonists.
- Diet: Salt restriction if hypertensive, potassium restrict if hyperkalaemia is a problem, ensure adequate calories and a reasonable protein intake, supplement vitamins and iron. Patients need to follow a low phosphate diet.
- Avoid nephrotoxic agents if possible, and review and adjust drug doses.

- Cardiovascular: Treat even mild hypertension and consider treating hyperlipidaemia. Encourage patients to stop smoking and take regular exercise. Oedema may respond to fluid restriction and/or diuretics.
- Early symptoms due to anaemia are often treated effectively by giving erythropoietin.
- Bone disease needs to be treated, with calcium and vitamin D (alfacalcidol) supplements, but aim to lower serum phosphate with reduced intake and phosphate binders.

Some patients will live out their life with the above treatments, and die of other causes. Others may not be fit for dialysis, or prefer conservative treatment. Dialysis is indicated when symptoms of uraemia develop, but before problems with fluid overload, hyperkalaemia or late-stage symptoms such as pericarditis ensue.

Prognosis

Treatment ameliorates some of the symptoms and biochemical disturbances; however, not all patients respond to treatment. Renal transplantation offers the best treatment, but is of limited availability.

Renal osteodystrophy

Definition

This term refers to the various bone diseases that develop due to chronic renal failure.

Pathophysiology

The main mechanism is that of secondary hyperparathyroidism:

1 Chronic renal failure causes reduced hydroxylation of $25(OH)D_2$ to the active vitamin D metabolite, $1,25(OH)_2D_3$. This leads to reduced absorption of calcium from the diet and therefore lowers serum calcium levels. In addition, phosphate levels rise, due to reduced renal excretion. This binds calcium, further lowering serum calcium levels and also causes calcium deposits in tissues.

2 In response to the low serum calcium, the parathyroid glands in the neck are stimulated to produce increased amounts of parathyroid hormone (i.e. secondary hyperparathyroidism).

3 Hyperparathyroidism leads to increased osteoclastic activity (to mobilise calcium from bone, and partially restore serum calcium levels to normal. Hyperparathyroidism also releases PO_4, which cannot be excreted and so contributes further to hyperphosphataemia.

Other mechanisms include:

- Metabolic acidosis also promotes demineralisation of bone.
- On long-term renal dialysis aluminium is retained, which deposits in bone, blocking calcification of the osteoid.

Clinical features

See Osteomalacia, Osteoporosis, Secondary and Tertiary Hyperparathyroidism for the clinical features and X-ray findings.

Osteosclerosis may also occur, where there are alternate stripes of sclerotic and osteoporotic bone. This affects the trabecular bone of the spine, to produce a 'rugger-jersey spine' appearance on X-ray.

Investigations

- Serum Ca^{2+} may be normal or low, PO_4^{2-} is high and often alkaline phosphatase is raised.
- Raised parathyroid hormone.
- $25(OH)D_2$ (Vitamin D_2) is normal but $1,25(OH)_2D_3$ (Vitamin D_3) is low.

Management

Serum PO_4^{2-} must be lowered by restricting dietary intake and taking phosphate binders such as calcium carbonate with meals. Vitamin D supplements (active analogues, e.g. alfacalcidol which do not require renal activation) are used in addition to ensuring an adequate calcium intake. The aim of treatment is to suppress the PTH to slightly higher than normal levels, control the parameters, avoid ectopic calcification and bone disease.

Glomerular disease

The glomerulus is an intricate structure, the function of which depends on all its constituent parts being intact (see Fig. 6.7).

1 Blood reaches the glomerular capillary system via the afferent arteriole. On the vascular side of the barrier between the blood and the filtrate is endothelium, fused to the glomerular basement membrane (GBM). On the filtrate side is an epithelium composed of podocytes, attached to the GBM by foot processes. The connective tissue, which supports the capillary network, is called 'mesangium'.

2 The pressure in the glomerular capillaries is higher than that in the urinary lumen, so that constituents of the blood are filtered into the urinary lumen. This 'ultrafiltrate' is almost an exact mirror of plasma except for proteins because the GBM is relatively impermeable to high molecular weight proteins such as albumin. It is also less permeable to negatively charged molecules.

There are three main types of glomerular disease:

- Glomerulonephritis describes a variety of conditions characterised by inflammation of glomeruli in both kidneys, which have an immunological basis.
- Vasculitis which can mimic glomerulonephritis, by damage to the glomerular vessels.
- Glomerular damage may also occur due to infiltration by abnormal material, such as by amyloid (see page 513).

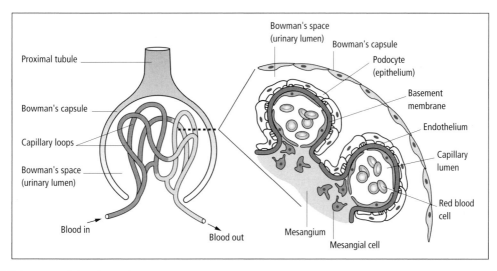

Figure 6.7 Structure of the glomerulus.

The type of damage caused to the structure of the glomerulus determines the pathological appearance, has a broad relationship to the effect on renal function and hence the clinical presentation. The disease process may be diffuse affecting all the glomeruli, or focal affecting only some of the glomeruli. Affected glomeruli may be completely damaged (global), or only a part may be damaged (segmental). Most glomerular diseases are either diffuse global or focal segmental.

Within the glomerulus itself, there are different appearances:

- Proliferation of endothelial cells and mesangial cells is common in diseases that cause nephritic syndrome (see Fig. 6.8). Endothelial cell proliferation leads to occlusion of the capillary lumen, reduced blood flow, oliguria and acute renal failure. Mesangial cell proliferation, which is usually associated with increased production of mesangial matrix, can lead to scarring (sclerosis) of all or part of the glomerulus. Increased matrix can lead to reduced blood flow and/or proteinuria.
- GBM thickening, which can be due to a number of mechanisms, tends to cause nephrotic syndrome, and can be due to a number of mechanisms (often co-existent) including deposition of immune complexes, over-synthesis of basement membrane material and in-growth of mesangium.
- More severe patterns may occur when the glomerular capillary walls are acutely and severely damaged.

Fibrinoid necrosis, where fibrin is deposited in the necrotic vessel walls. Crescents are formed when necrotic vessel walls leak blood and fibrin, so that macrophages and proliferating epithelial cells invade the Bowman's space, crushing the glomerulus. If there are crescents in most of the glomeruli, the term rapidly progressive glomerulonephritis is used, as severe rapid onset acute renal failure usually results.

Almost all forms of glomerulonephritis have a cellular or humoral immunological basis:

- Humoral response: Immune deposits (antibodies or antibody–antigen complexes) in the glomerulus fix and activate complement and a variety of other inflammatory mediators such as antioxidants, proteases and cytokines. The sites, number and type of deposits determine the type and extent of damage caused. Mesangial deposits cause mesangial cell proliferation and increased mesangial matrix. Subendothelial deposits are close to the glomerular capillary lumen, so excite marked inflammation which can lead to rapidly progressive glomerular nephritis, whereas subepithelial deposits excite less of an inflammatory response, because the glomerular basement membrane prevents the influx of cells from the capillaries. Circulating immune complexes filtered by the kidney tend to cause less injury than complexes formed *de novo* in the glomerulus.
- Cellular response: Some glomerular diseases (such as minimal change nephropathy and focal segmental

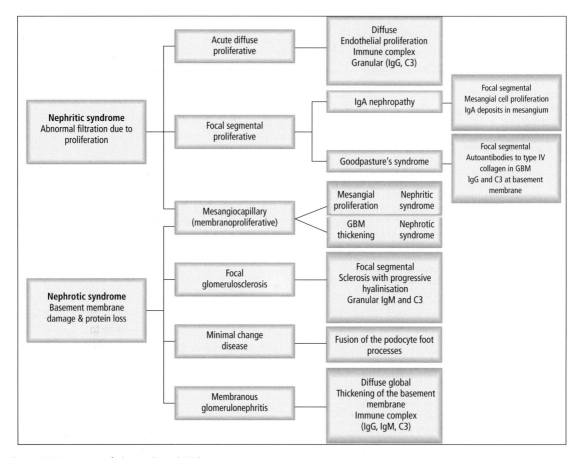

Figure 6.8 Summary of glomerulonephritides.

glomerulosclerosis) show little or no antibody deposition. It appears that lymphocytes, in particular T cells play a role in causing the functional changes.

- Macrophages: These may be involved in both humoral and cellular pathways.

Immunofluorescence and electron microscopy: The diagnosis of glomerular disease may not be possible with light microscopy only. Immunofluorescence is used to look for immune complex and C_3 and C_4 deposits and electron microscopy is also used.

Nephrotic syndrome

Definition

Nephrotic syndrome is defined as proteinuria (>3 g/24 hour), hypoalbuminaemia and oedema. See also proteinuria (page 227).

Aetiology

The most common causes of nephrotic syndrome in adults (apart from secondary causes) are membranous nephropathy and focal segmental glomerulosclerosis (see Table 6.7). In children, minimal change disease is more common, accounting for up to 90% of cases under the age of 10 years.

Drugs that can cause nephrotic syndrome include NSAIDs, gold and other heavy metals, and penicillamine.

Pathophysiology

The glomerular basement membrane (GBM) becomes more permeable than usual so protein leaks out into the urine. There is no acute inflammatory response either because there are no immune deposits (such as in minimal change nephropathy, focal segmental glomerulosclerosis and in amyloidosis) or the immune complexes are subepithelial (such as in membranous nephropathy).

Table 6.7 Causes of nephrotic syndrome

Cause	Approx. percentage
Secondary, e.g. DM, SLE, amyloidosis, drugs, pre-eclampsia etc.	35%
Membranous glomerulonephritis	20%
Focal segmental glomerulosclerosis (FSGS)	20%
Minimal change disease	10%
Any proliferative glomerulonephritis, e.g. IgA nephropathy	10%
Mesangiocapillary glomerulonephritis	5%

Haematuria and renal failure are therefore usually minor or absent. Albumin is the main protein lost, but clotting factors, transferrin and other proteins may be lost as well. The liver is able to synthesise enough albumin to compensate for the losses initially, but if protein losses are large, hypoalbuminaemia results. Peripheral oedema is the result of a fall in plasma oncotic pressure, so that fluid stays in the tissues, and also sodium retention by the kidney.

Clinical features
Gradual development of swelling of eyelids, peripheral oedema, ascites and pleural effusions. The urine may be frothy due to proteinuria. There may be relevant history of drugs, other past medical history or a family history of renal disease.

Complications
- Venous thrombosis and pulmonary embolism due to loss of antithrombin III in the urine, lowered plasma volume and increased clotting factors (II, V, VII, VIII and X).
- Renal vein thrombosis may occur particularly in patients with a very low serum albumin (<20 g/L) or membranous nephropathy. This is usually asymptomatic, the first sign may be a pulmonary embolus, or it may present acutely due to venous infarction with flank pain, haematuria and renal impairment.
- Infection, particularly streptococcal infections, possibly due to low levels of IgG.
- Hypercholesterolaemia is thought to occur due to increased hepatic lipoprotein synthesis as a response to decreased plasma oncotic pressure. Reduced metabolism also plays a part in hypercholesterolaemia and hypertriglyceridaemia.

- Acute renal failure may occur due to hypovolaemia (often diuretic-induced), or in some cases there is both glomerular and tubular damage. Most causes of nephrotic syndrome do not cause ARF.
- Loss of specific binding proteins, e.g. transferrin, leading to iron-resistant hypochromic anaemia.
- Protein malnutrition.

Investigations
- Measured or calculated creatinine clearance and total protein.
- Urine microscopy.
- Bence Jones protein (to look for myeloma).
- Blood for U&Es, albumin, cholesterol, FBC, ESR, CRP.
- A variety of other blood tests may be able to suggest a diagnosis, such as serum protein electrophoresis, ANA, anti-dsDNA, C_3, C_4.
- Renal biopsy is indicated in most cases, but children and teenagers without haematuria, hypertension or renal impairment are very likely to have minimal change disease, so if a trial of steroids leads to full remission, biopsy may be avoided.

Management
Treatment of the underlying cause.
- ACE-inhibitors are used to lower intraglomerular pressure. This reduces the proteinuria and slows progression of renal disease.
- Sodium restriction and diuretics are used to relieve oedema, but with care to avoid precipitating prerenal failure, due to intravascular hypovolaemia.
- Dietary protein must be sufficient to compensate for urinary losses.
- Treat complications: Hyperlipidaemia responds to treatment of the nephrotic syndrome, although HMG CoA reductase inhibitors (statins) are often needed. Consider anticoagulation and prophylactic penicillin.

Nephritic syndrome

Definition
Nephritic syndrome is characterised by hypertension, haematuria and acute renal failure.

Aetiology
- Acute diffuse proliferative, e.g. post-streptococcal glomerulonephritis.

- Goodpasture's disease (anti-Glomerular Basement Membrane (GBM) disease).
- Systemic diseases such as systemic lupus erythematosus (SLE), Henoch–Schönlein purpura (HSP), vasculitis (Wegener's granulomatosis, polyarteritis), malignant hypertension and haemolytic-uraemic syndrome (HUS).

Pathophysiology

Proliferation of endothelial cells and mesangial cells, or vasculitis, leads to occlusion of the capillary lumen, reduced blood flow, oliguria and acute renal failure. Damaged glomeruli leak red blood cells causing microscopic (occasionally macroscopic) haematuria. The low GFR also leads to activation of the renin–angiotensin system, exacerbating hypertension. Proteinuria may also be present.

- Focal nephritis: When less than 50% of the glomeruli are affected this usually manifests as haematuria with or without minor proteinuria. The majority of glomeruli are unaffected so renal failure is minimal or absent.
- Diffuse nephritis: If more than 50% of the glomeruli are affected then oliguria and acute renal failure results. If diffuse nephritis is severe (with crescents in most of the glomeruli) then rapidly progressive glomerulonephritis results.

Clinical features

The full nephritic syndrome includes haematuria, proteinuria, hypertension and oedema (from salt and water retention), oliguria and uraemia, but the features are variably present. Often, the patient is unwell and there may be features of the underlying illness, for example haemoptysis with Goodpasture's syndrome, rash, joint pains, a preceding infection, e.g. diarrhoea or a sore throat. Headache and loin pains are common non-specific features. Salt and water retention can lead to hypertensive encephalopathy and pulmonary oedema.

Macroscopy/microscopy

The kidneys are oedematous, swollen, with scattered petechiae sometimes seen. The microscopic appearances are described in greater detail in section on Glomerular Disease (see page 240) and under each individual condition.

Investigations

- Urine dipstick is positive for blood and may be positive for protein. Urine microscopy may demonstrate the dysmorphic red blood cells and red cell casts, which indicate a nephritic urine.
- Patients should be investigated as for acute renal failure (see page 234).
- Renal biopsy is required in most cases to help identify the underlying cause, deomonstrate the pattern of disease, indicate prognosis and guide management.
- FBC and peripheral blood film particularly to look for thrombocytopenia, and evidence of haemolysis.
- More specific tests which are useful in nephritic syndrome include:
  1 ANA and anti-dsDNA (anti-double stranded DNA antibody is specific for SLE)
  2 ANCA - Anti-neutrophil cytoplasmic Antibody (found in vasculitides such as Wegener's)
  3 Anti-GBM antibody
  4 Complement C_3 and C_4 – these are low in certain conditions.
  5 ASO and anti-DNAase – these are evidence of a preceding streptococcal infection
  6 Serum cryoglobulins

Management

This is as for acute renal failure. Urgent treatment of the underlying cause is often needed to prevent permanent loss of renal function and early referral to a renal physician is necessary.

Acute diffuse proliferative glomerulonephritis

Definition

A diffuse global glomerular disease, which is immune complex mediated and usually precipitated by a preceding infection.

Incidence

The commonest glomerulonephritis worldwide, falling in the United Kingdom.

Age

Any age, peak in schoolchildren.

Sex

M > F

Aetiology

The most common infectious agent is β-haemolytic *Streptococcus*, Lancefield Group A although other bacteria, viruses and malaria may be causative. A similar picture is seen in systemic lupus erythematosus.

Pathophysiology

There are subendothelial immune deposits of immune complexes, which may be derived from the circulation or formed *de novo* in the kidney. These result in complement activation and an inflammatory response, causing endothelial cell proliferation. Subepithelial deposits can lead to a variable degree of proteinuria.

Clinical features

The disease presents as acute nephritic syndrome (haematuria, oliguria and variable renal failure), with malaise and nausea 1–2 weeks after a illness such as a sore throat. Mild facial oedema and hypertension are variably present.

Macroscopy/microscopy

- All the glomeruli demonstrate endothelial, epithelial and mesangial cell proliferation, together with neutrophils. Crescents may be formed in severe cases.
- Immunofluorescence reveals granular deposits of C_3 and IgG.
- Electron microscopy shows subepithelial deposits (called humps or lumpy deposits).

Complications

Severe acute renal failure, rapidly progressive glomerulonephritis, hypertensive encephalopathy and pulmonary oedema.

Investigations

Renal biopsy is required to make a definitive diagnosis but may not always be necessary.

- Throat swabs, swabs of skin lesions, anti-streptolysin O titre, anti-DNAse B antibodies and other tests may identify recent infection.
- Low plasma complement especially C_3.

Management

- Antibiotics are usually given, although there is no evidence that they have an effect on the glomerulonephritis. There is no role for steroids or other specific treatments.
- General measures are as for acute renal failure and nephritic syndrome. Dialysis may be required.

Prognosis

Most patients, especially children, have complete clinical resolution over 3–6 weeks, even in those with crescents on biopsy.

- Up to 30% develop progressive renal disease, sometimes becoming manifest many years later with hypertension, recurrent or persistent proteinuria and chronic renal impairment. Late biopsy may show glomerulosclerosis, which is thought to be due to the loss of some glomeruli, leading to hyperfiltration through the remaining glomeruli, causing gradual changes to the glomeruli and ultimately renal failure. In other cases of persistent disease, the original glomerular disease may have been membranoproliferative glomerulonephritis.
- Adults are more likely to develop rapidly progressive glomerulonephritis (>80% glomeruli affected) and have incomplete resolution afterwards.

Focal segmental proliferative glomerulonephritis

Definition

Focal segmental proliferative glomerulonephritis is characterised by cellular proliferation affecting only one segment of the glomerulus and occurring in only a proportion of all glomeruli.

Aetiology

This histological pattern is caused by:

- Primary glomerular diseases such as IgA nephropathy (also called mesangial IgA disease or Berger's disease) and Goodpasture's disease (anti-GBM disease).
- Systemic diseases such as systemic lupus erythematosus (SLE), microscopic polyarteritis, Wegener's granulomatosis, infective endocarditis and Henoch–Schönlein purpura.

Pathophysiology

There are immune complexes deposited in the glomerular tuft. The reaction to this is localised inflammation and mesangial proliferation, causing reduction of renal blood flow, leading to haematuria and in some acute cases, nephritic syndrome. In severe cases, the necrosis of the glomerular cells stimulates crescent formation (rapidly progressive GN). Whereas IgA nephropathy tends to follow a slower, more benign course, a more florid form occurs in Goodpasture's disease and the systemic causes in particular.

IgA nephropathy

Definition

IgA nephropathy (also called mesangial IgA disease or Berger's disease) is a form of focal segmental glomerulonephritis usually presenting as recurrent haematuria associated with upper respiratory tract infections.

Incidence

The commonest glomerulonephritis in the developed world.

Aetiology/pathophysiology

Most cases are idiopathic. Associated with Henoch–Schönlein Purpura, cirrhosis, coeliac disease and dermatitis herpetiformis. There is a weak association with HLA-DR4. It is thought that the disease is related to abnormal IgA homeostasis.

Clinical features

One third of patients present with recurrent macroscopic haematuria during or after upper respiratory tract infections, one third have persistent microscopic haematuria and/or persistent mild proteinuria. The others may present with hypertension, or nephrotic or nephritic syndrome.

Macroscopy/microscopy

Typically there is mild, focal mesangial proliferation but histology is variable. Immunofluorescence shows extensive IgA and C_3 deposits in the mesangium.

Complications

Acute renal failure can occur with an episode of gross haematuria. It has a good prognosis with renal function returning to baseline. Chronic renal failure may also occur.

Investigations

Serum IgA levels are high in 50%. Renal biopsy is not always required. For those with recurrent macroscopic or microscopic haematuria but no evidence of significant proteinuria the course is usually benign and the diagnosis is made clinically. Those with deterioration in renal function or with persistent significant proteinuria are biopsied, as they may benefit from more aggressive treatment, or may have another diagnosis.

Management

Best treatment is poorly defined.
- Fish oil may slow progression.
- Hypertension should be treated. ACE-inhibitors are used even in those without hypertension to lower intraglomerular pressure to reduce proteinuria and slow progression. Angiotensin-II receptor antagonists may also be used to maximise the benefit.
- Corticosteroids are only used in selected patients, such as those with nephrotic syndrome, with little or no haematuria, few changes on renal biopsy, as these resemble minimal change disease in their course and response to treatment.
- More aggressive immunosuppression may benefit some patients, such as those with crescentic disease.

Prognosis

Patients with only haematuria have a good prognosis. Proteinuria, renal impairment and histological evidence of scarring, tubular atrophy and capillary loop deposits signify a worse prognosis. Approximately a third develop renal impairment, and a third reach end-stage renal failure (ESRF) and require renal replacement therapy. The disease recurs in approximately 50% of transplant kidneys.

Goodpasture's disease (anti-GBM disease)

Definition

Anti-GBM disease is a rare disease characterised by the development of autoantibodies to the basement membranes of the glomerulus and lung alveoli, resulting in glomerulonephritis.

Age
Young > old

Sex
M > F

Aetiology/pathophysiology
The pathogenic antibodies have been characterised as IgG autoantibodies to the $\alpha 3$ chain of type IV collagen. The response to the immune deposits is complement activation, polymorph infiltration and a proliferative glomerulonephritis. Crescents form as a result of epithelial cell proliferation and monocyte infiltration into Bowman's space, causing rapidly progressive glomerulonephritis (RPGN).

Clinical features
- The usual presentation is of acute renal failure with oliguria, an active urine sediment with dysmorphic red blood cells, red cell casts and proteinuria.
- Goodpasture's syndrome is defined as RPGN with pulmonary haemorrhage. Symptoms include haemoptysis, shortness of breath and symptoms of anaemia. Although this may occur in anti-GBM disease it is more commonly due to other causes (see Table 6.8).
- Pulmonary haemorrhage is more common in patients with underlying lung disease, lung infections, pulmonary oedema and in smokers.

Macroscopy/microscopy
On renal biopsy there are diffuse global proliferative changes on light microscopy, often crescentic. Immunofluorescence demonstrates linear IgG and C_3 deposits at the GBM.

Investigations
Initial investigation is as for acute renal failure and nephritic syndrome.
- Serum anti-GBM antibody can be detected by radioimmunoassay (ELISA). Up to 40% of cases have a

Table 6.8 Causes of Goodpasture's syndrome

ANCA-associated vasculitis including Wegener's
    granulomatosis
Anti-GBM disease (Goodpasture's disease)
Concurrent ANCA and anti-GBM antibodies
Systemic lupus erythematosus

positive ANCA as well as anti-GBM antibodies, which can cause a systemic vasculitis.
- Chest X-ray may demonstrate pulmonary infiltrates due to haemorrhage.
- Pulmonary function tests may be performed to look for increased transfer factor (evidence of alveolar haemorrhage).

Management
- Plasmapheresis is used to remove circulating anti-GBM, and high dose steroids and cyclophosphamide are used to switch off the production of antibody. Smoking, lung infection and pulmonary oedema all increase the risk of pulmonary haemorrhage.
- If patients are dialysis dependent at presentation, and have 100% crescents on renal biopsy, the chances of renal recovery are poor. The decision to treat these patients if they have no evidence of pulmonary haemorrhage or other vasculitis with aggressive therapy is difficult, as the risks of the above treatment are considerable.
- Anti-GBM disease only rarely relapses, so the cyclophosphamide can be stopped after 3 months, and the steroids are tailed off.

Prognosis
Patient survival and long-term renal function correlate well with the degree of renal impairment at presentation. Relapses occur particularly in those with ANCA and anti-GBM antibody, and it may occasionally recur after transplantation. Early diagnosis and treatment is the key to reducing morbidity and mortality.

Mesangiocapillary glomerulonephritis (membranoproliferative GN)

Definition
MCGN (or MPGN) is a descriptive term for a pattern of glomerular disease with mesangial proliferation and GBM thickening. It may be a primary disease (two types) but many cases are secondary (see Table 6.9).

Aetiology/pathophysiology
- Type I MCGN is almost certainly an immune complex mediated disease, perhaps caused by an unknown infectious agent.

Table 6.9 Important causes of secondary MCGN

Autoimmune
  Systemic lupus erythematosus
  Rheumatoid arthritis
Viral infection
  Mixed essential cryoglobulinaemia
  Hepatitis B and C infection
Chronic infection
  Infective endocarditis
  Infected ventricular shunts
  Leprosy, malaria, schistosomiasis (worldwide)
Malignancies, e.g. lymphoma, leukaemia, renal cell Ca
Cirrhosis

- Type II MCGN is also called 'dense deposit disease' because on electron microscopy, continuous ribbon-like deposits of C_3 are seen along the GBM, tubules and Bowman's capsule. The cause is unknown, but there is an association with partial lipodystrophy.

In type I, immune complexes activate complement, whereas in type II there is increased peripheral consumption of C_3 by a circulating IgG antibody (C_3 nephritic factor).

Clinical features

Patients usually present with haematuria and/or proteinuria and a variable degree of renal failure. In severe cases patients may present with nephrotic syndrome, nephritic syndrome or a mixed picture. Features of any underlying condition may also be present.

Investigations

Renal biopsy is required for diagnosis. Low C_3, with normal C_{1q} and C_4. C_3 nephritic factor positive in MCGN type II. Underlying causes should be looked for, particularly treatable infections, malignancies and cryoglobulinaemia.

Management

Treatment of any underlying cause may lead to partial or complete remission. In those without nephrotic syndrome, conservative management is probably indicated, as the prognosis is good. In those with nephrotic-range proteinuria, specific treatments such as steroids and antiplatelet agents may be tried with very variable benefit.

Prognosis

Idiopathic MCGN is typically progressive leading to end stage renal failure. It often recurs in transplanted kidneys.

Minimal change disease

Definition

Minimal change disease (MCD) is an important cause of nephrotic syndrome, characteristically the glomeruli look normal on light microscopy.

Age

Causes up to 90% of cases of nephrotic syndrome in those under age of 10, but only ~20% of cases in adulthood (more often in young adults).

Sex

M > F in childhood, and M = F in adults.

Aetiology/pathophysiology

Idiopathic in almost all cases. Very rarely secondary, e.g. to drugs, malignancy. It is thought to be a T lymphocyte mediated disorder, perhaps with production of a cytokine (permeability factor) which damages the glomerular epithelial cells. There is no evidence of an immune complex process. The damage to the epithelial cells is believed to cause a reduction in the fixed negative charge on the glomerular capillary wall, which permits protein (particularly albumin) to cross into the urinary space. Resultant hypoalbuminaemia causes a reduced blood oncotic pressure and hence oedema. Acute renal failure can occur in MCD due to hypovolaemia, ischaemic tubular necrosis, renal vein thrombosis and interstitial nephritis.

Clinical features

Patients present with gradual development of swelling of eyelids, hands and feet, ascites and pleural effusions. The urine may be frothy due to proteinuria. Hypertension and haematuria are rare. Renal function is usually normal in uncomplicated cases.

Macroscopy/microscopy

Electron microscopy reveals fusion of the foot processes of the podocytes, this is diagnostic if the light microscopy is normal.

Investigations

In adults, renal biopsy is normally needed for diagnosis. In children renal biopsy is only indicated in patients with atypical features or who do not respond to treatment.

Management

- The mainstay of treatment is with corticosteroids, with complete remission of proteinuria in over 90% of cases. Proteinuria may take up to 3 or 4 months to completely disappear. Relapse can occur when steroids are reduced. Cyclophosphamide, cyclosporine and other drugs have also been used to induce remission in steroid-resistant cases, or to reduce the steroid dose in those who are steroid-dependent.
- Patients may also require anti-coagulation and penicillin prophylaxis.

Prognosis

Progression to CRF is very rare in those with true MCD. Repeat renal biopsy may demonstrate another condition such as focal segmental glomerulosclerosis in those who do not respond to treatment.

Membranous glomerulonephritis

Definition

This is the one of the two most common causes of nephrotic syndrome in non-diabetic adults (together with focal segmental glomerulosclerosis). Also called membranous nephropathy (MN), glomerulonephropathy or glomerulopathy.

Incidence/prevalence

MN accounts for as many as 25–30% of cases of adult nephrotic syndrome. The idiopathic form causes ~20% of cases, although this varies by population.

Age

Peak age 30–50 years.

Aetiology

Eighty-five per cent are idiopathic. Secondary causes are shown in Table 6.10. Malignancies are an important cause – being present in 5–10% of cases, particularly in older persons.

Table 6.10 Major causes of membranous nephropathy

Malignancies	Lung, colon, breast cancer
	Haematological less often
Autoimmune disease	SLE
	Rheumatoid arthritis
Drugs	Penicillamine, gold
	NSAIDs
Infections	Hepatitis B, hepatitis C
	Malaria, schistosomiasis, syphilis
Miscellaneous	Chronic renal transplant rejection
	Sarcoidosis
	Other glomerular diseases

Pathophysiology

The mechanism is unknown. It is thought that antibodies directed against antigens in the subepithelial space form immune complexes. In idiopathic MN, these are probably autoantibodies, whereas in secondary causes circulating antigen is filtered by the kidney, leading to *de novo* immune complexes or possibly circulating immune complexes. Because the immune deposits are subepithelial there is usually no marked inflammatory response. The BM becomes more permeable to protein, leading to proteinuria and the nephrotic syndrome. Over many years, there is increase in mesangial matrix causing hyalinization of glomeruli and loss of nephrons.

Clinical features

Patients may present with asymptomatic proteinuria, or (in most cases) nephrotic syndrome. There may be features consistent with an underlying disease, particularly malignancies, which is usually overt at time of presentation.

Macroscopy/microscopy

Renal biopsy shows thickened capillary loops (ranging from mild in early disease, to marked in late disease), usually with mild to moderate mesangial proliferation. Silver stains classically show 'spikes' where basement membrane has grown between subepithelial deposits. Immunofluorescence shows immune complexes (IgG, IgM, C_3) deposited subepithelially in the BM in a diffuse global pattern.

Investigations

Renal biopsy is required for diagnosis. Complement is normal (low levels in SLE-associated and hepatitis B-associated MN).

Management

Any underlying cause should be treated. Where no cause has been identified, treatment is disputed, as the course is often slow and spontaneous remission may occur. There is evidence that intensive immunosuppression with corticosteroids and chlorambucil or cyclophosphamide for 6 months improves prognosis, but this has a significant risk of adverse effects. Other treatments include ACE inhibitors, NSAIDs and omega-3 fatty acids (fish oils).

Prognosis

Approximately 50% develop CRF over 10 years; 25% undergo remission; 25% have stable, persistent proteinuria. Some patients develop a rapidly progressive course to end-stage renal failure.

Focal (segmental) glomerulosclerosis

Definition

Focal segmental glomerulosclerosis (FSGS) is one of the two most common primary causes of nephrotic syndrome in adults and the second most common cause in children.

Incidence/prevalence

Causes ~20% of cases of nephrotic syndrome in adults and children.

Aetiology

There are several classifications of FSGS, for example by the likely cause:

- Primary FSGS: This is the idiopathic form, which tends to present with overt nephrotic syndrome in children and young adults.
- Secondary FSGS: This tends to present with proteinuria and renal insufficiency, without nephrotic syndrome, usually in older adults. It is thought to be part of a physiological response to glomerular hyperfiltration/hypertrophy (e.g. in unilateral renal agenesis, reflux nephropathy, diabetes, pre-eclampsia) or previous focal damage to the glomerulus and then healing by scarring such as following vasculitis or lupus nephritis.
- Specific causes such as drugs, toxins, HIV, heroin and familial forms.

Pathophysiology

The GBM is more permeable to proteins but the cause of this is unclear.

- Podocyte damage: The initial problem may be damage to the epithelial cells (podocytes), attached to the GBM, possibly due to a circulating factor.
- Glomerulosclerosis: Denudement of the basement membrane may lead to adhesion to the Bowman's capsule. Alternatively large plasma proteins may leak through the capillary wall, accumulate in the subendothelial space and compress the capillary lumen.
- Over time, the sclerosis affects more segments of the glomerulus, leading to global sclerosis and permanent loss of the function of that nephron.

Clinical features

In children and young adults with rapid onset of nephrotic syndrome, FSGS is suggested by atypical features such as non-selective proteinuria, haematuria, hypertension or renal impairment at the onset of nephrotic syndrome. These may develop later in the course of the illness. Steroid non-responsiveness in a patient with apparent minimal change disease also suggests FSGS.

Macroscopy/microscopy

Increase in the mesangial matrix in glomeruli in a focal segmental pattern, with collapse of the adjacent capillary loop. There may be tubular atrophy and interstitial fibrosis. Immunofluorescence usually shows a lack of immune deposits, apart from some non-specific binding of granular IgM and C_3 in the sclerosed areas of mesangium.

Investigations

Definitive diagnosis can only be made on renal biopsy. Because of the focal nature of the disease and the tendency for the juxta-medullary glomeruli to be affected first, the disease may be missed on renal biopsy (and hence a diagnosis of minimal change disease made).

Management

Almost all patients are treated with ACE inhibitors and cholesterol-lowering agents. ACE-inhibitors lower intraglomerular pressure and so reduce proteinuria (with a probable slowing of deterioration of renal function).

- In primary FSGS, approximately 50% may respond to steroids, although relapse is common and longer courses are generally required. Steroid resistant cases may respond to ciclosporin, and steroid-dependent cases may benefit from the addition of ciclosporin or cyclophosphamide.
- Secondary FSGS has no specific treatment. The FSGS may respond to withdrawal of any causative agent or treatment of any underlying cause.

Prognosis
Patients with marked proteinuria, tubular atrophy, interstitial fibrosis have a worse prognosis.

Tubular and interstitial diseases

Tubulointerstitial disease

Definition
Tubulointerstitial disease, also called tubulointerstitial nephritis or interstitial nephropathy, is the term used for inflammation of the renal parenchyma, i.e. the interstitium and tubules, with relative sparing of the glomeruli.

Aetiology
There are many causes, the most common being exposure to drugs, especially certain antibiotics and analgesics, and infections. Often the diagnosis is idiopathic, if no agent is discovered (see Table 6.11).

Table 6.11 Important causes of acute and chronic tubulointerstitial disease

Acute		Chronic
Drugs	Penicillins, cephalosporins	Lithium, Cisplatin
	Diuretics	Heavy metals e.g. lead
	NSAIDs	NSAIDs
Infection	Pyelonephritis	Pyelonephritis, e.g. TB, reflux
Metabolic/ Endocrine	Hyperuricaemic nephropathy (with haematological malignancies)	Juvenile gouty nephropathy
Ischaemic		Sickle cell disease Diabetes mellitus

Acute tubulointerstitial nephritis – drug-induced
The most common mechanism is a hypersensitivity reaction to the drug, with lymphocytes and eosinophils infiltrating the interstitium causing tissue oedema. The tubular epithelium undergoes acute necrosis.

Patients present usually within 3 weeks of exposure with acute renal failure and variable fever, joint pains and rashes. They often have haematuria and mild proteinuria. Urine volumes may be reduced or normal. Classically there is eosinophilia and eosinophils in the urine.

Withdrawal of the drug often leads to resolution. High dose steroids may be given.

Chronic tubulointerstitial nephritis
Drugs and toxins such as cisplatin and heavy metals cause chronic inflammation, characterised by fibrosis of the interstitium and atrophy of the tubules leading to chronic renal failure (CRF). This picture is also common in idiopathic interstitial nephritis.

Analgesic nephropathy is a particular form of tubulointerstitial disease caused by long-term use of NSAIDs. There is chronic inflammation and there may also be ischaemic necrosis of the renal papillae, which can slough off and cause obstruction. Analgesic nephropathy leads to CRF and there is also an increased risk of carcinoma of the urothelium.

Sickle cell disease and diabetic nephropathy can also cause ischaemic papillary necrosis.

Prognosis
This depends on the underlying cause. Acute tubulointerstitial nephritis has a good prognosis. Chronic renal failure may progress to end-stage renal disease and require renal replacement therapy.

Renal tubular syndromes

Definition
These are syndromes in which a metabolic disorder of tubular function is the main feature. They may be inherited or acquired.

Aetiology
They may be classified as single or multiple defects, or they can be grouped according to the part of the

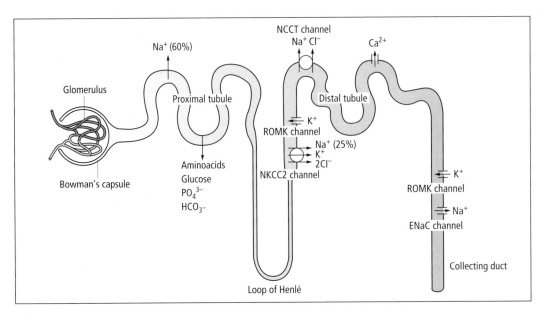

Figure 6.9 Renal tubular function.

nephron affected (see Fig. 6.9). See also Renal Tubular Acidosis (see below). The single defects are discussed here.

Proximal tubule: The proximal tubule is the site of maximal reabsorption of glucose and sodium. Water and anions such as aminoacids follow sodium. Osmotic diuretics and carbonic anhydrase inhibitors act at this site. Disorders of the proximal tubule may lead to one or more of the following syndromes:

- Renal glycosuria is an autosomal recessive inherited condition characterised by glycosuria with normal blood glucose. There is impaired reabsorption of glucose in the proximal tubules, with no clinical sequelae. Glycosuria is a normal response during pregnancy.
- Aminoaciduria may affect only one amino acid or several. The most important single defect is cystinuria, an autosomal recessive condition which predisposes to urinary stone formation (see page 270). Treatment is with high fluid intake and alkali ingestion, because the cystine is more soluble in alkaline conditions. Drugs such as penicillamine may be used to form complexes with the cystine. In Fanconi syndrome (which may be an inherited juvenile form or acquired in adults) there is defective reabsorption of most aminoacids, glucose, phosphate and bicarbonate. There may be potassium

depletion, polyuria and immunodeficiency secondary to immunoglobulin loss. Phosphate loss leads to vitamin D resistant rickets in childhood, and osteomalacia in adults.

- Phosphate transport defects: There are several types, usually X-linked, although occasional sporadic inherited or acquired cases do occur. They cause inappropriate loss of phosphate from the tubules and result in hypophosphataemia and vitamin D resistant rickets (VDDR). Treatment is with oral phosphate supplements with vitamin D or 1,25 dihydroxyvitamin D (calcitriol).

Thick ascending loop of Henle: Sodium is pumped out of the lumen in the ascending loop, water is drawn out of the descending loop by osmosis. This creates a concentration gradient within the medulla of the kidney, which draws water out of the collecting duct and hence concentrates the urine. Loop diuretics such as furosemide act from within the lumen of the ascending loop binding to the chloride site of the NKCC2 channel. This interferes with the pump reducing the concentration gradient resulting in more dilute urine.

- Bartter type I syndrome is an autosomal recessive defect in the gene encoding the NKCC2 pump. It results in high urinary sodium loss, dehydration, secondary hyperaldosteronism and hypokalaemic alkalosis. There is hypercalciuria and nephrocalcinosis.

- Bartter type II syndrome is an autosomal recessive defect in the gene encoding the ROMK channel. Decreased potassium excretion causes hyperkalaemia, which interferes with the action of the NKCC2 pump. This results in a similar syndrome of sodium loss, dehydration and hypercalciuria as Bartter type I; however, hypokalaemia only occurs after treatment with sodium supplements.

Distal convoluted tubule: Thiazide diuretics act from within the lumen of the distal tubule binding to the chloride site of the NCCT channel reducing sodium and water reabsorption. Calcium reabsorption is increased leading to hypercalcaemia.

- Gittleman syndrome is an autosomal recessive mutation in the gene encoding the NCCT channel. As there is increased sodium in the urine reaching the collecting duct there is exchange of sodium for potassium in the collecting duct resulting in a hypokalaemic metabolic alkalosis.

Collecting duct: At the collecting duct there is reabsorption of sodium in exchange for potassium excretion. This is under the influence of aldosterone which increases sodium (and hence water) reabsorption. Spironolactone and amiloride affect this exchange and hence increase urinary water and sodium loss. In contrast to other diuretics, these cause potassium reabsorption and are termed potassium-sparing diuretics. The permeability of the collecting duct is under the influence of anti diuretic hormone (ADH or vasopressin).

- In diabetes insipidus (see also page 445) the action of ADH is impaired. This results in excessive water loss in the urine.

Renal tubular acidosis

Definition

Renal tubular acidosis (RTA) is a metabolic acidosis of renal origin, characterised by hyperchloraemic metabolic acidosis with a normal anion gap.

Aetiology/pathophysiology

RTA may be inherited or acquired. Under physiological conditions, the kidneys help to maintain acid–base balance, together with the lungs (which remove carbon dioxide). RTA is classified into three main types each with differing pathophysiology.

- Type 1 (Distal RTA) causes include primary, idiopathic and connective tissue disorders such as Sjögren's and rheumatoid arthritis. Impaired H^+ secretion in the distal tubule leads to progressive accumulation of acid in the body. Even when bicarbonate levels fall to as low as 10 mmol/L or below, the urine remains relatively alkaline (pH $\geq$ 5.5). If untreated, persistent metabolic acidosis leads to increased mobilisation of calcium phosphate from bone, and this causes hypercalciuria promoting the formation of renal stones. Type 1 RTA is treated with bicarbonate replacement, with correction of hyperkalaemia.
- Type 2 (Proximal RTA) usually occurs in the context of a general proximal tubule disorder called Fanconi syndrome, which may be familial inherited, idiopathic or acquired, e.g. due to drugs, heavy metals or myeloma. The proximal tubule fails to reabsorb the HCO_3^-, so this passes to the distal tubules. Once plasma bicarbonate levels fall to about 12–16 mmol/L, the distal tubule is able to reabsorb the amount of filtered bicarbonate, so severe acidosis does not occur. The main problems occur due to the loss of other substances such as amino acids and phosphate. Type 2 is treated with bicarbonate, thiazide diuretic and potassium bicarbonate or potassium-sparing diuretics. Fanconi syndrome is treated with large doses of vitamin D.
- Type 4 is hypoaldosteronism or resistance to the effects of aldosterone such as caused by mild renal failure, interstitial nephritis or potassium-sparing diuretics like spironalactone. It appears that aldosterone deficiency causes hyperkalaemia, which is associated with a mild metabolic acidosis. Urinary pH usually remains appropriately low (<5.3). Mineralocorticoid deficiency is corrected using fludrocortisone. Hyperkalaemia may be life-threatening and the underlying disorder often shortens life expectancy.

Hyperuricaemic (gouty) nephropathy

Definition

Disorders of uric acid metabolism may cause renal disease due to a chronic nephropathy, an acute nephropathy or through the formation of uric acid stones.

Chronic Hyperuricaemic Nephropathy

- There is still a debate as to whether patients who have hyperuricaemia, gouty tophi, and chronic renal failure have gouty nephropathy as the cause for their renal impairment. Renal failure leads to raised uric acid levels and in some cases there may have been another cause for their renal failure. It is thought that urate crystals deposit in the renal interstitium, causing chronic inflammation, interstitial fibrosis and hence the development of chronic renal failure.
- There is a distinct autosomal dominant disorder of uric acid metabolism which is associated with early onset renal failure and hypertension. This is called familial juvenile gouty nephropathy, although it is still unclear whether uric acid deposition is the primary cause. Allopurinol may improve renal function, but rarely completely prevents deterioration.

Acute hyperuricaemic nephropathy

- This occurs when there is an acute rise in uric acid as in patients who have haematological malignancies or polycythaemia rubra vera. Prior to treatments such as chemotherapy or radiation which cause acute cell lysis, prophylactic treatment may be required. Acute hyperuricaemia may also occur in conjunction with tumour lysis syndrome (i.e. with hyperkalaemia, hyperphosphataemia and hypocalcaemia). Uric acid crystals precipitate in the collecting ducts, renal pelvis and ureters, causing obstruction.
- Patients present with acute oligoanuric renal failure, sometimes with loin pain or colic. There are very high uric acid levels and uric acid crystals may be seen on urine microscopy unless there is little or no urine production.
- This complication is prevented by pretreatment with high doses of allopurinol or rasburicase prior to chemotherapy or radiation, and giving intravenous fluids to lower the concentration of uric acid in the urine. Despite this, some patients still develop ARF in which case fluid and diuretics are given to try to flush out the crystals. Haemodialysis may be used to remove circulating uric acid.

Uric acid stones

See page 270.

Renal cystic disease

Adult polycystic kidney disease

Definition
Adult polycystic kidney disease is an autosomal dominant inherited condition characterised by gradual replacement of renal and occasionally other tissue by cysts.

Incidence/prevalence
1 in 1000. Accounts for 10% of chronic renal failure cases.

Age
Presents at any age.

Sex
M = F

Aetiology
Autosomal dominant; 90% of cases associated with PKD1 gene on chromosome 16, and 5–10% of cases with PKD2 on chromosome 4. PKD1 patients tend to develop renal failure earlier.

PKD1 encodes a protein called polycystin-1, which is found in plasma membranes of renal tubular epithelial cells, hepatic bile duct cells and pancreatic duct cells. Renal, liver and pancreatic cysts all occur in APKD. Abnormal polycystin-1 protein may affect cell adhesion, leading to inappropriate cell growth. This gene is closely related to the tuberous sclerosis gene in which renal cysts can also occur.

PKD2 encodes polycystin-2 protein, which is expressed in the distal tubules, collecting duct and thick ascending limb of Henle and appears to be involved in calcium signalling.

The mechanism of cyst formation is not yet understood, although it appears that there may need to be a second somatic mutation, because the disease variably affects tubules and individuals. There is evidence that the cysts arise from one progenitor cell (monoclonal). There also appear to be environmental effects, for example liver cysts are more common in women, which is thought to be an effect of oestrogen.

Pathophysiology
Cysts develop in both kidneys, progressing in size and number over the years. They gradually compress the renal parenchyma. There is also evidence of vascular

disease and interstitial fibrosis leading to gradual deterioration of renal function.

Clinical features

Around two thirds of patients have a positive family history and the disease may be detected due to radiological screening of family members. Patients may present with loin pain, lumbar pain, haematuria, an abdominal mass, hypertension or with chronic renal impairment. Pyelonephritis, an infected cyst or bleeding into cysts may occur, causing acute abdominal or lumbar pain and haematuria in some cases.

On examination, bilateral, irregular abdominal masses may be palpable. The liver may also be enlarged.

Macroscopy

Bilateral kidney enlargement with a mass of cysts ranging in diameter.

Complications

Cysts develop in the liver in 40%, also in the lung and pancreas. There is an association with berry aneurysms (10–30%) of the cerebral arteries, which together with hypertension, predisposes to subarachnoid haemorrhage (SAH). The risk of SAH may be as high as 20% in those with a positive family history of SAH.

Unlike other causes of renal failure, in APKD erythropoietin levels are often preserved, preventing the development of anaemia. In some cases polycythaemia may occur.

There is also an association with heart valve disease, diverticulosis and abdominal/inguinal hernias. Renal stones may develop.

There does not appear to be an increased risk of renal cell carcinoma, although the diagnosis of this is made harder by the presence of multiple cysts.

Investigations

Diagnosis is confirmed by renal ultrasound or IVU, which shows large kidneys with long 'spidery' calyces. In children and young adults, the diagnosis may be missed as the cysts develop with age. In older people without APKD, simple cysts may occur, so over the age of 60, four or more cysts in each kidney are needed to make the diagnosis. Genetic diagnosis is difficult because of multiple large genes with a diffuse spread of mutations.

Management

- Supportive. Control of infection with antibiotics and treat hypertension.
- Development of end stage renal failure means that dialysis or transplantation are needed.
- Some patients require cyst decompression for intractable pain, or even nephrectomy if very enlarged kidneys cause symptoms such as tiredness and loss of appetite.
- Screen family members and offer genetic counselling as appropriate.

Prognosis

Approximately 25% of patients need dialysis by the age of 50, 40% by age 60 and 50–75% by age 75. One third die from complications of hypertension, particularly heart disease and stroke. Poor prognostic indicators include younger age at diagnosis, Afro Caribbeans, males, hypertension, PKD1 gene and an episode of macroscopic haematuria.

Simple renal cysts

Definition

These are common, usually asymptomatic benign cysts of the kidney of unknown cause.

Incidence/prevalence

Related to age and sex, with about 1–2% of 30–50 year olds, but as many as 15–30% in over 70 years, having one or more cysts.

Age

Rare under the age of 30.

Sex

M > F (2:1)

Clinical features

Almost always asymptomatic and so tend to be found incidentally on ultrasound, IVU or CT. They have no effect on renal function, except rarely when they may induce hypertension. Occasionally they may become infected or develop haemorrhage and rarely may become malignant.

Macroscopy

There are single or multiple cysts up to 5–6 cm in diameter filled with clear watery fluid, which have a smooth lining.

Investigations

If there are multiple cysts, a diagnosis of adult polycystic kidney disease should be considered. If the cyst looks as if it may have any solid or mixed echogenicity components, a thickened wall, or appears loculated on ultrasound, then further investigation by CT may be indicated, to differentiate a cyst from a possible malignancy. Cyst aspiration/drainage is indicated for infected cysts as diagnosis and treatment.

Management

No specific treatment required, except for complications.

Renal tract obstruction

Urinary tract obstruction

Definition

Obstruction of the urinary tract at any level, whether partial or complete, can cause symptoms and renal impairment.

Aetiology

The likely causes depend on the age of the patient and the level of obstruction. In children, abnormal anatomy such as urethral valves or stenosis is most likely, whereas stones are more likely in adults. In older men prostatic hypertrophy or carcinoma are most common. With increasing age in both sexes retroperitoneal or pelvic malignancy should be suspected. See Table 6.12.

Pathophysiology

If urine continues to be produced, obstruction causes a rise in pressure and dilatation of the proximal part of the urinary tract. The effects of obstruction depend on the site, severity and rate of onset of obstruction.

- Renal obstruction usually causes loin pain, whereas bladder outflow obstruction may cause a sensation of a full bladder (see page 261).
- If both kidneys are completely obstructed (either at the level of the ureters (uncommon) or because of bladder outflow obstruction), or if there is only one functioning kidney which becomes obstructed, complete anuria may occur. More commonly partial obstruction can lead to renal impairment, despite continued passage of urine. Partial obstruction may also sometimes cause polyuria, due to loss of concentrating ability of the tubules.
- Acute obstruction is almost always associated with pain, but chronic progressive obstruction usually causes dilatation with little or no pain.

Clinical features

Renal obstruction should be considered as a diagnosis in all presentations of renal failure, as it is often asymptomatic. Loin pain, which may be dull, sharp, constant or intermittent, may occur. High intake of fluids may exacerbate the pain. Loin tenderness may be present, a distended bladder may be palpable and rectal and vaginal

Table 6.12 Causes of urinary tract obstruction

Level	Intrinsic	Wall	Extrinsic
Kidney and ureter	Clot Renal Tumour Cysts Casts, protein etc	Urothelial Tumour Stricture (Idiopathic hydronephrosis)	Tumour of pelvis Aortic aneurysm Idiopathic retroperitoneal fibrosis TB Radiation Fibrosis
Bladder	Tumour Foreign body		Prostate – BPH or carcinoma
Urethra	Tumour Foreign body	Urethral valve Stricture Tumour	

examination should be performed to look for pelvic disease.

Macroscopy
An acutely obstructed kidney is swollen, but chronic damage to the kidneys may make it small and shrivelled.

Complications
Infection above the level of obstruction can cause pyelonephritis (pyonephrosis is the term for an infected, obstructed hydronephrosis) or cystitis, and patients can become very unwell due to pain, fever and sepsis.

Investigations
The investigation of choice is a renal ultrasound (USS), as this will diagnose obstruction and its cause in most cases. If the kidneys are poorly visualised CT scanning is a useful substitute. In renal obstruction USS and CT will show a hydronephrosis, i.e. dilated renal pelvis and calyces (also called pelvicalyceal dilatation) and/or dilated ureters. However dilatation may not be seen if there is oligo-/anuria, in the first 72 hours before the systems have dilated, or if there is retroperitoneal fibrosis encasing the ureters. False positives may occur on USS or CT because of cysts, staghorn calculi or a dilated baggy low-pressure system, which may be mistaken for an obstructed system. Therefore, if there is doubt, one of the following may be required:

- Intravenous urogram (IVU). This is very useful, particularly in acute obstruction before there is dilatation, as it shows contrast 'held up' by the obstruction and may show the lesion as a space-filling defect such as a radio-lucent stone or a papilla. A plain film should be done first to look for radio-opaque stones. IVU should be avoided in renal failure.
- Radionuclide study such as MAG3 can show impaired uptake, delayed peak activity and delayed transit time on the side of the obstruction. This picture is also seen in any cause of renal impairment, but if it reverses with a dose of diuretics, then obstruction is not present.
- As part of the management percutaneous nephrostomy can be placed and then anterograde pyelography and ureterography can be performed through the nephrostomy. This avoids intravenous contrast. Alternatively retrograde ureterography can be performed, using a cystoscope. Catheters are introduced into the ureteric orifices and contrast injected. Cystoscopy may also visualise a cause of obstruction.

U&Es may demonstrate renal impairment. FBC may show a normochromic, normocytic anaemia of chronic disease.

Urine should be sent for microscopy and culture, urgently if infection is suspected.

Management
It is important to diagnose and treat urinary tract obstruction quickly, as delayed treatment can cause irreversible loss of renal function.
- Bladder catheterisation should be performed if bladder neck obstruction is suspected. Percutaneous nephrostomy is indicated for ureteric or pelvi-ureteric junction obstruction. Acute renal failure and its complications require appropriate treatment (see page 234).
- Infection of an obstructed system requires drainage of the system, together with high dose intravenous antibiotics.
- Relief of the obstruction can cause marked polyuria, as much as 500–1000 mL/hour. Some of this is due to loss of concentrating ability of the tubules, which may take a few days to recover, but often the patient is also fluid overloaded. Careful fluid balance monitoring is needed, to avoid hypotension or prerenal failure during this phase.

Pelviureteric junction obstruction (idiopathic hydronephrosis)

Definition
Narrowing of the pelviureteric junction (PUJ) which is a common cause of gross hydronephrosis.

Age
Likely to be congenital but may present at any age.

Aetiology/pathophysiology
The cause is unknown. There appear to be excessive collagen fibres around the muscle cells at the PUJ, which prevent their proper relaxation, so that there is a narrowed segment of the ureter at the exit of the renal pelvis. This causes gross dilatation 'hydronephrosis' of the renal pelvis.

Clinical features

Usually presents as a pain or ache in the back or abdomen which may be exacerbated by drinking large amounts of fluid, for example it may become symptomatic for the first time in students who drink large quantities of beer. There may be a palpable loin mass. Occasionally the hydronephrosis is so marked that it can mimic ascites.

In some cases, it is asymptomatic and diagnosed incidentally when an ultrasound is performed for another reason. Congenital cases may be found on antenatal ultrasound scan, or in childhood during investigation of urinary tract infections.

Complications

Infection of the dilated system due to urinary stasis, renal stones and renal failure.

Investigations

An IVU shows a dilated renal pelvis (often grossly) with normal, undilated ureters. There is delayed passage of contrast, which is not overcome by administration of diuretics. If obstruction is in doubt, further investigations as for urinary tract obstruction (see above) may be needed.

Management

If the PUJ obstruction is causing symptoms or renal impairment, reconstruction of the renal pelvis (pyeloplasty) can be undertaken so that the renal pelvis drains into the ureter, by excising the narrowed segment.

Prognosis

It is not possible to predict how much function will recover and a small proportion of patients continue to have pain.

The kidney in sytemic disease

- Hypertension: See page 73.
- Diabetes mellitus: This is a common cause of renal disease and accounts for a large number of patients who need dialysis. See page 451.
- Multiple myeloma: Many patients with multiple myeloma will develop renal complications such as proteinuria, acute or chronic renal failure and amyloidosis. There are several contributing factors to the

development of ARF, including hypercalcaemia and dehydration. The mechanism of development of 'myeloma kidney' is via a direct toxic effect on renal tubular cells and blockage of the tubules and collecting ducts by the paraprotein. In addition, patients may develop amyloidosis and renal tubular acidosis as complications of multiple myeloma. See page 490.

- Amyloidosis: This condition may be systemic or confined to the kidneys and is an important cause of glomerular disease. It can cause proteinuria, nephrotic syndrome and renal failure. See page 513.
- Henoch–Schönlein purpura (HSP): This systemic vasculitis causes a purpuric rash, abdominal pains, joint pains and a glomerulonephritis that is indistinguishable from IgA nephropathy. This is unsurprising, as HSP is characterised by tissue deposition of IgA containing immune complexes. See page 381.
- Systemic lupus erythematosus: This multisystem connective tissue disease commonly affects the kidneys. SLE is the great mimicker of almost every type of glomerulonephritis from minimal change disease, to membranous nephropathy, to proliferative glomerulonephritis. See page 365.
- Systemic sclerosis: This connective tissue disorder can cause acute or chronic renal disease due to the damage caused to the renal arterioles. The only treatment known to be of benefit is ACE inhibitors. See page 367.
- ANCA-associated vasculitis: This includes Wegener's Granulomatosis and Polyarteritis Nodosa which can cause rapidly progressive glomerulonephritis, with acute renal failure. Early treatment with immunosuppression regimes such as plasmapheresis, high dose steroids and cyclophosphamide can improve renal function. See pages 124 and 379.

Thrombotic thrombocytopenic purpura – haemolytic uraemic syndrome

Definition

Haemolytic uraemic syndrome (HUS) and thrombotic thrombocytopenic purpura (TTP) are probably two separate entities, but have such similar clinical presentations and findings that they are usefully considered together. When acute renal failure is predominant it is called HUS, and when neurological problems are predominant it is called TTP. Often both ends of the spectrum are present in the same patient. The characteristic features of TTP–HUS are microangiopathic haemolytic anaemia (MAHA) and thrombocytopenia, with variable renal and neurological abnormalities.

Incidence/prevalence
HUS is one of the commonest causes of ARF in children.

Age
More common in children and young adults.

Geography
Clusters and epidemic foci suggest an infective trigger.

Aetiology
There appear to be inherited and acquired forms of HUS and TTP.
- The epidemic form of HUS has been associated with a variety of bacterial and viral agents, including a verotoxin (also called Shiga toxin) produced by *Escherichia coli* (O157:H7).
- Many cases of TTP are idiopathic.
- There is an association of TTP–HUS with later stages of pregnancy, SLE and certain drugs.

Pathophysiology
There are several postulated mechanisms.
- It has been suggested that an initial toxic insult to the vascular endothelium may induce platelet activation. This results in intravascular coagulation and haemolysis of red blood cells. Certain individuals appear to be more susceptible, perhaps due to inherited or acquired abnormalities of their coagulation/platelet activation systems.
- In *E. coli* O157 associated HUS, the verotoxin appears to act by several mechanisms, including a direct platelet-aggregating effect, a toxic effect on the endothelium and neutrophil activation.
- In familial TTP patients have a hereditary deficiency of von Willebrand Factor (vWF) cleaving protease, and many patients with non-familial TTP have an antibody directed against this enzyme. vWF is produced by endothelial cells and forms Ultra Large (ULvWF) multimers which circulate in the plasma and promote aggregation of activated platelets. VWF cleaving protease breaks these multimers down rapidly; however, if there is a deficiency of this enzyme, ULvWF multimers accumulate and cause platelet aggregation.
- Lack of other inhibitors or antibodies against them have also been postulated.

Clinical features
Patients may present with some or all of the following.
- Haemolytic anaemia with mild jaundice, lethargy.
- Thrombocytopenia which may result in purpuric rash or bleeding.
- Acute renal failure (usually oligo-/anuric).
- Neurological abnormalities including headache and confusion, seizures and coma.
- Fever.

Microscopy
Thrombi mainly composed of platelets are found in arterioles and fibrin deposits are seen in the endothelium of glomerular capillaries. This causes a focal segmental glomerulonephritis. Widespread hyaline thrombi are seen in TTP.

Investigations
TTP-HUS should be suspected in any case of thrombocytopenia and microangiopathic haemolytic anaemia (without another clinically apparent cause)
- FBC and peripheral blood film: Anaemia, thrombocytopenia, film shows schistocytes and 'helmet cells' (fragments of red blood cells) and increased reticulocytes. Direct antiglobulin test must be negative (to exclude an immune cause). Clotting profile should be normal.
- U&Es to look for renal failure and hyperkalaemia.
- Dipstick may show some proteinuria and be positive for blood because of haemoglobinuria, but urine microscopy usually shows few red cells.
- Serum bilirubin and LDH are raised and haptoglobins are very low due to the haemolysis.

Management
Early diagnosis and treatment is needed to prevent irreversible renal failure and to reduce mortality. The treatment of choice is plasma exchange with fresh frozen plasma. Without this, TTP-HUS in adults had a ∼90% mortality. In contrast, HUS in children due to O157 often resolves spontaneously with supportive therapy, e.g.

for the renal failure, and plasma exchange is used for persistent or severe cases.

Plasma exchange appears to correct the coagulation/platelet abnormalities, either by replacing the lost vWF cleaving protease or removing the antibodies, or both.

Platelet transfusions should be avoided unless there is severe bleeding, as they may exacerbate the condition.

Prognosis
This has markedly improved with the advent of plasma exchange. Chronic renal failure occurs in a substantial number of patients.

Congenital disorders of the kidney

Congenital malformations of the kidney

Definition
Congenital malformations of the kidney are not uncommonly found on antenatal screening and in newborns.

Aetiology
Often associated with other congenital abnormalities and the risk is higher in those with a previous family history. Chromosomal abnormalities account for a proportion, but most are sporadic.

Normal fetal kidney development
The fetal kidneys develop when the ureteric bud comes into contact with the metanephric blastema caudally (in the 'pelvic' area), signalling it to form nephrons and the collecting system. This forms the 'metanephros', which becomes a functioning kidney and begins to produce urine by around 11 weeks. By 14–16 weeks, most of the amniotic fluid consists of fetal urine. Then the kidneys have to migrate rostrally, to lie in the lumbar region.

Renal agenesis
If the ureteric bud fails to develop properly, the ureter and kidney do not develop.
- Bilateral agenesis is rare and incompatible with life. It may present with oligohydramnios. About 50%

occur as part of Potter syndrome with a flattened facies, limb deformities and hypoplastic lungs, sometimes with developmental abnormalities of other organs.
- Unilateral agenesis is much more common and associated with other renal abnormalities such as reflux or strictures and unicornuate uterus. In some cases, the kidney may develop abnormally, with multiple cysts, then regress before or soon after birth. The remaining kidney undergoes compensatory hypertrophy. Some develop proteinuria later in life due to progressive glomerulosclerosis, occasionally leading to renal failure. However, the prognosis for these patients is excellent with no reduction in life expectancy.

Renal hypoplasia
- Simple renal hypoplasia is when the kidney is smaller than normal, but the structure and histology of the kidney is normal, although the nephrons may be slightly small.
- Oligonephronic renal hypoplasia (also called oligomeganephronia) is when there are far fewer nephrons than normal (about a quarter the usual number), fewer renal papillae and microscopy shows abnormally enlarged glomeruli and nephrons. The prognosis is poor for these patients, although there may be some initial improvement in renal function over the first few years of life, they develop progressive focal glomerulosclerosis with proteinuria and end stage renal failure.

Dysplasia (failure of differentiation)
The kidney develops abnormally with primitive tubules and cartilagenous components.
Abnormal migration of the kidneys:
- Horseshoe kidney – the kidneys remain fused at the upper (10%) or lower (90%) poles to form a horseshoe-shaped structure. Rarely, they remain fused at both poles to form a discoid kidney.
- Ectopic kidney – one or both of the kidneys may remain in the pelvis, or one of the kidneys may migrate to the other side.

These anatomical abnormalities may be symptomless, or problems with the flow of urine can cause obstructive uropathy and predisposition to urinary stones and infections. In pregnancy, low pelvic kidneys can interfere with labour. They are diagnosed by IVU or renal USS.

Congenital malformations of the ureter

Definition
Developmental abnormalities of the ureter are relatively common.

Aetiology
Often sporadic, but increased risk in those with a positive family history.

- Agenesis: This occurs with renal agenesis.
- Atresia: Failure of the ureteric bud to canalise, associated with renal dysplasia.
- Ectopic ureteric orifice: The ureter normally enters the bladder outside the area of the trigone. An ectopic ureter often arises from a duplex kidney, which may be associated with vesicoureteric reflux. Occasionally the ureter can drain into the vagina or seminal vesicle. Surgical re-implantation of the ureter may be indicated.
- Ureterocele: The ureteric orifice is tiny, so that the ureter dilates to form a cyst by the bladder wall. If not surgically dilated, the obstruction leads to hydronephrosis.
- Primary obstructive megaureter: The cause of this condition is unknown. The whole ureter becomes dilated, apart from the terminal segment. If the stenosis is causing obstruction, treatment is with surgical re-implantation of the ureter.

Clinical features
Many are asymptomatic. Obstruction is chronic and therefore usually painless. Urinary stasis or reflux can lead to repeated urinary tract infections, which in children may cause non-specific fevers, malaise, failure to thrive and abdominal symptoms.

Management and prognosis
In recurrent infections, renal scarring results unless the condition is diagnosed and treated with prevention and early detection of UTI's and surgical repair where indicated. Unrelieved obstruction can also lead to irreversible loss of renal function.

Disorders of the bladder and prostate

Bladder outflow obstruction

Definition
Obstruction to urinary flow from the bladder to the urethral meatus.

Incidence/prevalence
Common in men.

Age
Increases with age

Sex
M > F

Aetiology
The causes of bladder outflow obstruction are shown in Table 6.13.

Pathophysiology
A reduction of >70% in the urethral lumen or vesicourethral junction (VUJ) causes obstruction, leading to reduced flow, increased voiding pressure and

Table 6.13 Causes of bladder outflow obstruction

Mechanical		
Intrinsic	Foreign body, e.g. clot
	Stones (rare)
Wall	Urethral valve (male neonates)
	Stricture: fibrosis, usually after trauma or infection
	Bladder neck spasm
	Tumour
Extrinsic	Enlarged prostate (BPH or Ca)
	Prostatitis
	Pregnancy
	Constipation
Neuropathic	Trauma to spinal cord
	Parkinson's Disease
	Guillain-Barré Syndrome
	Multiple sclerosis
Drug induced	Anticholinergics
	Antidepressants

compensatory bladder hypertrophy. Over time, the bladder distends, then the ureters (causing hydroureters) and finally the renal pelvises. Often there may be an underlying chronic obstruction for example an enlarged prostate. Another factor may then cause acute urinary retention, e.g. constipation, bed rest (e.g. after surgery).

Clinical features

The symptoms depend on the speed of onset and degree of obstruction.

- Acute obstruction (acute urinary retention) causes severe discomfort, due to a wish to void urine, without the ability to do so. The bladder is tender, palpably enlarged. There is complete anuria, although there may be small amounts of urine voided due to overflow incontinence.
- Chronic obstruction causes three features: hesitancy, poor urinary stream (<10 mL/second) and terminal dribbling. Frequency and nocturia are not symptoms of obstruction. The symptoms usually develop over years, and if left untreated patients may present with renal failure. However, polyuria and/or nocturia may be symptoms of the loss of concentrating ability of the tubules, which can occur in long-standing obstruction.

Macroscopy

Dilation above the obstruction. Bladder trabeculation.

Complications

As a result of chronic obstruction, the bladder dilates and fails to empty fully, defined as >50 mL residual urine (normally 5–10 mL in young, fit person). Renal failure can be caused by both acute and chronic obstruction. Chronic urinary retention leads to:

- Reduced functional bladder capacity and therefore increased frequency.
- Recurrent UTI's.
- Stone formation can be caused by urinary stasis, UTI's predispose to stone formation, and also stones may predispose to infection.

Management

Relief of the obstruction is usually by insertion of a urinary catheter, followed by treatment of the underlying cause.

Benign prostatic hyperplasia

Definition

Hyperplasia of the prostate is a common cause of bladder outflow obstruction.

Incidence/prevalence

Common.

Age

Affects ∼50% of men age 50–60, >80% of men age >80.

Sex

Males

Aetiology

Thought to be due to increased androgen effects (dihydrotestosterone and its metabolites), or oestrogens. Functioning testes are important: castrati (before puberty) do not get BPH. Castration post-onset gives a 30% reduction in size only.

Pathophysiology

Androgens appear to act on the periurethral area of the prostate 'McNeal's transition zone' to stimulate hyperplasia. There is compensatory bladder hypertrophy. At 30–40 years there is microscopic evidence, by 50 years it is macroscopically visible, by 60 years the clinical phase begins.

The obstruction is due to both direct impingement of the enlarged prostate on the urethra and also the dynamic smooth muscle contraction of the prostate, prostatic capsule and bladder neck.

Clinical features

Usually a long history of bladder outflow obstruction, but may present as acute urinary retention or a UTI, or with frequency and urgency symptoms. Per rectum examination reveals a smoothly enlarged prostate, with intact median groove.

Macroscopy

There is hyperplasia of the transition zone. Nodules formed of hyperplastic glandular acini displace and compress the true prostatic glands peripherally forming a false capsule. Weight usually up to 200 g (normal is 15 g).

Microscopy
Benign epithelial proliferation with large acini, smooth muscle and fibroblast proliferation. Oedema and inflammation are common, as are areas of infarction.

Complications
Bladder decompensation – due to chronically increased residual volumes (urine retained after voiding), the bladder may become less contractile, lowering flow rates further. Obstruction may lead to dilated ureters and kidney (hydroureter, and hydronephrosis). It may also cause ARF or CRF.

Investigations
It is important to exclude other causes of bladder outflow obstruction or bladder instability.
- FBC, U&Es, serum prostate specific antigen (PSA) and urine microscopy and culture are routine.
- Urodynamics: Maximal urinary flow rates less than 10 mL/second are almost diagnostic of bladder outflow obstruction. Between 10 and 15 mL/second, combined pressure/flow studies may be done to exclude those with other problems, as resection of the prostate in these patients may not relieve symptoms. The disadvantage of the latter, is that urinary catheterisation is required.
- Bladder scan: This simple scan uses ultrasound to measure the post-voiding residual volume is useful. Patients with a high residual volume are at risk of bladder decompensation and UTIs.
- If there is evidence of renal impairment, renal USS should be performed to look for hydronephrosis.

Management
In patients with mild symptoms, monitoring may be advised, as symptoms often improve over time. For those with moderate to severe symptoms the choice is between a trial of medical therapy or surgical therapy.

Drugs are aimed at relaxing the contractile component and reducing the volume of the prostate.
- α-blockers such as doxazosin, terazosin and tamsulosin improve symptoms and bladder outflow rates in 60–90% of patients, but may cause unacceptable hypotension.
- Finasteride is a 5 alpha reductase inhibitor which inhibits the conversion of testosterone to dihydrotestosterone. It is also useful, but generally less effective for

symptoms than α-blockers. It seems to be more effective in those with very large prostates and its effects may improve with time.

Transurethral resection of the prostate (TURP) has been the standard treatment. The procedure involves removal of prostatic tissue using electrocautery via a resectoscope from within the prostatic urethra, under general or spinal anaethesia. Post-operatively patients require a three-way catheter and continuous bladder irrigation to reduce the risk of clot retention until haematuria is mild.
- Early complications: Post-op (immediate) haemorrhage, urethral blood clot and urinary retention. Antibiotic prophylaxis is usually given to prevent urinary tract infection. Hypervolaemia and hyponatraemia with a metabolic acidosis may occur (TURP syndrome) due to absorption of irrigating fluid (may be > 1 L).
- Later complications include: ≤14% become impotent, retrograde ejaculation, epididymo-orchitis, bladder neck contracture or urethral stricture requiring surgery or dilatation, incontinence. About 20% require further TURP within 10 years.

Other options (not widely available) include:
- Stent which is cost-effective in those with a short life-expectancy or temporarily for patients unfit for surgery, e.g. due to recent MI, and has less operative morbidity.
- Microwave ablation by transurethral catheter (TMT= transurethral microwave thermotherapy) or transrectally.
- Electrovaporisation utilises electrical energy to vaporise prostatic tissue, with the advantage of no further sloughing of tissue and less bleeding post-procedure.
- Endoscopic laser may result in less bleeding and shown to be as effective with similar costs to TURP.
- Radiofrequency 'needle' can be used, although further treatment is often required within 5 years.

Urinary incontinence

Definition
Urinary incontinence is the involuntary loss of urine from the urethra. It has a major physical, psychological and functional impact on the individual.

Incidence/prevalence

Even in young patients it is relatively common (up to 30% of women <65 years but only up to 5% of men <65 years). In older patients the age ratios approach 1–2F:1M. Rates are much higher in certain settings such as care of the elderly institutions (up to 45%) and psychiatric care of the elderly (90%).

Age

Increases with age.

Sex

F > M

Aetiology

Incontinence has been associated with many conditions and risk factors such as chronic cough, depression, dementia, pregnancy, vaginal delivery (particularly with episiotomy, forceps delivery), impaired mobility, drugs and chronic medical conditions such as heart failure, chronic lung disease, stroke, multiple sclerosis and diabetes.

Pathophysiology

Incontinence is multifactorial. To remain continent there must be:

- The ability to control micturition at the level of the urinary tract as well as neurological control.
- The ability to recognise the sensation of bladder filling and to be able to respond appropriately and sufficiently quickly to this.
- The ability to mobilise safely or the manual dexterity to use a container.
- The motivation to maintain dryness and hygiene.

Clinical features

Symptoms of incontinence may be grouped into those of specific syndromes:

- Stress incontinence occurs when intra-abdominal pressure is increased, e.g. on coughing, bending over, or running and jumping. The leak may occur at the time or just after. This is due to poor sphincter function.
- Urge incontinence is when the patient has an overwhelming urge to void leading to leakage. This may be precipitated by the sound of running water,

washing hands or even prematurely, e.g. on arriving home. This is mainly due to detrusor instability/overactivity.

- Mixed stress and urge incontinence is also common.
- Overflow incontinence is continual or unprecipitated leakage without urge. This may result from either the lack of sensation of a full bladder or sphincter incompetence. Bladder outflow obstruction may lead to overflow incontinence due to bladder decompensation. Rare causes include spinal cord compression affecting the sacral segments (S2, 3 and 4) or the conus medullaris. Patients may empty the bladder by straining or manual compression.

A comprehensive examination is important and can avoid the need for specialist tests. It is important to assess fluid balance, mobility, cognitive ability and relevant neurology. Rectal examination for constipation, rectal masses and vaginal speculum examination for atrophy, masses, cystocele or rectocele.

Complications

Increased risk of urinary tract infections (UTI's) and stones. Hydronephrosis, reflux damage to kidneys.

Investigations

- A voiding diary is useful to record the time, volume and relevant events, e.g. beverages, activities, sleeping and medications.
- In all patients with persistent incontinence, U&Es, glucose, calcium, vitamin B_{12} and urinalysis should be performed (with culture if indicated).
- Pad test (weighing a pad before and after various exercises).
- Post-void bladder volume should be assessed. Urodynamic investigations are rarely required.
- Occasionally, depending on the history and examination, other tests include X-rays, ultrasound renal tract and neurological testing for sacral evoked response.

Management

Treatment depends on the class of incontinence and the underlying cause:

Stress incontinence: Initially non-surgical options (e.g. exercises, medication) can be tried, but surgery is the main treatment.

- Pelvic floor (Kegel) exercises (with or without weighted cones) may be used but are dependent on the motivation of the patient. Systemic or topical oestrogen therapy may be of benefit. Imipramine (a mixed anticholinergic and α-agonist) has been used. Ring pessaries are useful for those with uterine prolapse.

- Surgery is effective but carries a significant morbidity. Using a transabdominal approach (but without entering the peritoneal cavity) stitches are placed through the fascia at the level of the bladder neck or urethra to hitch the urethra and bladder neck up and forwards. These are sutured either to Cooper's ligament (a Burch colposuspension or urethropexy) or to the periosteum of the pubic bone (a Marshall–Marchetti–Krantz colposuspension). For vaginal cystoceles (where the bladder herniates into the vaginal canal), a transvaginal approach may be used to repair the cystocele but this is generally less effective. Alternatively using both vaginal and transabdominal approaches a sling or sutures are used to lift the bladder neck or mid-urethra up to the rectus abdominis muscle.

Urge incontinence: unlike stress incontinence, behavioural and medical therapies are the main treatments. Surgery (clam cystoplasty to increase the size of the bladder using bowel) is rarely successful.

- Behavioural therapy can be more effective than medication. In patients with cognitive awareness of bladder filling and the ability to independently toilet, bladder training is used to learn methods of deliberately suppressing the urge to pass urine. In patients without cognitive awareness or lack of motivation to remain dry, scheduled or prompted voiding reduces the number of episodes of incontinence, as well as the volumes passed when incontinent.
- Drug therapy: Anticholinergics are the mainstay of drug treatment (e.g. oxybutynin, tolterodine). These tend to cause a dry mouth and may cause constipation and/or urinary retention. Imipramine may also be tried but tends to be avoided in the elderly due to side effects.

Combined stress and urge incontinence may be treated with behavioural therapy with or without medical therapy. Surgical treatment appears to be less effective than in pure stress incontinence. Overflow incontinence: Treatment is aimed at the underlying cause.

- If there is bladder outlet obstruction, either TURP or incision of the bladder neck (or external sphincter) is used to reduce outlet obstruction.

- In spinal cord compression emergency decompression is essential (see page 000). In other neuropathic conditions intermittent self-catheterisation is the preferred treatment.
- Patients who are unfit for TURP or are unable to self-catheterise may require a long-term indwelling catheter.
- Prevention of infection is important both by using sterile catheters and possibly using prophylactic antibiotics.

Urinary tract infections

Urinary tract infections (UTIs)

Definition
An infection of the urinary tract which may be further distinguished on the basis of anatomy, e.g. cystitis, pyelonephritis. In females, vaginitis is another syndrome which commonly overlaps.

Age
All ages

Sex
F > M

Aetiology
Most frequently due to bacteria, in particular *E. coli* and *Proteus mirabilis*. Hospital acquired infections may be due to other organisms such as *Staphyloccoccus, Enterococcus* and *Klebsiella*. Less commonly, fungi (*Candida* and *Histoplasma capsulatum*), parasites (the protozoan *Trichomonas vaginalis* and the fluke *Schistosoma haematobium*) and very rarely viruses can cause UTIs.

Pathophysiology
- Bacterial virulence factors: Critical to the pathogenesis of bacteria is adherence to the uroepithelium as infections ascend from the urethral orifice to the bladder and to the kidney in pyelonephritis. *E. coli* have special fimbriae (also called pili) which permit adhesion. Other virulence factors include flagellae (to permit mobility), production of enzymes such as haemolysin (*E. coli* and *Proteus*) which induces pore formation

in cell membranes. *E. coli* also inhibits phagocytosis. Urease is produced by some organisms (e.g. *Proteus*), it hydrolyses urea and increases ammonia, which facilitates bacterial adherence.

- Host predisposing factors include any functional or anatomical abnormality of the urinary tract such as urinary stasis, reflux or stones. Other important risk factors include sexual intercourse, diabetes mellitus, immunosuppression, instrumentation (including catheterisation) and pregnancy.
- Urine itself is inhibitory to the growth of normal urinary flora (non-haemolytic *Streptococcus corynebacteria*, *Staphylococcus*) through its pH and chemical content.

Clinical features

Acute cystitis typically presents with dysuria (a burning pain on passing urine), urgency and frequency. Fever and other systemic features are variable. Macroscopic haematuria is not uncommon, although this should prompt further investigation for any other underlying disease such as urinary stones or a bladder malignancy. Pyelonephritis may present with few lower urinary tract symptoms, but more commonly causes systemic upset with fever, rigors, chills, and loin pain or tenderness. Prostatitis causes fever, malaise and pain in the perineum and lower back as well as dysuria and frequency. Both pyelonephritis and prostatitis may be due to ascending or haematogenous infection (usually ascending).

- UTIs in pregnancy, the elderly and those with indwelling catheters may be asymptomatic, or may present nonspecifically with fever, falls, vomiting, or confusion etc.

Macroscopy

The urine is cloudy due to the pyuria (pus cells) and bacteriuria, and may contain visible amounts of blood (macroscopic haematuria). Sterile pyuria (pus cells without a positive culture) may be caused by antibiotic treatment, stones, drugs such as NSAIDs and occasionally tuberculosis.

Complications

- Recurrent infections which may be relapses or a reinfection. Over time, recurrences can cause chronic inflammatory changes in the urinary tract (bladder, prostate).

- Urinary stones for example, *Proteus*, through the production of urease, causes the alkalinisation of urine, so that phosphate, carbonate and magnesium are more likely to precipitate to form struvite stones.
- Bacteraemia can lead to septicaemia and in vulnerable hosts, infective endocarditis.

Investigations

Mid-stream urine for urinalysis (dipstick testing), microscopy, culture and sensitivity. A culture is regarded as positive if $>10^5$ of a single organism per mL.

Patients with systemic symptoms should have a blood culture, FBC and differential, U&Es and creatinine to look for dehydration and any evidence of renal impairment. Further investigations are required in children (see page 268), males and females with recurrent infections.

Management

Empirical antibiotic therapy is used in symptomatic patients, until culture and sensitivity results are available. Uncomplicated cystitis in a woman usually only requires 3 days of oral antibiotics, whereas longer courses are required in complicated cases, e.g. those with urinary stasis, indwelling catheters, pyelonephritis and prostatitis. Intravenous antibiotics should be used in those who are systemically unwell or those who are vomiting.

- Commonly used drugs include trimethoprim, amoxycillin and co-amoxiclav (as many infections are caused by β-lactamase producers). Quinolones such as ciprofloxacin are useful as resistant *E. coli* and *Proteus* are uncommon, but they do not adequately cover gram-positive organisms.
- Intravenous therapy is often with a cephalosporin with or without gentamicin.

Oral fluids should be encouraged where possible to prevent dehydration and relieve symptoms. Cranberry juice may also have a role in reducing symptoms, but has not been shown to be effective in treatment or prevention of UTIs.

Recurrent UTIs may be reduced, e.g. by passing urine after intercourse, treatment of stones and in some cases prophylactic antibiotics. These may cause microbial resistance, and some centres advise a 'cycling regime', e.g. of three different antibiotics, each used for 1 month to prevent this.

Acute pyelonephritis

Definition
Acute upper urinary tract infection, which causes inflammation of the interstitium of the kidney.

Aetiology
Bacterial infection, either ascending from the lower urinary tract or, less commonly due to haematogenous spread in bacteraemia or septicaemia. The most common organism is *E. coli*, as for other UTIs.

Pathophysiology
Predisposing factors to ascending infection include pregnancy (progesterone dilates the ureters), diabetes mellitus (does not increase incidence of UTI's but does seem to make them more likely to be severe), urinary stasis due to obstruction, dilatation or neurological causes and reflux.

Clinical features
Fever >38°C, rigors, loin pain and tenderness with or without lower urinary tract symptoms. Nausea and vomiting are common. Features may be less specific in the elderly.

Macroscopy/microscopy
The kidneys appear hyperaemic, and tiny yellow-white spherical abscesses may be seen in the cortex. There is neutrophilic infiltration, and bacteria may be seen.

Complications
- Gram negative septicaemia causing shock is uncommon in young, otherwise healthy patients, but may lead to multiorgan failure. Necrotic renal papillae due to inflammatory thrombosis of the vasa recta, can be shed, causing obstruction and acute renal failure.
- Recurrent infections cause renal scarring and impaired renal function, which may cause hypertension.
- See also perinephric abscess (see below).

Investigations
- Urine microscopy and culture. Urinalysis is usually abnormal, but may not be grossly so.
- FBC and differential. U&Es and creatinine (assess hydration and renal function).
- Blood culture.
- Renal USS and plain KUB X-ray may be performed if response to treatment is slow, or in suspected complicated cases, to exclude any underlying renal tract abnormality, and the presence of stones. If there is any evidence of obstruction this requires rapid drainage (see page 256). Some stones are not radio-opaque, and will be missed with these tests, in which case an IVU or CT scan is more definitive.

Management
Mild cases may respond to oral antibiotics as for urinary tract infection, but many require intravenous therapy such as gentamicin and ciprofloxacin. In hospitalised patients, once clinically improving and able to tolerate oral medications, i.v. antibiotics and fluids can be converted to oral. Antibiotics should be tailored to the sensitivity and specificity, and continued for 10–14 days (longer courses in patients who were more unwell, complex, immunosuppressed or responded slowly).

Renal or perinephric abscess

Definition
An abscess that forms in the kidney, or in the perinephric fat, as the result of ascending infection or haematogenous spread. These have become less common, due to more effective antibiotic treatment of pyelonephritis.

Aetiology
As with other urinary tract infections, the most common organisms are *E. coli* and *Staphylococcus*.

Pathophysiology
Commonly the infection ascends via the lower urinary tract to cause pyelonephritis. In most cases, there is an underlying renal abnormality such as reflux, stone(s) or a polycystic kidney that predisposes to a focal area becoming walled off to form an abscess. Haematogenous spread accounts for ~25% of cases, e.g. in infective endocarditis, or other cause of bacteraemia. Perinephric abscesses may arise due to infection spreading from the kidney into the perinephric fat, or by direct haematogenous spread.

Clinical features

Symptoms are initially as for pyelonephritis. The diagnosis of renal abscess should be suspected in those patients who are seriously unwell, who have a known underlying renal abnormality and in those who do not improve after 5 days of appropriate antibiotic treatment.

Investigations

- Urine microscopy and culture. Urinalysis may be normal if the abscess does not communicate with the urinary collecting system.
- FBC and differential. U&Es and creatinine.
- Blood culture.
- Renal ultrasound scan or CT will demonstrate a thick-walled cavity, often filled with necrotic material. It may not be possible to differentiate it from a renal cell carcinoma. CT with contrast usually shows increased contrast in a ring around the abscess. USS or CT-guided aspiration and/or drainage are useful to provide a specimen for microscopy and culture, and may be useful therapeutically.

Management

Antibiotic choice is as for pyelonephritis, until culture results are known. In large abscesses (>3 cm) medical therapy alone is often insufficient, and percutaneous drainage or even partial or total nephrectomy may be required. Longer courses of antibiotics are usually required, often 1–2 months.

Chronic pyelonephritis (reflux nephropathy)

Definition

Chronic pyelonephritis is the damage caused to the kidneys by persistent or recurrent infection. The term should largely be replaced by 'reflux nephropathy', the most common form.

Incidence/prevalence

Accounts for about 15% of cases of end-stage renal failure and is an important cause of hypertension in later life.

Aetiology

The development of chronic pyelonephritis requires there to be infections in a kidney with an underlying anatomical abnormality, such as reflux or stones.

Vesicoureteric reflux (VUR) where urine refluxes back up from the bladder into the ureter, due to an incompetent vesicoureteric junction, is common, affecting 1% of neonates and 30–45% of young children who present with a urinary tract infection (UTI). Reflux due to high pressure can also develop in patients with obstruction due to urethral valves and after spinal cord injury. The severity of the VUR predicts the risk of developing renal damage.

There is a strong familial incidence of VUR, siblings may have a 30–40% risk of also being affected, and infants born to mothers with VUR may have an even higher risk.

Pathophysiology

In reflux nephropathy, the papillae are damaged, and the calyces become dilated and 'clubbed'. As areas of the kidney are chronically or recurrently infected, they become scarred, leading to loss of nephrons. As renal function deteriorates, hypertension may follow, which accelerates the renal damage by hypertensive-induced vascular change. Unilateral chronic pyelonephritis does not cause renal impairment, as long as the other kidney is normal an adequate GFR is maintained. However, hypertension may lead to damage to the single functioning kidney.

Clinical features

A single proven UTI in early childhood should be investigated for any underlying congenital abnormality predisposing to reflux, to assess the degree of VUR and any scarring which has already occurred. Recurrent UTI's in adults should also be investigated. If the diagnosis is missed (often the UTI's are asymptomatic), then patients present later in life with hypertension, proteinuria and/or renal impairment.

Macroscopy

The kidneys are smaller than normal, with an irregular, blunted, distorted pelvicalyceal system and areas of scarring 1–2 cm in size. The poles tend to be more affected.

Microscopy

Areas of interstitial fibrosis with chronic inflammatory cell infiltration. The tubules are atrophic or dilated and the glomeruli show periglomerular fibrosis. Some may be hyalinized in response to damage.

Investigations

The scarring of reflux nephropathy is best visualised by DMSA scans. Intravenous pyelogram and renal ultrasound may also identify damaged kidneys (but are less sensitive) and dilated ureters. Infants and young children are screened for VUR following a single UTI, as should siblings, and infants of mothers with proven VUR. Screening may involve renal ultrasound, DMSA scan, micturating cystourogram (MCUG) or MAG3 scan with indirect cystourogram dependant on age.

Management

Patients with chronic renal failure require appropriate treatment (see Chronic Renal Failure page 237). Patients with VUR should be treated with prophylactic antibiotics until reflux is shown to have resolved or puberty. Previously severe reflux was treated with surgical re-implantation of the ureters, this has now been shown to have no additional benefit and risks urinary obstruction.

Urinary schistosomiasis (bilharzia)

Definition

Schistosomiasis is the disease caused by the parasitic flukes, schistosomes.

Incidence/prevalence

Schistosomiasis affects 200 million people worldwide.

Geography

Urinary schistosomiasis occurs in Africa, the Middle East, Spain, Portugal, Greece and the Indian Ocean, particularly in rural areas where the snail vectors are present. Travellers may pick up the infection, even with brief exposure to contaminated water.

Pathophysiology

The eggs of *S. haematobium* are excreted through the bladder wall into the urine causing haematuria. Eggs that are trapped in tissue cause local inflammation, scarring and fibrosis in the bladder and ureters, which can lead to obstruction, calcification and hydronephrosis.

Clinical features

Patients with *S. haematobium* may be asymptomatic, or have frequency, dysuria, haematuria (microscopic or macroscopic) and incontinence. Secondary anaemia may occur. Complications include hydronephrosis and renal failure, and chronic inflammation predisposes to squamous cell carcinoma of the bladder. *S. mansoni* and *japonicum* can cause proteinuria and nephrotic syndrome by immune complex deposition and may cause other systemic features.

Investigations

Dipstick urine to look for blood. Urine microscopy to look for eggs with a terminal spine. Anti-schistosomal antibodies can be measured, although these take a month to become positive.

Managment

Praziquantel is the treatment of choice.

Acute epididymo-orchitis

Definition

Acute primary infection of the epididymis and the testis.

Age

Normally under 40 years.

Sex

Male

Aetiology/pathophysiology

The most common causes are *N. gonococcus*, *Chlamydia trachomatis*, *E. coli* and other gram-negative bacilli. Orchitis is also an important complication of mumps. TB is an important differential. The infection starts in the lower genital tract either as a sexually transmitted infection or as a urinary tract infection. Resolution is usually accompanied by healing and scarring, there may be permanent damage to the tubules risking infertility.

Clinical features

Patients present with a greatly enlarged and very tender testis, the pain usually comes on quickly (30–60 minutes) and is sometimes released by supporting the scrotum. Other causes of a painful scrotal swelling are shown in Table 6.14.

Table 6.14 Causes painful scrotal swelling

Torsion of testis or testicular appendage
Incarcerated hernia
Infarcted germ cell tumor
Scrotal cellulitis and fasciitis
Post-traumatic causes

On examination the swelling is confined to one side and the swelling is hot and very tender.

Microscopy

There is extensive infiltration of the seminiferous tubules and interstitium with neutrophils, initial oedema is considerable and there is often patchy haemorrhage.

Complications

Infertility is an important complication.

Investigations

Urine (first catch is best, rather than MSU, under these circumstances) and any urethral discharge should be cultured.

Management

Treatment is with antibiotics, bed rest and scrotal support. In young adults, erythromycin (to cover *Chlamydia*) is probably best, whereas in older individuals or where there is a good history of UTI, suggested antibiotics are the same as those for UTI, e.g. trimethoprim.

Urinary stones

Urinary stones

Definition

The development of stones in the urinary tract or urolithiasis.

Incidence/prevalence

Affects about 10% of the population at some time in their lives.

Age

Peaks age 20–50 years.

Sex

M > F (4:1)

Aetiology

Risk factors include: dehydration, urinary tract infections, disorders of calcium handling (hypercalcaemia, hypercalciuria), hyperuricaemia, small intestinal disease or resection, renal tubular acidosis, hereditary conditions (such as cystinuria) and drugs in particular sulphonamides at high doses and indinavir (a protease inhibitor used to treat HIV).

Pathophysiology

Stone formation usually occurs because compounds of low solubility are present in the urine in high concentrations. There are inorganic inhibitors of crystal formation, such as magnesium, citrate and organic inhibitors such as glycoseaminoglycans and nephrocalcin. Uric acid appears to interfere with this inhibition, so when present in high concentrations it predisposes to the formation of both uric acid and non-uric acid stones.

Stones commonly contain calcium oxalate (80%) but about half of these also contain hydroxyapatite. ~10% are struvite (magnesium ammonium phosphate) stones which consist of struvite and calcium carbonate-apatite), with the remainder formed of calcium phosphate, uric acid or cystine (see Table 6.15).

Clinical features

Renal or ureteric colic is the most common presentation. The pain is characteristically in sharp, intense waves over a background pain, occurring in the loin, radiating to the groin and testes or labia. Patients feel sick and often

Table 6.15 Types of Urinary Stones

Type of stone	Pathogenesis	Features
Calcium	30% have hypercalciuria Idiopathic (most common)	1. Absorptive (primary increased intestinal absorption)
		2. Renal (primary renal loss of calcium compensated by ↑ absorption)
		3. Resorptive (primary increased skeletal resorption)
	Hypercalcaemia	Less commonly
Oxalate	↑ urinary oxalate levels	
Uric acid	Hyperuricosuria	↑↑ uric acid stones ↑ calcium oxalate stones
Cystine	Cystinuria	Autosomal recessively inherited condition

vomit. They are restless and move around trying to relieve the pain. Bladder or urethral stones may cause pain on passing urine, inability to pass urine or the sensation of passing gravel. Ninety per cent have haematuria, some may have proteinuria.

Infection may present as an acute, recurrent or chronic cystitis, pyelonephritis or pyonephrosis (obstruction with a stone can lead to hydronephrosis, which if this then becomes infected, can make the patient very unwell).

If the stone obstructs a single functioning kidney, postrenal acute renal failure results.

Investigations

- Plain AXR: Most stones are radio-opaque and show up on plain abdominal X-rays. Calcium oxalate stones look spiky, calcium phosphate stones are often smooth and can be large. Uric acid stones are radiolucent and cystine stones only slightly radio-opaque.
- IVU: i.v. contrast with AXR at 5 and 20 minutes to show exactly where the stone is in relation to the kidneys and ureters. This should be avoided if there is significant renal impairment because excretion is poor so that images are less informative and there is an increased risk of contrast causing acute renal failure.
- Renal ultrasound may show stones inside kidney and demonstrate hydronephrosis due to obstruction. CT is often more sensitive.
- Serial X-rays to see if stone is moving.
- Urine microscopy and culture. Strain all urine to try to catch the stone so that it can be analysed. Crystals may be seen in urine which can help identify the type of stone.

Management

Treat pain, e.g. with opiates and/or NSAID such as diclofenac (useful i.m. or as a suppository). Some recommend anti-spasmodic drugs. Ensure adequate fluid intake. Stones $\geq$5 mm in diameter are less likely to pass, stones <5 mm especially in the lower half of ureter are more likely to pass without intervention.

Surgical techniques are needed if the stone does not pass. It may be necessary to relieve obstruction urgently, if there is obstruction or infection. Obstruction can be relieved by retrograde stent insertion (usually requires general anaesthetic), or percutaneous nephrostomy insertion under local anaesthetic.

- Lithotripsy (external ultrasound shock waves), US guided, no need for anaesthetic. Stones within calyces cannot be broken up this way.
- Lasertripsy, electrical.
- Open surgery (nephrolithotomy or ureterolithotomy), or percutaneous removal via a nephrostomy. Alternatively perurethral by cystoscopy with a Dormia basket for low stones.

Subsequent management

To reduce the risk of recurrence, all patients should be advised to drink plenty of fluid, especially at night and to treat urinary infections early.

- Patients with calcium stones should avoid calcium intake and vitamin D supplements. Potassium citrate may also be given to increase urine levels of citrate which inhibits calcium stone formation.
- Oxalate is found in tea, chocolate, nuts, strawberries, spinach, rhubarb and beans.
- Uric acid excretion can be reduced using allopurinol.
- Cystine stones can be reduced using oral sodium bicarbonate to alkalinise the urine, or D-penicillamine.

Consider looking for predisposing factors such as plasma calcium and parathyroid hormone (if radio-opaque stone), phosphate, urate if radiolucent stones, and 24 hour collection of urine for components of stones.

Prognosis

Despite preventative strategies recurrence rates are as high as 75%.

Stag horn calculus

Definition

A urinary stone which fills the calyces and pelvis of a kidney, these are usually associated with infection and are formed of struvite.

Aetiology/pathophysiology

Stag horn calculi are struvite stones (i.e. formed of struvite and calcium carbonate-apatite). Infection with *Proteus* or *Klebsiella* causes increased amounts of ammonia, due to the presence of urease (which breaks down urea into ammonia and carbon dioxide). This increases the amount of ammonium, but also alkalinises the urine, decreasing the solubility of phosphate. Infection can also be a complication of stones.

Clinical features

May be asymptomatic in early stages. Later, pain, haematuria and impaired renal function.

Investigations

As for urinary stones. Assess the kidney function with radionuclide imaging. If <10% renal function the kidney should be removed. If there is >25% function in a younger patient many would probably try to preserve the kidney.

Management

Open surgery, or very slow gradual breaking up of the calculus using 'perc-bang' combination therapy, which involves placing a stent from the kidney to the bladder for stones to descend, then debulking the stone with repeated lithotripsy. Nephrectomy is advised for a symptomatic stag horn calculus in a poorly functioning kidney.

Disorders of the male genital system

Torsion of the testis

Definition

Twisting of testis on its pedicle is a surgical emergency.

Age

Most occur in young children and peri-pubertally, less common over 25 years.

Sex

Male

Aetiology

Torsion occurs if the testis is insufficiently fixed by its lower pole to the tunica vaginalis by the gubernaculum testis, so allowing it to twist.

Pathophysiology

Twisting of the testis on the spermatic cord leads to venous/haemorrhagic infarction.

Clinical features

Characteristically the patient presents with an acutely tender swollen testis of sudden onset, there may be a history of minor trauma or recent vigorous exercise. Nausea and vomiting are common associated symptoms. There may be history of previous self-resolving episodes of pain, particularly at night in young boys (can be associated with nocturnal sexual arousal that occurs during REM sleep). Examination classically reveals a red hemiscrotum, with an asymmetrically high, swollen testis (pulled up by the shortened, twisted spermatic cord). However, it may be difficult to examine due to pain. The cremasteric response is absent in torsion (stroking or pinching the inside of the thigh should cause the ipsilateral testis to rise), but this response is not reliable below the age of 30 months or over 12 years.

The main differential is epididymo-orchitis in which the tenderness may be localised to the epididymis and pain may be relieved by support of the scrotum, but it can be difficult to distinguish particularly as the testis can also swell in this condition.

Complications

If surgery is delayed beyond 12–18 hours the blood supply is compromised and infarction occurs requiring surgical orchidectomy.

Investigations

Diagnosis is clinical and surgery should not be delayed. However, in dubious cases, colour Doppler USS may be performed to look for blood flow, if absent torsion is very likely.

Management

The scrotum is explored, the twist is reversed and if the testis is viable *both* testes are fixed in position as the condition is a bilateral defect. If surgical fixation is performed promptly fertility is unimpaired.

Hydrocele

Definition

Collection of fluid within the coverings of the testes.

Incidence/prevalence

Common.

Age

Congenital hydroceles occur in childhood, secondary are more common age 20–40 years.

Aetiology

Most hydroceles are idiopathic but may occur secondary to trauma, infection or neoplasm.

Pathophysiology

Fluid accumulates between the two layers (parietal and visceral) of the tunica vaginalis. It is thought to occur due to imbalance of secretion/reabsorption of peritoneal fluid from these layers. Congenital hydrocele is caused by the persistence of the processus vaginalis and can be associated with herniation of abdominal contents into the sac.

Clinical features

Patients present with an increase in the size of the testis or a swelling in the scrotum, which can be massive before becoming uncomfortable. Idiopathic hydroceles generally develop very slowly, whereas secondary hydroceles develop rapidly. Usually the hydrocele covers the testis, so that it is difficult to palpate. In the upper part of the swelling, a normal spermatic cord should be palpable (this differentiates a hydrocele from an inguinal hernia). A simple hydrocele transilluminates well, but if there is blood (a haematocele) or it is chronic and the wall is thickened, it does not.

Investigations

If there is any doubt an ultrasound scan confirms the diagnosis and is useful to exclude an underlying testicular tumour.

Management

1 Any secondary cause should be identified and treated.
2 Treatment is by surgical excision or plication of the sac. Aspiration should not be attempted as there is a risk of infection and bleeding.
3 If the hydrocele fluid becomes infected or contains blood, incision and drainage of pus are necessary, and examination of the scrotal contents to exclude an underlying tumour may be performed at that time.

Varicocele

Definition

Varicoceles are dilated veins (pampiniform plexus) along the spermatic cord.

Incidence/prevalence

As common as 1 in 5 post-pubertal males, but often asymptomatic.

Aetiology/pathophysiology

These are the equivalent of varicose veins, due to the valve leaflets becoming incompetent, blood flows back down towards the testis. Varicoceles occur more commonly on the left side due to the perpendicular drainage of the left spermatic vein into the renal vein, which is compressed between the aorta and superior mesenteric artery. Isolated right-sided varicocele should raise the suspicion of a thrombus in the IVC or right renal vein, possibly associated with renal cell carcinoma, because on the right the spermatic vein drains directly into the IVC and should remain competent.

Varioceles are commonly found in men who are infertile, but many also have normal sperm counts. The cause of infertility is not clear. Testicular atrophy is thought to occur due to the slightly raised temperature triggering germ cell apoptosis.

Clinical features

Patients may complain of a dragging sensation or aching pain in the scrotum, particularly on standing. Infertility may be a presenting feature. On palpation there is a soft swelling like 'a bag of worms' along the spermatic cord, which is compressible and disappears on lying flat.

Management

Surgery is indicated in boys and young males with asymmetrical growth of the testes/testicular atrophy, and seems to improve testicular growth. However, in infertile men with a varicocele, surgery has not been shown to improve sperm counts. Ligation of the spermatic vein can be either by open or laparoscopic surgery. In older males who no longer wish to have more children, treatment with scrotal support and analgesia may be sufficient.

Phimosis

Definition
Narrowing of the penile orifice due to contraction of the foreskin.

Aetiology/pathophysiology
Normally the foreskin does not retract at birth and it may be months to years before it becomes retractile. In congenital phimosis, the orifice is too small from birth causing difficulty in micturition. If the foreskin is not retractable beyond childhood, there may be difficulty in cleaning under the foreskin predisposing to infection (balanitis) and carcinoma of the penis.

Clinical features
- A young child with congenital phymosis may have difficulty with micturition, with ballooning of the prepuce as it becomes full of urine.
- In adolescence and adulthood, if the foreskin does not retract fully, pain may be felt on erection and with sexual intercourse.

Complications
- Recurrent balanitis may occur due to secretions collecting under a poorly retractile foreskin. Balanitis causes pain and a purulent discharge.
- If a poorly retracting foreskin remains retracted after an erection it can act as a tight band causing oedema and engorgement of the glans (paraphimosis) due to disruption of venous blood flow.
- Phimosis increases the rate of penile cancer by at least 10-fold.

Management
Symptomatic phimosis is treated by elective circumcision. Circumcision is not required in asymptomatic young children, unless for religious reasons. In cases of acute paraphimosis, the band is excised under general anaesthetic if the foreskin cannot be drawn forwards and circumcision is advocated.

Epididymal cysts

Definition
Epididymal cysts are fluid filled swellings connected with the epididymis that occur in males. If the fluid contains sperm, it is called a spermatocele.

Aetiology/pathophysiology
They arise from the collecting tubules of the epididymis, as a thin-walled cyst containing watery or slightly milky fluid.

Clinical features
A swelling in the scrotum located above and behind the testes, thus some patients attend saying they have developed a third testis. Cysts may be small, multiple, and are frequently bilateral and transilluminate brightly.

Management
As the cysts are totally benign, they are best left alone. Surgery to remove the cyst(s) risks damaging the spermatic pathway, such that bilateral operations can cause sterility, and more conservative removal often leads to recurrence.

Impotence

Definition
Inability to achieve or sustain a sufficiently rigid erection in order to have sexual intercourse. Occasional episodes of impotence are considered normal, but if erectile dysfunction precludes more than 75% of attempted intercourse, a man is considered 'impotent'. Also called male sexual dysfunction.

Incidence/prevalence
This has been underestimated in the past, due to the reluctance of men to discuss this and the assumption that impotence is inevitable with advancing age. With greater understanding, increased availability of treatment and more widespread discussion of the problem, 40% of men aged 40 are recognised to have some degree of sexual dysfunction, increasing by approximately 10% with each decade.

Aetiology
The cause is pyschogenic in 25% of cases, drugs (25%) and endocrine abnormalities (25%). The other 25% are caused by diabetes, neurological and urological/pelvic disease.

Psychogenic causes can be divided into following:
- Depression, causing loss of libido and erectile dysfunction. Many impotent men also become depressed.

- Performance anxiety occurs in men who, after one or more episodes of erectile dysfunction, become so anxious that subsequent attempts at intercourse fail, leading to escalation of the problem.
- Distraction or loss of focus, e.g. by work issues or other tasks that need to be done, can cause loss of erection during sexual intercourse.

Drugs:

- Commonly used drugs can cause impotence such as antihypertensives, in particular thiazide diuretics, anti-depressants and drugs used to treat peptic ulcer disease. Barbiturates, corticosteroids, phenothiazines and spironolactone may reduce libido.
- Nicotine and alcohol. Recreational drugs such as cocaine and hallucinogenic drugs can cause impotence with long-term use.

Endocrine:

- Testosterone not only acts to increase libido, but is needed for a rigid erection, by maintaining nitric oxide synthase levels in the penis. Oestrogen therapy (e.g. for prostate cancer) can also result in impotence.
- Hyperprolactinaemia, hyperthyroidism and hypothyroidism.
- Diabetes lowers intracavernosal levels of nitric oxide synthase, and these patients also have increased atherosclerosis which can impair blood supply. Autonomic neuropathy is also an important factor.

Central sexual impulses (e.g. caused by images or sounds) pass to T11-L2, which then sends signals to the pelvic vessels, to increase blood supply to the penis. There is also a reflex arc at S2–S4 which means that genital stimulation increases vascular flow. Neurological disease at any level can therefore interfere with sexual function.

Clinical features

Some features in the sexual history, medical history or examination may point towards a cause. Complete loss of erections, including nocturnal erections, suggests a neurological or vascular cause. Sudden loss of sexual function without any previous history of problems, or major genital surgery, suggests performance anxiety, stress or loss of interest in the sexual partner. Ability to generate an erection, but then inability to sustain it may be due to anxiety or to a problem with vascular supply, or nitric oxide synthase levels, e.g. in diabetes. It is important to take a drug history and enquire about possible features of depression, smoking, alcohol or drug abuse.

Investigations

Simple hormonal tests for prolactin levels, thyroid function tests, testosterone levels are sometimes useful. Diabetes mellitus should be looked for by urine dipstick/blood sugar levels.

Management

- Oral treatments include Sildenafil (Viagra) is a type 5 phosphodiesterase inhibitor, which allows cyclic GMP to accumulate (nitric oxide induced vasodilatation is mediated by cyclic GMP which is catabolised by type 5 phosphodiesterase), so increasing the ability to generate and maintain an erection. It needs to be taken 1 hour before sex, and its effects last for 4 hours. Its vasodilation effects can cause headache, dizziness, a blue tinge to vision (reversible) and even syncope. It is contraindicated with concomitant nitrate use (including sublingual and GTN patch) within 24 hours, as profound hypotension can result. There are now two newer similar drugs – vardenafil and tadalfil, which have a more rapid onset, but longer duration of action, allowing more spontaneity.
- Anti-depressants such as selective serotonin reuptake inhibitors may be useful, particularly for premature ejaculation.
- Penile self-injection with vasoactive drugs such as papaverine, or alprostadil suit some individuals. An important side-effect is priapism – a prolonged erection which may need surgical intervention to remove clot.
- Vacuum devices can be used to 'suck' blood into the penis and then a ring is applied at its base to maintain the erection. Ejaculation is not possible with these devices.
- Surgical intervention involves the implantation of a prosthesis into the corpus cavernosa.
- Psychological counselling is useful for those with a psychological cause.

Genitourinary oncology

Kidney tumours

Benign tumours are commonly found incidentally at post-mortems or on imaging.

- Renal adenomas are derived from renal tubular epithelium. Tumours less than 3 cm in diameter are arbitrarily termed benign adenomas, but histologically they are similar to renal cell carcinomas and have the potential to metastasise.

- Oncocytomas are uncommon. Microscopically they contain only large well-differentiated cells with eosinophilic cytoplasm filled with mitochondria.
- Angiomyolipomas are associated with tuberose sclerosis, and are hamartomas: tumours composed of smooth muscle, fat and large blood vessels.
- Renal fibromas are derived from spindle cells, usually less than 1 cm in diameter and in the medulla.
- A rare tumour of the juxta-glomerular cells may present as hypertension in young patients.

Malignant tumours

- The most common is renal cell carcinoma (85–90% in adults).
- Transitional cell carcinomas of the renal pelvis account for only 5–10%. These share the same pathology as in bladder cancer.
- Wilm's tumour is the most common renal tumour in children.

Renal cell carcinoma

Definition
Adenocarcinoma of the kidney, which arises from the renal tubular epithelium. (Previously also called hypernephroma or Grawitz tumour).

Prevalence
2% of all visceral tumours; 85–90% of primary renal malignancies in adults.

Age
Increases with age, most over age 50 years.

Sex
M > F (3:1)

Aetiology
Predisposing factors include smoking, carcinogens such as asbestos and petrochemical products, obesity and genetic factors.

In von Hippel–Lindau (vHL) syndrome (an autosomal dominant inherited condition with familial haemangioblastomas in the CNS) one third of patients develop clear cell renal cell carcinoma (CCRCC). In tuberose sclerosis, most renal lesions are benign angiomyolipomas, but there is also an increased risk of papillary renal cell carcinoma.

Pathophysiology
- The VHL gene is a tumour suppressor gene. More than 75% of sporadic CCRCC have loss of or inactivation of both VHL alleles.
- Papillary renal cell tumours may have trisomy of Chr 17 (adenomas) or with additional trisomy of 16, 20 or 12 (carcinomas).

Clinical features
Presenting symptoms may include haematuria, fever, night sweats, anorexia, abdominal or loin mass, loin pain and weight loss. Systemic features or paraneoplastic syndromes are relatively common:

- A normochromic, normocytic anaemia is common, but polycythaemia, i.e. increased red cell mass, occurs in up to 5% of patients, due to the overproduction of erythropoietin.
- Hypercalcaemia is common, either due to bony metastases or the production of parathyroid hormone-related protein (PTHrP).
- Polymyalgia-like symptoms with aching proximal muscles may occur, which are unresponsive to steroid therapy.

Many patients remain asymptomatic until advanced local disease or metastases develop, so may present with the symptoms of complications and increasingly lesions are diagnosed incidentally.

On examination, occasionally a palpable loin mass may be found and lymphadenopathy, hepatosplenomegaly, ascites, a varicocele (which does not collapse when supine) in the scrotal sac and any evidence of metastases should be looked for.

Other features which may raise the suspicion of renal cell carcinoma include hypertension, raised ESR, or abnormal liver function tests despite a lack of liver metastases.

Macroscopy
There is a rounded mass, usually in the upper pole, with a soft, yellow-grey cut surface with haemorrhage and necrosis. It is often surrounded by a pseudocapsule.

Microscopy

Sheets of clear or granular cells with small or normal looking nuclei and cytoplasmic glycogen or fat. They are similar in appearance to adrenal cortical cells, hence 'hypernephroma'. Different histological subtypes have been described, the most common of which are clear cell (75–85%) and papillary/chromophilic (15%).

Complications

Local spread especially into the renal vein, and may grow as far as the inferior vena cava and right atrium. Tumour may also spread into neighbouring tissues, such as the adrenal gland and other abdominal organs. Lymphatic spread is common. Distant spread occurs as cannonball metastases in bone, lungs, brain or liver.

Investigations

Urinalysis shows haematuria in ~40%. Blood tests including FBC, U&Es, ESR, LFTs and calcium.

Renal ultrasound scan is usually the diagnostic imaging method. A solid tumour >3 cm is diagnostic, but sometimes a cyst is seen which needs to be differentiated between a simple benign cyst, a complex cyst or solid tumour. Doppler USS should be performed to look for renal vein thrombus.

Abdominal CT scan will show in more detail any suspicious features: thickened, irregular walls, multiloculated mass and contrast enhancement. CT will also demonstrate any local invasion, lymph node and renal vein involvement.

Staging tests include chest X-ray and CT chest, bone scan.

Management

Surgical removal is the treatment of choice for those without metastases (if there is a single metastasis this can be resected along with the primary tumour). The tumour is very resistant to chemotherapy or radiotherapy. In the past, radical nephrectomy with removal of the kidney, perinephric fact, together with the ipsilateral adrenal gland and hilar and para-aortic lymph nodes was routinely performed. Some now perform either total nephrectomy (without removal of the adrenal or lymph nodes), or more conservative surgery, i.e. wide resection or partial nephrectomy, for tumours <5 cm in size, but these techniques may have a greater risk of recurrence.

Palliative radiotherapy is used for symptomatic painful bone or skin metastases.

Highly vascular metastases, e.g. in lung or bone may cause pain or haemorrhage which can be treated effectively by local arterial embolisation.

Hormonal therapy and immunotherapy are being investigated on a trial basis.

Prognosis

If confined to renal capsule 10-year survival is 70%. Very poor if metastases present, 25% of patients present with metastases and they have a 45% 5-year survival.

Bladder cancer

Definition

Bladder cancer is the most common urological malignancy, ~90% of cases are transitional cell carcinoma, with the rest being squamous cell carcinoma, adenocarcinoma or mixed/undifferentiated tumour.

Incidence/prevalence

Common malignancy; 1 in 5000 in United Kinddom.

Age

Peak age 50–70 years.

Sex

M > F

Geography

Increased in the Middle East and industrialised areas.

Aetiology

There are several risk factors for the development of bladder cancer.

Environmental:

- Exposure to certain carcinogens and industries cause as many as 20% of cases. Aromatic amines, or derivatives, which are strongly carcinogenic are commonly found in the printing, rubber, textile and petrochemical industries. Diesel exhaust fumes also modestly increase the risk (e.g. for taxi and bus drivers).
- Smokers are two to three times more likely to have bladder cancer than non-smokers.

- Chronic cystitis, bladder stones and schistosomiasis through chronic inflammation and squamous metaplasia predispose to squamous cell carcinoma.

Genetic:

- Through polymorphisms of various cytochrome P450 enzymes, some individuals appear to oxidise arylamines more rapidly, which makes them more prone to malignancy, as this is the first step towards activation of these carcinogens.
- Acetylator status also affects predisposition. Slow acetylators de-activate carcinogens more slowly, increasing the risk of cancer.
- Half of Caucasians inherit the complete lack of the Glutathione S transferase M1 allele. This enzyme detoxifies carcinogens and these individuals have almost twice the risk of bladder cancer compared to those with one or two copies of the GSTM1 allele.

Radiotherapy, for example for pelvic tumours, predisposes to later development of bladder cancer. Cyclophosphamide is an important cause of bladder cancer. It generally appears within a decade of treatment and is dose-related, but the risk is reduced by the concomitant use of Mesna.

Pathophysiology

It is thought that in most cases, the bladder and ureters become exposed to carcinogenic agents which are excreted in high concentrations in the urine. This may explain why, in many cases, there is a 'field change' to the whole of the urothelium from renal pelvis to urethra, so that multiple and recurrent tumours occur. However, an individual's tumours have also been shown in many cases to be monoclonal, so that local spread may also be partly the cause. Adenocarcinoma arises from the urachal remnants in the dome of the bladder.

Clinical features

The most common presenting feature is painless frank haematuria. Other symptoms include pain and symptoms such as increased urinary frequency, dysuria and/or urgency. Whilst all these symptoms are most commonly caused by other conditions such as urinary tract infection, if they persist, bladder carcinoma should be suspected. Pain may be felt in the loin when there is obstruction, or suprapubically if there is invasion through the bladder wall. Haematuria over the age of 40 should be considered to be due to bladder cancer, until proven otherwise.

Macroscopy

Low-grade tumours have a papillary structure and look like seaweed. T2 is coral-like. Higher grade tumours appear more solid, ulcerating lesions. TNM staging is used which requires cystoscopy and examination under anaesthesia (EUA):

Ta Papillae projecting into the bladder lumen.

Tis Transitional cell carcinoma in situ: intraepithelial tumour with a flat, red appearance.

T1 Started invading bladder wall: in mucosa or submucosa (not palpable at EUA).

T2 Superficial muscle involved (rubbery thickening on EUA).

T3 Deep muscle involved, through bladder wall (mobile mass).

T4 Invading adjacent structures (fixed mass).

Microscopy

Transitional cell carcinomas are graded from I to IV or G1 to G3, according to the cellular and nuclear pleomorphism and mitoses.

G1 Well-differentiated.

G2 Moderately well differentiated.

G3 Poorly differentiated/anaplastic.

Complications

Tumours of stage >T3 metastasise, but this is uncommon. There is spread to lymph nodes and vascular spread to liver and bone.

Investigations

Cystoscopy is the main investigation, although all patients should also have a renal US or CT to exclude renal tumour or obstruction. IVU is useful at showing any filling defects in the ureters, as well as the bladder. If IVU is not possible (e.g. due to renal impairment), then ureteroscopy and/or retrograde contrast studies should be performed from the bladder upwards.

Management

Depends on stage:

i Tis or Ta, and T1 are initially treated by cystoscopic transurethral resection of the bladder tumour

(TURBT). Follow-up 3 months later has a 50% recurrence rate and regular follow-up is needed, usually for 5–10 years. Those at higher risk of recurrence, e.g. rapid recurrences, multiple, large and in particular flat lesions, and stage Tis or T1, require further treatment with adjuvant intravesical therapy. Bacillus Calmette-Guerin (BCG), i.e. the live attenuated form of *Mycobacterium bovis*, instilled into the bladder at intervals is very effective, although other agents are also used.

ii Localised, muscle-invasive disease (T2, but also high-grade T1) is optimally treated by a radical cystectomy – males are treated by cystectomy with proximal urethral and prostate removal, females require cystectomy with the whole urethra removed and an ileal conduit with urinary diversion (ureters to ileum). In males it is possible to use a piece of ileum to form a bladder substitute 'substitution urethroplasty' because the sphincter is below the prostate. However this is a major operation and patients may be medically unfit.

iii Locally advanced disease (T3 and T4) is life threatening and requires radical cystectomy in combination with radiotherapy or chemotherapy.

- Radical radiotherapy may be used where surgery is contraindicated, or post-surgery. Morbidity results from radiation cystitis and proctitis leading to a small fibrosed rectum. In females radiation vaginitis and/or an asensate vagina, and in males impotence occurs due to nerve damage.
- Chemotherapy is increasingly used with surgery, or may be used alone as a palliative measure. Neoadjuvant chemotherapy (i.e. chemotherapy before surgery) may be advised in those thought to be non-resectable (as they may render the tumour resectable), or more conventional post-surgery chemotherapy or radiotherapy. Most regimens are cisplatin based.

Prognosis

Depends on stage and grade at presentation and the age of the patient. Recurrence is common and may be of a higher grade (25%). Some patients appear to have a few, minor recurrences, whereas others have widespread, invasive recurrences. T1 has an 80% 5-year survival and T4 has 10% 5-year survival (but very age dependent).

Prostate cancer

Definition
Adenocarcinoma of the prostate.

Prevalence
Second most common malignancy in men. Causes 11% of cancer deaths (>8000 pa).

Age
>50 years (40% > 70 years, 60% > 80 years)

Sex
Male

Geography
Varies by population (90x). Most common in Afro Caribbeans, common in Europe, rare in Orientals.

Aetiology
Predisposing factors include age, ethnicity, family history, genetic factors and diet, with a diet high in animal fat, low in vegetables showing an increased risk, but omega fatty acids (found in oily fish), selenium and vitamin E appear to be protective.

Pathophysiology
The cancer is commonly androgen-dependent, but there is no evidence that its growth is driven by a hormone imbalance in an individual. However, population studies have shown that men with higher testosterone levels appear to be at greater risk of prostate cancer.

Clinical features
- Bladder outflow obstruction occurs late, when tumour has extended to the transurethral area. The tumour may cause irritative as well as obstructive symptoms, i.e. urinary urgency, frequency, nocturia, hesitancy and slow flow.
- In most cases it is diagnosed either on rectal examination as the finding of an asymmetric prostate, a nodule or a hard, irregular craggy mass, often altering the median groove. Increasingly, prostate cancer is diagnosed because of the finding of a raised prostate specific antigen (PSA).

Table 6.16 TNM staging

T1	Impalpable	24%	N0–N3 Regional node status
T2	Organ confined	13%	M0–M1 Metastases
T3	Through capsule	52%	
T4	Locally invasive	11%	

- Occasionally, it may present with haematospermia, especially in older men, or as metastatic disease with an occult primary.

Macroscopy

The tumours usually are in the peripheral zone of the prostate and appear as hard yellow-white gritty tissue (see Table 6.16).

Microscopy

Most are well differentiated and consist of small acini in a glandular pattern. Immunohistochemical techniques have also been developed, which can help identify whether cells are malignant and if they are of prostatic origin (e.g. if found in bone or lymph node biopsies).

Gleason score: The biopsy material is examined under a microscope and a Gleason grade 1–5 (grade 1 being most differentiated, grade 5 the least) is assigned to the two most commonly occurring patterns of cells. These two grades are then added together to give the Gleason score (2–10). A combined Gleason score of $2 + 3 = 5$, means that there is predominantly grade 2 and 3 disease present in the biopsy.

- 2, 3, 4 – Well differentiated, low grade.
- 5, 6, 7 – Moderately differentiated.
- 8, 9, 10 – Poorly differentiated, high grade.

Complications

Urinary tract infection and renal tract obstruction may occur, which can lead to renal failure.

Spread may be local or distant:

- Local spread is usually outward through the capsule.
- Lymphatic spread to pelvic and para-aortic nodes.
- Vascular spread, mainly to bone (classically sclerotic lesions), lung and liver.

Investigations

- TRUS (Transrectal ultrasound) and biopsy: Needle biopsy of the outer prostate by transrectal route is more sensitive than transurethral route. The tumour may be hyper, iso- or hypo-echogenic.
- Raised serum PSA: >4 ng/mL is abnormal. Benign prostatic hypertrophy, inflammation or biopsy of the prostate may also cause a raised PSA.
- CT abdomen and pelvis to look for local invasion and lymph node involvement, and a bone scan to look for bony metastases.
- Serum alkaline phosphatase (ALP) is usually raised when there are bony metastases.

Management

This depends on the tumour staging, grade and also on the patient's age and co-morbidity, as many of the treatments have significant side effects.

Organ-confined, low-grade disease:

- These tumours tend to grow slowly, in older patients (>70 years) and those likely to die of co-morbidity before the cancer causes significant symptoms or metastasises, it may be reasonable to 'watch and wait'.
- Younger patients should have radical treatment with the intent to cure: radical prostatectomy and/or radiotherapy to the prostate and local nodes. However, radical surgery is a major operation, with a 60% incidence of impotence (compared to 16% preoperatively) and an increase in urinary incontinence. Radiotherapy can also cause complications such as acute and chronic radiation proctitis (diarrhoea, urgency, bleeding), and impotence in 40–50%.

Locally advanced (T3 or T4) disease:

- For local symptom control TURP, radical prostatectomy or radiotherapy (external or brachytherapy) may be used, but recurrence and spread will almost certainly occur, so hormone therapy (see below) is generally advised with or without surgery.

Metastatic or high grade local disease:

- Treatment is for symptoms only (palliative). The aim is to deplete the cancer of circulating androgens:
  i Bilateral orchidectomy is often declined by patients due to psychological reasons and there are now other medical alternatives.
  ii LHRH agonists are given parenterally and are equally effective as orchidectomy, the second choice is the use of oral anti-androgens, e.g. cyproterone, flutamide, or the two classes may be combined.
  iii Oestrogen therapy is less popular now, due to the excess risk of cardiovascular deaths.

iv Chemotherapy is not as effective and is used mainly for non-responsive disease.

- Throughout treatment a multidisciplinary approach is needed with regard to palliation of symptoms. Bisphosphonates are used for bone pain and to prevent fractures. Localised radiation is used for bone pain and recently bone-targeting radioisotopes have been developed for those with multiple metastases.

Prognosis
Depends on grade, volume of primary and TNM staging; 50% present with incurable disease. If confined to prostate: 80% have 5-year survival and 60% have 10-year survival. If metastases are present: 20% have 5-year survival and 10% have 10-year survival.

Introduction to testicular tumours

Definition
Tumours of the testis may be classified broadly into those arising from the germ-cell line and those arising from non-germ cells.

Incidence
Relatively uncommon (~3–6/100,000 per annum), but still the most common solid organ tumour in young men and increasing in recent years.

Age
Depends on type, peak 25–40 years.

Sex
Males

Aetiology
Maldescent of the testis has a 10–15-fold risk. Ten per cent of all testicular tumours develop in testes which are or were cryptorchid, some contra-laterally. A family history is also a known risk factor as is infertility.

Pathophysiology
It is currently thought that the precursor of most germ cell tumours is intratubular germ cell neoplasia (sometimes called testicular carcinoma in situ), where the seminiferous tubules have atypical germ cells.

It appears that these atypical cells are formed early in gestation and may be influenced by events in utero. They then lie dormant, until puberty, when they spread non-invasively. In some individuals, they become malignant and either develop along the seminomatous or teratomatous line.

Classification
The main components of the testis are the germ cells (spermatogonia), the sex cords or seminiferous tubules (Sertoli cells) and stroma (Leydig cells). Germ cell tumours are the most common (90–95%) testicular tumours. Germ cells are multipotent, i.e. can form many tissue types, as normally they are involved in reproduction and may form both embryonic and extra-embryonic tissue. Therefore many different cell types may coexist in a germ cell tumour (see Fig. 6.10).

Non-germ cell tumours (see Fig. 6.11) include those arising from Sertoli and Leydig cells, of which only ~10% behave malignantly. Leydig cells normally produce testosterone, so Leydig cell tumours have the potential to produce steroid hormones at levels high enough to have systemic effects. Both Leydig cell and Sertoli cell

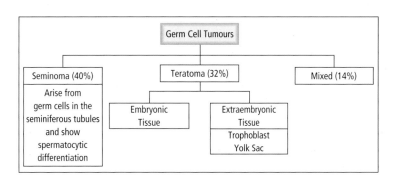

Figure 6.10 The British Testicular Tumour Panel Classification of Germ cell tumours (% are as a proportion of all testicular tumours).

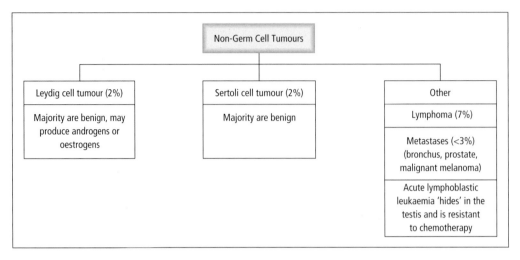

Figure 6.11 The British Testicular Tumour Panel Classification of Non-germ cell tumours (% are as a proportion of all testicular tumours).

tumours are uncommon. Other tumour types include lymphoma and metastases.

Clinical features

Testicular tumours usually present as slow, painless, smooth or irregular enlargement of a testis. A dull ache or dragging sensation in the lower abdomen or perineal/scrotal area is common. Acute pain occurs as a presenting feature in 10%, which may be attributed to trauma. Malignant tumours may present with metastatic disease before the primary is noticed and occasionally the tumour secretes hormones, causing symptoms such as gynaecomastia or precocious puberty.

On examination, there may be a concomitant hydrocele, making examination more difficult. The testes should be soft, smooth and mobile. Suspicious features include a hard, fixed mass, which may have smooth or irregular borders. If the mass transilluminates, this suggests a hydrocele, but it is not possible to exclude an underlying tumour without imaging. Associated gynaecomastia or lymphadenopathy should be looked for, as well as any evidence of metastases, e.g. to the liver.

Complications

Spread is generally initially through the lymphatics, to iliac and para-aortic lymph nodes via the spermatic cord, then the mediastinal lymph nodes. Haematogenous spread leads to metastases most commonly in the lungs, liver and bone.

Investigations

USS of the scrotum, especially if there is clinical doubt. Scrotal biopsy should be avoided, as this increases the risk of local spread and recurrence.

Other tests are directed at the staging of the tumour:
- Tumour markers – Alpha-fetoprotein (αFP), beta-human chorionic gonadotrophin (β–HCG) and lactate dehydrogenase (LDH) should be measured before treatment. These are raised in ∼50% of patients and are useful for follow-up after treatment.
- A chest X-ray, CT abdomen and pelvis are generally needed. CT thorax/head may be indicated, if metastases to these areas are suspected.
- Staging is from I to IV see Fig. 6.12 but the TNM staging is also used.

Management

Testicular cancer is now one of the most curable solid organ tumours. Radical orchidectomy via an inguinal incision, with occlusion of the spermatic cord before mobilization (to reduce risk of intraoperative spread) is needed for all patients, to establish the histology, grade and staging (TNM). A testicular prosthesis may be placed at the time of surgery. Retroperitoneal lymph node dissection at the same time is indicated in low stage

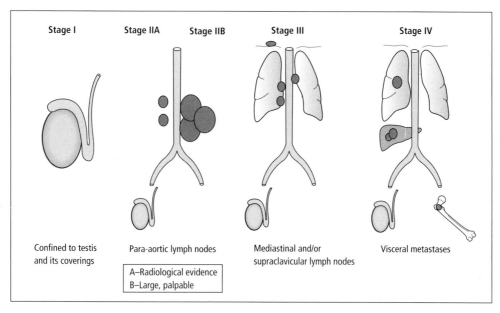

Figure 6.12 Staging of testicular tumours.

(I or IIA) disease, as CT scan is often falsely negative. However in higher stage disease, this may be postponed until the response to chemotherapy has been assessed. Chemotherapy and radiotherapy are both used in treatment. Seminomas are more radiosensitive.

Seminoma

Definition
These are testicular tumours of germ-cell origin which have differentiated along the spermatocytic line.

Incidence/prevalence
Most common testicular tumour (40%); ~2/100,000 p.a.

Age
Peak age 35–50 years.

Sex
Male

Aetiology
As for testicular tumours. Seminoma is the most common type to occur in maldescended testes.

Clinical features
As for testicular tumours. Bilateral involvement is rare.

Macroscopy/microscopy
The tumour appears as a homogeneous firm white mass, amidst normal, brown testis. Usually there is no evidence of haemorrhage or necrosis. There are three histological subtypes of seminoma, termed classic, anaplastic and spermatocytic (British Testicular Tumour Panel) depending on the microscopic features:

- Classic seminoma (85% of seminomas). Sheets of large, polygonal cells with clear cytoplasm (vacuolated and glycogen containing) and small central dark-staining nuclei. The presence of fibrous septa containing prominent lymphocytic infiltration is a favourable prognostic factor.
- Anaplastic seminoma (5–10% of seminomas). This type is more aggressive than classical seminoma. It shows marked pleomorphism and increased mitotic activity.
- Spermatocytic seminoma (4–6% of seminomas). This is a rare neoplasm which occurs in slightly older patients. It is not associated with intratubular germ cell neoplasia. The cells are pleomorphic, have a high

mitotic rate and contain abundant eosinophilic cytoplasm. They do not contain glycogen. Amongst the larger cells, are small cells which resemble spermatocytes. Despite the apparent histological features of aggressiveness they have an indolent growth and show virtually no tendency to metastasise.

Around 10% of seminomas contain trophoblastic giant cells, and these produce human chorionic gonadotrophin, which may be detectable in the blood. However, this does not appear to affect prognosis, or response to treatment.

Complications

i Seminomas tend to spread via the lymphatics initially, to the iliac and para-aortic lymph nodes.
ii Bloodstream spread is a late feature.

Management

All patients undergo radical orchidectomy as an initial measure.

- Stage I: Localised radiotherapy or 1–2 cycles of carboplatin chemotherapy reduce relapse to around 1–3%.
- Stage II and above (metastatic disease): Generally advised to have combination chemotherapy, usually with cisplatin/etoposide/bleomycin. Residual tumour is treated with further chemotherapy or radiotherapy.
- All patients should be regularly followed up with tumour markers and imaging, e.g. chest X-ray +/− abdominal USS or CT as indicated.

Prognosis

More than 99% of cases stage I disease have a normal lifespan. Even with metastatic disease 90% of these fall into the good prognosis category and they have an 86% 5-year survival. There is a higher risk of contralateral cancer, but this usually responds well to treatment.

Teratoma (non-seminomatous germ cell tumours)

Definition

Testicular germ cell tumour which has differentiated along embryonal and extra-embryonal lines.

Incidence/prevalence

32% of testicular tumours; $\sim$1–2/100,000 per annum.

Age

Any. Peak 20–30 years.

Sex

Males

Aetiology

As for other testicular tumours.

Pathophysiology

Teratomas are more aggressive than seminomas, although this is dependent on the tumour histology. The range of teratoma subtypes reflects the totipotency of the germ cells, which may develop along either embryonic or extra-embryonic cell lines. It has prognostic value.

Clinical features

As for testicular tumours.

- Teratoma differentiated (TD): This is a relatively uncommon and usually occurs in infants. The tumour consists of epithelial-lined cysts and stroma containing fully differentiated cells of many types with no features of malignancy. It is associated with a good prognosis.
- Malignant teratoma intermediate (MTI): This is a partly solid and partly cystic with some areas appearing more like TD (muscle, stromal cells with epithelial-lined spaces) and other areas which show pleomorphism. Fifty per cent of patients have an elevated serum βhCG or αFP level.
- Malignant teratoma undifferentiated (MTU) or embryonal carcinoma (WHO classification): Typically, these are small, poorly demarcated grey-white lesions which have a variegated appearance due to foci of fleshy and necrotic areas. Microscopically, they appear pleomorphic, with many mitoses and primitive epithelial cells forming irregular sheets, tubules, alveoli and papillary structures. Ninety per cent of patients have elevated serum βhCG or αFP levels.
- Malignant teratoma trophoblastic (MTT): Tumours containing any area of syncytiotrophoblast and cytotrophoblast arranged in a villous pattern behave

aggressively, invading blood vessels. Blood-borne metastases are a common early feature. βhCG and αFP are commonly found in the serum and can be detected in cells by immunocytochemistry.

- Yolk sac Tumour. Pure yolk sac tumours tend to be found in young children, with yellow-white mucinous lesions. Yolk sac elements are often found with other germ cell tumour elements, when they form solid and papillary lesions which consists of micro-sheets and cords of cells with vacuolated cytoplasm. These are highly malignant and confer a worse prognosis.
- Mixed germ-cell tumour: Tumours may consist of any combination of teratoma, seminoma, yolk sac tumour and hCG-containing giant cells (trophoblastic). 'Teratocarcinoma' in the WHO classification indicates neoplasms containing both teratoma and embryonal carcinoma (MTU).

Complications

Spread occurs via the blood stream to lung, liver, brain and bone. Nodal spread also occurs (iliac and para-aortic lymph nodes).

Management

After radical orchidectomy:

- Stage I: Retroperitoneal lymph node dissection is often needed if the tumour staging (TNM) showing risk for metastasis. It is often positive, i.e. turning the patient into Stage II.
- Stage II and above (metastatic disease): Chemotherapy (triple agent, e.g. cisplatin, etoposide, bleomycin) is used for metastatic disease. If there is residual tumour, with normal markers, surgical resection is indicated to remove tumour bulk, which often is only mature teratoma. If tumour markers do not respond, second choice chemotherapy is tried. Radiotherapy is generally ineffective.

Prognosis

Apart from higher stage disease, the worst prognosis is in those with very high tumour markers and histologically in those which are undifferentiated, vascular invasive or if containing trophoblastic or yolk sac elements. Even for metastatic disease modern treatment has improved the 5-year survival rates significantly to over 90% if all prognostic markers are good, down to 48% for poor prognostic markers. However, when salvage chemotherapy is needed for relapse, response is generally less good although new agents such as paclitaxel and gemcitabine appear to be giving better results.

Leydig cell tumour

Definition

This is a non-germ cell tumour of the stroma of the testis, derived from the Leydig cells.

Incidence/prevalence

Less common than germ-cell tumours.

Age

Two peaks 5–10 years and 30–35 years.

Sex

Male only

Aetiology

As for all testicular tumours.

Pathophysiology

Leydig cells are cells contained in the interstitium which normally produce testosterone. Leydig cell tumours may produce levels of steroid hormones (e.g. testosterone, oestrogens, corticosteroids) sufficient to cause systemic effects. Approximately 15% of adult tumours are malignant (in children they are invariably benign).

Clinical features

Local features as for testicular tumours, but they more commonly present with secondary effects such as gynaecomastia and loss of libido in adults. In pre-pubertal cases, precocious puberty and gynaecomastia may occur.

Macroscopy/microscopy

Circumscribed, yellow-brown, uniform tumour which ranges from 1 cm to a bulky mass. Microscopically, the cells resemble normal Leydig cells – sheets or nests of large, polygonal cells with round nuclei and abundant granular eosinophilic cytoplasm. Vacuolated cytoplasm, or pinkish crystals of Reinke may be seen.

Complications, investigations, treatment
As for testicular tumours.

Sertoli-cell tumour

Definition
This is a non-germ-cell tumour of the testis, derived from the Sertoli cells which are part of the seminiferous tubules (sex cords). Also called androblastoma.

Incidence/prevalence
Less common than germ-cell tumours.

Age
Any. Peak at 40 years.

Sex
Male only

Aetiology
As for all testicular tumours.

Pathophysiology
The Sertoli cells form the testicular tubules and when stimulated by follicle-stimulating hormone from puberty, they are capable of supporting the maturation of spermatogonia. Normally they do not secrete sex hormones, but tumour cells may secrete low levels of androgens or oestrogens, but these are very rarely high enough to cause systemic effects. About 90% are benign.

Clinical features
As for testicular tumours.

Macroscopy/microscopy
Homogeneous grey-white to yellow masses of variable size, which are well circumscribed. Normal Sertoli-like cells with tall columnar cytoplasm, often forming cords like seminiferous tubules. Certain histological features predict metastasis; for example multiple mitoses and large cell calcifying cell type.

Complications, investigations, treatment
As for testicular tumours.

Nervous system

7

Clinical

Symptoms

Headache

Headache is a very common symptom. Most headaches do not have a serious cause. The history is the most important diagnostic tool.

As with most types of pain, specific features that must be enquired about include: Site, Onset, Character, Radiation, Associated symptoms, Timing, Exacerbating and relieving factors, and Severity (SOCRATES). The site of pain is sometimes generalised, but if focal may be described as frontal, occipital, temporal and either unilateral or bilateral. See Table 7.1.

Drugs, including recreational drugs and substances such as alcohol, nicotine and caffeine, can lead to headaches, either directly or during withdrawal.

Features that suggest a serious underlying disease:
- Sudden onset
- Severe pain
- Associated neurological abnormalities
- Impaired consciousness
- Seizures
- Previous head injury or history of fall or trauma
- Signs of systemic illness

Fits and faints

Transient loss of consciousness may occur in the context of fits (seizures) or faints and falls. The major causes can be classified into cardiovascular, neurological or metabolic. Cardiovascular causes are described under Syncope (see page 24).

Seizures: Features that suggest a seizure include witnessed convulsions (one or both sides of the body), post-ictal (post-seizure) confusion, drowsiness and headache. Loss of consciousness is not invariable. Biting the side of the tongue and urinary incontinence (due to relaxation of the bladder sphincters) and other injuries such as shoulder dislocation are very suggestive. If there are warning signs prior to the seizure, e.g. a certain smell, a feeling, visual phenomena, these are described as an 'aura' and are in fact a type of seizure, which may then be followed by convulsions. Auras are unusual in other types of fits and faints except for in migraine which does not result in loss of consciousness or seizure.

Absence seizures (previously called petit mal) are found only in children – the individual appears briefly unresponsive to onlookers but without seizures and without loss of muscle tone.

Not all seizures are due to epilepsy – intracranial lesions such as tumours, stroke and haemorrhage, or extracranial causes such as drugs and alcohol withdrawal are important underlying causes.

Metabolic causes that must be excluded in any suspected fit or faint include hypoglycaemia and hypocalcaemia.

- Hypoglycaemia is most common in previously diagnosed diabetic patients and is often associated with hunger, sweating and shaking, but may be asymptomatic until loss of consciousness occurs.

Table 7.1 Important causes of headache

Diagnosis	Symptoms
Subarachnoid haemorrhage	This is classically a sudden onset, very severe headache 'as if kicked by a horse.' There may be signs of meningeal irritation (vomiting, photophobia and neck stiffness) and loss of consciousness. The headache may subside or persist, but is typically at its worst at the dramatic onset.
Meningitis	A generalised headache classically associated with fever and neck stiffness. Vomiting and photophobia are common. The speed of onset may be over minutes, hours or even days.
Tension type headache	This is a common cause of chronic, constant headaches. Usually a throbbing, tight band or pressure sensation around the head. Care is required to exclude temporal arteritis in patients over the age of 50 years if a short history.
Headaches due to raised intracranial pressure	A headache that is worst on waking (due to the increased cerebral oedema from lying flat) or exacerbated by coughing, straining or sneezing (as these increase CSF pressure). Vomiting may be present. When due to an underlying tumour, the time course may be short, or over months to years depending on the site and any associated complications such as haemorrhage or hydrocephalus.
Migraine	Classical migraine has an aura (a prodrome of symptoms such as flashing lights) lasting up to an hour preceding the onset of pain, frequently accompanied by nausea and vomiting. The headache is often localised, becoming generalised and persists for several hours.
Cervical spondylosis	Pain in the suboccipital region associated with head posture and local tenderness relieved by neck support.
Temporal arteritis	Severe headache and scalp tenderness over the inflamed, palpably thickened superficial temporal arteries with progressive loss of the pulse. They may complain of pain in the jaw on eating or talking (jaw claudication). Patients are over 50 years and may have a history of polymyalgia rheumatica.

- Hypocalcaemia may cause a tonic-clonic seizure associated with paraesthesia, numbness, cramps and tetany.

Hysteria may lead to non-epileptic attacks (pseudoseizures) with or without feigned loss of consciousness. The patient will drop to the ground in front of witnesses, without sustaining any injury and have a fluctuating level of consciousness for some time with unusual seizure-like movements such as pelvic thrusting and forced eye closure. There may be a history of previous psychiatric illness or other functional symptoms. This is a diagnosis of exclusion and should be made with caution.

Dizziness and vertigo

Vertigo is defined as a hallucination of movement. It is the sensation experienced when getting off a roundabout and as part of alcohol intoxication. Patients may complain of dizziness, giddiness, nausea, vomiting and finding standing and walking impossible.

Vertigo may result from peripheral lesions (disease of the labyrinth or the vestibular component of the VIIIth

nerve), or central lesions (brain stem). In both types motion, particularly of the head, can exacerbate the sensation. With a chronic lesion such as a tumour, adaptive mechanisms reduce the sensation of dizziness over a period of weeks.

Labyrinth disorders (peripheral lesions)

Peripheral lesions tend to cause a unidirectional horizontal nystagmus enhanced by asking the patient to look in the direction of the fast phase. When the patient walks, they tend to veer to one side, but walking is generally preserved except in the acute stages (see Table 7.2).

- Vestibular neuronitis (acute labrynthopathy) – The most common cause of acute vertigo with nystagmus but without tinnitus or hearing loss. The cause is not known. Symptoms last days to weeks and can be reduced with vestibular sedatives (useful only in the short term), but may recur.
- Positional vertigo – vertigo and nystagmus lasting a few seconds which is prompted by head movement. One type is benign paroxysmal positional vertigo (BPPV) which may follow vestibular neuronitis

Table 7.2 Peripheral lesions causing vertigo

Causes	Characteristics of vertigo	Hearing loss and tinnitus
Acute vestibular neuronitis	Acute onset, lasting 2–5 days	None
Benign paroxysmal positional vertigo (BPPV)	Postural, lasting <1 min	None
Ménière's disease	10 min to 10 h	Yes
Barotrauma & perilymphatic fistula	Inducible by pressure changes	Yes
Drugs such as aminoglycosides		Some cases

or head trauma. Positional testing with the Hallpike manoeuvre is diagnostic.

- The Hallpike manoeuvre (see Fig. 7.1): The patient is swung rapidly from a sitting position to lying with the neck extended and turned to one side (so that the head hangs over the end of the bed). The patient's eyes are closely observed for nystagmus for up to 30 seconds, then sat upright and nystagmus looked for again. This is repeated on the other side. This test can provoke intense nausea, vertigo and even vomiting, particularly in peripheral lesions. In BPPV nystamus appears after a few seconds (latency), lasts less than 30 seconds (transience), and disappears with repeated testing (fatigable).

Any atypical features suggest a central lesion.

- Ménière's disease is a triad of episodic vertigo lasting a 10 minutes to 10 hours, tinnitus and hearing loss. It responds poorly to vestibular sedatives.

Central lesions

A central lesion due to disease of the brainstem, cerebellum or cortex should be suspected if the history and examination are atypical for a peripheral lesion. For example, risk factors for cerebrovascular disease, previous history of migraine, demyelination, or the presence of any other neurology. Deafness and tinnitus do not occur with central lesions.

Causes include multiple sclerosis, migraine, stroke particularly cerebellar infarction or haemorrhage, vertebrobasilar ischaemia (posterior circulation TIA), tumour of the cerebellopontine angle, cerebellum, fourth ventricle or acoustic neuroma.

Altered sensation or weakness in the limbs

Altered sensation in the limbs is often described as numbness, pins and needles ('paraesthesiae'), cold or hot sensations. Painful or unpleasant sensations may be felt, such as shooting pains, burning pain, or increased sensitivity to touch (dysaesthesia). There may be a precipitating cause, such as after trauma, or exacerbating features.

The distribution of the sensory symptoms, and any associated pain (such as radicular pain, back pain or neck pain) can help to determine the cause.

Muscle weakness (loss of power) may occur in specific muscles or muscle groups.

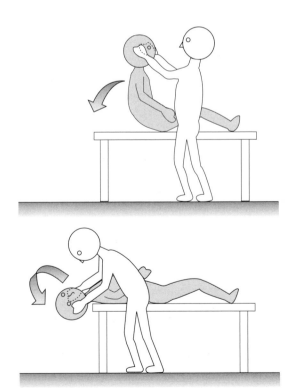

Figure 7.1 The Hallpike maneouvre.

- It should be differentiated from general symptoms of weakness such as fatigue.
- Muscle weakness due to lack of use develops rapidly, for example in the legs due to a painful hip or following surgery or a debilitating illness.
- Distribution of the weakness, onset and any associated pain, e.g. back pain may point to a cause.

Although formal assessment of muscle weakness takes place in the examination, certain questions to assess the *functional* ability of the patient are required:

- Can you carry and lift objects as you could before? (assesses hand and upper limb power).
- Can you get up from a chair easily? Do you need to use your arms to help you get up from a chair or to climb up stairs? (assesses lower limb power).

Patterns of neurological disorders
See Fig 7.2.

Upper motor neurone signs

The motor pathway originates in the precentral gyrus, with corticospinal tracts which pass down through the internal capsule, then into the brainstem, where they cross over (the pyramidal decussation) and then pass down to the contralateral spinal cord. Any lesion along this pathway can lead to upper motor neurone signs (UMN). Depending on the level of the lesion the weakness may be ipsilateral or contralateral to the lesion. Signs include:

- Pronator drift (downward drift and inward rotation of the upper limb with pronation).

 Mononeuropathy, e.g. ulnar nerve lesions. Usually associated with motor lesions.

 Dermatomal loss occurs in dorsal root. All modalities of sensation are lost.

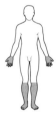 Glove and stocking sensory loss in all modalities (pain, temperature, vibration and joint position sense) occurs in peripheral neuropathies. These affect the longest nerves first, hence the distribution. They may have peripheral muscle weakness, which is also bilateral, symmetrical and distal.

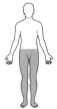 Bilateral symmetrical loss of all modalities of sensation occurs with a transverse section of the cord. These lesions are characteristically associated with lower motor neurone signs at the level of transection and upper motor neurone signs below the level. Cervical lesions lead to a quadriplegia, thoracic lesions to paraplegia.

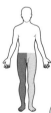 Hemisection of the cord causes an ipsilateral loss of vibration and proprioception and contralateral loss of pain and temperature termed 'Brown–Séquard Syndrome'. There are also ipsilateral upper motor neurone signs below the level of the lesion and lower motor neurone signs at the level of the lesion. This arises due to the level at which the different pathways decussate.

Figure 7.2 Patterns of sensory loss.

- Increased tone (spasticity).
- Decreased power in a pyramidal distribution (i.e. affecting extensors more than flexors in the upper limbs, but affecting flexors more than extensors in the lower limbs).
- Increased tendon reflexes, absent abdominal reflexes and up-going (extensor) plantar reflexes.
- No muscle wasting or fasciculations (wasting may occur in long standing lesions due to disuse atrophy).

Patterns of UMN weakness

Depending on the severity, the weakness may be described as a 'plegia' = total paralysis, or a 'paresis' = partial paralysis, but these terms are often used interchangeably (see Table 7.3).

Cerebral hemisphere disease may occur either in the cortex or the internal capsule. Common causes are strokes (vascular occlusion or haemorrhage) and tumours.

- Internal carotid artery occlusion may cause a hemiparesis.
- Occlusion of the middle cerebral artery territory may cause UMN signs more in the arms than the legs.
- Occlusion of the anterior cerebral artery (ACA) territory may cause UMN signs more in the legs than the arms.

Lower motor neurone signs

Lower motor neurone (LMN) signs are due to lesions of the anterior horn cell (or cranial nerve nucleus), the motor nerve root leaving the spinal cord, or of the peripheral nerves):

- Decreased tone (flaccidity).
- Decreased power in the distribution of the affected nerves or nerve roots (not pyramidal).

- Decreased or absent reflexes. Plantars remain downgoing (or are absent).
- Wasting develops within 3 weeks of a lesion.
- Fasciculations, which are small local contractions of muscle motor units, due to spontaneous discharge of muscle fibres innervated by a single motor nerve filament.

Patterns of LMN weakness

The pattern depends on which nerves or roots are affected, and at what level.

- Anterior horn cell lesions occur as part of motor neurone disease, polio or other viral infections, and can affect multiple levels.
- Spinal root damage is often due to compression for example, a disc protrusion causing compression at T1 will cause weakness and wasting of the small muscles of the hand.
- The brachial and lumbosacral plexus can be affected by inflammation or trauma.
- Single or multiple peripheral nerve lesions cause weakness in the distribution of that nerve or as part of a multiple neuropathy.

Patterns of sensory loss

Cerebellar signs

- Nystagmus: This is usually horizontal and the fast phase is towards the side of the lesion.
- Dysarthria: Scanning speech, which is when the speech is heard syllable by syllable. Ask the patient to say 'British Constitution' or 'West Register Street'. It occurs when both lateral lobes are affected.

Table 7.3 Patterns of upper motor neurone weakness

Term	Area of lesion
Diplegia	A type of cerebral palsy affecting the lower limbs predominantly.
Quadriplegia/tetraplegia	Affecting all four limbs. Usually due to a cervical spinal cord lesion, occasionally bilateral cerebral lesions.
Hemiplegia	Weakness of one half of the body (sometimes including the face) caused be a contralateral cerebral hemisphere lesion, a brainstem lesion or ipsilateral spinal cord lesion (unusual).
Paraplegia	Affecting both lower limbs, and usually caused by a thoracic or lumbar spinal cord lesion e.g. cord compression. Bilateral hemisphere (anterior cerebral artery) lesions can cause this but are rare.
Monoplegia	Contralateral hemisphere lesion in the motor cortex causing weakness of one limb, usually the arm.

- Rebound: Hands and arms outstretched, eyes closed, push down each hand in turn, and look for rebound (overshooting).
- Finger-nose test: Intention tremor and past-pointing.
- Dysdiadochokinesis: Tapping alternately with the palmar and dorsal aspects of the hand is poor.
- Heel-shin test: Poorly performed, the patient is unable to keep heel on shin.
- Truncal ataxia: Also called central ataxia. Test the ability of the patient to sit on the edge of the bed with their arms crossed.
- Gait: Wide-based gait, with a tendency to drift towards the side of the lesion. Stopping and turning is difficult. If there is no obvious abnormality, ask the patient to walk heel to toe. Even a mild cerebellar problem makes this very difficult.

Causes include the following:
- Multiple sclerosis
- Trauma
- Endocrine: Hypothyroidism.
- Vascular: Cerebellar haemorrhage, cerebellar ischaemic stroke.
- Drugs: Phenytoin, carbamazepine.
- Metabolic: Alcohol (acute, reversible or chronic degeneration)
- Neoplastic: Tumour, paraneoplastic syndrome, e.g. lung carcinoma
- Congenital: Arnold–Chiari malformation, Friedreich's ataxia

Extrapyramidal signs (Parkinsonism)

- Appearance: Expressionless face. Drooling saliva. Resting tremor which is slow and classically pill-rolling (abduction-adduction of thumb with flexion–extension of the fingers). The tremor is improved with action, but worse on concentration (ask the patient to count backwards from 100 in serial 7's).
- Speech: Monophonic, quiet. Tendency to peter out.
- Tone: Cogwheel rigidity due to increased tone together with tremor. Power, reflexes, sensation and coordination are normal.
- Bradykinesia (slowness in movements) is noticeable when doing alternate hand tapping movements, or touching the thumb to each finger in turn. Micrographia (small, spidery handwriting).
- Gait and posture: A flexed position with head drooped, shoulders and spine flexed, knees slightly flexed. Initiation of movement is impaired (hesitancy) with the appearance of falling into walking. The gait is slow and shuffling with reduced arm swing. A festinating gait is when the patient looks as though they are shuffling in order to keep up with their centre of gravity, and then has difficulty in stopping and turning round.

Tremor

The three groups of tremor are distinguished by observation (see Table 7.4).

Gait

- Spastic gait: This is a sign of upper motor neurone disease. The gait is stiff, one or both legs are kept extended. If unilateral, the leg is swung out to the side to move it forwards (circumduction). If bilateral, the pelvis has to alternately tilt and the gait often becomes scissor-like. The patient can stand on tip-toe, but often not on their heels.

Table 7.4 Types of tremor

Type of tremor	Description	Causes
Resting Positional tremor (only appears when hands and arms out-stretched)	Pill-rolling	Parkinsonism
	Fine	Physiological Hyperthyroidism Drugs: e.g. salbutamol, lithium, sodium valproate
	Coarse	Alcohol Benign essential tremor (often familial)
Action (intention tremor and past-pointing)	On purposeful movement	Cerebellar

- Foot-drop: This is caused by weakness of ankle dorsiflexion, usually a feature of a lower motor neurone disease such as a peripheral neuropathy. The knee is lifted high and as the ankle cannot dorsiflex, the foot tends to slap on the ground. If bilateral, it is called a high-stepping gait.
- Ataxic: This is the typical gait of a person with cerebellar disease. The gait is broad-based, and there may be a tendency to veer to the side of the lesion in unilateral disease. Even if mildly affected the patient is unable to walk heel-toe in a straight line.
- Parkinsonian: There is hesitancy, that is slowness in initiating movement, and turning. The steps are small and shuffling, and the patient tends to be flexed or stooped. 'Festination' is the hurrying steps which appear to be the only way the patient can remain upright. In the upper limbs, there is reduced arm swing, and increased tremor may be apparent. In Parkinson's disease, this pattern tends to be asymmetrical, whereas it is symmetrical in other causes of parkinsonism.
- Waddling gait: Proximal muscle weakness such as occurs in myopathies leads to difficulty in rising to an erect position and then the pelvis tends to drop on the side of the lifted leg.
- Antalgic gait: Pain around the joints or within the muscles may give rise to abnormalities in gait (the classical limp).

Investigations and procedures

Electroencephalography

An electroencephalogram (EEG) is a recording of the electrical activity of the brain. It is obtained by placing electrodes on the scalp, using a jelly to reduce electrical resistance. A recording of at least half an hour is usually needed, to maximise the chances of picking up transient abnormalities. The patient needs to lie still, as electrical changes due to movement can interfere with the recording.

Its main use is for the classification of epilepsy, but is it may also be useful in the diagnosis of other brain disorders such as encephalitis. In epilepsy, different waveforms may be seen. The EEG is often normal between seizures, and anti-convulsant medication can alter the EEG.

- Characteristic abnormalities are described under Epilepsy, but include spikes and spike and wave discharges.
- Photic stimulation and hyperventilation are routinely performed to increase the sensitivity if the resting EEG is normal.
- Sleep-deprived EEG, which allows recordings when the patient dozes and wakes.
- EEG recording in status epilepticus is useful at demonstrating whether seizure activity is suppressed by medication, particularly in a paralysed, ventilated patient.
- The EEG is abnormal post-ictally, which can be helpful in the diagnosis of epilepsy.
- Focal abnormalities, e.g. localising abnormal electrical activity to the frontal lobe can suggest an underlying epileptogenic focus, e.g. a tumour or area of infarction or encephalitis, as well as occurring in focal status epilepticus.

Encephalitis, cortical necrosis (e.g. in stroke or post-anoxic damage), metabolic brain disorders including drug-induced delirium, and tumours can cause either focal or generalised EEG abnormalities. EEG changes are seen even before MRI changes are evident.

Electromyography (EMG) and nerve conduction studies (NCS)

These are tests of the function of muscles (EMG) and the peripheral nerves (NCS). They are useful in the diagnosis of muscle disease, diseases of the neuromuscular junction, peripheral neuropathies and anterior horn cell disease.

Electromyography

A needle electrode is placed into muscles and insertional, resting and voluntary electrical activity is studied, using a computer screen and a speaker.

- Denervated muscle shows prolonged insertional activity, fibrillation potentials and positive sharp waves.
- Peripheral neuropathies and anterior horn cell disease lead to a reduced number of motor units, which fire rapidly.
- Anterior horn cell disease – large motor units form, causing visible fasciculations, which can also be shown by EMG.

- Myotonic discharges can be seen, e.g. in myotonic dytrophy, and myopathic changes may occur with any primary muscle disorder. However, a normal EMG does not exclude a muscle disorder.

Nerve conduction studies

Surface electrodes or occasionally needles are used both for stimulation and recording:

- Motor and sensory conduction velocities (slow in demyelinating disorders).
- Action potential size – in axonal neuropathies, the conduction velocity and latencies are normal, but the total action potential is reduced in amplitude.
- F wave latencies and velocities are also useful – these are like an 'echo' which occurs as a nerve that is stimulated peripherally, the action potential travels up to the spinal cord, and back down – it allows the evaluation of brachial and lumbosacral plexus and nerve roots.
- Repetitive stimulation is useful in the diagnosis of neuromuscular junction disorders – see myasthenia gravis, Eaton–Lambert syndrome.

Lumbar puncture

This is the procedure by which cerebrospinal fluid (CSF) is aspirated by an approach between the lumbar vertebrae.

Indications

When any of the following are suspected:

- Infection (meningitis, encephalitis, fungal infections or neurosyphilis).
- Multiple sclerosis.
- Subarachnoid haemorrhage (with a normal CT head).
- Guillain–Barré syndrome.
- Meningeal carcinomatosis (malignant meningitis) including lymphoma.

CSF pressure measurement is useful – particularly in the diagnosis of idiopathic (benign) intracranial hypertension, where CSF removal may be a therapeutic manoeuvre.

Lumbar puncture (LP) is also required for intrathecal administration of contrast media (in myelography), and drugs such as antimicrobials and chemotherapy.

Contraindications

- Infection at the site of LP.
- Suspected intracranial mass lesion – focal neurology or depressed GCS should lead to a CT brain scan prior to LP.
- Suspected raised intracranial pressure or papilloedema before CT evaluation.
- Suspected spinal cord compression.
- Bleeding disorders should be corrected first (including a platelet count of $<40 \times 10^9$/L, anti-coagulant drugs such as heparin or warfarin).
- Congenital lumbosacral lesions such as meningomyelocele, because the cord may be tethered or low.

Procedure

After giving consent, the patient is positioned on their left side on a firm surface, with the back at the edge of the couch. The knees are drawn up as far as possible and the neck flexed, to open up the spinous processes of the lumbar vertebrae.

The aim is to insert the needle between L3–L4 or L4–L5 in adults (below the level of the spinal cord). L4 normally lies at the level of the iliac crests. The area is cleaned and infiltrated with lidocaine.

The lumbar puncture needle is inserted in the midline with its stylet in place aiming slightly towards the umbilicus. The needle is advanced slowly ~4–5 cm, and a slight give is often felt as it penetrates the dura mater. The stylet is withdrawn and if no CSF appears, it is re-inserted and the needle advanced slightly – this is repeated until CSF appears. If the needle encounters firm resistance, it should be withdrawn and another approach tried.

Sometimes the patient will feel a pain radiating into the leg or back – this is due to the needle touching a root – if it persists, the needle will have to withdrawn and a slightly different angle attempted.

Once CSF appears, the CSF pressure can be measured by attaching a manometer (normal 6–15 cm H_2O). CSF is collected in three sterile tubes (sent for microscopy and culture, protein and cytology) and an additional sample is sent for glucose measurement. A simultaneous blood sample for glucose should be sent. Oligoclonal bands are identified using paired CSF and serum samples.

Complications

The most common complication is headache, which may be treated by lying flat and adequate hydration.

Bleeding, infection, arachnoiditis, exacerbation of spinal cord compression, cerebral herniation and spinal cord or root injury are all recognised risks, but occur rarely.

CT head

Computed tomography detects differences in X-ray density between bone, brain, blood and CSF. There is a difference in healthy tissue and infarcted, infected or oedematous tissue. It may be possible to differentiate between old lesions and acute lesions – including infarcts and bleeds.

Indications

- Space-occupying lesions: cerebral tumours (may miss low-grade astrocytomas), abscesses.
- Cerebral infarction.
- Extracerebral or intracerebral haematomas.
- Subarachnoid haemorrhage (may miss up to 15%).
- Pituitary for tumours, pituitary infarction (although MRI is preferred if available).

Intravenous contrast injections show areas of increased blood supply, breakdown of the blood-brain barrier and oedema.

Lesions under 1 cm in diameter may be missed, although improvements in technology are increasing the sensitivity of scans. Small lesions close to the skull may be missed.

CT of the skull is also useful for detecting minor fractures particularly basal skull fractures, which may be difficult to see on skull X-ray.

Newer CT scanners are able to diagnose cerebellar lesions more reliably than in the past, but MRI is still preferred if brainstem or cerebellar lesions are suspected.

Faster scans are now possible – particularly helpful for patients unwilling or unable to lie flat for long, although in some cases general anaesthetic may be necessary for unco-operative patients.

MRI brain and spinal cord

Magnetic resonance imaging uses the magnetic properties of protons to generate images of tissues.

It has the advantage of not exposing the patient to ionising radiation (particularly important in young infants, children and pregnant mothers). It is very versatile due to various processing which may be performed on the data. However, the main disadvantage is that any metal in the patient not only causes interference, but can become dislodged. Pacemakers may be reprogrammed by the electromagnetic pulses, and the magnetic field may induce a large current leading to burns so MRI is contraindicated. The MRI scanner can also be claustrophobic, and in the case of sick patients, is relatively unaccessible – although some units have facilities for ventilation in the MRI scanner.

MRI differentiates soft tissues much more clearly than CT.

- T1 weighted images: Fat, brain tissue and old haematomas have high signal strength. Bone, CSF, cartilage and calcium have low signal strength (i.e. look darker).
- T2 weighted images: High water content tissues and CSF have high signal strength (i.e. look white).

Tumours as small as 5 mm are clearly seen, even in the brainstem and cerebellum (these areas with a lot of surrounding bone are often poorly seen on CT). Acute infarction is seen earlier than on CT, at 6–12 hours. With new techniques (diffusion weighted MRI) changes can appear even earlier than this. MRI is excellent at detecting white matter lesions such as demyelination in multiple sclerosis, or intracerebral small vessel disease. Spinal cord MRI is useful for tumours, cord compression and vascular malformations. Intravenous gadolinium is used as a contrast to demonstrate areas of increased vascular supply and oedema. It is also useful in MR angiography (MRA), for example when looking for AV malformations.

Cerebrovascular disease

Stroke

Definition

A stroke is defined as a sudden onset of non-traumatic focal neurological defect of a vascular aetiology, that either causes death or lasts more than 24 hours.

Incidence

Third commonest cause of death in Western World (1–2 per 1000 per year).

Age
Uncommon under 40 years.

Sex
M > F, but mortality twice as high in females.

Geography
Black community, Japanese more common.

Aetiology
20% of strokes are haemorrhagic and 80% are ischaemic, of which two-thirds arise from extracranial lesions and one-third arise from intracranial lesions. Strokes may also be due to subarachnoid haemorrhage. Risk factors for stroke can be divided into

- Intra- or extra-cranial atherosclerosis: In particular hypertension, smoking, hyperlipidaemia, family history of stroke or ischaemic heart disease and diabetes mellitus.
- Heart disease: Valvular heart disease such as mitral stenosis, infective endocarditis, and any condition which predisposes to mural thrombus such as atrial fibrillation or myocardial infarction.
- Less common causes: Hyperviscosity or prothrombotic states, e.g. polycythaemia, oral contraceptive pill; vasculitis; clotting disorders.

Pathophysiology
Haemorrhagic strokes are discussed elsewhere. Ischaemic strokes are due to the interruption of arterial blood supply, and the clinical picture depends on the size of artery and hence extent of territory affected, the area affected, and whether there is temporary or permanent ischaemia and hence infarction.

Clinical features
Anterior circulation (carotid territory) strokes are the most common, in particular those involving a branch of the middle cerebral artery. This causes infarction of the motor pathways (at the level of the motor cortex or the internal capsule) and usually results in a contralateral hemiparesis. This is an upper motor neurone (UMN) deficit, i.e. increased tone, reduced power and brisk tendon reflexes, although acutely there may be a flaccid, areflexic paralysis. The arm tends to be affected more than the leg (the motor cortex for the leg is supplied by the anterior cerebral artery).

- Other features of an MCA territory infarct include an ipsilateral UMN lesion of the face (weakness of the lower facial muscles), hemianopic visual field loss and if the dominant hemisphere is affected dysphasia may occur due to infarction of areas governing speech (Wernicke's and Broca's areas).

Posterior circulation (the vertebral, basilar arteries and their branches) strokes affect the brainstem, cerebellum and occipital lobes. One characteristic but uncommon pattern is lateral medullary syndrome which can be caused by thromboembolism of the posterior inferior cerebellar artery (PICA) or the vertebral artery. It causes sudden vertigo and vomiting. On examination there is ipsilateral ataxia (loss of co-ordination), contralateral loss of pain and temperature sensation and there may be nystagmus, diplopia and an ipsilateral Horner's syndrome.

- If the pontine reticular formation is involved in brainstem infarcts, important basic functions such as alertness, breathing and circulation may be affected leading to coma and death.

Lacunar infarcts are small (<1 cm) often slit-shaped areas of infarction usually in the basal ganglia, internal capsule and pons caused by hyaline arteriosclerosis within the small fine perforating arteries of the brain. They are predisposed to by hypertension and diabetes, are often asymptomatic but may cause focal neurological defects such as weakness of a single limb, or limited ataxia.

- Multiple lacunar or larger infarcts can result in a multi-infarct dementia with a picture of loss of intellect occurring in a step-wise pattern. The final picture may include dementia and a shuffling gait which resembles Parkinson's Disease.

In clinical situations a full neurological examination should be performed and a careful cardiovascular examination in order to reveal any source of embolus or other predisposing disease.

Macroscopy/microscopy
- In the first 24 hours, there is little macroscopic change. The tissue may look paler and lose differentiation between white and grey matter.
- The normal pattern of tissue change within the brain following a stroke is liquifactive necrosis. Structural breakdown takes place, the infarcted tissue becomes soft and is at risk of reperfusion haemorrhage.

Macrophages enter the infarct and remove the dead tissue, whilst around the edges astrocytes proliferate and healing takes place by scarring (gliosis). Large infarcts cannot be completely replaced and heal as spaces surrounded by gliosis.

Investigations

- CT brain scanning is used to differentiate between haemorrhage, infarction and a space occupying lesion. The scan may be normal in the first 24–48 hours, although large infarcts normally show due to oedema and loss of differentiation between white and grey matter. MRI scans are more sensitive.
- Investigation of underlying cause
  Full blood count: Haemoglobin and platelets for polycythaemia, anaemia or thrombocytopenia/ thrombocytosis, ESR for vasculitis/arteritis.
  Urinalysis and blood glucose for diabetes mellitus.
  Cardiac investigation: Blood pressure measurement, chest X-ray, ECG for recent infarct/arrhythmia. Transthoracic is indicated and transoesophageal echocardiography may also be required.
  Carotid doppler studies to examine for carotid vascular disease particularly in younger patients or if signs dictate. Further investigation such as carotid and vertebral angiography may be indicated.

Management

- Patients who present within 3 hours of onset of symptoms who have no evidence of haemorrhage or large infarct on CT head scan should be considered for thrombolysis.
- Acutely, treat any exacerbating factors such as hypotension, hypoglycaemia, hyperglycaemia, or severe hypertension (with caution, to prevent sudden loss of perfusion pressure, particularly in the acute stages, when the brain is unable to autoregulate BP well). Prevent and treat any complications such as deep vein thrombosis due to immobility, aspiration pneumonia due to disordered swallow, pressure sores and limb contractures.
- Inpatient or outpatient rehabilitation is used to regain maximal functional improvement, and so reduce the impact on the patient's life, including physiotherapy, speech therapy, and occupational therapy. Patients who are admitted to a dedicated stroke unit have

been shown to have improved functional outcome and reduced mortality.

- Prevention of recurrence: Any risk factors present should be treated. All patients with ischaemic (not haemorrhagic) stroke should ideally be on an antiplatelet agent such as aspirin. Cholesterol-lowering agents (statins) and anti-hypertensive agents have also been shown to reduce recurrence. Anti-coagulants are indicated in certain conditions such as atrial fibrillation and valvular heart disease, but only after approximately 2 weeks and when blood pressure is controlled, to reduce the risk of haemorrhage into infarcted tissue.
- Internal carotid endarterectomy is not justified unless there have been unequivocal transient ischaemic attacks or stroke within 6 months with good recovery and significant ipsilateral carotid artery stenosis (>70%). There is a 1–5% risk of stroke or death due to the surgery. The artery is clamped with cerebral blood flow maintained by collateral supply or by a shunt. The stenosing plaque is shelled out and the artery repaired by suture or a patch. The procedure is increasingly being done under local anaesthesia or by endovascular stenting.

Prognosis

Overall, 40% of patients die as the result of their stroke (mainly in the first month), 40% are left significantly disabled and 30% have reasonable recovery.

Transient ischaemic attack (TIA)

Definition

Non-traumatic focal neurological deficit due to cerebral ischaemia lasting less than 24 hours with a complete clinical recovery. TIAs may recur or precede a stroke.

Aetiology/pathophysiology

90% of transient ischaemic attacks are caused by extracranial thromboembolic disease within the great vessels, the carotid or vertebral arteries, or mural thrombi following a myocardial infarction.

Clinical features

The onset of a TIA is identical to that of a stroke, but tends to last minutes or hours. The site of the lesion is often suggested by the clinical pattern. Common symptoms include weakness, numbness, and transient monocular loss of vision (amaurosis fugax) or other visual disturbance. Evidence of vascular disease such as bruits, valvular heart disease, and other risk factors such as hypertension, arrhythmias, hypercholestrolaemia or diabetes mellitus should be sought. Important differentials include hypoglycaemia, focal epilepsy (usually with a preceding jerking of one or more limbs, and a post-ictal phase) and migraine (symptoms may precede or follow the onset of headache).

Investigations
These are as for stroke. CT head may distinguish between TIA, stroke and haemorrhage. However, <24 hours after a stroke, the CT may still be normal.

Management
All patients should be on an antiplatelet agent such as aspirin. Other treatments include antihypertensives, statin cholestrol lowering agents, and management of cardiac arrhythmias, heart disease or diabetes mellitus.

In patients with symptomatic TIAs with an underlying significant carotid stenosis (>70%), surgery is indicated with carotid endarterectomy (see above).

Prognosis
Five years after a transient ischaemic attack
- 1 in 6 patients will have had a stoke.
- 1 in 4 patients will have died usually from a stroke or heart disease.

Hypoxic ischaemic brain injury

Definition
The global brain damage resulting from a failure of tissue perfusion.

Aetiology
Generalised failure of blood flow or oxygenation may result from cardiac or respiratory arrest, severe hypoglycaemia, drowning or carbon monoxide poisoning.

Pathophysiology
The generalised loss of perfusion results in diffuse death of neurones. The blood flow through the brain is subject to autoregulation. Within the range of 80–170 mmHg systolic pressure the cerebral blood flow is independent

of the perfusion pressure; however, a low oxygen concentration or a blood pressure outside the range will result in tissue damage. Shorter periods or less severe episodes lead to 'watershed infarction' of the junctional areas between the cerebral arteries, in particular the visual cortex and cerebellum. The hippocampus is also at risk of damage as it has a high metabolic demand.

Clinical features
Mild cases tend to have an impaired intellect with memory loss and cortical blindness. Severe cases have a prolonged comatose state with variable outcome including the persistent vegetative state.

Macroscopy
There is loss of cortical mass mainly from the white matter leading to an atrophic brain. Neurones are replaced with gliosis by astrocytes.

Management
The underlying cause requires rapid identification and management to limit the extent of necrosis. Long term care requires multidisciplinary input and may necessitate ongoing residential care.

Intracerebral haemorrhage

Definition
Spontaneous haemorrhage may occur within in the basal ganglia, internal capsule, cerebellum or pons presenting as a stroke.

Incidence
Accounts for 15% of strokes.

Age
Occurs most commonly in the elderly.

Aetiology/pathophysiology
- Prolonged uncontrolled hypertension is the most common cause. Pseudoaneurysms form on fine perforating arteries, these have a tendency to rupture leading to haemorrhage.
- Arteriovenous malformations may haemorrhage especially in younger patients.

- Cerebral hemisphere haemorrhages may be caused by cerebral amyloid (accounting for 10% of haemorrhages in people over 70 years of age).
- Other causes include bleeding into a tumour, disorders of coagulation and rarely, vasculitis.
- Intracranial venous thrombosis may be complicated by intracerebral haemorrhage (see page 300).

Clinical features

Clinical signs are unreliable in distinguishing ischaemic stroke from a haemorrhagic stroke, hence this is a diagnosis made following a CT brain scan. Headache and coma are more common in intracerebral haemorrhage.

Macroscopy

Blood clot which causes compression to the surrounding brain. If the patient survives the haematoma is removed by phagocytosis, and replaced by gliosis.

Management

- Resuscitate as necessary with management of the airway, breathing and circulation.
- Reverse any clotting deficiency and avoid aspirin.
- Hypertension needs to be treated cautiously, in the early stages, to prevent hypoperfusion.
- Neurosurgery is rarely indicated, but is often required in cerebellar bleeds which may cause obstructive hydrocephalus.
- Rehabilitation, ideally on a stroke unit, includes physiotherapy, speech therapy, and occupational therapy to gain maximal resolution of the neurological deficits. Any risk factors present, particularly hypertension, should be managed to help prevent recurrence.

Sub/extradural haemorrhage

Definition

Bleeding from vessels either outside or inside the dura mater.

Aetiology

Tearing of blood vessels which may be traumatic or spontaneous. Extradural haemorrhage results from tearing of the middle meningeal artery. Subdural haemorrhage is caused by traumatic tearing of an epiploic vein. Risk factors include a tendency to fall and clotting abnormalities (including anti-coagulant therapy).

Pathophysiology

- Extradural bleeds may result from a skull fracture (usually the temporal bone with which the middle meningeal artery is closely associated), causing the rapid accumulation of a haematoma in the potential space between the skull and the dura.
- Acute subdural haematomas may be seen after a head injury, the large bleed causes a rise in intracranial pressure and neurological deterioration.
- Chronic subdural haematoma usually occurs as a result of minor trauma, particularly in the elderly and alcohol abusers. Blood accumulates over days or weeks causing a slow growing haematoma. There may be further accumulation of fluid due to the osmotic pressure of the degenerating blood, or further acute bleeds.

Clinical features

- Extradural: There is generally a history of head injury. Classically the patient has a brief loss of consciousness at the time of injury, then a lucid interval followed by development of headache, progressive hemiparesis and loss of consciousness. Cerebellar herniation (coning) causes an ipsilateral dilated pupil, followed by bilateral fixed dilated pupils, tetraplegia and death
- Subdural: The onset may be indolent, and symptoms may fluctuate. Headache, drowsiness, and confusion (dementia if chronic) are common. Focal signs may be present and epilepsy may occur.

Investigations

The diagnosis is confirmed by a CT brain scan.

Management

Extradural bleeds usually require emergency neurosurgery. Subdural haematomas may require surgery, but are often managed conservatively with serial CT scans in patients without an acute history.

Subarachnoid haemorrhage

Definition

Spontaneous intracranial arterial bleeds into the subarachnoid space.

Incidence

15 per 100,000 per year. Accounts for 5–10% of cerebrovascular disease.

Aetiology

In most cases spontaneous subarachnoid haemorrhage results from an underlying lesion:

- Saccular (berry aneurysms), 85%
- Arteriovenous malformations, 10%
- No lesion found, 5%

Saccular or berry aneurysms arise due to defects in the internal elastic lamina of arteries and occur in 2% of the population. They may be multiple, and tend to occur at junctions of arteries on the circle of Willis or with its adjacent branches. Common sites include the anterior communicating artery, the posterior communicating artery and the middle cerebral artery. Most are idiopathic, but they are associated with diseases such as arteritis, coarctation of the aorta, Marfan's syndrome and adult polycystic kidney disease.

Arteriovenous malformations (AVM) are developmental abnormalities of blood vessels.

Clinical features

Sudden onset of a very severe headache, often followed by vomiting and/or loss of consciousness. There are signs of meningeal irritation with neck stiffness and a positive Kernig's sign (pain in back on flexing the hip). Neurological signs, papilloedema and retinal haemorrhages may be present.

Macroscopy

A layer of blood is present over the brain in the subarachnoid space and in the cerebrospinal fluid.

Complications

The blood acts as an irritant, causing vascular spasm leading to further ischaemia, infarction and cerebral oedema. It also interferes with CSF resorption, causing hydrocephalus which may be acute or chronic.

Investigations

CT brain scanning will demonstrate the bleed in most cases, but is falsely negative in up to 15% (less >8 hours after onset), therefore a lumbar puncture to demonstrate the presence of blood in the CSF space may be required. To differentiate from a 'bloody tap', i.e. trauma from the spinal tap needle, xanthochromia (yellowness of the CSF due to blood pigments) is looked for. It appears 12 hours post SAH, and may persist for 1–2 weeks.

If the patient is suitable for surgical intervention, carotid and vertebral angiography is used to demonstrate the site of the aneurysm or AVM.

Management

1 Patients should be resuscitated as necessary.
2 Oral nimodipine (a calcium-channel blocker) has been shown to reduce mortality. It is thought to work by reducing vascular spasm. Severe hypertension may need to be controlled but hypotension must be avoided to prevent further loss of perfusion pressure, so patients are kept well hydrated with intravenous saline.
3 In suitable patients surgical or radiological intervention for aneurysms takes place a few days later in a neurosurgical centre:
   - The neck of the aneurysm is clipped, and in some cases the aneurysm is wrapped in gauze to induce a fibrous reaction.
   - An alternative method is to obliterate the lumen of the aneurysm by intra-arterial embolisation using metallic coils.
4 AVMs can be treated with microembolism or focal radiotherapy.

Prognosis

50% of patients with a subarachnoid haemorrhage die prior to or soon after arrival In hospital, and a further 10–20% die in the first few weeks from rebleeding. Without intervention the risk of rebleeding is 30% in the following year from a berry aneurysm, 10% for AVMs.

Intracranial venous thrombosis

Definition

Venous thrombosis of either cerebral cortical veins or dural venous sinuses, which may result in focal signs.

Aetiology

Causes include trauma, dehydration and sepsis, infection of adjacent foci in the head (e.g. middle ear or skull air sinuses) and it has been associated with thrombophillia, oral contraceptives, pregnancy and puerperium.

Pathophysiology

Impairment of venous drainage due to thrombosis may lead to venous infarction as tissue congestion may compromise the arterial blood supply. The high pressure in small vessels may cause rupture and haemorrhage.

Clinical features
Fever and headache are often features.
- Cortical vein thrombosis results in a stroke and seizures.
- Cavernous sinus thrombosis causes headache, fever and eye signs (diplopia, proptosis, chemosis, opthalmoplegia, papilloedema) which usually become bilateral.
- Lateral venous sinus thrombosis has a sub acute onset of fever, earache, headache, nausea and vomiting. Papilloedema may be seen. This condition arises from mastoiditis and is now rare.
- Sagittal sinus thrombosis causes headache, papilloedema, focal signs, confusion and epilepsy.

Investigations
CT head may show occluded veins, oedema or haemorrhage but is often normal, the best investigation is MRI with venography (MRV). Investigations to identify underlying causes should also be performed.

Management
Anti-coagulation (despite evidence of haemorrhage), anti-convulsant drugs and treat the underlying cause wherever possible.

Infections of the nervous system

Meningitis and encephalitis

Bacterial meningitis

Definition
Bacterial infection of the meninges (the tissues lining the brain and spinal cord).

Aetiology
The likely organism changes with age. In adults, the most common are *Neisseria meningitidis*, *Streptococcus pneumoniae*, and *Haemophilus influenzae*. Less common organisms include gram-negative bacilli (particularly as a hospital acquired infection) and *Listeria* in the elderly and immunocompromised. Predisposing factors include predisposition to streptococcal infection (e.g. asplenic patients), otitis media, alcoholism, skull fracture, neurosurgery or immunosuppression.

Pathophysiology
The organisms may spread directly from the nasopharynx, middle ear, the skull vault or haematogenously then crossing the blood-brain barrier. Once within the cerebrospinal fluid (CSF), the bacteria multiply rapidly. There is an acute inflammatory response to the bacteria with neutrophils and cytokine release, then endothelial dysfunction causing disruption of local blood flow, oedema, and ischaemia and cell death. Hydrocephalus, raised intracranial pressure, cranial nerve palsies or other neurological problems such as seizures may occur as a result. *Neisseria meningitidis* may cause meningitis, septicaemia or both simultaneously.

Clinical features
- Meningitis should be considered in all patients with a headache and fever. Patients may have a prodromal illness resembling 'flu'.
- The symptoms may progress rapidly over hours, or a few days. The headache is generalised, and increases in intensity to severe. Associated symptoms include photophobia, confusion and non-specific symptoms such as malaise, nausea and vomiting, and neck pain.
- Examination often demonstrates neck stiffness (an inability to touch chin to chest passively or actively). Other signs of meningism are a positive Kernig sign (when the hip is kept flexed at 90°, knee extension causes pain or is resisted) or Brudzinski sign (spontaneous flexion of the hip when the neck is flexed). Patients are examined for a petechial rash which suggests *N. meningitidis*.
- There may be evidence of an underlying cause or origin for the infection.

Complications
Neurological and cerebrovascular complications include intracranial venous thrombosis, cerebral oedema and hydrocephalus. Septic shock and disseminated intravascular coagulation occur in 8–10% of patients with meningococcal meningitis. *N. meningitidis* is also associated with adrenal haemorrhage (Waterhouse–Friderichsen syndrome) which is rapidly fatal.

Table 7.5 CSF findings in meningitis

	Normal	Bacterial	Viral	Tuberculous
Appearance	Clear	Cloudy	Clear	Opalescent
Cells/mm^3	0–5	10–100,000	15–2000	250–500
Cell type	Lymphocytes	Neutrophils	Lymphocytes	Lymphocytes
Glucose	>60% blood	<60% blood	>60% blood	<60% blood
Protein (g/L)	0.15–0.35	0.5–5	0.15–1.25	0.45–5.0

Macroscopy/microscopy

Inflamed arachnoid mater, with exudate in the subarachnoid space which is rich in neutrophils. There may be oedema, focal infarction and congested vessels in the underlying brain tissue.

Investigations

If there is no evidence of intracranial mass lesion, focal neurology, papilloedema or reduced consciousness, a lumbar puncture can be performed otherwise a CT brain is indicated prior to LP. CSF is sent urgently for protein, glucose, microscopy and culture (see Table 7.5). CSF pressure is characteristically raised. Other important tests include blood culture (up to 50% positive, if taken before antibiotics given), coagulation screen and blood glucose levels for comparison with CSF glucose. Low inflammatory markers (CRP and ESR) and low white blood counts do not exclude the diagnosis and are associated with a worse prognosis. PCR, ELISA and antigen testing are increasingly used.

Management

Treatment delay may be fatal, if the patient is severely unwell treatment should be commenced before performing LP/CT brain. CSF taken soon after antibiotics are given still demonstrates the causative organism in many cases.

- A broad-spectrum antibiotic such as a cephalosporin at high doses is initially recommended due to the increasing emergence of penicillin-resistant streptococci. Once cultures and sensitivities are available, the course and choice of agent can be determined (ceftriaxone/cefotaxime for *Haemophilus influenzae* and *Streptococcus pneumoniae*, penicillin for *N. meningitidis*, and ampicillin for *Listeria*).
- Dexamethasone for 2–4 days which is commenced shortly before or at the time of giving antibiotics may

reduce mortality and overall morbidity in adults and may reduce the incidence of hearing loss in children.
- Nasopharyngeal clearance may be recommended for the patient and household 'kissing contacts', e.g. with a quinolone or rifampicin. Cephalosporins provide good clearance of nasal carriage in the patient, but penicillins do not.
- Any underlying cause may need to be treated.

Vaccination

Vaccination with the *H. influenzae B* (HiB) vaccine has dramatically reduced this as a cause of meningitis in children. It is recommended in asplenic patients.

Meningococcal meningitis is most commonly of the type B meningococcus, for which there is no vaccine. However, the type C vaccine is used to reduce the chance of an epidemic when clusters occur and is now a routine childhood immunisation.

Conjugate *Strep. pneumoniae* vaccine (Prevenar®) is given to infants with chronic diseases, and Pneumovax® (live attenuated) is used in at risk patients.

Prognosis

Despite the advent of antibiotics, the mortality is still as high as 15–20%, with a significant proportion of survivors having persistent neurological abnormality. Poor prognostic markers include hypotension, confusion and seizures.

Viral meningitis

Definition

Acute viral infection of the meninges is the most common cause of meningitis. It often occurs as combined meningo-encephalitis and in many cases it is a diagnosis of exclusion after investigating for bacterial or tuberculous meningitis.

Aetiology

A variety of viruses may infect the meninges including enteroviruses, mumps, herpes simplex (see page 400), HIV and Epstein–Barr virus.

Pathophysiology

In viral meningitis there is a predominantly lymphoid immune reaction without the formation of pus or adhesions, there is no cerebral oedema unless encephalitis occurs.

Clinical features

Patients present with headache usually over 1–2 days, fever, nausea, photophobia, malaise and neck stiffness. Rash, upper respiratory symptoms and occasionally diarrhoea may be present. There may be evidence of genital ulcers in those with primary HSV-2 infection, but these are absent in recurrent infections.

Investigations

A lumbar puncture should be performed if meningitis is suspected. The cerebrospinal fluid (CSF) is usually clear, with predominant lymphocytes, but early in the illness, polymorphs may predominate.

Culture is possible, but rarely useful clinically as it takes up to 2 weeks. PCR has been used in some cases to speed diagnosis and hence stopping antibiotics.

CT brain is normal.

Management

If bacterial meningitis is suspected, broad-spectrum antibiotics must be given without delay. Analgesia is given for headache but no specific treatment is indicated in most forms of viral meningitis. Generally, it is a benign self limiting condition lasting 4–10 days.

Tuberculous meningitis

Definition

Infection of the meninges with *Mycobacterium tuberculosis*.

Incidence

It is seen in 1% of all cases of TB.

Age

May occur at any age.

Geography

Rare in the developed world but a major problem in developing countries.

Aetiology

May arise as a complication of miliary tuberculosis or in primary or post primary infections. In the Western world, TB occurs most often as part of a reactivation process due to immune deficiency, e.g. secondary to ageing, alcoholism, HIV or immunosuppression. Tuberculous meningitis is rare after BCG vaccination.

Pathophysiology

If a tuberculous focus develops in the brain, meninges or skull and ruptures into the subarachnoid space, a hypersensitivity reaction occurs leading to intense inflammation. This inflammation can directly involve the cranial nerves, particularly at the base of the brain; it can lead to a vasculitis which causes strokes; and it can cause communicating hydrocephalus by impeding cerebrospinal fluid (CSF) flow and resorption.

Clinical features

The onset is usually insidious over days or weeks, although it may present as an acute illness.

Stage I: Vague headache, lassitude, anorexia and low-grade fever.

Stage II: Signs of meningism (headache, vomiting, confusion, neck stiffness). Focal neurology may develop at this time including cranial nerve signs and hemiparesis.

Stage III: Untreated, the patient becomes comatose.

Macroscopy/microscopy

The subarachnoid space is filled with a viscous green exudate, the meninges are thickened and tubercles and chronic inflammation may be seen in the brain and on the meninges.

Investigations

A lumbar puncture should be performed and the CSF should be stained with Ziehl Nielson stain, and then undergo prolonged culture. The CSF is typically cloudy, with a predominance of mononuclear cells (250–500 lymphocytes/mm^3) with raised protein and lowered glucose. Repeated LP cultures increase the diagnostic sensitivity, as a single sample is only positive in less than 50%.

CT and MRI imaging may demonstrate hydrocephalus and basilar meningeal enhancement – both together are strongly suggestive of TB, MRI may demonstrate a focal vasculitis.

Polymerase chain reaction (PCR) testing is useful but not reliable, with only 60% positive in proven cases.

In addition, suspected cases should be screened with a chest X-ray, sputum culture and in confirmed cases an HIV test should be performed.

Management

A minimum of 12 months therapy with rifampicin and isoniazid supplemented by pyrazinamide and a fourth drug for at least the first 2 months is recommended. The fourth drug may be ethambutol or streptomycin but these only penetrate the CNS adequately in the early stages, whilst the meninges are inflamed. Treatment should be initiated on clinical suspicion, before confirmation, as deterioration can occur within days, and even when treated mortality is as high as 15–40%.

Corticosteroids have been shown to reduce vascular complications, and improve survival and neurological function. High dose prednisolone is used in cases with rapid progression, cerebral oedema, hydrocephalus or basilar enhancement on CT, with high levels of CSF protein (>0.5 g/L) and in cases where there is a clinical deterioration with the onset of therapy, due to the increase in inflammatory response which may occur.

Other causes of meningitis

Definition

In some cases of clinical meningitis, initial investigations may demonstrate meningeal inflammation but routine blood and CSF cultures are negative.

Aetiology

The differential diagnosis for these cases of 'aseptic meningitis' is wide (see Table 7.6).

Investigations/management

In many cases of aseptic meningitis, the diagnosis is of a self-limiting, benign viral meningitis. However, it is important to consider these other causes, particularly if

Table 7.6 Differential diagnosis of aseptic meningitis

	Examples
Bacterial	Partially treated bacterial meningitis
	Parameningeal bacterial infection e.g. subdural abscess, sinusitis
	Mycobacterium tuberculosis
	Leptospirosis
	Lyme disease (*Borrelia burgdorferi*)
	Syphilis
Viral	Echovirus
	Enteroviruses
	HIV
	HSV
	Mumps
	Polio
Fungal/Parasitic	Particularly in immunocompromised patients –
	Cryptococcus, Candida, *Aspergillus*
	Toxoplasmosis, Amoeba
Malignancy	Lymphoma
	Leukaemia
	Metastatic carcinoma and adenocarcinomas
Auto-immune/ Inflammatory	Systemic lupus erythematosus
	Behçêt's disease
	Sarcoid
Drugs	Particularly nonsteroidal anti-inflammatory drugs

the patient does not improve. Further investigations may include:

- CT/MRI scanning of the brain and sinuses.
- Repeated lumbar punctures, including further fluid for cytology, specific CSF antibody. titres, e.g. for mumps, and PCR for, e.g. TB, HSV, enterovirus.
- CSF staining for acid-fast bacilli, fungi.
- TB cultures, viral cultures and fungal cultures (although these take days to weeks).
- Serum serology (acute and convalescent samples).
- HIV testing.

If it is not clear whether the process is bacterial or viral, antibiotics may be given empirically whilst awaiting further investigation.

Acute viral encephalitis

Definition

Inflammation of the brain parenchyma caused by viruses.

Aetiology

This is an uncommon disease, but the most common cause in the United Kingdom is the herpes simplex virus (HSV). Other viruses causing encephalopathy include echovirus, coxsackie virus, other members of the herpesviruses (e.g. varicella zoster, cytomegalovirus, Epstein–Barr virus). Around the world, arthropod-borne viruses cause epidemics and rabies causes an almost invariably fatal encephalitis.

Pathophysiology

HSV tends to cause a temporal encephalitis. Immuno-compromised individuals, children, teenagers and the elderly have an increased risk. Inflammation affects the meninges and parenchyma causing oedema and hence raised intracranial pressure, diffuse and focal neurological dysfunction.

Clinical features

The main triad of symptoms is headache, fever and altered level of consciousness. It is an important differential of bacterial meningitis. In HSV type I encephalitis nausea, vomiting, and meningism (neck stiffness) affect over two-thirds and up to half develop focal symptoms and signs, e.g. hemiparesis or dysphasia. Seizures (particularly temporal lobe seizures) are also a presenting feature.

Macroscopy/microscopy

The meninges are hyperaemic, the brain is swollen, sometimes with evidence of petechial haemorrhage and necrosis. There is cuffing of blood vessels by mononuclear cells and viral inclusion bodies may be seen.

Investigations

- CT scanning may show areas of oedema (a normal scan does not exclude the diagnosis, but is indicated before lumbar puncture (LP) in cases with altered consciousness or focal neurological signs). MRI is more sensitive.
- LP – the cerebrospinal fluid commonly shows lymphocytosis and raised protein levels. Glucose is uncommonly reduced (a sign of bacterial infection). CSF may be sent for HSV PCR and antibody tests for HSV, EBV, CMV and VZV. CSF cultures are usually unhelpful.

- EEG may be helpful in the diagnosis in over 90% of cases of HSV-I.
- In systemic illnesses, serum viral antibody titres can be helpful.

Management

In all cases except herpes simplex encephalitis there is no effective treatment apart from supportive management. Seizures are treated with anticonvulsants. Suspected cases of herpes encephalitis are treated urgently with high dose i.v. acyclovir for 10 days, with up to 5% of cases relapsing after treatment.

Prognosis

Herpes simplex encephalitis has a mortality of 20% despite treatment, with poor prognostic factors including older age, GCS $\leq$10 at onset of therapy. Persistent neurological deficits occur in 50%, particularly memory impairment, personality change, dysphasia and epilepsy.

Miscellaneous infective or post-infective CNS disorders

Tetanus

Definition

Tetanus is a toxin mediated condition causing muscle spasms following a wound infection.

Aetiology

Clostridium tetani (the causative organism), an anaerobic spore forming bacillus, originates from the faeces of domestic animals. It is found widely in the soil.

Pathophysiology

The bacteria enter the body at the site of a wound and if there is an anaerobic environment (e.g. if there is a foreign material present in the wound) they replicate and produce a neurotoxin, tetanospasmin. This toxin travels along the sheaths of peripheral nerves to the CNS and acts by blocking the release of inhibitory mediators in the spinal motor synapses. The result is an overactivity of both the motor system and the sympathetic nervous system, causing spasms and autonomic dysfunction.

Clinical features

The incubation period can be days to weeks and the wound may be so slight as to be unnoticed.

- Generalised tetanus is the most common presentation, with lockjaw (trismus), caused by masseter spasm. The facial muscles may contort to cause a typical expression (risus sardonicus). Any sensory stimulation such as noise results in generalised muscle spasms including arching of the back (opisthotonos). Spasms of the larynx can impede respiration, and autonomic dysfunction causes arrhythmias, sweating and a labile blood pressure.
- Localised tetanus can occur around the contaminated wound, full recovery is usual.
- Cephalic tetanus is uncommon but invariably fatal. It occurs when *C. tetani* is inoculated from the middle ear.

Investigations

The diagnosis is essentially clinical, bacteria are rarely isolated.

Complications

Muscle spasms may lead to injury, in severe cases respiratory failure, cardiac arrest or aspiration leading to death.

Management

Following contaminated injury patients require with early wound debridement and the administration of human tetanus immune globulin (passive immunisation) if their immunisation status is unknown or they have not had a booster in the last 5 years.

- A booster dose with tetanus toxoid (which is an inactivated toxin which induces active immunisation), or course of three injections, should additionally be given, as the protection from antitetanus immune globulin only lasts 2 weeks. Antibiotics may also be indicated.

Active tetanus: Patients should be nursed in a quiet, dark area to reduce spasms. Surgical wound debridement should be performed where indicated and intravenous penicillin and high doses of human tetanus immune globulin should be given i.m. (some around the wound). However, the immunoglobulin can only neutralise circulating toxin, it has no affect on bound toxin.

Large doses of diazepam may be needed to reduce spasms and cardiovascular instability is controlled with β blockers. Tracheostomy and ventilatory support may be necessary for severe laryngeal spasm.

Children are routinely vaccinated against tetanus from age 2 months.

Poliomyelitis

Definition

Infection of a susceptible individual with poliovirus type 1, 2 or 3, which can lead to a mild meningitic illness with acute paralysis and subsequently post-polio syndrome.

Age

Mainly a disease of childhood.

Sex

No sexual preponderance.

Geography

Acute poliomyelitis has been eradicated in developed countries, apart from rare cases due to the live, attenuated oral polio vaccine. Serotype 2 has been completely eradicated worldwide (announced by WHO in 1999).

Aetiology

Poliovirus is a ssRNA, non-encapsulated, icosahedral virus 25–30 nm in size. It is an enterovirus, i.e. it spreads by the faeco–oral route.

Pathophysiology

The virus is neurotropic, with propensity for the anterior horn cells of the spinal cord and cranial nerve motor neurones. The virus enters via the gastrointestinal tract, then migrates up peripheral nerves.

Clinical features

The incubation period is 7–14 days, a number of patterns occur:

- Subclinical infection occurs in 95% of infected individuals.
- Acute polio presents with a mild self-limiting fever with or without meningism.
- Paralytic poliomyelitis occurs in about 0.1% of individuals. This form is predisposed to by male sex;

exercise early in the illness; trauma, surgery, or intramuscular injection which localises the paralysis, recent tonsillectomy (bulbar poliomyelitis).

i After an initial febrile illness, symptoms subside for 4–5 days.

ii Symptoms then reoccur with greater severity and signs of meningeal irritation and muscle pain, followed by paralysis typically affecting one arm and the opposite leg.

iii Bulbar poliomyelitis is characterised by cranial nerve involvement commonly with palsies of the soft palate, pharyngeal and laryngeal muscles. Dysphagia and dysarthria result, with the risk of aspiration pneumonia.

iv Respiratory involvement may lead to the need for ventilatory support.

Complications

Post-polio syndrome – this is progressive, often painful weakness in the territories originally affected by the acute illness which can occur many years later (usually 20–40 years) in about a quarter of patients. More suffer from pain, but without progressive weakness. It appears to be a failure of the compensatory mechanisms which occur to bring about the original recovery – those with a greater original recovery tend to have the greatest decline, and those who were younger at the age of acute polio appear to be relatively protected.

Investigations

Diagnosis is clinical but laboratory confirmation is by viral culture. In post-polio syndrome, polio virus is not found in the CNS, but muscle EMG and biopsy show evidence of motor unit loss.

Management

- Acute treatment is supportive with bed rest, respiratory support where indicated.
- Post-infection:
  i Occupational and physical therapy should be used to maximise function.
  ii Splinting and even tendon transfer or arthrodesis may be required for weakness or joint deformity.
  iii Shortening: Leg length inequality of up to 3 cm may be treated by built up shoes, larger differences may require leg lengthening (or shortening of the opposite leg) procedures.

- Post-polio syndrome management is non-specific, with the treatment of limb and joint deformities, management of pain, and maximisation of function and strength by not overworking muscles. Sleep disorders, including nocturnal hypoventilation, need to be treated with non-invasive ventilation.
- Prophylaxis: Live attenuated (Sabin) or killed (Salk) polio vaccine.

Abscesses of the nervous system

Cerebritis and cerebral abscess

Definition

A focal infection within the parenchyma of the brain – cerebritis – can lead to the formation of a cerebral abscess.

Aetiology

Often the causative organism cannot be identified, or a mixed growth of bacteria is found. Bacteria that cause cerebral abscesses include various *Streptococci*, *Bacteroides*, *Staphylococci* and *Enterobacteria*. Immuno-suppressed patients are predisposed to fungal abscesses such as *Candida*, *Aspergillus* and *Toxoplasma*.

Pathophysiology

The organism may enter the brain by direct extension from meningitis, otitis media or sinusitis, or by haematogenous spread, e.g. from infective endocarditis. Surgery or trauma may also inoculate organisms through an open wound. Multiple lesions suggest haematogenous seeding.

Clinical features

The onset of symptoms is usually insidious, with headache as the most common symptom, variable neck stiffness, fever, and possible focal signs, seizures or confusion.

Macroscopy/microscopy

In the first 1–2 weeks, there is inflammation and oedema (cerebritis). Later, necrosis and liquefaction lead to formation of a cavity filled with pus. There are acute inflammatory cells (neutrophils), surrounded by gliosis and fibroblasts.

Investigations

Leucocytosis and a raised ESR are common.

- The diagnosis is made by CT or MRI scanning, but there may be non-specific oedema in the early stages. Later, ring-enhancement demonstrates the breakdown in blood-brain barrier.
- In most cases lumbar puncture is contra-indicated due to risk of brain-stem herniation (coning), but aspiration or excision biopsy of the abscess may be carried out by a neurosurgeon if the organism is in doubt. Fungi and mycobacteria must be looked for.

Management

Frequently treatment is by a combination of antimicrobial therapy and surgical drainage.

Prognosis

25% mortality despite treatment, epilepsy is common in survivors.

Tuberculoma

Definition

A tuberculoma is a localised caseous abscess within the brain caused by *M. tuberculosis*. It is rare in the West, but the commonest single intracranial lesion in India.

Aetiology/pathophysiology

A tuberculoma is a chronic caseating intracranial granuloma, which may arise from haematogenous spread during primary TB, e.g. miliary TB.

Clinical features

The condition is often asymptomatic as they are rarely large enough to cause symptoms of an intracranial mass lesion. Rupture into the subarachnoid space may cause tuberculous meningitis. A tuberculoma in the brainstem may cause hydrocephalus by obstruction.

Investigations

Lesion may be seen on X-ray as an area of internal calcification, or on CT/MRI. Skin testing, e.g. Mantoux is not reliable.

Management

Anti-tuberculous therapy as for tuberculous meningitis should be used (see page 303) but is often unsuccessful, in which case surgical drainage may be used.

Disorders of conciousness and memory

Epilepsy

Definition

Epilepsy is a recurrent tendency to seizures. Seizures are due to paroxysmal discharge of cerebral neurones.

Incidence

Approximately 2% have two or more seizures during their lives.

Age

Any

Sex

M = F

Aetiology

A cause for epilepsy is found in less than 25% of cases. Most of the others are thought to be genetically determined.

- About 30% have an affected first degree relative.
- Head trauma: minimal risk if <30 minutes concussion, high risk if there is contusion, haemorrhage or prolonged amnesia.
- Surgery to the cerebral hemispheres is followed by epilepsy in 10%.
- Perinatal trauma and fetal anoxia are common causes of seizures in childhood.
- Intracranial mass lesions affecting the cerebral cortex e.g tumours.
- Vascular malformations.
- Cerebral infarction particularly in the elderly.
- Drugs, alcohol, drug withdrawal.
- Inborn errors of metabolism.

Clinical features

Epilepsy is most often diagnosed on the history, from witnesses (see Table 7.7). Features suggestive of a fit are described under Fits and Faints (see page 287).

Table 7.7 Types of seizures

Type of seizure	Description
Partial seizures	
Simple partial (consciousness maintained)	Motor: usually twitching or jerking of one side of the face, or one limb. Sensory, e.g. auditory or somatosensory. Autonomic: pallor, sweating, etc. There may be a Jacksonian March, with the epilepsy progressively involving more of a limb, e.g. hand, then elbow, then shoulder.
Complex partial (impaired conciousness)	May begin as a simple partial then become complex, or be complex from the start. Often with disturbance of higher cerebral function, e.g. sense of fear. Semi-purposeful movements may occur. The patient has little or no recall of the episode.
Secondary generalised	Partial seizures (simple or complex) can progress to secondary generalised seizures.
Generalised seizures	
Nonconvulsive (absence)	Impaired conciousness but without falling, although there may be involuntary movements. Usually last less then 20 s. EEG shows characteristic 3 per second spike and wave discharges
Convulsive (usually followed by post-ictal confusion)	
Myoclonic	Sudden shock-like jerks affecting one part or the whole body
Clonic	Generalised jerking
Tonic	Rigidity, increased tone, respiration ceases
Tonic–clonic	Initial rigid tonic stage during which respiration ceases, then generalised jerking Micturition, salivation and tongue-biting may occur. If this lasts >30 min, it is called status epilepticus.
Atonic (drop attacks)	Loss of muscle tone causing patient to fall to ground

The main terms used to describe seizures are:

Partial (focal, localised seizure)

- A partial seizure may be simple (no loss of consciousness) or complex (impaired consciousness).

Generalised (diffuse, whole brain affected)

- A generalised seizure may be convulsive (jerking, with motor involvement) or non-convulsive (absence, motor tone unaffected).

Investigations

The urgency of the tests depends on the clinical findings.

- Blood tests – FBC, U&Es, glucose, calcium, magnesium, LFTs and thyroid function tests.
- ECG.
- EEG may be normal even in genuine epilepsy.
- MRI (or CT where MRI is not available) is increasingly used in all patients to look for an underlying lesion.

Management

With a first seizure, it is important to exclude any underlying cause such as a biochemical disturbance, menin-

gitis, stroke etc which may need urgent treatment. It is also important to decide if the patient is likely to have further seizures.

- If the seizure lasts <10 minutes with full recovery, with no neurological or systemic disorder the patient can usually be discharged home after a period of observation. They should be accompanied and be advised not to drive (see below).
- If unwell, pyrexial, persisting neurology or prolonged confusion post-seizure – urgent investigation with imaging, blood test, possibly lumbar puncture is required.
- Prolonged seizures or recurring seizures require inpatient admission for monitoring and initiation of treatment to control seizures.

Status epilepticus

This is defined as a prolonged single attack or continuing attacks of epilepsy without intervals of consciousness. The duration at which status is diagnosed is variable, most classically 30 minutes; however, treatment is started at 15 minutes in order to avoid brain damage or death. Status epilepticus is a medical emergency which carries a 10–15% mortality.

General measures include airway protection, oxygen and intravenous access.

Urgent blood tests as above, including clotting, arterial blood gas and save 50 mL serum (for later analysis of anti-epileptic drugs (AEDs) levels, drug screen, alcohol for example).

Ensure any usual AEDs given.

Consider i.v. glucose (and i.v. thiamine).

- Lorazepam or diazepam are first-line treatment
- If no response, intravenous phenytoin loading dose of 15 mg/kg is given.
- If still in 'refractory status' (more than 60 minutes of seizures, or >30 minutes after phenytoin) thiopentone or propofol are used (anaesthetic agents) preferably with EEG monitoring to demonstrate effectiveness, and endotracheal intubation and transfer to an intensive care unit is required.
- Following recovery from status epilepticus, long-term anti-epileptic medication should be reviewed or initiated.

Initiation of treatment

Anti-epileptic drugs (AEDs) should be tailored to the individual (see Table 7.8).

Neurosurgery is rarely undertaken except in selected patients, with persistent, frequent seizures where there is a significant adverse impact on quality of life, with poor control by medication and a clear electrical focus. Procedures include local resection, lobectomy, hemispherectomy and in some cases, less invasively by stereotactic radiosurgery.

Prognosis

Most people with epilepsy are able to lead a normal active life with medication to control their seizures, and continue their education and work. The management of epilepsy should include the discussion of social issues such as support at home, relationships, employment and psychological issues such as depression. Women who wish to become pregnant need special advice, but there is no reason why they should not have children. There are support groups available.

Table 7.8 Choice of AEDs in different types of epilepsy

Type of seizure	1st choice drugs	2nd choice drugs
Generalised tonic–clonic	Sodium valporate Carbamazepine* Lamotrigine	Phenytoin* Levetiracetam
Generalised Nonconvulsive (Absence)	Sodium valporate Lamotrigine	Ethosuximide Lamotrigine
Myoclonic	Sodium valproate	Clonazepam Lamotrigine
Partial seizures	Carbamazepine* Sodium valproate Lamotrigine	Phenytoin* Gabapentin Topiramate Tiagabine Levetiracetam

*High dose oral contraceptive pill should be used and high dose folic acid for women of child-bearing age as these and phenobarbitone are enzyme-inducing AEDs. Avoid valproate in women planning pregnancy. Women on enzyme-inducing AEDs should also have vitamin K in the month prior to delivery to reduce the risk of neonatal haemorrhage caused by inhibition of vitamin K transplacental transport.

General advice includes avoidance of certain sports such as rock-climbing, unless seizures are well-controlled; swimming is safe as long as supervised; and bathroom doors should be left unlocked.

Driving: If a patient has had one or more seizures they are not allowed to hold an ordinary Category 1 UK driving licence until seizure-free for 1 year. However, if attacks only occur whilst asleep and this pattern is established for 3 years, patients can drive even if seizures continue. Following a provoked seizure, e.g. due to head injury, stroke, cranial surgery but excluding drugs or alcohol, the suspension may be shorter. Patients should be advised to contact the DVLA. The DVLA also advise patients not to drive whilst any reduction of their medication takes place for 6 months after each change.

Depending on any underlying cause and absence of EEG changes, anticonvulsant therapy can be discontinued if they have been free of an attack for 2–3 years.

Acute confusional state (delirium)

Definition

Rapid onset of global but fluctuating confusion with an underlying toxic, vascular, ictal (seizure) or metabolic defect.

Aetiology

- Predisposing factors: The very young and very old, hearing loss or visual difficulty, those with diffuse brain disease such as dementia or taking drugs with anticholinergic properties such as tricyclic antidepressants, unfamiliar environment (e.g. hospital, nursing home).
- Precipitating factors can be divided into intracranial and extracranial (see Table 7.9).

Clinical features

- Disorientation and impaired conscious level – especially worse at night.
- Poor cognition, incoherent thought and speech.
- Mood and affect labile with depression, irritability, paranoia and aggression.
- Hallucinations – auditory and visual.
- Delusions are common.
- Motor activity may be increased but is often purposeless.
- Autonomic overactivity: Sweating, tachycardia and dilated pupils.

Table 7.9 Causes of acute confusional state

Extracranial/systemic	
Infection	Sepsis, e.g. UTI, pneumonia
Toxic	Alcohol intoxication, withdrawal
Drugs	Prescribed/illicit drugs, including overdose or withdrawal
Endocrine	Hyper- or hypothyroidism, hyper- or hypoglycaemia
Metabolic	Uraemia, hyper- or hyponatraemia, hypercalcaemia
	Hepatic failure
Hypoxia	Hypoxia and/or hypotension
Vitamin deficiency	Vitamin B_{12}
	Thiamine (Wernicke–Korsakoff)
Intracrania	
Trauma	Head injury
Vascular	Transient ischaemic attack, stroke, any intracranial bleed or space-occupying lesion
Epilepsy	May be post-ictal (after a seizure) or nonconvulsive status
Infection	AIDS, syphilis, meningitis, encephalitis, brain abscess
Tumour	Astrocytoma, etc

A detailed history including pre-morbid cognitive state, alcohol and drugs is essential, fluctuation helps separate delirium from dementia, examination should look for focal neurological signs and any evidence of other illness. Patients with dysphasia may appear confused, and require careful assessment.

Investigations

- Blood: FBC, U&E, ESR, CRP, calcium, glucose, thyroid function, syphilis serology, LFTs and clotting screen.
- Blood cultures if pyrexial.
- Urine for microscopy and culture. Consider saving urine for toxicology screen.
- ECG for possible acute myocardial infarction, arrhythmia, signs of hyperkalaemia.
- Imaging includes CXR, and where indicated CT or MRI.

Management

- Detection of the underlying cause of the confusional state and relevant treatment.
- Supportive therapy including rehydration, correction of electrolyte imbalance, improved lighting at night, facilitation of orientation, and avoidance of conflict.
- Cautious use of short-acting sedatives may be useful for restlessness and agitation, but can exacerbate the problem. Severe cases may require benzodiazepines, haloperidol or one of the newer anti-psychotics such as risperidone or olanzapine.

Prognosis

Where recovery occurs it is usually rapid with return to a premorbid functional level. The prognosis is dependent on the underlying cause and co-morbid features.

Coma

Definition

Coma is a state of unrousable unconsciousness.

Aetiology

The causes are mainly those of acute confusional state (see Table above), although there are other causes as well. Examples include:

- Systemic causes such as hypoglycaemia, hypothyroidism, hypoadrenalism, hypopituitarism,

Table 7.10 The Glasgow Coma Scale

Eye opening	
Spontaneously	4
To speech	3
To pain	2
No response	1
Best verbal response	
Orientated	5
Disorientated	4
Inappropriate words	3
Incomprehensible sounds	2
No response	1
Best motor response	
Obeys verbal commands	6
Localizes painful stimuli	5
Withdrawal to pain	4
Flexion to pain	3
Extension to pain	2
No response	1

respiratory failure with carbon dioxide retention, and hypothermia.
- Intracranial causes such as stroke, space-occupying lesions or haemorrhage tend not to cause coma unless there is extensive cerebral involvement or brainstem involvement (either directly or by raised intracranial pressure).

Clinical features

It is important to establish the level of consciousness. A useful way of grading this is the Glasgow Coma Scale (GCS – see Table 7.10).

1 The first priority is resuscitation – stabilise airway, breathing and circulation and check the glucose level (BM). Hypoxia, hypoglycaemia or hypotension are reversible causes of coma and will exacerbate any other cause. If the GCS is ≤8 the patient is at increased risk of aspiration because they are unable to protect their airway, thus intubation and ventilation should be considered.

2 Examination of the patient for clues to a systemic cause, e.g. needle-marks in intravenous drug users, evidence of liver failure, abnormal rate or pattern of respiration and evidence of an intracranial cause, e.g. external evidence of head injury, meningism (meningitis, subarachnoid haemorrhage) and neurological signs.

Investigations

These are as for acute confusional state. In many cases, if early assessment and investigations do not suggest a systemic cause, urgent CT brain is indicated, followed by lumbar puncture if the CT scan is normal.

Management

Following resuscitation treatment of the underlying cause is the main priority.
- If hypoglycaemia is possible, intravenous glucose should not be delayed. In at-risk patients such as alcoholics and in pregnancy, intravenous thiamine should be given prior to any intravenous glucose as there is a small risk of precipitating irreversible Wernicke–Korsakoff's syndrome.
- Continued monitoring, regular GCS assessments.
- Empirical use of naloxone (reverses opiates), flumazenil (reverses benzodiazepines) should be considered.
- Seizures should be controlled.
- Supportive care – coma patients require special treatment with a multi-disciplinary approach to avoid complications such as aspiration pneumonia, pressure sores, contractures, and they will require nasogastric or parenteral feeding.

Head Injury

Definition

Head injury is one of the most common causes of death and disability in young men, mainly due to road traffic accidents.

Incidence

Common; based on hospital attendances and admissions the incidence is ∼250 per 100,000 population.

Age

Young > old

Sex

M > F

Aetiology

The main aetiological causes of head injury are road traffic accidents and alcohol:
- Non-penetrating trauma: As a result of acceleration/deceleration to the head, rotational and shearing forces act on the brain.

- Penetrating trauma: Penetration of the skull by an external object such as a bullet.

Pathophysiology

The pathology of head injury can be divided into two groups:

- Primary brain damage:
  - i Cerebral contusions occur as the brain moves within the skull, causing bruising of the brain, particularly on the side of the trauma (coup lesion) and on the opposite side of the brain (contrecoup). Contusions heal by gliosis stained with haemosiderin.
  - ii Diffuse axonal injury due to shearing forces causing damage to cortical white matter tracts. Patients who survive such injury may have severe brain damage.
- Secondary brain damage occurs after the initial trauma, and is the result of problems in maintaining blood and oxygen supply to the brain due to hypoxia (e.g. airway obstruction, respiratory failure) or mass effect from haematoma. The degree of secondary brain damage can be influenced by medical or surgical treatment, whereas primary brain damage occurs at the time of injury and therefore can only be influenced by other factors such as car design to reduce pedestrian injury. Following trauma, the brain is much more susceptible to hypoxia and hypotension due to disruption of autoregulation and impaired vascular supply.

Clinical features

In a mild injury the patient is stunned or dazed for a few seconds or minutes. Loss of consciousness is transient and following this the patient remains alert with no amnesia. In more severe injuries, there is persistent posttraumatic amnesia. Neurological signs including papilloedema (although rare) and any evidence of penetrating injury or skull fracture should be looked for. Patients may have other injuries depending on the nature of the accident or trauma. The Glasgow Coma Scale is used to assess the level of consciousness (see Table 7.10).

Macroscopy/microscopy

- Early contusions appear as petechial haemorrhages. Over a period of several hours there is oozing of blood and the contusions become haemorrhagic with swelling of the brain. Petechial haemorrhage may occur in the corpus callosum and brain stem.
- Axonal damage appears as swollen torn ends of the axon.

Complications

Short term: Vascular, e.g. meningeal artery tear, causing extradural haematoma, or dural vein tear causing a subdural haematoma. Subarachnoid and intracerebral haemorrhage may also occur. Headache, dizziness and depression are common after a head injury.

Long term:

- Posttraumatic epilepsy.
- Chronic traumatic encephalopathy (the punch drunk syndrome seen in professional boxers).
- Benign positional vertigo.
- Hydrocephalus.

Management

- Resuscitation including intubation and ventilation as required. If neck injury is suspected, the patient should be immobilised until a spinal cord injury or unstable cervical spine has been excluded.
- Assessment of the severity of coma by the Glasgow Coma Scale, and full neurological and general examination. The decision to admit for observation is based on the history and assessment at presentation. In these cases, it is important to continue at least hourly neurological observations (vital signs, GCS and pupillary sizes/responses). Osmotic diuretics such as mannitol may also be used to reduce brain oedema.
- Investigations including routine investigations (FBC, U&Es and clotting) and a CT brain where indicated.
- In severe cases initial management may include admission to intensive care for intracerebral pressure monitoring and management, e.g. with mannitol and diuretics.

All patients require close monitoring to check for development of complications that require urgent treatment. CT brain is urgently indicated if

- level of consciousness depressed (A GCS score of <8 following resuscitation).
- the GCS score falls despite initial management.
- presence of skull fractures.
- the patient is difficult to assess, e.g. due to alcohol or drug intoxication.

Urgent neurosurgical assistance is required in the case of a depressed skull fracture, or expanding intracranial haemorrhage, particularly extradural haematomas or acute subdural haematomas.

Prognosis

Recovery may take weeks to months. Prolonged coma can still be followed by good recovery. 10 per 100,000 people die annually and the prevalence of survivors with a persisting disability or impairment is 100 per 100,000.

Dementia

Definition

A syndrome of acquired cognitive impairment, with progressive global loss of cognitive function in the context of normal arousal.

Incidence

1% of those aged 65–74 years, 10% of those over 75 and 25% of those over 85 years.

Aetiology

There are numerous causes of dementia, including
- Alzheimer's disease (most common >60%).
- multi-infarct dementia caused by multiple small infarctions, decline may be step-wise (~20%).
- dementia with Lewy bodies (5%).
- fronto-temporal dementias (~10%) such as cortical atrophy.
- alcohol.
- hydrocephalus, subdural haematoma, previous head injuries (punch-drunk syndrome).
- infections such as syphilis, HIV or prion diseases (Creutzfeld Jacob disease).

Clinical features

See also under specific causes of dementia. Patients may have impairment of the following cognitive functions:
- Learning and retaining new information, e.g. remembering recent events.
- Impaired reasoning, judgement.
- Ability to carry out complex tasks, e.g. managing household finances.
- Language skills, e.g. word finding.

- Spatial memory and orientation (e.g. wandering, getting lost).
- Personality and behaviour, loss of social skills, sometimes with aggression or sexual disinhibition.

Apathy and/or depression are common, there may be disturbances of sleep, confusion of day & night, with nocturnal restlessness and wandering. Auditory or visual hallucinations and delusions are particularly common in dementia with Lewy bodies. Other neurological signs such as hemiparesis, seizures tend to occur very late in dementia.

Generally, in the early stages, the patient is aware of a loss of their memory and may become very frustrated and anxious. It may at first be attributed to 'old age'. They lose the ability to function in daily life gradually, and in later stages they become more apathetic, with little spontaneous effort and therefore require full personal care such as feeding, washing, dressing and toiletting.

A collateral history from a relative or close carer who has known the patient for a long time is essential. The carer is often the one most emotionally affected by the changes wrought by dementia.

Investigations

These are to exclude any treatable causes of chronic confusion.
- Bloods: FBC, U&Es, calcium, LFTs, Vit B_{12}, thyroid function tests, blood glucose, syphilis serology.
- Chest X-ray.
- CT or MRI brain to look for cortical atrophy and exclude hydrocephalus, subdural haematoma or a space-occupying lesion such as a cerebral metastasis. There may be specific changes of specific dementias.

Management

The specific management strategies are covered under specific causes but general treatment includes the following:
- Multidisciplinary assessment.
- Family support responding to the changing needs of carers.
- Home care/day care/respite care/residential care/ hospital care.
- Behavioural problems may respond to phenothiazines or atypical neuroleptics.

- Antidepressants may improve functional level in those with low mood.
- Psychological therapy.
- For mild to moderate Alzheimer's dementia, multi-infarct dementia and dementia with Lewy bodies, cholinesterase inhibitors such as donepezil have been shown to be of benefit, in delaying the need for nursing home care.

Alzheimer's disease

Definition
A primary degenerative cortical dementia.

Incidence
Most common neurodegenerative disorder and cause of dementia.

Age
The onset can be in middle age, but the incidence rises with age. The annual risk of developing Alzheimer's disease (AD) is 1% in people aged 70–74 years, 2% in those aged 75–79 years and then steeply rises to 8% in those over 85 years.

Aetiology/pathophysiology
- Risk factors include family history, Down's syndrome and previous head injury.
- Molecular analysis of the amyloid found in the brains of patients with AD shows that it is derived from a family of normal cell membrane proteins called amyloid precursor proteins (APP) encoded on Chr 21. When APPs are cleaved by specific enzymes called secretases, a highly amyloidogenic protein is produced which is referred to as β-amyloid protein or Aβ42 protein. It is thought that these plaques then cause inflammation and hence neurotoxicity and apoptosis.
- Mutations on Chr 21 in Down's syndrome cause over-production of APP.
- Some cases of early onset AD are due to an autosomal dominant disorder with mutations on Chr 14 or 21 – these cause increased activity of the secretases.
- Apolipoprotein ε4 (apoε4) genotype on Chr 19 is over-represented in AD patients compared with the other alleles ε2 and ε3. Heterozygotes have approximately twofold relative risk for developing AD and homozygotes have a fourfold or 50% risk.

- Neurochemical analysis reveals that patients with Alzheimer's disease have widespread neurotransmitter defects, particularly loss of acetylcholine esterase and acetylcholine from the cortex/subcortical structures.

Clinical features
The features are those of dementia, but with an insidious onset and progressive decline in memory and at least one of:
- Dysphasia: Loss in language skills, especially with names and understanding speech.
- Apraxia: Inability to execute a skilled or learned motor act, e.g. inability to brush teeth, write, get dressed despite intact muscle function and comprehension.
- Agnosia: Loss of ability to recognise objects, people, sounds, shapes or smells despite normal sensory functions. Usually classified by the sense affected, e.g. visual agnosia.
- Disturbance in executive functioning (higher mental functions such as planning, abstract thought, organisation).

With progression over a number of years patients become immobile and emaciated. Death is commonly due to a complication of immobility or other diseases.

Macroscopy
The brain is small, with shrinkage of the gyri and widening of the sulci. Temporal lobe atrophy is prominent, particularly in the parahippocampal gyrus but also in the frontal and parietal lobes.

Microscopy
There are several abnormalities.
- Senile plaques in the cerebral cortex – spherical deposits with a central core of amyloid composed of β (A4) protein. Amyloid is also seen deposited in cerebral arteries causing amyloid angiopathy.
- Neurofibrillary tangles – intraneuronal inclusions comprising bundles of abnormal filaments. The tangles are composed of a microtubule binding protein called Tau protein, and are frequently flame shaped and occupy much of the space within the neuronal cytoplasm.
- Cortical nerve processes become twisted and dilated (neuropil threads) due to the accumulation of the same fibres that cause the tangles.

- Lewy bodies – eosinophilic cytoplasmic neuronal inclusions, in some cases. These are also seen in Lewy body dementia.
- Neuronal loss is seen from the cortex particularly in patients under the age of 80 years.

Investigations

The diagnosis is clinical although investigations to exclude other causes of dementia are necessary. AD cannot be definitively diagnosed until brain tissue is obtained, e.g. at post-mortem, but in most cases a clinical diagnosis is accurate.

Management

The management of AD includes those used for all types of dementia.

In addition, for early AD, acetylcholinesterase inhibitors such as donepezil, have been shown to improve cognitive function and delay decline by the equivalent of 2 months per year.

The gene of one of the enzymes which cleaves APP (β secretase) has been cloned, leading to hopes of other targeted therapies.

Prognosis

Most patients die within 5–10 years of diagnosis. Younger patients appear to progress more slowly.

Creutzfeld–Jakob disease

Definition

Rapidly progressive dementia caused by a prion (proteinaceous infectious agent), described in 1982 by neurologist Stanley Prusiner

Incidence

One case per million worldwide.

Geography

More common in certain parts of the world due to familial cases, e.g. Israel and North Africa.

Aetiology

Caused by a transmissable proteinaceous particle which is a modified version of a normal human protein. It does not contain any nucleic acid. It is resistant to many of the normal methods of sterilisation including heat.

- Sporadic CJD remains the most common type.
- Iatrogenic CJD (iCJD) results from transplantation of tissue from an infected individual, such as corneal grafts, cadaveric pituitary hormones and contaminated neurosurgical instruments. No cases have been shown from blood transfusion products.
- Variant CJD (vCJD) –1996 saw the identification of a 'new' form of CJD primarily affecting younger people. There is reasonable evidence that this may be due to the ingestion of Bovine Spongiform Encephalopathy (BSE) infected beef. There have been reported cases of person-to-person transmission by blood transfusion.

Pathophysiology

Prion diseases appear to have a long incubation period, but once clinically apparent, show rapid progression. Neither the transmission nor the mechanism of action of the prion in CJD is clearly understood. There are other prion diseases such as

- Kuru – which used to be prevalent in Papua New Guinea and is believed to have been spread by ritual cannibalism.
- Scrapie in sheep and BSE in cattle.
- Hereditary prion diseases due to mutations in the gene (PRNP) on chromosome 20 can cause several clinical entities within the same kindred including CJD, Gerstmann–Straussler–Sheinker syndrome and fatal familial insomnia.

It is currently thought that a normal glycoprotein in the brain (the function of which is unknown) undergoes conformational change to become prion protein (PrP). This abnormally conformed protein is resistant to digestion by proteases and tends to form polymers. The disease appears to be propagated further by the abnormally conformed protein inducing normal protein to conformationally change, leading to further polymer formation. In familial cases, it appears that the abnormal protein arises spontaneously due to a mutation of the gene encoding PrP, whereas in other cases there appears to be inoculation or ingestion of the prion, which is transported to the nervous system and can then cause prion disease in susceptible individuals.

Clinical features

CJD presents as a rapid onset of dementia, characteristically with myoclonic jerks (in ∼90% of patients, but not in vCJD). Extrapyramidal signs and upper motor neurone signs occur frequently. Sensory signs and symptoms and psychiatric symptoms occur in vCJD, but are uncommon in other forms.

Microscopy

Neuronal loss, increase in glial cells, lack of inflammation and small vacuoles in the neuropil which has lead to the term 'spongiform encephalopathy'.

Investigations

CT brain scans are usually normal, but serial scans may show rapidly progressive ventricular enlargement and cortical atrophy. MRI in vCJD only shows increased T2 signal in the basal ganglia.
EEG is often abnormal in sporadic CJD.
CSF is unremarkable and has normal protein levels. There are raised levels of a normal intraneuronal protein (14-3-3 protein) detectable in the CSF of patients with CJD, which may simply imply rapid neuronal death, but can be a useful marker.

There is no reliable method of confirming diagnosis except by brain biopsy or postmortem. vCJD may be suggested by the finding of prion protein on tonsillar biopsy, although this is not yet a reliable clinical test.

Prognosis

The disease is fatal within 1 year of onset of symptoms for most forms, but 2 years in vCJD.

Wernicke–Korsakoff syndrome

Definition

Wernicke's encephalopathy is a triad of confusion, ophthalmoplegia and ataxia. Korsakoff syndrome is a loss of short-term memory and disinhibition, leading to confabulation. These result from thiamine (vitamin B_1) deficiency.

Aetiology

Usually seen in alcoholics, but may also be seen in starvation, malnutrition, parenteral feeding without vitamin supplements and chronic vomiting, e.g. hyperemesis gravidarum. Thiamine is present in fortified wheat flour (the natural thiamine is removed by milling, so it is replaced by law in most countries), fortified breakfast cereals, milk, eggs, yeast extract and fruit.

Pathophysiology

Thiamine is an essential factor for the maintenance of the peripheral nervous system and the heart. It is involved in glycolytic pathways, mediating carbohydrate metabolism. Deficiency leads to ischaemic damage to the brainstem.

If patients are given a large dose of sugar, the increased thiamine requirement to process this may precipitate the syndrome, so thiamine should be given together with intravenous glucose in a hypoglycaemic alcoholic.

Clinical features

Wernicke's presents with confusion, double vision and unsteadiness, with an acute or chronic onset of nystagmus. Other signs include ptosis, abnormal pupillary reactions and altered consciousness. It may present with headache, anorexia, and vomiting. Untreated Wernicke's can lead to irreversible Korsakoff's syndrome and/or death with coma within 2 weeks.

Occasionally, patients present with Korsakoff's, with a relatively selective although profound deficit in ability to acquire new memories. This leads to confabulation. Other intellectual functions are relatively well-preserved. Patients may have a peripheral neuropathy due to other nutritional deficiencies.

Investigations

Diagnosis is usually clinical, and on response to thiamine. Erythocyte transketolase activity and blood pyruvate are increased, but treatment should not be delayed whilst waiting for results.

Management

Urgent thiamine i.v. or p.o. Treatment of Wernicke's encephalopathy may unmask Korsakoff's syndrome.

Prognosis

Recovery is prompt in most cases, occurring within 24–48 hours. There is more residual impairment in chronic cases when the diagnosis is delayed.

Brain death

Definition
This is defined as 'irreversible loss of the capacity for consciousness combined with the irreversible loss of the capacity to breathe'.

Aetiology
The brainstem is the seat of consciousness and of respiratory drive. Any intracranial cause or a systemic cause such as severe, prolonged hypoxia or hypotension can lead to brainstem death.

In view of the fact that many patients may be established on a ventilator prior to brain death being diagnosed, ways of assessing brain death have been developed, to allow the withdrawal of ventilation. Although patients who fulfil these criteria can be kept alive by ventilation, eventually they will die from other causes.

Clinical features
In order to diagnose brainstem death several criteria must be met.

Prior to brainstem testing, the following preconditions must be fulfilled:

- There must be a diagnosis for the cause of the irreversible brain damage, e.g. head injury, subarachnoid haemorrhage or anoxic, ischaemic damage.
- The patient must be unresponsive (GCS = 3), and have no spontaneous respiratory efforts on the ventilator.
- There must be no possibility of drug intoxication, including any recent use of anaesthetic agents or paralysing agents.
- Hypothermia should be excluded and body temperature must be >35°C.
- There must be no significant metabolic, endocrine or electrolyte disturbance causing or contributing to the coma.

Brainstem testing
This should be carried out by two experienced clinicians (one a consultant, another an experienced registrar or consultant) on two separate occasions 12 hours apart. These tests are designed to show that all brainstem reflexes have been lost completely.

- Pupils fixed and unresponsive to light.
- Absent corneal reflexes.

- Absent vestibulo-ocular reflexes on ice-cold water being instilled into each ear.
- Absent cough and gag reflexes on pharyngeal, laryngeal or tracheal stimulation.
- No motor response within the cranial nerve distribution (eye, face, head) elicited by stimulation of any somatic area such as nail bed pressure, supraorbital pressure and Achilles tendon pressure.

Apnoea testing
The patient is pre-ventilated with 100% oxygen and continuous oxygen administered via a tracheal catheter (to prevent hypoxia during the test) and then the ventilator is disconnected and the pCO_2 is allowed to climb to 6.65 kPa. No respiratory effort should occur.

If all the above criteria are fulfilled, the patient is diagnosed as brainstem dead, and ventilation may be withdrawn. They may be suitable for organ donation, if the family consent.

Patients with some evidence of brainstem activity may still have a very poor prognosis. Death may occur due to cardiovascular collapse, e.g. sepsis, cardiac arrhythmia. However, if the patient remains stable, but with very little brain function, it may be appropriate to withdraw life prolonging treatment, but this may require application to the courts.

Parkinson's disease and other movement disorders

Parkinson's disease

Definition
A common degenerative disease of dopaminergic neurones characterised by tremor, bradykinesia, rigidity and postural instability.

Incidence
1 in 1000 adults and 1 in 200 over the age of 65.

Age
Prevalence increases sharply with age.

Sex
M slightly > F

Geography
Common worldwide

Aetiology
There is little known about the aetiology
- Nicotine: Some epidemiological evidence suggests a decreased risk in smokers, but that may be due to younger death in this group.
- There are some familial forms, particularly early-onset Parkinson's.

Pathophysiology
The substantia nigra is one of the nuclei of the basal ganglia. In Parkinson's disease there is progressive cell loss and the appearance of eosinophilic inclusion bodies (Lewy bodies) in the dopamine-rich part of the substantia nigra (called the pars compacta). Biochemically there is a loss of dopamine and melanin in the striatum which correlates with the degree of akinesia. Degeneration also occurs in other brain stem nuclei. The basal ganglia project via a dopaminergic pathway to the thalamus and then to the cerebral cortex, where it integrates with the pyramidal pathway to control movement. Hence it is sometimes called the extrapyramidal system.

Clinical features
The features are asymmetrical.
- The tremor is slow 4–6 Hz, typically pill-rolling and may involve the whole limb, legs and trunk. It is increased by emotion and decreased on action.
- Increased tone and tremor together cause a cog wheeling rigidity. Increased tone alone may cause lead-pipe rigidity.
- The movement disorder consists of bradykinesia (slowness of movement) and hypokinesia (reduced size of movement). For example, tapping one hand on the other is slow, of reduced amplitude and frequency.
- The gait is characteristic, with difficulty initiating movement (hesitancy), then difficulty in stopping (festination), slowness or freezing when asked to turn. When walking there may be a reduced arm swing and increased pill-rolling tremor. The posture is usually stooped, flexed and the person has difficulty in keeping balance (postural instability), falling whilst standing or walking. There is a loss of postural reflexes.
- Other features include facial masking, dribbling of saliva, dysphagia, dysphonia and dysarthria – quiet monotonous speech with a tendency to peter out with continued effort. There is an increased incidence of dementia in Parkinson's disease.

Macroscopy/microscopy
Loss of pigment from the substantia nigra due to the death of melanin-containing dopaminergic neurones. Surviving cells contain spherical inclusions called Lewy bodies – hyaline centres with a pale halo.

Investigations
Clinical diagnosis, but other parkinsonian syndromes should be considered.

Management
This includes a multidisciplinary approach for this chronic disease, including education, support, physiotherapy and physical aids.
- Levodopa, a dopamine precursor, is the most important agent used. It is given with an peripheral dopa-decarboxylase inhibitor (such as carbidopa or benserazide) to prevent the conversion of l-dopa to dopamine peripherally, and so to reduce side-effects of dopamine such as nausea and hypotension. Levodopa exerts most effect on bradykinesia and rigidity (less on tremor).
  i After several years of treatment, patients develop 'on' periods when they have a good response to the medication, lasting a few hours, then an 'off' period, when they freeze. They may also have involuntary movements called dyskinesias, or painful dystonias (abnormal posturing – which may be an early feature). These appear to be due to the progressive degeneration of the neuronal terminals, such that dopamine is not taken up properly. It is speculated that they may be prevented by using other drugs to treat mild symptoms, and using drugs which may have a 'neuroprotective' action, e.g. by blocking free radicals, and preserve neuronal function.
  ii 'On/off' phenomenon may be treated by increasing the frequency of doses, or using catechol-O-methyl transferase (COMT) inhibitors such as entacapone which inhibit the peripheral and central metabolism of l-dopa and dopamine, so giving a more stable level.

- Dopamine agonists (such as bromocriptine, pramipexole, cabergolide and apomorphine) act directly on dopamine receptors, and are useful in patients who responded to l-dopa, but have developed l-dopa related dyskinesias. These may be considered first-line treatment in young patients. They have a neuroprotective effect *in vitro*.
- Anticholinergic agents may improve symptoms. In PD there is a relative overstimulation at the basal ganglia by cholinergics compared to dopamine. This can be redressed by anticholinergic drugs such as benztropine and procyclidine. They tend only to be used in mild tremor, and they do not help with akinesia or gait.
- Selegiline is a monoamine oxidase B inhibitor which slows the catabolism of dopamine. It is useful in early Parkinson's.
- Amantadine is an antiviral agent, which is thought to act by increasing dopamine release and having NMDA receptor antagonist properties. It may be of value in mild early cases and has the advantage of few side-effects.
- Depression is common, difficult to treat and makes Parkinson's disease worse. Hallucinations due to medication and insomnia also occur frequently.

Surgery: These procedures are reserved for advanced cases.

- Stereotactic placement of small lesions in the ventrolateral nucleus of the thalamus can help tremor, but does not help bradykinesia. Unilateral pallidotomy (removal of or lesions made in the globus pallidus) can help tremor, rigidity, bradykinesia and postural instability. However surgery carries the risk of haemorrhage or infarction in 4%, with a 1% mortality.
- High frequency deep brain stimulation suppresses neuronal activity. Bilateral subthalamic nucleus stimulation or globus pallidus stimulation is most useful in those with difficulty with the on-off phenomenon, as it can improve motor function whilst off medication and dyskinesias whilst on medication. There is a risk of infection from the equipment.

Prognosis

The course of Parkinson's disease is very variable. The average survival is ~10 years from onset of symptoms. Drugs appear not to prolong life but levodopa has greatly improved quality of life.

With initial treatment:
~1/3 improve markedly;
1/3 show some improvement;
1/3 show no significant improvement, which should prompt the search for another cause of the symptoms, as other causes of parkinsonism do not usually respond to the treatment for idiopathic Parkinson's disease.

Other causes of Parkinsonism

Definition

There are certain disorders that mimic idiopathic Parkinson's disease, i.e. with tremor, bradykinesia and rigidity but do not respond to the usual treatments.

Aetiology

The main causes are cerebrovascular disease, antidopaminergic drugs such as neuroleptic drugs, e.g. haloperidol, reserpine and the anti-emetic metoclopramide.

There are also specific 'Parkinson's plus' syndromes where there is evidence of other neurological deficit:

- Multiple system atrophy (MSA) is parkinsonism in association with autonomic failure in particular postural hypotension and urinary dysfunction. It groups together the syndromes previously known as olivopontocerebellar atrophy, Shy–Drager syndrome and striatonigral degeneration.
- Progressive supranuclear palsy (PSP) is parkinsonism with downward gaze palsy (a loss of the ability to look downwards). It tends to cause a rapid deterioration, with marked postural instability, frequent falls and difficulty swallowing. In later disease, behavioural changes such as emotional lability and personality changes, disordered sleep and cognitive loss are features, which may lead to the initial diagnosis of dementia.

Pathophysiology

Cerebrovascular parkinsonism is likely to be due to progressive loss of dopaminergic neurons due to small vessel disease. Drugs which interfere with the dopamine pathway tend to cause bradykinesia and rigidity, but with less tremor, and the symptoms reverse on stopping the medication.

Clinical features

Features that suggest other causes of parkinsonism include:

- Symmetry of signs (Parkinson's disease is usually asymmetrical).
- History of drug use, in particular dopamine antagonists.
- Additional neurology such as upgoing plantars or cerebellar signs.
- Early dementia, prominent hallucinations, autonomic neuropathy and axial rigidity are signs of Parkinson's plus syndromes:

Management

Levodopa and other treatments used in Parkinson's disease tend to have little or no effect, therefore withdrawal of the causative drug, or supportive treatment. PSP and MSA may respond to dopamine agonists, but postural hypotension tends to be exacerbated by medication.

Benign essential tremor

Definition

An action tremor without features of parkinsonism.

Aetiology/pathophysiology

Often inherited as an autosomal dominant trait. It tends to present in the teens or in the elderly and affects males and females equally.

Clinical features

A symmetrical, flexion-extension tremor, affecting the hands and head in particular, and sometimes the voice. Oscillations are not usually present at rest, but occur posturally, e.g. holding a newspaper, and are increased by anxiety and movement.

Management

Treatment is often unnecessary, small doses of a β adrenergic blocker such as propranolol or primidone often reduce the tremor. The condition is slowly progressive and may cause some disability.

Huntington's disease

Definition

Genetically inherited progressive chorea and dementia.

Incidence

1 in 20,000

Age

Peak presentation in middle age.

Sex

M = F

Geography

Worldwide

Aetiology

Huntington's disease is an autosomal dominant condition with full penetrance.

Pathophysiology

There is an expanded trinucleotide repeat sequence (CAG) mutation on the short arm of chromosome 4. Normally, the number of repeats is less than 35, but once this increases to over 36, the gene product called huntingtin causes the disease. The more repeats there are, the earlier and the more severe the disease is, and the expansion tends to increase in subsequent generations (genetic anticipation). It is not clear how the abnormal protein causes the neuropathological effects, but it is thought that the mutant protein may cause biochemical effects, increase apoptosis and also (by interfering with the normal protein) downregulate neuronal growth factors:

- There is atrophy of the caudate nucleus and putamen in particular (these basal ganglia nuclei are important in control of movement). There is also diffuse cerebral atrophy (which would account for dementia).
- There are neurochemical effects, such as a depletion of acetylcholine and GABA but an increase in somatostatin and other hormones in the striatum. This results in a loss of inhibition of the dopaminergic pathway, i.e. release of dopamine which leads to chorea.

Clinical features

The disease usually manifests as progressive cognitive impairment and increasing movement disorder. Chorea consists of jerky, quasi-purposeful and sometimes explosive movements, following each other but flitting from one part of the body. When seen in middle age

Huntington's disease should be suspected. The family history may be concealed or unknown.

Macroscopy/microscopy

Marked loss of small neurones in the caudate nucleus and putamen.

Investigations

Genetic analysis is becoming available for pre-symptomatic testing but this raises an ethical dilemma, as there is no treatment. However, it is important, as many young adults wish to know their status before embarking upon having a family.

Management

No treatment arrests the disease but dopamine-blocking drugs such as haloperidol and dopamine-depleting drugs such as tetrabenazine may help to control the chorea. Patients and their families should be offered genetic testing and counselling where appropriate.

Prognosis

There is a relentless progression of dementia and chorea with death usually occurring within 20 years from the onset of symptoms.

Multiple sclerosis

Definition

An immune-mediated disease characterised by discrete areas of demyelination in the brain and spinal cord.

Incidence/prevalence

About 60 per 100,000 in England.

Age

Peak onset is between the ages of 25 and 40 years, uncommonly presents over the age of 60.

Sex

Women slightly more than men (1.7:1).

Geography

The disease shows strong geographical variation, with whites having twice the risk of non-whites and those in higher latitudes (i.e. colder climates) having higher risk.

Aetiology

There are several factors postulated.
- It is thought that there is an abnormal immune response, possibly triggered by an unknown viral antigen.
- Genetic predisposition to the disease – monozygotic twins have a 20–40% concordance, whereas siblings and dizygotic twins have a 3–5% risk.
- There is an association with HLA-A3, B7, DR2 and DR3.
- Childhood exposure to some environmental factor – migration before the age of 15 years leads to the risk of MS becoming that of the new country.

Pathophysiology

Discrete areas of demyelination called 'plaques' ranging in size from a few millimetres to a few centimetres. They are often perivenous and common sites in the brain include the optic nerve, around the lateral ventricles and in the brainstem and cerebellar peduncles. The cervical spinal cord is also commonly affected, but any part of the central white matter may be involved. The myelin of the peripheral nerves is not affected.

Initial oedema around the soft patches of white matter leads to symptoms that partially resolve as the oedema subsides.

The areas of demyelination are disseminated in time and place.

Clinical features

There are several patterns of the course of MS.
- Relapsing-remitting MS affects about 20–30% of patients, with lesions (and symptoms and signs) affecting different areas of the CNS at different times, with full or partial recovery between episodes, but no progression between.
- Primary-progressive MS affects 10–20% (particularly older patients), the pattern is that of chronic progressive deterioration from the time of onset.

- Secondary-progressive MS (about 40%) when the initial onset is of relapsing-remitting, then after several years this becomes a chronic progressive form of the disease.

Examples of clinical features include the following:

- Optic neuritis – usually unilateral visual loss which progresses over days, which may be mild or severe. Pain in or behind the eye, exacerbated by movement, is common. On examination there is loss of visual acuity and colour vision, a central scotoma and fundoscopy may demonstrate a swollen optic disc (in retrobulbar neuritis, where the optic nerve is affected, the disc looks normal). In an initial presentation of unilateral optic neuritis, only about half of patients will go on to develop MS.
- There may be motor, sensory, bladder, bowel or sexual disturbances. There may be hemiparesis, paraparesis or monoparesis. On examination, upper motor neurone signs are found (i.e. increased tone, pyramidal distribution of weakness, brisk reflexes, upgoing plantars and loss of abdominal reflexes).
- Lhermitte's phenomenon is suggestive of MS – lightning like pains going down into the spine or limbs which occurs on neck flexion.
- Visual disturbances such as diplopia due to VIth nerve palsy or internuclear ophthalmoplegia. Internuclear ophthalmoplegia is a horizontal gaze palsy resulting from a lesion affecting the medial longitudinal fasciculus (MLF) in the brainstem or pons. When a patient attempts lateral gaze there is an inability to adduct the eye which is ipsilateral to the MLF lesion and the contralateral eye fully abducts but with nystagmus.
- Cerebellar involvement may also cause other cerebellar signs may occur.
- Depression and intellectual impairment are common in long-standing MS, especially with widespread cerebral hemisphere involvement.

The diagnosis may be made clinically if there are two or more attacks separated in time with, clinical evidence of lesions in different areas. Following a single attack or clinical evidence of only one lesion area the diagnosis may still be made if there is radiological evidence of two or more lesions in time or space (McDonald Criteria).

Microscopy

Loss of myelin associated with lymphocytic cuffing of small vessels. In fresh lesions, increased numbers of macrophages phagocytose the damaged myelin and form foam cells. Old lesions are firm, grey-pink 'burnt-out plaques' that have very few inflammatory cells and are dominated by astrocytes.

Investigations

- MRI brain and spinal cord shows increased intensity lesions on T2-weighted images, gadolinium will cause enhancement of an acute lesion on T1-weighted images.
- CSF shows oligoclonal bands of IgG only within the CNS (i.e. not found in serum). This test is only positive in ~90% and false positives can occur.
- Electrophysiological tests: visual brainstem, somatosensory and auditory evoked responses may demonstrate previously subclinical lesions.

Management

Supportive management and counselling, physiotherapy as indicated. Bladder symptoms, muscle spasms, pain and other problems are treated appropriately.

- Short course, high-dose oral or intravenous steroids are used in acute relapses. These cause more rapid improvement, but do not appear to reduce the residual neurological deficit. They are therefore usually reserved for disabling visual or motor disease.
- Recently β interferon has been used in clearly relapsing-remitting MS to reduce relapse rate by 1/3 and it reduces the number of lesions seen on MRI. However, it is not widely available and its effects are limited.
- The progressive forms of the disease are more difficult to treat, and immunosuppressive drugs have been used. β interferon may be useful in secondary-progressive MS.

Prognosis

The prognosis of multiple sclerosis is very variable, the relapsing-remitting pattern having a better prognosis than the progressive forms. Death eventually occurs after late-stage disease (optic atrophy, spastic quadriparesis, brain-stem and cerebellar disease) typically from complications of immobility.

CNS causes of headache

Hydrocephalus

Definition
The term hydrocephalus is used to describe conditions in which there is enlargement of the cerebral ventricles due to an increase in the CSF volume within the ventricles and CSF spaces.

Aetiology
Hydrocephalus can be divided into obstructive/non-communicating hydrocephalus, in which there is a blockage of the passage of the CSF within or between the ventricles, and communicating hydrocephalus, in which there is impaired resorption of the CSF in the subarachnoid space.

Obstructive hydrocephalus: One or more cerebral ventricles may be dilated, depending on the site of obstruction.
- Primary or secondary tumours of the posterior fossa or brain stem.
- Subarachnoid haemorrhage, head injury and meningitis.
- Aqueductal stenosis.
- Cerebral haemorrhage, abscesses or cysts.

Communicating hydrocephalus:
- Normal pressure hydrocephalus – there is interference with the normal flow and resorption of CSF in the subarachnoid space. It may be associated with previous subarachnoid haemorrhage or meningitis, but usually there is no cause found.
- Intracranial venous thrombosis
- Basilar meningeal disease affecting the subarachnoid space.

Pathophysiology
Normally, CSF produced in the choroid plexus of the lateral ventricles flows through the foramen of Monro into the slit like third ventricle and then through the narrow aqueduct of the upper brain stem. It then flows into the fourth ventricle, where there are three apertures which allow the CSF to drain into the subarachnoid space. It flows over the surface of the brain and spinal cord and is normally reabsorbed through the arachnoid villi into the cerebral veins.

Clinical features
- In acute hydrocephalus the raised intracranial pressure results in headache, vomiting, gait apraxia and disturbance in consciousness.
- In chronic or less acute hydrocephalus signs and symptoms include headache (typically present on waking, made worse by coughing, straining or sneezing), vomiting and papilloedema. Any shift in the cranial contents can produce a variety of signs and symptoms including focal neurological signs, e.g. sixth nerve palsy.
- Normal pressure hydrocephalus presents with one or more of dementia, ataxia and urinary incontinence.

Complications
Raised intracranial pressure may lead to cerebral oedema, bradycardia and hypertension. Compression of the medulla due to cerebral herniation (coning) causes impaired consciousness, respiratory depression and death.

Investigations
Lumbar puncture is contraindicated in obstructive hydrocephalus due to the risk of coning. CT brain should be performed in attempt to identify the enlarged ventricles and to differentiate between communicating and non-communicating hydrocephalus. In normal pressure hydrocephalus, if removal of CSF by LP improves symptoms and signs, patients may benefit from CSF shunting.

Management
In all cases, treatment is aimed at the underlying cause. However, emergency treatment to reduce intracranial pressure and maintain cerebral perfusion may be required:
- General measures include ensuring good oxygen supply, avoiding hypercapnia, and maintaining systemic blood pressure. Steroids and mannitol are used in certain circumstances.
- Drainage of the ventricles is achieved by a frontal burr hole and extraventricular drain, which also allows intracranial pressure monitoring.
- If the blockage is not amenable to surgical correction a ventricular shunt may be inserted. A catheter is introduced into the lateral ventricle and tunnelled

subcutaneously into the neck and into the peritoneal cavity. The shunt has a one way valve but blockage leads to an acute hydrocephalus. Shunts may become infected.

Idiopathic intracranial hypertension

Definition
A syndrome of raised intracranial pressure without obvious cause.

Aetiology
A condition mainly affecting overweight young women. A similar condition is seen secondary to endocrine abnormalities, polycystic ovaries, vitamin A toxicity, steroids and other drugs.

Clinical features
Patients present with headache, visual obscurations and may have tinnitus. On fundoscopy they have papilloedema. In more advanced cases an enlarged blind spot, visual field loss or a sixth cranial nerve palsy may occur. Severe untreated disease may result in ischaemia of the optic nerve presenting with progressive blindness.

Investigations
CT brain is normal (there are no mass lesions or ventricular dilatation). CSF examination is normal although there is increased CSF pressure. MRI may be performed to exclude intracranial venous thrombosis. Repeated formal visual field assessment is required.

Management
No treatment is of proven benefit; however, therapies aim to conserve vision.
- The acute stages can be managed with repeated lumbar puncture and diuretics.
- If the pressure is severe and vision threatened optic nerve sheath decompression/fenestration may be indicated.
- Recurrence prevention includes weight reduction; however, a lumboperitoneal shunt may be appropriate in patients requiring repeated CSF drainage.

Migraine

Definition
Episodic headache which may be associated with visual and gastrointestinal disturbance.

Incidence
10% of the population.

Age
Usually starts around puberty.

Sex
F > M

Aetiology
The cause is unknown although there is a familial tendency. Precipitating factors include:
- Emotion: anxiety, depression, shock, excitement.
- Alcohol, chocolate, coffee are reported as potential triggers.
- Migraine is common premenstrually and around the menopause.

Pathophysiology
The exact pathophysiology is unclear:
- It has been suggested that migrainous headaches are due to vasodilatation, with auras due to preceding vasoconstriction.
- A second theory suggests that there is a primary neurological dysfunction, probably originating in the brainstem, which then causes secondary neurovascular changes. The primary event appears to cause a wave of cortical hypoperfusion and hence neurological dysfunction (associated with the aura phase) which then precipitates the headache by activating the trigeminal nerve which leads to pain by neuroinflammatory changes (release of pain-causing peptides and vasodilatation) at the meninges.
- Serotonin (5-hydroxytryptamine (5-HT)) plays an important role probably via effects on the vasculature and on neurological function. Serum levels of hydroxytryptamine rise at the onset of the prodromal symptoms and fall during the headache.
- Ischaemia and/or depression of cortical function may cause focal neurological symptoms, e.g. hemiplegic migraine.

Clinical features

Can be divided into prodromal symptoms, aura and headache.

- Prodromal symptoms may last a few days and include mood and appetite changes.
- The aura is usually visual, e.g. visual obscurations, flashing lights, distortion, but may involve other senses, motor or speech dysfunction. Each symptom lasts up to an hour.
- The headache begins as the aura fades. It is unilateral in two-thirds of cases, bifrontal or generalised in others. It may be unilateral, then become generalised. The pain may be dull or pulsating and is usually exacerbated by movement, coughing or sneezing. Associated symptoms include photophobia, nausea and vomiting. The headache typically lasts several hours and may last up to several days.
- Migraine without aura occurs in 80% of migraine sufferers.

Investigations

In most cases, none are necessary. If there are neurological abnormalities on examination CT or MRI brain may be performed.

Management

General measures include reassurance and avoidance of precipitating factors.

- Treatment of the headache involves the use of simple analgesics especially NSAIDs which are most effective if taken early. The 5-hydroxytryptamine agonists (triptans) may be very effective. Anti-emetics may be of value.
- Prophylactic agents are used in patients with frequent headaches. They include pizotifen (a 5-hydroxytryptamine antagonists), propranolol, tricyclic antidepressants such as amitryptiline and anticonvulsants such as sodium valproate.

Tension headache

Definition

Recurrent headaches which are usually feel like a band or tight sensation around the head.

Aetiology/pathophysiology

The most common type of headache. The aetiology of tension headache is not known although possible factors include stress, concentrated visual effort, previous head injury and analgesia abuse. It appears that the mechanisms of tension headache are similar to migraine, although to a lesser degree.

Clinical features

Some patients have almost daily headaches, with the pain constant or waxing and waning. They complain of a band around the head, pressure behind the eyes and a dull or throbbing headache. The presence of a long history of such headaches is very suggestive of tension headache.

Investigations

CT brain is not usually indicated. In acute cases in older patients, an ESR should be sent to exclude temporal arteritis.

Management

Reassurance, avoiding any precipitating factors and treatment with analgesics such as paracetamol or NSAIDs. Combination drugs which include caffeine, codeine or ergotamine should be avoided, as they can cause rebound headaches and substance dependency. Chronic tension headaches may be relieved by the use of amitryptiline.

Trigeminal neuralgia

Definition

Intermittent excruciating pain in the distribution of one or more branches of the trigeminal nerve.

Aetiology/pathophysiology

Trigeminal neuralgia is generally idiopathic. There appears to be demyelination of the trigeminal nerve root, in some cases it is hypothesised that this occurs due to compression by a vessel, tumour or cyst. Multiple sclerosis is a well-described cause.

Clinical features

Severe, brief stabbing or electric shock-like pain, usually unilateral, and affecting part of the face (ophthalmic, maxillary or mandibular branch(es)). Severe pain may lead to facial grimacing ('tic doloureux'). It may be precipitated light touch in the distribution of the affected nerve, or other actions such as chewing, talking, exposure to cold air. If there are neurological signs on examination then an underlying pathology should be suspected.

Investigations
The diagnosis is clinical. In certain patients, MRI to exclude MS, or an underlying tumour is indicated (i.e. under the age of 40, bilateral symptoms, no response to conservative therapy, sensory loss).

Management
Carbamazepine can be effective. Combination therapy, by adding other anti-epileptic drugs or clonazepam may be useful. Refractory neuralgia may require surgical treatment such as microvascular decompression or alcohol injection into the Gasserian ganglion.

Prognosis
Remissions for months or years may occur, often followed by recurrence.

Temporal arteritis
See page 378 in Chapter 8 (Musculoskeletal System)

Motor neurone disease

Definition
Progressive neurodegenerative disorder of upper and lower motor neurones.

Incidence/prevalence
1–2 per 100,000 per annum with a prevalence of 6 in 100,000.

Age
Onset usually in middle age.

Sex
Men slightly more common than females.

Aetiology
Unknown cause, although in about 5% of cases, there is autosomal dominant inheritance and the condition has been localised to chromosome 21.

Clinical features
Motor neurone disease causes mixed upper and lower motor neurone signs. The ocular movements are not affected, there are never sensory, cerebellar or extrapyramidal signs, awareness is preserved and dementia is unusual. Three patterns are recognised depending on which group of motor neurones is lost first; however, most patients progress to a combination of the syndromes.
- Amyotrophic lateral sclerosis is disease of the lateral corticospinal tracts. Amyotrophy means atrophy of muscle. The clinical picture is that of a progressive spastic tetra or paraparesis with additional lower motor neurone signs. Typical clinical findings include spasticity, reduced power, muscle fasciculation and brisk reflexes with upgoing plantars.
- Progressive bulbar palsy is a disease of the lower cranial nerve nuclei and their supranuclear connections. The features are those of a bulbar and pseudobulbar palsy with upper and lower motor neurone signs, i.e. progressive loss of power in the muscles of facial expression, muscles of mastication, articulation and swallowing. The tongue appears wasted and fasiculating. There may be nasal regurgitation and an increased risk of aspiration pneumonia.
- Progressive muscular atrophy starts with muscle wasting in the small muscles of one hand and spreads throughout the arm. It often becomes bilateral over time. There is wasting and weakness with fasciculations and variable reflexes (increased if upper motor neurones affected at the level of the reflex, decreased or absent if lower motor neurones are affected).

Microscopy
There is loss of motor neurones from the cortex, brain stem and spinal cord. There is gliosis with secondary degeneration of the motor tracts. Inclusion bodies containing ubiquitin (a protein involved in the removal of damaged cell proteins) are found in the surviving neurones.

Complications

Weakness of respiratory muscles with risk of pneumonia and respiratory failure. Swallowing difficulties predispose to aspiration pneumonia.

Investigations

There are no specific diagnostic tests. Denervation may be confirmed by electromyography, the CSF is usually normal although protein may be raised. MRI of the cervical spine is indicated if there are predominantly upper limb signs with or without lower limb upper motor neurone signs.

Management

Supportive measures such as splints and crutches may be useful, and communication aids for dysarthria. Riluzole, a glutamate antagonist has been shown to improve prognosis by a few months.

Prognosis

Remission is unknown, the disease progresses gradually and causes death, often from bronchopneumonia. Survival for more than 3 years is unusual although there are rare 'benign' forms of the condition with prolonged survival.

Disorders of the spinal cord

Spinal cord lesions

Spinal cord lesions usually produce upper motor neurone signs with associated sensory deficit (see Fig. 7.3). Nerve roots at the level of the lesion may also be affected resulting in some lower motor neurone signs.

- The motor pathways and vibration and proprioception cross in the medulla, so that lesions in the spinal cord cause ipsilateral deficits.
- Pain and temperature nerves enter the spinal cord, ascend a few segments and then cross the centre of the cord to ascend in the contralateral anterior horn, so that lesions in the spinal cord cause contralateral deficits.

Transverse section of the spinal cord

Injury at a cervical level causes quadriplegia and total symmetrical anaesthesia. Injury at thoracic or lumbar levels causes paraplegia and bilateral symmetrical anaesthesia below the level of the lesion.

Motor: LMN signs at level, UMN signs below the level.

Sensory: The sensory level, below which there is loss of cutaneous sensation, indicates the site of a spinal cord lesion.

Sphincter control: Loss of bladder and bowel control.

Causes include fracture dislocation of vertebrae, penetrating trauma, transverse myelitis or compression due to a tumour.

Hemisection of the spinal cord Brown–Séquard syndrome

Motor: Ipsilateral LMN signs at level and UMN signs below.

Sensory: Below the level of the lesion there is ipsilateral vibration and proprioceptive loss, and contralateral loss of pain and temperature sensation. Light touch is often reduced.

Causes include multiple sclerosis, trauma, tumour (angioma) and degeneration due to radiation.

Posterior columns

Disease of the posterior columns causes an unsteady gait (sensory ataxia) due to loss of position sense in the legs and uncertainty of foot position. Sensation to light touch and proprioception are lost.

Causes include:

- Subacute combined degeneration of the cord (vitamin B_{12} deficiency): There are UMN signs in the lower limbs due to the disease also affecting the lateral corticospinal tracts. There may be an associated peripheral neuropathy which may reduce or abolish tendon reflexes, masking the expected UMN findings.
- Multiple sclerosis.
- Tabes dorsalis (3° syphilis): Degeneration of the dorsal roots initially followed by posterior column involvement. It is characterised by shooting pains, with loss of proprioception, numbness or paraesthesia.
- HIV infection.

Central cord lesion (syringomyelia)

Syringomyelia is a fluid-filled cavity in the spinal cord associated with Arnold–Chiari malformations, spinal cord

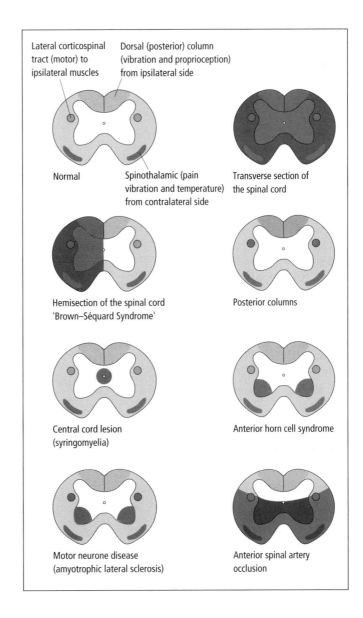

Normal

Lateral corticospinal tract (motor) to ipsilateral muscles

Dorsal (posterior) column (vibration and proprioception) from ipsilateral side

Spinothalamic (pain vibration and temperature) from contralateral side

Transverse section of the spinal cord

Hemisection of the spinal cord 'Brown–Séquard Syndrome'

Posterior columns

Central cord lesion (syringomyelia)

Anterior horn cell syndrome

Motor neurone disease (amyotrophic lateral sclerosis)

Anterior spinal artery occlusion

Figure 7.3 Spinal cord lesions.

tumours and trauma. Usually localised to a few segments, commonly affecting the cervical canal.

Motor: (Early) anterior horn cells compressed at that level causing wasting and reduced reflexes; (late) corticospinal tracts involved, causing UMN signs below that level.

Sensory: (Early) decussating spinothalamic tracts affected, causing reduced pain and temperature sensation, only in the affected segments (or just below). Sensation in the lower limbs is preserved.

Late posterior column involvement, when all levels below are affected.

Anterior horn cell syndrome

Motor: LMN signs, which may be unilateral (ipsilateral to the lesion) or bilateral.

Specific loss of these cells occurs in motor neurone disease (see also below) and poliomyelitis.

Motor neurone disease – 'amyotrophic lateral sclerosis'

The commonest pattern of MND affects the anterior horn cells and the lateral corticospinal tracts. It is characterised by mixed UMN and LMN signs. Patients often present with spastic quadriparesis, brisk reflexes and upgoing plantars (UMN signs), fasciculation may be present. With progression, muscle wasting and fasciculation may become more obvious. No sensory signs, although sensory symptoms may be reported.

Anterior spinal artery occlusion

Motor: Flaccid paraplegia, urinary retention.
Sensory: Loss of pain and temperature sensation (the dorsal column sensory pathways may be totally or only partly spared).

It is associated with atherosclerosis and dissecting abdominal aortic aneurysm. Total loss of blood flow causes an acute presentation, milder UMN & LMN symptoms may occur in 'transient ischaemic attacks', which may partially recover.

Spinal cord compression

Definition

Spinal cord compression is a medical emergency, as without rapid relief of the compression, permanent neurological deficit results.

Aetiology

Causes are shown in Table 7.11.

Clinical features

Patients may present with clumsiness, weakness, loss of sensation, loss of bowel or bladder control which may begin as urinary hesitancy and urgency progressing to painless urinary retention. Back pain may precede the presentation with cord compression for many months and there may be radicular pain at the level of compression (radiating around the chest for thoracic lesions and into the limb(s) for cervical and lumbar lesions). On examination there may be a spastic paraparesis or tetraparesis with weakness, increased reflexes and upgoing

Table 7.11 Causes of spinal cord compression

Lesion	Examples
Tumours	
Vertebral	Metastases or myeloma
Extradural	Lymphoma, metastases (lung, breast, prostate)
Extramedullary	Meningioma, neurofibroma
Intramedullar	Glioma, ependymoma
Disc lesions	Trauma, chronic degenerative, prolapse
Infections	Epidural abscess, tuberculosis, granuloma
Epidural haemorrhage	Spontaneous or traumatic

plantars. There is variable sensory loss below the level of the lesion.

- Conus medullaris: Compression of the sacral segments of the cord causes early disturbance of bladder and bowel control, there is reduced sensation over the perianal region.
- Cauda equina lesion: Compression below L1 affects the spinal nerves and cauda equina resulting in a flaccid, asymmetrical paraparesis. Reflexes are loss and there is loss of sensation over the perianal region (saddle anaesthesia). However, bladder and bowel control are preserved until relatively late.

Investigations

Plain spinal films may show bone disease, urgent MRI spine or myelography (injection of water-soluble contrast into the lumbar subarachnoid space) is required in acute cases. MRI is most useful as it can demonstrate most causes of spinal cord compression.

Management

Identification and treatment aimed at the underlying cause. In as many as 20% of cases, the cord compression is the initial presentation of an underlying malignancy. Radiotherapy is used for metastases, in other causes urgent neurosurgical decompression is required to maximise return of function.

Prognosis

Prognosis is related to the degree of damage and speed of decompression. Bladder control that has been lost for more than 24 hours is usually not regained.

Syringomyelia and syringobulbia

Definition
A syrinx is a fluid filled slit like cavity developing in the spinal cord (syringomyelia) or the brain stem (syringobulbia).

Age
Usually presents aged 20–40 years.

Sex
M = F

Aetiology
The cavity or syrinx is in continuity with the central canal of the spinal cord. It is associated with a history of birth injury, bony abnormalities at the foramen magnum, spina bifida, Arnold–Chiari malformation (herniation of the cerebellar tonsils and medulla through the foramen magnum) or hydrocephalus.

Pathophysiology
The expanding cavity may destroy spinothalamic neurones in the cervical cord, anterior horn cells and lateral corticospinal tracts.

Clinical features
Mixed upper and motor neurone signs, sometimes in an odd distribution, it is usually bilateral, but may affect one side more than the other.

- Syringomyelia: There is typically wasting of the intrinsic muscles of the hand, with loss of upper limb reflexes and spastic weakness in the legs. The sensory changes are loss of pain and temperature sensation in the affected levels, e.g. C5 to T1 with preservation of touch. Neuropathic joints, neuropathic ulcers and accidental trauma and burns may result.
- Syringobulbia: When the cavity extends into the brain stem the lower cranial nerves are affected – the tongue is atrophied and fasciculates, there may be nystagmus, dysarthria, Horner's syndrome. Involvement of the fifth nerve nuclei causes loss of facial sensation, classically in a circumferential pattern, and the VIIIth nerve nucleus may be affected causing hearing loss.

Investigations
Diagnosed by CT or MRI scanning.

Management
Decompression of the foramen magnum, aspiration of the syrinx, sometimes with placement of a shunt may halt progression.

Prognosis
Condition is intermittently progressive over a number of decades.

Transverse myelitis

Definition
Acute inflammation of the spinal cord.

Aetiology
Causes include syphilis, viral and mycoplasma infections, multiple sclerosis, systemic lupus erythematosus and post-radiation therapy. Some cases have been reported post-vaccination. Many cases are idiopathic.

Pathophysiology
Inflammation may be due to vasculitis, or the preceding infection. There is oedema of the cord, which causes upper motor neurone signs below the level of the lesion, usually a paraparesis, and sensory loss up to the level of the lesion. Sphincter dysfunction may occur.

Clinical features
Spinal shock, i.e. a flaccid weakness may initially occur, which then becomes a spastic paraparesis. The patient may complain of a tight band around the chest, which may suggest the level of the lesion. Upper motor neurone signs are found below the lesion. Occasionally lower motor neurone signs are found at the level of the lesion, due to involvement of the anterior horn cells.

Investigations
MRI may show oedema and excludes a space-occupying lesion. CSF may be normal, or show increased protein content and pleocytosis. Other investigations are directed at the underlying cause, e.g. syphilis serology, mycoplasma titres, anti-dsDNA (for SLE).

Management
Steroids may be used, once infection has been excluded, to speed recovery. Vasculitis may need aggressive

management. Supportive management, including physiotherapy.

Prognosis
Most idiopathic and post-infectious cases improve with time.

Disorders of muscle and neuromuscular junction

Muscular dystrophies

Myotonic dystrophy

Definition
Inherited disease of adults causing progressive muscle weakness. Myotonia is a continued muscle contraction after the cessation of voluntary contraction.

Incidence
Affects 1 in 8000 of the population.

Age
Onset 20–50 years.

Sex
M = F

Aetiology/pathophysiology
Autosomal dominant condition with variable penetrance. Most patients have an amplified trinucleotide (CTG) repeat sequence in the DM(1) gene on chromosome 19. Myotonic dystrophy demonstrates genetic anticipation. Each generation has increased numbers of repeats resulting in an earlier onset and more severe disease. The gene codes for a protein kinase, which is present in many tissues, the mechanism by which this causes the observed clinical features is unknown.

Clinical features
Patients develop ptosis, weakness and thinning of the face and sternomastoids. They have myotonia, delayed muscle relaxation after contraction, e.g. slow relaxation of grip after shaking hands. Other features include cataracts, frontal baldness in males, mild intellectual impairment, dementia, cardiomyopathy and conduction defects, and weakness of distal limb muscles, which may

be severe in late stages. There is an increased risk of diabetes mellitus.

Investigations
EMG shows myopathic potentials and myotonia. The diagnosis can now be confirmed by genetic testing.

Microscopy
Affected muscles show abnormalities of fibre size, with fibre necrosis, abundant internal nuclei and replacement by fibrofatty tissue.

Complications
Patients show neurofibrillary tangles of Alzheimer's disease in the brain with ageing. Infants born to mothers with myotonic dystrophy may have profound hypotonia, feeding and respiratory difficulties, clubfeet and developmental delay.

Management
Phenytoin or procainamide may help the myotonia. Supportive splints and foot braces help distal limb weakness. Complications such as diabetes mellitus and cardiac failure should be regularly screened for. Patients should be offered genetic counselling as appropriate.

Prognosis
The condition is gradually progressive with a variable prognosis.

Neuromuscular junction disorders

Myasthenia gravis

Definition
Acquired disorder of the neuromuscular junction characterised by muscle fatiguability, ptosis & dysphagia.

Incidence
4 in 100,000.

Age
Peaks in women aged 20–40 and in men over age 60.

Sex
2F : 1M

Aetiology/pathophysiology

80–90% of cases have an autoantibody directed at the acetylcholine receptor. The thymus appears to be involved in the pathogenesis, with 25% of cases having a thymoma and a further 70% have thymic hyperplasia.

- There also appear to be genetic factors, such as an association with HLA-B8, DRw3 and it is associated with other autoimmune conditions including thyroid disease, rheumatoid arthritis, systemic lupus erythematosus (SLE) and pernicious anaemia.
- Myasthenic syndromes can be caused by D-Penicillamine, lithium and propranolol.

At the neuromuscular junction, immune complexes are deposited at the postsynaptic membrane causing interference with and later destruction of the acetylcholine receptor.

Clinical features

Fatiguability is the single most characteristic feature. Exercise increases the degree of muscle weakness, and rest allows recovery of power. Acute exacerbations are triggered by stress including surgery, and by drugs.

- It affects the extraocular muscles, causing variable ptosis (typically worse at the end of the day) and unusual abnormalities of eye movements. This causes diplopia and blurred vision. The pupils are spared.
- The muscles of mastication, speech and facial expression are affected. This can cause difficulty with swallowing and eating – the chin may need support whilst chewing, and a 'myasthenic snarl' when smiling.
- The proximal limb muscles show fatiguability on repeated use. The respiratory muscles may be affected in a myasthenic crisis requiring ventilatory support. Initially the reflexes are preserved but may be fatiguable, muscle wasting is a sign of late disease.

Complications

Transplacental passage of ACh-R antibodies can cause neonatal myasthenia gravis in 10–20% of neonates, which manifests with flaccidity, poor feeding and respiratory difficulties within the first 48 hours. It can last up to 3 weeks.

Investigations

- Edrophonium (anticholinesterase) – Tensilon test – injected i.v. as a test dose provides improvement within seconds lasting for 2–3 minutes.

- Serum acetylcholine receptor antibodies are present in 90% and are specific.
- Nerve stimulation shows characteristic decrement in evoked muscle action potentials following repetitive stimulation of the motor nerve.
- Scanning for thymic masses.
- Screening for associated disease such as hyperthyroidism, SLE and rheumatoid arthritis is useful.

Management

Oral anticholinesterases such as pyridostigmine treat the weakness but do not affect the course of the disease. Overdosage can cause weakness, probably due to excessive depolarization of the ACh receptor or desensitisation. Care should be taken when prescribing other medications as they may exacerbate the disease.

- Thymectomy improves symptoms and prognosis in those under the age of 60. Complete removal of the thymus is important. Thymectomy in older patients with hyperplasia alone is more controversial, tumours should however be removed. Increased weakness may occur acutely post-operatively, which can be managed by plasmapheresis.
- Corticosteroids can be used with good results in 70% despite risk of an initial relapse.
- In steroid resistant cases, azathioprine or ciclosporin may be added.
- Plasmapheresis and intravenous immunoglobulin are usually reserved for severe acute exacerbations.

Prognosis

Severity fluctuates but most have a protracted course, exacerbations are unpredictable but may be brought on by infections or drugs.

Eaton–Lambert syndrome

Definition

A rare paraneoplastic syndrome usually associated with small-call carcinoma (SCC) of the bronchus, causing muscle weakness.

Aetiology/pathophysiology

Antibodies directed against the presynaptic voltage-gated calcium channels have been detected. Around 70% have an underlying tumour, almost always SCC of the lung.

Clinical features

Proximal muscle weakness, particularly of the hips, later affecting the shoulders. Ptosis may occur. The ocular and bulbar muscles are typically spared. Unlike myasthenia gravis, weakness tends to be worst in the morning and improve with exercise. Reflexes are reduced, but normalise with exercise.

Investigations

- Nerve conduction studies show an incremental response when a motor nerve is repetitively stimulated, in direct contrast to the findings in myasthenia gravis (where there is a decremental response).
- Chest X-ray and CT screening for an underlying tumour.
- Specific serum antibodies can be detected.

Management

Treatment of the underlying tumour can lead to improvement. Plasmapheresis and intravenous immunoglobulin may be used, and drugs which increase acetylcholine release from presynaptic terminals appear to have symptomatic benefit.

Disorders of cranial and peripheral nerves

Cranial nerves

Olfactory nerve (I) lesion

Anatomy

The olfactory receptors lie in the olfactory epithelium in the upper part of the superior turbinate and the nasal septum. The axons form bundles which pass through the cribiform plate (ethmoid bone) to the olfactory bulb. The bundles are wrapped in meninges. The olfactory bulb neurones project through the olfactory tract to the frontal cerebral hemispheres, the medial temporal lobe and the basal ganglia.

Function

Smell

Specific causes

Trauma, frontal lobe tumour, meningitis.

Clinical features

Diminished sense of smell and taste (closely linked to smell) although this may be found in elderly patients without olfactory nerve lesions. Test ability of each nostril to detect several common smells.

The optic nerve

Anatomy

The optic nerve carries information from the retina via the optic chiasm, the lateral geniculate bodies and optic radiation to the occipital lobe where the visual cortex is situated.

Function

Vision

Clinical features

These depend on the location of the lesion (see Fig. 7.4).
Field loss:

- Eye lesions include diabetic retinal vascular disease, glaucoma, retinitis pigmentosa.
- Optic nerve lesions include multiple sclerosis, compression, syphilis, ischaemia, B_{12} deficiency.
- Optic chiasm lesions commonly caused by pituitary neoplasm, rarely secondary neoplasm.
- Optic tract lesions alone are rare but commonly occur as part of a middle cerebral artery stroke.
- Optic cortex lesions (macula spared) caused by posterior cerebral artery infarction. Widespread bilateral occipital damage, e.g. posterior circulation infarction causes cortical blindness (Anton's Syndrome) in which the patient lacks insight and denies blindness.
- Tunnel vision occurs in other conditions, e.g. in glaucoma or late retinitis pigmentosa.

Diseases affecting the optic nerve and the rest of the optic pathways may also affect visual acuity.

Abnormalities of the optic disc

Definition

The optic disc is where the retinal fibres meet to form the optic nerve. Diseases affecting the optic nerve may cause the disc to look abnormal:

1 Swollen, i.e. less cupped – papilloedema, optic neuritis (sometimes called papillitis)
2 Pale due to loss of axons and vascularity – optic atrophy

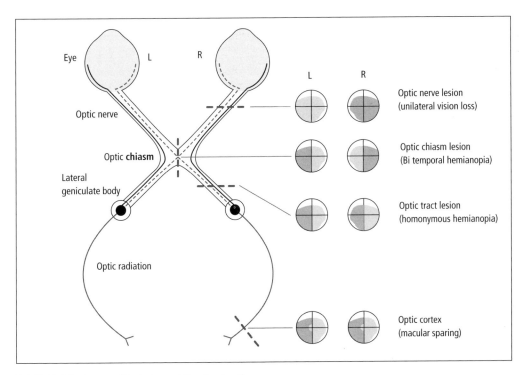

Figure 7.4 Field defects caused by lesions of the visual pathway.

Papilloedema

This term should be reserved to describe swelling of the optic disc due to raised intracranial pressure (or pressure behind the eye). The increased pressure causes axonal transport to become abnormal, causing swelling of the nerves. Papilloedema is usually (not always) bilateral, there is loss of venous pulsation, visual acuity is preserved (but with constriction of visual fields and an enlarged blind spot).

The term is often used to cover all causes of a swollen disc, but this is the differential diagnosis of papilloedema (see Table 7.12).

Optic atrophy

Optic atrophy may follow any damage to the optic nerve, particularly after ischaemia, optic neuritis and optic nerve compression. It may also be hereditary.

Clinical features

The degree of visual loss depends on the underlying cause. Optic neuritis and ischaemic neuropathy typically cause early visual loss.

Management

Directed at the underlying cause.

Horner's syndrome

Definition

A lesion of the sympathetic supply to one eye causing unilateral miosis (small pupil), slight ptosis, and anhydrosis.

Aetiology

Causes are given in Table 7.13.

Clinical features

The condition presents with unilateral pupillary constriction (miosis) with a slight ptosis and anhydrosis. The conjunctival vessels may be injected. Associated features may include a hoarse voice (due to either recurrent laryngeal nerve palsy or lower cranial nerve involvement), or signs in the neck, chest or hands pointing to the level of the lesion.

Table 7.12 Causes of papilloedema and other causes of a swollen optic disc

Causes of papilloedema	Causes
Space-occupying lesion	Tumour, abscess
Idiopathic (benign) intracranial hypertension	
Hydrocephalus	Obstructive or communicating
Other causes of a swollen disc	**Examples**
Optic nerve compression	Retro-orbital tumour – meningioma, metastases Graves' disease
Optic neuritis (inflammation of the optic nerve)	Multiple sclerosis, sarcoidosis, postviral, infectious
Ischaemic optic neuropathy	Temporal arteritis, retinal artery thrombosis, severe hypotension
Malignant hypertension	
Venous congestion	Cavernous sinus thrombosis, central retinal vein occlusion
Toxic	Ethambutol, methanol, alcohol, chloroquine
Metabolic	Vitamin A intoxication, hypercapnia, hypocalcaemia
Hereditary optic neuropathy	

Table 7.13 Causes of Horner's syndrome

Location of lesion	Examples
Sympathetic chain injury in the neck	Carotid artery aneurysm or dissection (most common)
	Iatrogenic, e.g. post-carotid artery surgery
	Malignancy, e.g. thyroid
	Trauma
Apex of the lung (T1 root)	Lung cancer, tuberculosis
Cervical cord lesions	Syringomyelia, cord tumours (rare)
Brainstem lesions	Vascular, especially lateral medullary syndrome
	Tumour
	Syringobulbia
Miscellaneous	Cluster headache

Investigations and management

A chest X-ray or MRI brain may be indicated to identify the underlying lesion. Treatment is directed at the underlying cause.

Oculomotor nerve (III) lesion

Arises anteriorly from the midbrain and passes between the posterior cerebral and superior cerebellar arteries, pierces the arachnoid dura and runs forward in the lateral wall of the cavernous sinus, then divides into:

- Superior ramus which enters orbit via the lower part of superior orbital fissure within a tendinous ring. It supplies superior rectus and levator palpebrae superioris muscles.
- Inferior ramus travels with superior ramus, but gives branches to inferior rectus and medial rectus muscles. It gives off a branch to the inferior oblique muscle, which carries parasympathetic nerve fibres to the ciliary ganglion, and thence to the pupillary sphincter and ciliary muscle.

Function

Full retraction of the upper eyelid, looking medially, pupillary constriction.

Specific causes

Affecting III alone (not IV and VI) – trauma, diabetes mellitus, giant cell arteritis, aneurysm of posterior communicating artery, idiopathic, raised intracranial pressure causing temporal lobe herniation, basal meningitis.

Clinical features

Ptosis, dilated unreactive pupil, eye turned down and out (divergent strabismus).

Trochlear nerve (IV) lesion

Anatomy

This motor nerve supplies superior oblique. It exits posteriorly from the brainstem and winds around to the front, then passes in the lateral wall of the cavernous sinus as far as the superior orbital fissure.

Function
Supplies superior oblique (moves the eye down and in).

Specific causes
Rare as isolated lesion, Generally occurs as a combined III, IV and VI nerve palsies (see below) when the eye is also intorted.

Clinical features
Diplopia on looking down or in.

Abducent nerve (VI) lesion

Anatomy
Supplies lateral rectus. It exits from the brainstem and runs through the subarachnoid space into the cavernous sinus, then passes through the superior orbital fissue.

Function
Lateral rectus deviates the eye laterally.

Specific causes
Particularly at risk from raised intracranial pressure or trauma due to its long course. Often occurs as a combined III, IV and VI nerve palsies

Clinical features
Diplopia on looking to the side. III, IV and VI combined nerve palsies are seen in stroke, tumours, Wernicke's encephalopathy, aneurysms and cavernous sinus thrombosis.

Trigeminal nerve (V) lesion

Anatomy
Emerges as two roots (large sensory and small motor root), passes out forwards the pons into the posterior cranial fossa and across the temporal lobe in the middle cranial fossa. The nerve expands to form the trigeminal ganglion, at the petrous temporal bone, and gives off 3 branches: ophthalmic (V_1), maxillary (V_2) and mandibular (V_3).

Function
The motor components supply the muscles of mastication and tensor tympani.

Table 7.14 Causes of trigeminal nerve (V) lesions

Location	Examples of causes
Brainstem (pons, medulla, upper cervical cord)	Infarct, tumour, multiple sclerosis, syringobulbia
Posterior fossa	Aneurysm, tumour, meningitis
Petrous temporal bone	Acoustic neuroma, trauma (fracture of bone), meningioma or other tumour
Cavernous sinus (only V_1 branch of V and usually III, IV and VI also affected)	Tumour, cavernous sinus thrombosis, aneurysm of the internal carotid.

The sensory components supply the sensation of the face:
1 V_1 supplies the forehead, the upper eyelid and eyeball.
2 V_2 supplies the lower eyelid, the side of the nose, the upper teeth and the upper lip.
3 V_3 supplies the mandible, the ear and the skin and mucous membranes of the lower jaw.

Pain and temperature fibres are also carried on the three divisions back to the trigeminal ganglion, but then dive down into the medulla to the spinal nucleus of V which extends as far as the upper cervical cord.

Specific causes
Causes are shown in Table 7.14. Herpes zoster can infect the trigeminal nerve (see page 326).

Clinical features
Sensory: Complete loss of sensation on one side of the face – if all branches are affected the lesion must be at the level of the ganglion or above. The earliest sign is loss of the corneal reflex. Dissociated sensory loss (i.e. loss of pain but touch intact) suggests only the spinal nucleus is affected, e.g. by syringobulbia or a foramen magnum tumour. If touch is lost, but pain and temperature intact, the lesion has to be in the pons or medulla.
Motor: When the mouth is opened, the lower jaw deviates to the side of the lesion.

Facial nerve (VII) lesions

Anatomy
The facial nerve has motor and sensory components. The motor nerve cell bodies are in the facial nerve nucleus in the pons. The nerve enters the internal auditory meatus and passes laterally within the petrous temporal bone to

the medial wall of the middle ear. Here the sensory nerve cell bodies cause a swelling called the geniculate ganglion and give off the nerve to stapedius and chorda tympani (taste and lacrimation) before exiting the skull through the stylomastoid foramen.

Each facial nucleus supplying the forehead muscle (frontalis) receives some innervation from each hemisphere, so that unilateral upper motor neurone lesions cause sparing of the forehead, whereas unilateral lower motor neurone lesions cause forehead involvement.

Function
Muscles of facial expression and taste of the anterior two third of the tongue.

Specific causes
- Lower motor neurone (all of one half of the face affected) – Bell's palsy, herpes zoster, polio, otitis media, skull fracture, parotid tumours.
- Upper motor neurone (forehead spared) – stroke, tumours.

Clinical features
The features of facial nerve palsy depend on the level of the lesion. If both lacrimation and taste are unimpaired, the lesion is below the stylomastoid foramen. Hyperacusis (hearing sounds louder than normal) suggests a lesion proximal to the stapedial branch.

Bell's palsy

Definition
Idiopathic weakness of the muscles of facial expression.

Clinical features
Spontaneous unilateral weakness of the muscles of facial expression. As it is a lower motor neurone deficit, the forehead is affected and the eye may not be able to close completely. It usually begins to improve spontaneously after about 10 days, but may take months to recover completely.

Investigations
Electrophysiological tests may help to predict outcome: lack of evoked potential after 3 weeks has a poor prognosis.

Management
If the patient is unable to close their eye completely, artificial tears should be used and the eye taped shut at night to prevent corneal ulceration. The evidence for steroid treatment is weak but may have an effect if given within a day of onset. In cases that do not resolve tarsorrhaphy (suturing of upper to lower lid, laterally) may be necessary. Cosmetic surgery and/or reinnervation using a lingual nerve transfer for example, can be used for chronic cases.

Prognosis
A significant proportion do not completely resolve and it occasionally recurs.

Vestibulocochlear nerve (VIII) lesion

Anatomy
The VIIIth nerve carries sensory information from the cochlear and vestibular apparatus. The auditory fibres arise from the cochlea and pass to the pontine auditory nucleus. These then project to the temporal lobes. The vestibular nerves arise from the semicircular canals and pass to the vestibular nuclei in the pons, and the cerebellum.

Function
Hearing (cochlear nerve) and movement/position of head in space, for balance and head–eye coordination (vestibular nerve).

Specific causes
Ménière's disease, acoustic neuroma, lead, aminoglycosides, furosemide, Paget's disease, herpes zoster.

Clinical features
Sensorineural deafness, tinnitus, vertigo, nystagmus.

Glossopharyngeal (IX) and vagus (X) lesions

Anatomy
Nerve fibres arise from nuclei in the medulla to form these two nerves, which pass out via the jugular foramen.

Function

They have motor, sensory and autonomic functions. Glossopharyngeal receives taste and common sensation from the posterior third of the tongue, the oropharynx via the pharyngeal plexus, and the tonsillar fossa and soft palate.

Vagus carries motor fibres to the muscles of the palate, pharnyx and larynx. It also carries autonomic innervation to the heart, respiratory tract and gut.

Specific causes

Central causes include vascular lesions of the medulla, tumours, syringobulbia and motor neurone disease. Aneurysms and tumours in the posterior fossa and meningitis may affect the nerves. The left recurrent laryngeal nerve (a branch of the vagus) may be damaged in head and neck surgery, or compressed by hilar lymph nodes from lung tumours.

Clinical features

Impaired gag reflex (IX forms the sensory component, X the motor), a hoarse voice and abnormal swallow.

Accessory nerve (XI) lesions

Anatomy

Spinal accessory branch arises from upper cervical cord segments and passes through the foramen magnum to join the cranial accessory branch. They leave the skull separately through the jugular foramen.

Function

Cranial nerves join the pharyngeal plexus and supply the muscles of the palate, pharynx and larynx. The spinal part supplies trapezius and sternocleidomastoid.

Specific causes

Polio, syringomyelia, tumours near the jugular foramen.

Clinical features

Weakness of lifting ipsilateral shoulder and turning head against resistance towards the contralateral side.

Hypoglossal nerve (XII) lesions

Anatomy

This arises from the hypoglossal nucleus in the medulla, and is a motor nerve supplying the muscles of tongue except palatoglossus.

Function

Speech, swallowing.

Specific causes

Stroke, bulbar palsy, polio, trauma and tuberculosis.

Clinical features

Tongue deviates to side of lesion when patient is asked to stick tongue out. The tongue may appear wasted.

Peripheral nerves

Lesions of peripheral nerves

Lesions of one or more peripheral nerves cause a characteristic motor and sensory loss. In some cases there is a pure motor or pure sensory deficit, but in most there is a combination of both.

A neuropathy means a pathological process affecting a peripheral nerve. Damage to the peripheral nerves are caused by a number of mechanisms, principally

- demyelination,
- axonal loss,
- compression or traumatic sectioning of a nerve,
- ischaemia and
- infiltration.

Mononeuropathies: Involvement of a single nerve. Traumatic peripheral nerve injuries may result from compression, penetrating trauma or closed fractures and dislocations. Traumatic nerve damage may result in:

- Neuropraxia, a transient loss of physiological function with no loss in continuity and no degeneration. Acute compression of the nerve causes focal (segmental) demyelination, but once the compression is relieved, recovery is usual within 6 weeks.
- Axonotmesis, which follows more severe compression or traction damage, with Wallerian degeneration of the nerve distal to the injury. The time taken to recover

depends on the length of nerve needed to regrow down the nerve sheath. Excessive fibrosis (scarring) hinders growth.

- Neurotmesis is division of a nerve, following which there is distal Wallerian degeneration. The nerve bundle is interrupted, in-growth of fibrous tissue prevents re-innervation, so that surgical repair is needed if function is to be restored. Ideally, immediate repair with end to end suture is undertaken with a reasonable prognosis. However if there is contamination the nerve ends are marked with non-absorbable sutures and after 2–3 weeks the nerve is surgically repaired – good recovery of function is rare.

Any cause of mononeuritis multiplex may also present initially as a mononeuropathy.

Mononeuritis multiplex: An uncommon form of neuropathy where two or more peripheral nerves are affected either together or sequentially. If symmetrical nerves are affected it may mimic a polyneuropathy. The main causes are diabetes mellitus, malignancy, amyloidosis, polyarteritis nodosa, connective tissue disorders, HIV infection and leprosy (commonest cause worldwide).

Peripheral neuropathy: A symmetrical disorder of peripheral nerves, usually distal more than proximal. It excludes cranial nerve palsies, mononeuropathies, mononeuritis multiplex and bilateral single nerve lesions. The commonest causes are

- Diabetes mellitus.
- Malignancy (e.g. lung, leukaemia, lymphoma, myeloma).
- Vitamin B deficiency (Thiamine (B_1) deficiency in alcoholics, Vitamin B_{12} deficiency).
- Drugs (e.g. isoniazid, phenytoin, nitrofurantoin, vincristine, cisplatin).

Other rare causes include uraemia; hypothyroidism; systemic diseases and vasculitis, e.g. sarcoid, systemic lupus erythematosus, amyloidosis, polyarteritis nodosa; toxins such as lead (motor), arsenic & thallium (initially sensory); infections such as leprosy, diphtheria; Guillain–Barré syndrome (acute inflammatory or postinfective polyneuropathy).

Radiculopathy: Damage to one or more nerve roots or a nerve plexus. The most important causes are trauma, compression (e.g. prolpased intervertebral disc, cervical or lumbar spondylosis or neurofibroma), malignant infiltration and herpes zoster.

Guillain–Barré syndrome

Definition
An acute inflammatory poly-radiculo-neuropathy characterised by progressive muscle weakness and areflexia.

Incidence
Although rare (~1–2 per 100,000 population per annum), it is the commonest cause of acute flaccid paralysis in healthy people. It affects all ages and both sexes equally.

Aetiology/pathophysiology
Immune mediated demyelination of peripheral nerves typically 2–4 weeks after a mild respiratory or gastrointestinal illness. It is thought that antibodies to the infecting organism cross-react with components of myelin. In particular, recent infection with *Campylobacter jejuni* is associated with a worse prognosis. Remyelination occurs over a period of 3–4 months and is associated with recovery in most cases.

Clinical features
Patients complain of distal paraesthesiae and numbness followed by weakness of distal limb muscles. This ascends over hours or days (up to 4 weeks) causing weakness, areflexia and sensory loss in the legs and arms, cranial nerve involvement with difficulty swallowing and respiratory muscle weakness in 20%. There may be backache or shooting pains down the back of the leg early in the course. Over the following weeks to months, the condition slowly improves.

Miller–Fischer syndrome, a clinical variant of Guillain–Barré syndrome, causes ophthalmoplegia, facial weakness, ataxia and areflexia.

Microscopy
Nerves show infiltration by lymphoid cells with phagocytosis of myelin by macrophages.

Complications
Respiratory insufficiency or aspiration risk (due to swallowing difficulties) may necessitate intubation and positive pressure ventilation. Autonomic involvement may occur at any stage, causing sweating, bladder dysfunction, hypo- or hypertension, arrhythmias and even sudden death by asystole.

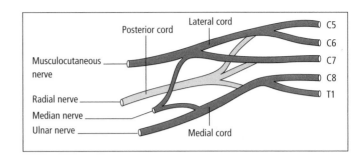

Figure 7.5 Anatomy of the brachial plexus.

Investigations

The diagnosis is essentially clinical but can be confirmed by EMG/ nerve conduction studies, which show slowing or blockage of conduction of nerve impulses. CSF analysis may be normal initially, but usually protein levels are high after the first week. Serial forced vital capacity (FVC) measurement is necessary to monitor respiratory muscle function. Oxygen saturations are of minimal value as they only fall late in respiratory failure.

Management

- Patients should have cardiac monitoring and in some cases may be admitted to an intensive care unit, if ventilation is likely.
- Intravenous immunoglobulin or plasma exchange reduces the duration and severity. They are generally used for moderate to severe cases (i.e. those who are unable to walk without assistance, or who require ventilation).

Prognosis

Recovery though gradual over many months is usual but is sometimes incomplete, leaving patients with distal neurological symptoms such as paraesthesiae or footdrop. Mortality is ∼5% despite intensive care. Prolonged (>2 months) of disability or recurrence should prompt the search for another cause.

Brachial plexus injuries

Definition

The brachial plexus is formed from the nerve roots of C5–T1, which form into the medial, lateral and posterior cords. These then form the median, ulnar, radial and musculocutaneous nerves supplying the arm (see Fig. 7.5). Lesions of the upper plexus (C5/6) cause Erb's palsy and lesions of the lower plexus (C8/T1) causes a Klumpke's palsy.

Aetiology

- Trauma: By severe traction with the arm in abduction (usually after a motorcycle accident), or penetrating trauma. Traction injury during a difficult labour may damage the brachial plexus most commonly causing an Erb's palsy.
- Cervical rib: A bony or fibrous protrusion from the transverse process of C7 can stretch the lower roots of the brachial plexus.
- Malignant infiltration.

Clinical features

- Erb's palsy (C5/6 lesions) with failure of abduction and external rotation of the arm. The arm is held in adduction and internal rotation (waiter's tip position).
- Klumpke's palsy (C8/T1 lesions) The intrinsic muscles of the hand are paralysed (ulnar nerve) resulting in wasting of the small muscles, a claw hand (flexor digitorum muscles supplied by the median nerve) and loss of ulnar sensation.
- In a total plexus lesion the entire arm is paralysed and numb.
- Pain is characteristic of infiltration.

Investigations

Chest X-ray may show an apical lung lesion (Pancoast tumour) or a cervical rib. MRI is the most useful imaging to investigate brachial plexus lesions.

Management

Treatment of the underlying cause. In traumatic injuries open wounds should be explored and clean cut nerves repaired or grafted if possible. Pain relief may be required.

Median nerve lesions

Definition
The median nerve arises from the brachial plexus and supplies the flexor aspect of the forearm and the following short muscles of the hand (LOAF) – the Lateral two lumbricals, Opponens pollicis, Abductor pollicis brevis and Flexor pollicis brevis).

Aetiology/pathophysiology
Median nerve injuries tend to occur near the wrist or high up the forearm. Where the median nerve passes through the anterior cubital fossa under the biceps aponeurosis into the forearm it is vulnerable to damage by forearm fractures and elbow dislocations (high lesions). It then passes under the flexor retinaculum (through the carpal tunnel) into the hand – low lesions are caused by compression in carpal tunnel syndrome (see below), cuts to the wrist or carpal dislocation.

Clinical features
- Low lesions: There is loss of muscle bulk in the thenar eminence, abduction and opposition of the thumb are weak and sensation is lost over the radial three and a half digits on the palmar surface.
- High lesions: In addition to the clinical findings of a low lesion, the long flexors of the thumb, index and middle fingers are paralysed.

Management
If the nerve is severed suture or grafting should be attempted.

Carpal tunnel syndrome

Definition
Syndrome of compression of the median nerve as it passes under the flexor retinaculum.

Age
Usually 40–50 years.

Sex
F > M (8:1)

Table 7.15 Causes of carpal tunnel syndrome

Hormonal	Pregnancy, oral contraceptive pill, periods, hypothyroidism, diabetes mellitus, acromegaly
Peripheral Oedema	Cardiac failure
Mechanical/degenerative	Fractures of the lunate, rheumatoid arthritis

Aetiology
Often idiopathic (for other causes see Table 7.15).

Pathophysiology
The carpal tunnel is a tight space through which all the tendons to the hand and the median nerve pass. Any cause of swelling is therefore likely to cause compression of the medial nerve. The condition is commonly bilateral.

Clinical features
Tingling and numbness in the thumb, index finger and middle finger. Characteristically the pain wakes the patient at night and the patient shakes the wrist or hangs it over the side of the bed to relieve symptoms (unlike in cervical spondylosis). Symptoms are also induced by repetitive actions, or when the wrists are held flexed for some time, for example whilst knitting or reading a newspaper, and this latter can be used as a test (Phalen's test), with the wrist hyperflexed for 1–2 minutes. Alternatively, tapping on the carpal tunnel (Tinel's sign) may reproduce the symptoms although both tests are unreliable. Usually the dominant hand is affected first, but the condition is normally bilateral.

Clumsiness and weakness may occur in late cases, when there is often wasting of the thenar eminence and decreased palmar sensation.

Investigations
Median nerve conduction studies show impaired conduction at the wrist.

Management
Splinting the wrist in extension, particularly at night is useful prior to surgery, during pregnancy, or in those who wish to avoid surgery. Diuretics may help. Corticosteroid injection provides temporary relief. Definitive treatment is by surgical division of the flexor retinaculum, usually

under local or regional anaesthetic. Treatment of underlying cause may relieve symptoms.

Ulnar nerve lesions

Definition
The ulnar nerve arises from the brachial plexus and supplies most of the intrinsic muscles of the hand.

Aetiology/pathophysiology
Most injuries occur at the elbow, although open wounds can arise anywhere. The ulnar nerve passes down the anterior medial aspect of the upper arm and wraps posteriorly round the medial epicondyle of the humerus where it is vulnerable to fracture of the elbow or chronic pressure. It enters the hand on the ulnar side, and can be damaged by pressure or lacerations at the wrist.

Clinical features
- Low lesions (at wrist): There is wasting of all the small muscles of the hand except the thenar eminence and there is a clawing of the ring and little fingers. Sensation is lost over the ulnar one and a half fingers.
- High lesions (at elbow): The claw deformity is less due to paralysis of the ulnar side of flexor digitorum profundus.

Management
If the ulnar nerve is severed, repair is may be attempted, stretching can be avoided by transposing the nerve to the front of the elbow. Failure of recovery can be overcome by tendon transfer. Nerve entrapment is treated with decompression and transposition of the nerve.

Radial nerve lesions

Definition
The radial nerve supplies the extensor muscles of the upper arm and forearm. It is a branch of the brachial plexus.

Aetiology
Injuries to the radial nerve may occur due to elbow fracture/dislocations, in the upper arm due to humerus fractures or prolonged pressure due to hanging an arm over the back of a chair (Saturday night palsy), or in the axilla (crutch palsy). Radial nerve lesions cause weakness in the brachioradialis and triceps muscles.

Clinical features
Wrist drop and sensory loss over the back of the hand at the base of the thumb (the anatomical snuffbox). If there is paralysis of triceps (weakness of elbow extension), this is evidence of a lesion above the upper third of the upper arm, e.g. in the axilla. Low lesions, i.e. at the elbow result in failure to extend the metacarpophalangeal joints.

Management
Compression due to crutch palsy or Saturday night palsy may take up to 3 months to recover. Open wounds should be explored immediately with nerve repair or graft. Other trauma should be given 6 weeks, with surgery if there is no sign of recovery.

Prognosis
Lesions that do not recover can often be overcome by suitable tendon transfers.

Sciatic nerve lesions

Definition
The sciatic nerve (L4–5, S1–3) is a branch of the lumbosacral plexus and the largest nerve in the body. It supplies most of the muscles and cutaneous sensation of the leg, so that sciatic nerve lesions cause serious disability.

Aetiology/pathophysiology
Division of the sciatic nerve occurs occasionally in penetrating injuries. Traction injuries occur more commonly in association with fractures of the pelvis or hip dislocations. It is most frequently injured by badly placed intramuscular injections in the gluteal region (avoided by injecting into the upper outer quadrant of the buttock). It supplies all the muscles of the lower leg, some of the hamstrings, and most of the sensation of the calf, as well as the skin on the sole and lateral side of the foot.

In most sciatic nerve lesions, the common peroneal nerve component is most affected, probably because its nerve fibres lie most superficial in the sciatic nerve trunk.

Clinical features

Flexion of the knee is markedly impaired and all the muscles below the knee are paralysed, causing drop foot. The calf is wasted. Sensation is absent in most of the skin below the knee.

Management

In traumatic damage, exploration and repair of the nerve should be carried out. A footdrop splint is worn to keep the ankle in a safe position, but the lower leg is very vulnerable to neuropathic ulceration and development of Charcot's joint, which may necessitate a below-knee amputation.

Femoral nerve injuries

Definition

The femoral nerve is a branch of the lumbar plexus, from nerve roots L1–4, and it supplies flexors of the hip and extensors of the knee.

Aetiology/pathophysiology

Complete division of the femoral nerve is rare. It may be injured by a gunshot wound, traction in an operation or bleeding into the thigh.

In the abdomen, the femoral nerve is related to the psoas muscle and supplies iliopsoas. It enters the thigh lateral to the femoral to supply the hamstring muscles in the thigh. Its two divisions, then supply all the anterior compartment muscles of the thigh, namely quadriceps femoris, which is a powerful extensor of the knee, and the skin of the medial and anterior surfaces of the thigh.

Clinical features

Weakness of knee extension and numbness of the medial and anterior aspect of the thigh, the medial aspect of the lower leg and the medial border of the foot. The knee jerk is depressed or absent. Hip flexion is only slightly affected and adduction is preserved.

Management

Evacuation of a haematoma or direct suturing or grafting of a cut nerve.

Prognosis

This is a disabling injury. In walking, quadriceps weakness can be compensated for to some extent by the adductor muscles.

Peroneal nerve lesions

Definition

The common peroneal nerve is the smaller terminal branch of the sciatic nerve which supplies muscles which act on the ankle joint.

Aetiology/pathophysiology

This nerve is easily damaged because it runs down in the popliteal fossa, then winds laterally around the neck of the fibula. It can be compressed by a plaster cast, in compartment syndrome, by lying unconscious with the leg externally rotated or it may be stretched when the knee is forced into varus with lateral ligament injuries.

It has two terminal branches, the superficial and deep peroneal nerves. The superficial nerve supplies peroneus longus and peroneus brevis, which plantarflex and evert the foot, and the skin on the lower, lateral side of the leg and foot. The deep nerve supplies muscles which dorsiflex the ankle and a small area of skin on the dorsum of the foot around the first web space.

Clinical features

Common peroneal nerve injury: Drop foot, both dorsiflexion of the ankle and eversion of the foot are weak but not plantarflexion (gastrocnemius and soleus are much more powerful plantarflexors of the foot). Sensation is lost over the front and outer leg and the dorsum of the foot.

Superficial branch injury: Foot eversion is lost, but dorsiflexion is intact. Sensation is lost over the outer side of the leg and foot.

Deep branch injury: This tends to occur in anterior compartment syndrome. There is weakened dorsiflexion and a small area of sensory loss on the dorsum of the foot.

Management

Most cases resolve spontaneously if due to compression. Compartment syndrome however requires emergency decompression. If the nerve is cut or torn, it should be repaired. A splint can be worn to keep the foot in a neutral position. If nerve damage is permanent, tendon transfers or arthrodesis of the foot can help.

Hereditary and congenital disorders

Cerebral palsy

Definition
Cerebral palsy (CP) is a heterogeneous group of conditions arising from a non-progressive lesion occurring in the developing brain. Although the lesion is non-progressive, the brain is still maturing and the clinical picture is therefore not static.

Incidence
3 per 1000 live births.

Aetiology
The precise cause of the damage may be difficult to identify and is often multifactorial. About 10–15% acquire the lesion at birth, and a similar proportion occur after the neonatal period. Most occur pre-natally. Causes include:
- Cerebral malformation.
- Hypoxia in utero and or peripartum.
- Stroke in the perinatal period – cerebral haemorrhage or infarction.
- Infection – intrauterine or post-natal.
- Trauma at birth or post-natal.
- Prolonged convulsions or coma in infancy.
- Kernicterus (severe jaundice leading to brain damage and seizures in the newborn).

Pathophysiology
As the lesion of CP arises early in development it interferes with normal motor development. The main handicap is usually one of disordered movement and posture but it is often complicated by other neurological and cognitive problems. CP is classified according to the clinical picture:
- Spastic CP accounts for 70% involving damage to the cerebral motor cortex or its connections. The features are clasp like hypertonia, brisk reflexes, ankle clonus and extensor plantar responses. The condition may be a hemiparesis (one side of the body, arm more than leg), quadriparesis (both sides, arms more than legs) or diplegia (legs affected).
- Dystonic (athetoid) CP accounts for 10%, and is characterised by irregular involuntary movements of some or all muscle groups. These may be continuous or occur only on voluntary movement.
- Ataxic CP accounts for 10% and is characterised by hypotonia, weakness uncoordination and intention tremor.
- Mixed CP makes up the remaining 10%.

Clinical features
Infants may present with poor sucking ability, increased or decreased tone, abnormal reflexes, convulsions or drowsiness in the neonatal period. However many such infants will develop normally. Usually CP can only be diagnosed after a few months when it becomes obvious that motor development is delayed. The persistence of primitive reflexes is also suggestive. The characteristic features described above may not present until later in childhood.

Complications
Mental retardation in 60%, epilepsy in 30%, visual impairment in 20%, hearing loss in 20%, orthopaedic deformities and osteoarthritis may result even with physiotherapy.

Investigations
Diagnosis is clinical.

Management
Multidisciplinary assessment and supportive treatment:
1 Medication may be needed to control fits and hyperactivity. Muscle relaxants such as dantrolene or baclofen may be used for spasticity, and botulinum toxin injections may delay deformity due to muscle shortening.
2 Physical therapy is started in the first year of life, before abnormal motor patterns have become established.
3 Splintage is often required to counteract spastic deformities.
4 Persistent deformities may require corrective orthopaedic surgery with post operative physiotherapy
   - Soft tissue procedures to improve muscle balance by re-routing or dividing tendons and muscles

- Bone operations to correct position and stabilise joints

5 Neurosurgical techniques are occasionally used for severe deforming spasticity to reduce spasm.

Prognosis

Most children with cerebral palsy survive to adulthood. Longer-term survival depends on their degree of disability, with those who never manage to feed or mobilise doing much worse, and often dying of aspiration pneumonia.

Neurofibromatosis type 1

Definition

An inherited disorder characterised by multiple skin neurofibromas, also called Von Recklinghausen's disease.

Incidence

1 in 3500 making it the most common autosomal dominant condition.

Aetiology/pathophysiology

Autosomal dominant condition caused by a group of mutations in the NF1 gene on the long arm of chromosome 17 (product neurofibromin). It has complete penetrance, but variable expression. It is thought that NF1 is a tumour supressor gene.

Clinical features

Diagnosis when two or more of
- six or more café-au-lait spots.
- two or more neurofibromas of any type or 1 plexiform (nerve root) neurofibroma.
- freckling of axillary or inguinal regions.
- optic glioma.
- two or more Lisch nodules (iris hamartomas).
- distinctive osseous lesions (focal kyphoscoliosis, pseudoarthrosis and dysplasia or thinning of the long bone cortex).
- a first degree relative with NF1 diagnosed as above.

Complications

There is an increased rate of benign and malignant tumours, particularly CNS tumours. Plexiform neurofibromas may undergo malignant change (called schwannomas or neurofibrosarcomas). Note that cutaneous neurofibromas do not undergo malignant change.

Epilepsy or mental retardation occur in up to 5% of patients; 30–40% of patients develop a scoliosis which may require surgical intervention

Investigations

It is a clinical diagnosis. MRI scanning is used if root pain or focal neurology develops, to look for malignant change in a neurofibroma or to assess if a neurofibroma is amenable to superficial resection.

Management

Surgery for cosmetic reasons and to correct bone deformity.

Neurofibromatosis type 2

Definition

Autosomal dominant condition characterised by the development of bilateral acoustic neuromas.

Incidence

1 in 100,000 individuals.

Aetiology

An autosomal dominant condition caused by a mutation in the NF2 gene on chromosome 22 which codes for a protein termed schwannomin or merlin. This protein acts as a tumour suppressor gene by an unknown mechanism.

Pathophysiology

Schwannomin has similarities with cytoskeletal components that link to the actin/spectrin complex, it is therefore suggested that the cell–cell interaction is abnormal and hence contact inhibition is prevented.

Clinical features

Patients may have a few, large café au lait spots. Unlike NF1 the main feature is bilateral acoustic neuromas. The earliest presenting symptom is unilateral hearing loss or tinnitus. Hearing loss may be sudden, vertigo is rare, patients with large tumours experience headaches, visual disturbances, and ataxia.

Complications

Patients also have a tendency to form other brain tumours such as meningiomas and gliomas.

Investigations

Pure tone audiometry reveals unilateral or asymmetrical sensorineural hearing loss, electric response audiometry shows characteristic prolonged I–V latency differentiating the hearing loss from cochlear deafness. CT and MRI are definitive.

Management

Surgical resection is the preferred treatment via neurosurgical-otological approach by translabyrinthine or suboccipital approach with facial nerve monitoring. Radiotherapy is used in patients unfit for surgery.

Tuberose sclerosis

Definition

Rare autosomal dominant phacomatosis (hereditary diseases characterised by hamartomas). Also known as tuberous sclerosis.

Incidence

1–5 per 10,000 live births.

Aetiology/pathophysiology

Autosomal dominant inherited condition – two different loci have been found, TSC1 gene one on chromosome 9 which codes for hamartin and the TSC2 gene on chromosome 16 which codes for tuberin – both are tumour suppressor genes. There is incomplete genetic expression and hence variable severity and a variable family history. Hamartomas appear in many different organs, including the brain which shows characteristic nodules (tubers) on the walls of the ventricles.

Clinical features

- Skin manifestations: de-pigmented patches which fluoresce with Wood's light, shagreen patches – roughened patches of skin, amelanotic naevi, angiofibromas (adenoma sebaceum) in butterfly malar distribution occurring after the age of 3.
- Neurological manifestations: infantile spasms, mental retardation, partial seizures.
- A minority of patients develop cardiac or renal tumours and polycystic kidneys.

Complications

Cardiac failure, arrhythmias including Wolf Parkinson White syndrome, renal cell carcinoma in less than 1%, liver angiomas (25% of patients but rarely symptomatic)

Investigations

Multiple intracranial nodules can be seen on CT or MRI, after 1 year these calcify and can be seen on skull X ray. Renal ultrasound and echocardiogram may be required.

Management

Annual review is recommended to assess seizure control and screen for development of new symptoms or complications. Skin lesions may respond to argon lasers and pulsed dye lasers (vascular lesions) or CO_2 lasers (fibrous lesions).

Friedreich's ataxia

Definition

Progressive degenerative spastic cerebellar ataxia occurring in the young.

Incidence

Rare, but it is the most common hereditary ataxia.

Age

Difficulty in walking occurs around age 12.

Aetiology/pathophysiology

It is an autosomal recessive condition. In most cases there is an abnormal expanded sequence of tri-nucleotide (GAA) repeats in the gene for frataxin. These repeats result in lower expression of the gene product, a mitochondrial protein. The number of repeats tends to elongate in subsequent generations which results in a worse clinical picture (genetic anticipation). Frataxin appears to protect against oxidative damage particularly in the brain, heart and pancreas. The neuropathological change is of degeneration of the posterior columns, corticospinal and spinocerebellar tracts.

Clinical features

- Progressive ataxia of all four limbs and trunk.
- Pyramidal weakness and extensor plantars.

- Absent joint position and vibration sense in the lower limbs.
- Absent reflexes in the lower limbs.
- Pes cavus.
- Cerebellar dysarthria.
- Nystagmus in 25%.
- Optic atrophy in 30%.
- Cardiomyopathy with T-wave inversion, left ventricular hypertrophy, arrhythmias.
- Diabetes mellitus occurs in about a third.

Investigations
Genetic testing and counselling.

Management
Cardiac arrhythmias should be controlled and ACE inhibitors may improve left ventricular hypertrophy. Diabetes may require dietary change, oral hypoglycaemics or insulin. Physiotherapy and orthopaedic intervention for skeletal deformity may be of benefit.

Prognosis
Death is usual before the age of 40, mainly due to complications of diabetes and heart disease.

Hereditary motor and sensory neuropathy (Charcot–Marie–Tooth disease)

Definition
Peroneal muscular atrophy or Charcot–Marie–Tooth Disease is a degenerative disorder of the peripheral nerves, motor nerve roots and spinal cord.

Aetiology
Inherited condition in which both autosomal dominant and recessive and X-linked patterns are seen.

Pathophysiology
Various forms are recognised including the following:
- HMSN type I is a demyelinating neuropathy with dominant inheritance.
- HMSN type II is an axonal neuropathy with variable inheritance pattern.
- HMSN type III is an autosomal recessive demyelinating sensory neuropathy with very high CSF protein levels.

Clinical features
- Syndrome in which there is distal limb wasting and weakness that slowly progresses over many years with variable loss of sensation and reflexes.
- The typical deformities are pes cavus, peroneal wasting, and claw hand.
- In severe cases the wasting begins in early childhood and results in complete disability with legs resembling 'inverted champagne bottles'.
- Mild cases present in adolescence or middle age usually with pes cavus.

Management
Custom shoes, foot orthoses or leg braces may improve gait. Corrective orthopedic foot surgery may help maintain mobility. Splinting, exercise, physiotherapy and surgery can help maintain hand function.

Tumours of the nervous system

Primary intracranial tumours

Definition
Primary tumours arise from the neuronal or support cells of the central nervous system.

Incidence
Primary brain tumours account for only 2% of all tumours (although metastases are the most common intracranial tumour). The incidence appears to be rising, only partly due to increased detection.

Age
The age of presentation depends on the underlying histology. Overall, tumours peak around the age of 50–60 years, but most medulloblastomas and other embryonal tumours occur before the age of 20 years.

Aetiology/pathophysiology
The only known risk factors for primary tumours are high-dose radiation, e.g. in atomic bomb survivors, following radiation treatment for childhood leukaemia, and genetic factors, such as in neurofibromatosis (acoustic neuromas). Most tumours grow slowly and many malignant tumours probably arise from benign tumours (see Table 7.16).

Table 7.16 Primary intracranial tumours and their frequency

Type	Tumour	Approximate frequency (%)
Primary malignancy	Low-grade astrocytoma	5–8
	Malignant astrocytoma	40
	Oligodendroglioma	5
	Ependymoma	10% in childhood, 1% in adults
	Medulloblastoma	4
	CNS lymphoma	3–5
	Total (in all ages)	~**55**
Benign	Meningioma	20
	Schwannoma (acoustic neuroma)	5–10
	Pituitary tumour	10–20
	Other, e.g. craniopharyngioma	7
	Total (in all ages)	~**45**

Clinical features

Mass lesions within the skull produce signs and symptoms by three mechanisms:

- Direct effect of the mass causing compression or infiltration of the surrounding nervous tissue causes focal neurological signs. This may also occur secondary to surrounding oedema or arterial or venous compromise, i.e. a stroke. Headache with focal neurology is a typical presentation.
- Raised intracranial pressure (ICP) usually develops slowly, so does not normally cause the typical triad of headache, vomiting and papilloedema. However, brainstem, floor of the third ventricle and cerebellar lesions tend to present initially with raised ICP:
  - i Distortion of the upper brain stem causes impaired consciousness.
  - ii Compression of the medulla due to herniation (coning) causes a third nerve lesion (due to compression of the ipsilateral third nerve) and sixth nerve lesion (due to stretching of the contralateral sixth nerve), ipsilateral hemiparesis, impaired consciousness, respiratory depression, bradycardia and death.
- Partial or generalised tonic clonic seizures are characteristic of many cerebral mass lesions.

Investigations

CT scanning will detect over 95% of intracranial tumours. MRI scanning, angiography is used for surgical planning. Biopsy is required for histological diagnosis, although a radiological diagnosis may be sufficient. Stereotactic biopsy has a high diagnostic yield and lower morbidity and mortality than standard open biopsy.

Management

- Surgical debulking may be performed. Complete resection of benign tumours is preferred; however, if close to vital structures, e.g. brainstem lesions, this is not always possible.
- Radiotherapy is used post-operatively, for unresectable lesions or in patients unfit for surgery.
- Cerebral oedema is treated with corticosteroids.
- Chemotherapy is used for malignant astrocytoma, to try to prolong survival by a few months.
- Seizures are treated with anticonvulsants.

Prognosis

Prognosis correlates with histologic type and grade, postoperative size, extent of the tumour and by the patient characteristics (age, performance status, and duration of symptoms).

Meningioma

Definition

Slow growing tumour arising from the meningeal covering of the brain and spinal cord.

Incidence

They account for ~20% of all intracranial tumours.

Age

Peak age 40–70 years.

Sex

F > M (2.5:1)

Pathophysiology

Meningiomas may grow to a large size over a period of years. Most are benign, with 10% behaving in a malignant fashion. If they arise close to the skull they may erode the bone. Meningiomas often occur along venous sinuses.

Clinical features

Most are asymptomatic and detected incidentally on neuroimaging. The most common presentation is a seizure or slowly progressive focal neurology. Visual or hearing abnormalities may be present, depending on the site. Frontal tumours cause changes in personality. A parasagittal (falx) meningioma causes a characteristic pattern of bilateral leg weakness mimicking a spinal cord lesion. Spinal meningiomas cause limb weakness and numbness.

Investigations

CT or MRI scans show an enhancing tumour adjacent to dural structures. There may be areas of calcification. Angiography may be used for surgical planning, which shows a delayed 'vascular blush' due to arterial supply from the meninges.

Macroscopy/microscopy

Meningiomas are rounded, rubbery lesions, composed of meningothelial cells with small foci of calcification (psammoma bodies).

Prognosis

Depends on histological features.

- The vast majority are typical (WHO grade 1) meningiomas, which are slow growing and have a low risk of recurrence after surgical removal.
- A small proportion are atypical (WHO grade 2–3) meningiomas with increased mitoses, nuclear pleomorphism and focal necrosis. These have a higher rate of recurrence.
- There is a rare group of malignant (WHO grade 4) meningiomas which are locally invasive and may metastasise.

Gliomas (astrocytomas and oligodendrogliomas)

Definition

Tumours with histological appearances of glial cells – the scaffolding cells of the CNS.

- Astrocytomas have predominantly astrocytic cells. They are categorised according to their histological appearance into low grade astrocytoma (WHO grade 2), anaplastic astrocytoma (WHO grade 3) and glioblastoma multiforme (WHO grade 4).
- Oligodendromas arise from the oligodendrocytes (CNS myelinating cells) and usually behave as low-grade tumours.
- Mixed glial tumours with astrocytic and oligodendroglial components occur and are termed oligoastrocytoma.

Aetiology

Astrocytomas occur anywhere in the brain. Oligodendrogliomas tend to arise in the cerebral hemispheres. Glioblastomas are the most aggressive pleomorphic type of glial cell tumour. Oncogene defects seen in astrocytomas are shown in Table 7.17.

Pathophysiology

Tumours do not metastasise but can spread locally by infiltration. There is also a risk that a low grade tumour may become more aggressive.

Clinical features

Most patients present with focal neurological signs and headache or signs of raised intracranial pressure. Convulsions may occur. The rapidity of onset of symptoms is often an indication of the aggressiveness of the tumour.

Table 7.17 Oncogene defects seen in astrocytomas

Low grade	p53 mutation, loss of alleles from chromosome 22
Anaplastic astrocytoma	p53 mutation, loss of alleles from chromosome 9, 13 and 19
Glioblastoma multiforme	p53 mutation, loss of alleles from chromosome 10 and EGFR (epidermal growth factor receptor) or PDGF (platelet derived growth factor) amplification.

Investigations

- Neuroimaging with CT or MRI – the latter is more sensitive and provides greater anatomical detail. Astrocytomas are usually highly vascular and enhance with contrast in over two-thirds of cases (less often in low-grade astrocytoma). Surrounding oedema is commonly seen, but due to the diffuse infiltration, the limits of oedema often demarcate the limits of the tumour spread. For this reason, prior use of corticosteroids can reduce the appearance of the size of the tumour. Oligodendromas commonly calcify. CT is less useful then MRI.
- Biopsy – stereotactic biopsy (linking information for CT and MRI to guide surgery via surface landmarks or a frame to achieve accuracy to within 1 mm) is used which increases sensitivity, and reduces morbidity and mortality.

Macroscopy/microscopy

- Astrocytomas are ill-defined pale areas which are not clearly demarcated from the adjacent brain. The cells look like astrocytes and there are different histological patterns.
- Oligodendrogliomas are macroscopically similar to astrocytomas, arising as greyish white lesions that are not clearly differentiated from the surrounding tissue. The cells have round nuclei and pale vacuolated cytoplasm (fried egg appearance).
- Glioblastoma muliforme tumours may be necrotic, haemorrhagic masses due to rapid growth. They are composed of pleomorphic cells.

Management

- It is still unclear whether early complete surgical removal of low-grade tumours that cause little or transient neurology improves the prognosis; although surgery is helpful for reducing the need for treatment of seizures, it has the disadvantage of often causing major neurological deficit.
- For astrocytomas, complete surgical removal is difficult due to the diffuse nature and difficulty in determining the limits of the tumour. For high-grade astrocytomas, in many cases the tumour is unresectable. Even if the tumour is resectable, the high risk of recurrence, together with the major morbidity of surgery may mean debulking surgery only and treatment with radiotherapy and/or chemotherapy.
- Hydrocephalus can be treated with a shunt. Seizures are treated with anti-epileptic drugs.

Prognosis

Low-grade tumours grow slowly over many years while glioblastoma multiforme causes death within months.

Musculoskeletal system
8

Clinical

Symptoms

Joint pain

Joint disorders often have pain as their presenting feature. Joint pain is described as arthralgia if there is no accompanying swelling or as arthritis if the joint is swollen. The pattern of joint involvement, its symmetry, onset, timing and provoking and relieving factors are important in establishing the diagnosis. Arthritis may involve a single joint (monoarticular), less than four joints (oligo or pauciarticular) or mutiple joints (polyarticular). The relationship to exercise may be important, as inflammatory disorders are often worse after periods of inactivity and relieved by rest, whereas mechanical disorders tend to be worse on exercise and relieved by rest. Joint pain tends to radiate distally and may be associated with local tenderness. A full systems enquiry is necessary as many disorders have multisystem involvement. Changes in sensation including tingling or numbness are often due to abnormalities in nerve function. This may be due to pressure, ischaemia or neuropathies. Establishment of the distribution helps to differentiate peripheral nerve damage from nerve root damage. Loss of function is important as therapy aims to both relieve pain and establish necessary function for daily activities.

Joint swelling

Swelling may be within the joint, the bone or the surrounding soft tissue. Joint swelling following an injury may be acute due to a haemarthrosis or appear more slowly due to an effusion.

Arthritis describes painful swollen joints. Again this may be a mono, oligo/pauci or polyarthritis. The distribution of joint involvement should be elicited including whether it is distal or proximal, symmetrical or asymmetrical. The nature of the onset, duration, timing and exacerbating factors should be noted. Any other associated features such as joint instability should be enquired about. This may be due to ligament damage.

Joint stiffness

Joint stiffness is another presentation usually associated with the other cardinal features of pain and swelling. Morning stiffness and stiffness after periods of inactivity are characteristic of rheumatoid arthritis but may occur with other forms of arthritis. Less than 10 minutes of stiffness is common in osteoarthritis compared with more than 30 minutes in inflammatory arthritis. Sacroiliac stiffness is a particular feature of ankylosing spondylitis. Locking of a joint is a sudden inability to complete a movement, such as extension at the knee caused by a mechanical block such as a foreign body in the joint or a torn meniscus.

Investigations and procedures

Laboratory investigations

Although some of the available tests used in diagnosis of rheumatological conditions are diagnostic, most have limited value as they may be present in multiple conditions (non-specific), or they may only be present in some of the patients with the disease (non-sensitive). Combining tests may allow a clinical diagnosis to be confimed (see Table 8.1).

Rheumatoid factor: These are antibodies of any class directed against the Fc portion of immunoglobulins. The routine laboratory test detects only IgM antibodies, which agglutinate latex particles or red cells opsonised with IgG. It is the presence of these IgM rheumatoid factor antibodies that is used to describe a patient as seropositive or seronegative. Seventy to eighty per cent of patients with rheumatoid arthritis have IgM rheumatoid factor; however, it may also be detected in a number of other conditions. Seropositivity allows prediction of severity and the need for earlier aggressive therapy and increases the likelihood of extra-articular features.

Antinuclear and anticytoplasmic antibodies: Antibodies against multiple cellular components have been characterised and may be detected.

Joint aspiration

Unexplained joint swelling may require aspiration to aid diagnosis. The aspiration itself may be of therapeutic value lowering the pressure and relieving pain. It is often coupled with intra-articular washout or instillation of steroid or antibiotic as appropriate. Examination of the synovial fluid may be of diagnostic value (see Table 8.2).

Table 8.1 Antibodies detectable in rheumatological conditions

Antibody type	Antigens	Condition associations
Antinuclear antibodies	Double stranded DNA	SLE highly specific
	Centromere	Systemic sclerosis
	High titre speckled pattern	Suggests antibodies to extractable nuclear antigens
Extractable nuclear antibodies	Ro (SSa)	Sjögren's syndrome
		Systemic lupus erythematosus
	La (SSb)	Sjögren's syndrome
		Systemic lupus erythematosus
	Sm	Systemic lupus erythematosus
	Ribonuclear protein	High in various connective tissue disease and overlap syndromes
Others	Jo-1 (histidyl tRNA synthetase)	Polymyositis with pulmonary fibrosis
	Scl 70	Scleroderma
Antineutrophil cytoplasmic antibodies	cANCA (proteinase 3)	Wegener's granulomatosis
	pANCA (myeloperoxidase)	General vasculitis, inflammatory bowel disease

Table 8.2 Synovial fluid analysis

Fluid	Normal	Non-inflammatory	Inflammatory	Septic
Colour	Straw	Straw yellow	Off white	Variable
Clarity	Clear	Clear	Opaque	Opaque
Viscosity	High	High	Low	Variable
WCC number	<200	200–2000	3000–75,000	>50,000
% PMN	<25	<25	>50	>90

Crystal arthropathies such as gout and pseudogout can be differentiated on examination of the crystals with polarised light microscopy. The crystals of gout are negatively birefringent, whereas the crystals of pseudogout are positively birefringent.

Diagnostic imaging

Many modalities of joint imaging and direct visualisation are used to diagnose and follow the course of musculoskeletal disorders and are often used in combination. The findings in individual conditions will be described later.

- X-ray: Many musculoskeletal disorders have characteristic X-ray findings. In acute inflammatory and infectious disorders X-ray changes may be delayed. Comparison of X-ray changes over time is especially useful in monitoring disorders that have a degenerative course.
- Ulrasound is of value in examining the joint and surrounding soft tissue. For example it may be useful in diagnosing the cause of a painful hip not amenable to palpation. It may be coupled with diagnostic aspiration or therapeutic joint injections.
- Magnetic resonance imaging (MRI) is of increasing value in the diagnosis of musculoskeletal disorders. It can demonstrate both bone and soft tissue disorders; in specialist centres dynamic MRI scanning can examine moving joints.
- Radioisotope bone scan shows the level of bone vascularity and remodelling. It is of use in inflammatory and infectious conditions prior to X-ray changes, it is of great value in identifying malignant bone infiltration and sites of infection.

Bone and joint infections

Acute osteomyelitis

Definition
Acute bacterial infection of bone.

Age
Normally seen in children and adults over 50 years.

Aetiology
Most infections result from haematogenous spread of organisms. Local spread from a soft tissue infection may also occur. Acute osteomyelitis is normally seen in children but may also occur in malnourished or immunocompromised adults.

- Haematogenous spread: *Staphylococcus aureus* and *Streptococci* are the common organisms. Previously *Haemophilus influenzae* was seen in young children, but it is now rare due to vaccination. Patients with sickle cell anaemia are prone to osteomyelitis due to *Salmonella*.
- Direct spread from local infection may occur with *Streptococcus*, *Staphylococcus*, anaerobes and gram-negative organisms.

Pathophysiology
In children the long bones are most often involved; in adults, vertebral, sternoclavicular and sacroiliac bones are more commonly involved than are long bones. Infections from a distant focus spread via the blood stream and settle in the bone. In children the organisms usually settle in the metaphysis because the growth disc (physis) acts as a barrier to further spread. In infants the infection tends to spread to the epiphysis and in adults the infection may occur anywhere in the bone.

Acute inflammation occurs accompanied by a rise in pressure leading to pain and disruption of blood flow. Pus forms within the medulla of the bone and forces its way to the surface along the Volkmann's canals forming a subperiosteal abscess. The infection then spreads locally and in infants may enter the joint. In children the physis acts as a physical barrier to intra-articular spread. Necrosis of the bone due to pressure and disrupted blood supply may cause pieces of bone to separate (sequestra).

Clinical features
Presentation ranges from an acute illness with pain, fever, swelling and acute tenderness over the affected bone, to an insidious onset of non-specific dull aching and vague systemic illness. A history of preceding infection may indicate the source and suggest the organism.

Complications
- As the bone heals and new bone is formed, infected tissue and sequestrated bone fragments may be enclosed.

Sinuses form in the presence of continuing infection, resulting in a chronic osteomyelitis.

- In children growth disturbance may result if the physis is damaged with resultant limb shortening or deformity.
- Infection may spread to the joint causing a septic arthritis or to other bones causing metastatic osteomyelitis.

Investigations

- The X-ray finding may take 2–3 weeks to develop. A raised periostium is an early sign that may be seen before any abnormality of the underlying bone. Later there is rarefaction (diminution in the density) of the metaphysis. With healing there is sclerosis and sequestrated bone fragments may be visible.
- CT scanning (MRI in spine) is accurate at demonstrating cortical damage and periosteal reaction to infection.
- There may be a leucocytosis and raised inflammatory markers (ESR, CRP). Blood cultures are positive in 50%.
- Radioisotope bone scanning can show increased activity before X-ray changes are evident.

Management

- Surgical drainage should be used if there is a subperiosteal abscess, if systemic upset is refractory to antibiotic treatment or if there is suspected adjacent join involvement.
- Antibiotics: Initially treat on the basis of likely pathogen then change depending on sensitivity. Parenteral treatment is often required for a prolonged period (2–4 weeks) prior to a long course of oral antibiotics to ensure eradication. All antibiotic therapies should be rationalised once culture and sensitivity are known.
  1 Infants and young children may need treatment with a third-generation cephalosporin to cover for *Haemophilus* infection.
  2 Older children and previously fit adults are treated with flucloxacillin and fucidic acid (*Staphylococcus*).
- Adequate analgesia is essential and may be improved with splints to immobilise the limb (which also helps to avoid contractures). Physiotherapy is required early to reduce associated muscle disuse atrophy and to maintain joint mobility.

Chronic osteomyelitis

Definition

Chronic osteomyelitis occurs when there is ongoing or relapsing infection resulting from encasement of infected dead bone during the healing of an acute osteomyelitis.

Aetiology

Previously, chronic osteomyelitis resulted from poorly treated acute osteomyelitis. It now occurs more frequently in post-traumatic osteomyelitis. Multiple organisms are often isolated from the pus.

Pathophysiology

Normally in an acute osteomyelitis, new bone is formed beneath the raised periosteum, which is termed involucrum. If the new bone formed encloses infected tissue and sequestrated bone fragments, pus discharges through perforations (cloacae) and sinuses. Bacteria in the bone may remain dormant for years giving rise to recurrent flares of acute infection.

Clinical features

The clinical course is typically ongoing chronic pain and low-grade fever following an episode of acute osteomyelitis. There may be pus discharging through a sinus. However, if the pus is retained within the bone or the sinus becomes obstructed, rising pressure leads to an acute flare of pain, redness, local tenderness and pyrexia (similar to an acute osteomyelitis).

Investigations

There is often no leucocytosis; however, the ESR is normally raised. X-ray shows areas of decreased density (rarefaction) surrounded by sclerotic bone and sometimes sequestra. The periostium may be raised with underlying new bone formation. Bone scans may be used to reveal the focus of infection.

Management

Discharging sinuses require dressing, and if an abscess persists despite antibiotic therapy it should be incised and drained. Prolonged combined parenteral antibiotics are required. Surgical intervention proves difficult but may involve debridement of necrotic tissue, dead space obliteration, provision of soft tissue coverage of the bone and stabilisation of bone.

Tuberculous bone infection

Definition
Spread of an infection by *Mycobacterium tuberculosis* to the bone and joints.

Incidence
Patients with tuberculosis have a 5% lifetime risk of developing bone disease.

Age
Usually children or young adults.

Geography
Major illness in developing countries, with increasing incidence in the developed world.

Aetiology
Tuberculous osteomyelitis is usually due to haematogenous spread from a primary focus in the lungs or gastrointestinal tract (see pages 105 and 154). HIV has increased the incidence of tuberculosis and tuberculous bone infections.

Pathophysiology
The disease starts in the intra-articular bone. The lumbar and lower thoracic spine is commonly involved (Pott's disease). A chronic inflammatory reaction occurs leading to caseation and later abscess formation (cold abscess). Abscesses may cause a mass effect on local structures. Weakened vertebrae are prone to collapse.

Clinical features
The onset of symptoms is insidious and often missed. The patient complains of pain and later swelling due to pus collection. Muscle spasm and wasting occur with limitation of movement and rigidity. In spinal tuberculosis, pain may be mild and presentation delayed until there is a visible abscess or vertebral collapse causing pain and deformity.

Investigations
- X-ray shows soft tissue swelling and decreased density (rarefaction) of the bone. In early stages the joint space is preserved, but later there is narrowing and irregularity with bone erosion and calcification within adjacent soft tissue.
- The ESR is usually raised and the Mantoux test is positive in 90% of immunocompetent patients.
- Synovial biopsy for histological examination and culture is often necessary.

Management
Chemotherapy with combination anti-tuberculous agents for 12–18 months (see page 105). Rest and traction may be useful; if the articular surfaces are damaged, arthrodesis or joint replacement may be required.

Septic arthritis

Definition
Inflamed painful joint caused by infection with a pyogenic organism.

Aetiology
Joint infection arises most commonly from haematogenous spread. Other mechanisms include local trauma or an adjacent infective focus such as osteomyelitis. It can also occur as a complication of joint surgery, although this is minimised by the use of laminar flow theatres and sterile techniques. The commonest causative organism is *Staph. aureus*.
- Toddlers and children: *Staph. aureus*, *Streptococci*, *Haemophilus* (rare since vaccination).
- Adults: *Staph. aureus*, *Streptococci*, *Neisseria gonorrhoea*.
- Immunosuppressed: Gram-negative bacteria, mycobacterium, fungi.
- Patients with sickle cell anaemia are particularly prone to infections with *Salmonella*.

Pathophysiology
Bacteria are initially found in the synovial membrane but quickly spread to the synovial fluid. Cytokine-mediated inflammation and a rise in intra-articular pressure follow the spread of bacteria. The pressure may cause compression of the blood vessels leading in the hip to avascular

necrosis of the femoral head especially in young children. Erosion of the articular cartilage results from the release of proteolytic enzymes from neutrophils within the inflammatory exudate. Prolonged exposure to these enzymes can result in chondrocyte and bone damage. Pus may find its way out of the joint causing an abscess, which may drain via a sinus.

Clinical features

The classical features of septic arthritis are a red, hot, painful monoarthritis associated with fever. Overall the knee is the most commonly affected joint, but hips are often the site in children. There may be evidence of the source of infection such as a urinary tract infection, skin or respiratory infection. On examination the joint is held immobilised in the position that maximises the intra-articular volume (e.g. a hip is usually held flexed, abducted and externally rotated). Movement of the joint is very painful and often prevented by pain and muscle spasm (pseudoparesis).

Complications

- If treatment is delayed there is severe articular destruction, which may heal by fibrosis with permanent restriction of movement, deformity or bony union.
- A tense joint effusion may result in dislocation.
- In children extensive destruction of the epiphysis may occur causing growth disturbance and deformity.

Investigations

- X-ray of the affected joint may show widening of joint space and soft tissue swelling but are of little diagnostic value.
- Blood tests may reveal a leucocytosis, raised ESR and CRP. Blood cultures should be taken and may be positive in a third of cases.
- Diagnosis is confirmed by aspiration of joint fluid for urgent microscopy, culture and sensitivities. The fluid often appears purulent at time of aspiration. Depending on the joint involved and available facilities, aspiration may be blind, ultrasound guided, CT guided or surgical.

Management

- Patients require adequate analgesia.
- Antibiotics should start immediately after synovial fluid and blood cultures have been taken. Initial therapy is dependent on the suspected organism. In previously healthy children and adults, penicillin (*Streptococcus* cover) and flucloxacillin (*Staphylococcus* cover) are used. A third-generation cephalosporin is used if *gonococcus* is suspected and in the immuno-compromised gentamicin is added to cover for anaerobic organisms. Antibiotic therapy is reviewed in the light of culture and sensitivities.
- Splintage and resting of the joint is essential. If the hip is infected it should be held abducted and 30° flexed. Drainage of pus and arthroscopic joint washout under anaesthesia can be performed.
- Surgical drainage may be indicated if the infection does not resolve with appropriate antibiotics or if percutaneous drainage is not possible. Arthroscopic procedures allow visualisation of the interior of the joint, drainage of pus and debridement.
- Surgery may also be required for the removal of foreign bodies or infected prosthetic material.
- If there is no cartilage damage, gentle mobilisation should begin once inflammation has settled.

Prognosis

Outcome is related to immune status of the host, virulence of the organism and the speed at which adequate antibiotic therapy is started. In *Staphylococcal* infections involvement of multiple joints carries a significant mortality (>90% if more than three joints involved).

Osteoarthritis

Definition

Previously thought of as a degenerative joint disorder of ageing, osteoarthritis is now considered to be a joint disorder resulting from damage and repair to cartilage and reaction in the surrounding bone.

Prevalence

Radiological changes universal in old age, symptomatic disease occurs in 20%.

Age

Peak onset 45–60 years.

Sex

F > M

Table 8.3 Causes of secondary osteoarthritis

Structural change	Intra-articular fracture, joint malalignment, joint hypermobility, congenital dysplastic hips, Perthes' disease
Inflammatory joint damage	Septic arthritis, rheumatoid arthritis, repeated haemarthrosis in haemophilia
Genetic collagen disorders	Mutations in type II collagen genes resulting in increased susceptibility to damage
Calcium deposition disorders	Chondrocalcinosis

Aetiology

- Primary osteoarthritis: Risk factors include obesity, increasing age, female sex, wear of cartilage through repeated trauma.
- Secondary osteoarthritis: Osteoarthritis may result from damage to the joint or changes to the way forces are transmitted through the cartilage (see Table 8.3).

Pathophysiology

Normal cartilage consists of chondrocytes, collagen and extracellular matrix. The damage seen in osteoarthritis is initiated by trauma, which may be a single event or repeated microtrauma. Any underlying collagen defect will predispose to damage. There is resultant increased proliferation and activity of chondrocytes under the influence of monocyte-derived growth peptides. Once the process of osteoarthritis has begun a number of factors are involved in the continued disease process:

- Mechanical forces can be causative, preventative or therapeutic.
- Proteases that are involved with cartilage degradation. It has been suggested that protease activation is important.
- Cytokines including IL-1 and TNF-α, have a role in cartilage degradation. Growth factors mediating collagen repair include insulin-like growth factor and transforming growth factor β (TGF-β), which reduces the activity of proteases and therefore limits cartilage degradation.
- Other factors implicated include crystals and nitric oxide.

Clinical features

Patients tend to present with gradual onset of joint pain, which is exacerbated by exercise and relieved by rest. As the disease progresses, pain occurs with less activity and eventually occurs at rest. Stiffness occurs after a period of rest, but is less severe than rheumatoid arthritis and lasts 5–15 minutes in morning. On examination there may be joint line tenderness, joint effusion, crepitus and bony enlargement due to osteophyte development. There is gradual limitation of movement with resultant muscle wasting and deformity.

- Hands: An enlargement of the distal (Heberden's nodes) and proximal interphalangeal (Bouchard's nodes) joints results in a square appearance of the hands. The development of Heberden's nodes appears to have a genetic predisposition.
- Feet/ankles: The first metatarsophalangeal joint is commonly affected; subtalar joint involvement may cause difficulty with walking.
- Knees: The medial part of the knee joint may be affected more than the lateral causing a genu varum. Knee involvement often results in osteophyte formation, joint effusion, crepitus and a Baker's cyst palpable in the popliteal fossa.
- Hips are commonly affected, although some apparent hip pain may be referred from other areas.
- Spine: Particularly the cervical and lumbar region.

Investigations

The first radiological finding is narrowing of the joint space. In weight-bearing joints narrowing is maximal in the areas subjected to the greatest pressures. As the cartilage is worn away, friction causes the exposed subchondral bone to become sclerotic (subarticular bony sclerosis). The presence of bone cyst formation is a common finding. Later findings include bony collapse and the formation of osteophytes (bony outgrowths that are seen at the margins of the joint). Inflammatory markers and autoantibodies are negative.

Management

1 Non-pharmacological management includes weight loss, physiotherapy, walking aids and hydrotherapy to rebuild lost muscle bulk.
2 Medical treatments are used for pain relief. Simple analgesia and nonsteroidal anti-inflammatory drugs are the mainstay of treatment supplemented by intra-articular steroid injection. See also indications for Cox II antagonists under rheumatoid arthritis (page 360).

3 Surgical: The aim of surgery is to relieve pain not treated by medical management and to increase useful function.

- Osteotomy is the surgical realignment of a joint (normally hip or knee), which may produce benefit for 1–10 years post-surgery. It allows alteration of the muscle use, the contact areas and the blood dynamics within the joint. It is of most use in younger patients with a good range of movement and relative preservation of the intra-articular cartilage.
- Arthroscopic procedures include synovectomy (removal of the synovium), irrigation of joints and debridement.
- Arthroplasty (joint replacement) is the treatment of choice in older patients. Hip and knee replacements are the most successful; however, there is a risk of failure after about 10 years. In the upper limb, although the joints are not weight bearing, the normal range of movement is difficult to achieve and the prostheses are prone to failure.
- Arthrodesis (joint fusion) can be useful for pain, but can only be used if the loss of function is acceptable.

Prognosis

The disease may show a slow progression, little or no change over years, or a stepwise deterioration. There are some genetically inherited disorders with early onset osteoarthritis, which have a much worse prognosis.

Seropositive arthritis

Rheumatoid arthritis

Definition

Rheumatoid arthritis is a chronic multisystem, inflammatory disorder with a characteristic symmetrical polyarthritis.

Prevalence

One to two per cent of the adult population affected.

Age

Peak age of onset 30–55 years.

Sex

2–3 F : 1 M

Geography

Prevalence varies across the world from 0.1–5%.

Aetiology

It is thought that one or more environmental trigger factors occur in a genetically susceptible individual setting up a sustained inflammatory response.

- Twin studies demonstrate a significantly higher concordance in monozygotic compared with dizygotic twins.
- Hormonal factors are implicated, possibly the effects of oestrogen on T cell function, as females are affected more than males and there is a tendency for the disease to become quiescent during pregnancy. This sex difference diminishes after the menopause reinforcing the possibility of a role for sex hormones.
- The DR region of HLA appears particularly important in the susceptibility to rheumatoid arthritis. Sixty per cent of patients who develop rheumatoid arthritis have DR4. Conversely certain HLA patterns appear to be protective.
- Infective agents have been suggested as triggering stimuli, including *Proteus mirabilis*, *Mycoplasma*, Epstein–Barr virus, parvovirus and various retroviruses.

Pathophysiology

- T cells: Antibody-mediated activation of T cells triggers a more generalised T cell activation. This may cause an inflammatory response to self-antigens (type II collagen, gp39) within the synovium in the presence of co-stimulatory factors found in abundance in rheumatoid tissue. Cytokine cascades result in a combination of angiogenesis and cellular influx, leading to transformation of the synovium with the ability to invade cartilage and connective tissue. The transformed synovium may also activate osteoclast-mediated bone erosion.
- Synovitis: Early disease is characterised by synovial inflammation and a cell-rich effusion within the joint causing swelling and pain. Neutrophils predominate within the effusion and release high levels of proteolyic enzymes, causing significant damage.
- Rheumatoid factors are autoantibodies to the Fc portion of IgG; they may be of any antibody class. Routine serological testing detects IgM rheumatoid factor. These factors undergo a maturation of affinity for Fc and tend to form lattice-like complexes found

throughout the tissues of the rheumatoid joint. It is thought that they provoke further inflammation and activate the complement system. Patients who test positive for IgM rheumatoid factor have a more severe pattern of joint damage.

- Long-standing inflammation and effusion distends the joint capsule causing laxity of the ligaments. The overall result is joint instability and continued use leads to joint deformity.
- After a variable period, synovial inflammation may become quiescent. Deformities, if already present, may continue to deteriorate through secondary degenerative changes.

Clinical features (articular)

Classically, rheumatoid arthritis presents as an insidious, progressive, symmetrical polyarthritis with pain, and stiffness particularly after periods of inactivity, swelling and limitation of joint movement. Occasionally a more rapid onset and progression is seen. Fifty per cent of patients presenting with episodic monoarthritis (palindromic rheumatism) will develop rheumatoid arthritis over the subsequent months or years.

- Hands and wrists: Initially there is muscle wasting and involvement of metacarpophalangeal and proximal interphalangeal joints. Later there is subluxation at metacarpal phalangeal joints and ulnar deviation of fingers. Characteristic fixed flexion (Boutonnière) or hyperextension (swan neck) deformities develop at the proximal interphalangeal joints. Tender swelling of the ulnar styloid, subluxation and deviation of the hand may occur. Carpal tunnel syndrome can occur.
- Feet and ankles: These are affected in 50% of cases, usually developing a few years after onset. Swelling of the metatarsal phalangeal joints progresses to hammer toe deformities with associated ulceration due to pressure over the metatarsal heads.
- Knees are affected with severe effusions, Baker's cyst formation, quadriceps wasting, flexion deformities and lateral angular deviation.
- Cervical spine inflammation and bone damage results in joint instability and risks atlantoaxial subluxation with resulting cervical myelopathy.
- Other joints involved include the temporomandibular joint causing a stiff painful jaw and the cricoarytenoid joint causing hoarse voice and inspiratory stridor.

- There is often associated muscle weakness and generalised osteopenia due to immobility, which may be further exacerbated by treatment with steroids.

Clinical features (extra-articular)
See Fig. 8.1.

Investigations
- Blood: Anaemia (usually normochromic normocytic), with raised inflammatory markers (ESR, CRP).
- Immunology: IgM rheumatoid factor is present in 70%.
- X-ray: Early changes include soft tissue swelling, periarticular osteopenia and marginal erosion of bone. Later there is progressive loss of joint space, more extensive erosive changes and bone destruction, joint subluxation and secondary degenerative changes.

Management
Treatment strategies are multimodal and include physical interventions, symptom-controlling drugs, steroids, disease modifying antirheumatic drugs (DMARD), anticytokines and surgery.

- Non-pharmacological interventions include patient education, physical therapy, psychological support (e.g. patient support groups), occupational therapy, nutritional and dietary advice, appliances and footwear.
- Symptom control is generally with nonsteroidal anti-inflammatory drugs, which reduce pain and stiffness (ibuprofen, indomethacin, diclofenac, etc.) These have not been shown to prevent joint erosions but they can result in greater joint movement.
- Cox II inhibitors should be used in preference to standard NSAIDs in patients who are at high risk of developing serious gastrointestinal adverse effects (e.g. patients over 65 years of age, those using other medications that increase the risk of upper GI bleeding or those requiring a prolonged course of maximal dose NSAIDs). Cox II inhibitors are relatively contraindicated in patients with cardiovascular disease, a previous history of peptic ulcer disease or previous GI bleeding.
- Oral, intravenous or intra-articular steroids are used to suppress inflammation, and may be administered. High doses may be required at times of exacerbation,

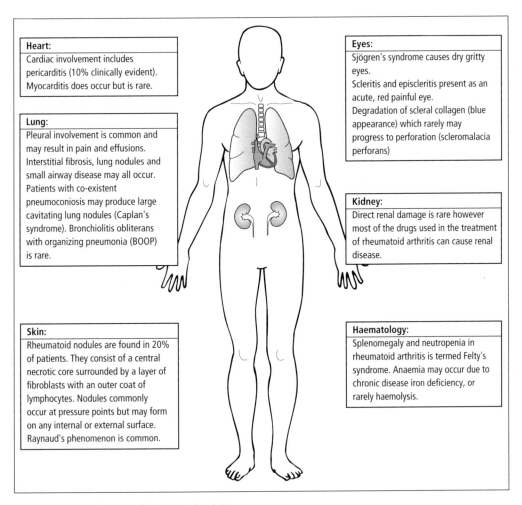

Heart:
Cardiac involvement includes pericarditis (10% clinically evident). Myocarditis does occur but is rare.

Lung:
Pleural involvement is common and may result in pain and effusions. Interstitial fibrosis, lung nodules and small airway disease may all occur. Patients with co-existent pneumoconiosis may produce large cavitating lung nodules (Caplan's syndrome). Bronchiolitis obliterans with organizing pneumonia (BOOP) is rare.

Skin:
Rheumatoid nodules are found in 20% of patients. They consist of a central necrotic core surrounded by a layer of fibroblasts with an outer coat of lymphocytes. Nodules commonly occur at pressure points but may form on any internal or external surface. Raynaud's phenomenon is common.

Eyes:
Sjögren's syndrome causes dry gritty eyes.
Scleritis and episcleritis present as an acute, red painful eye.
Degradation of scleral collagen (blue appearance) which rarely may progress to perforation (scleromalacia perforans)

Kidney:
Direct renal damage is rare however most of the drugs used in the treatment of rheumatoid arthritis can cause renal disease.

Haematology:
Splenomegaly and neutropenia in rheumatoid arthritis is termed Felty's syndrome. Anaemia may occur due to chronic disease iron deficiency, or rarely haemolysis.

Figure 8.1 Extra-articular features of rheumatoid arthritis.

but because of side effects, doses should be gradually reduced and stopped if possible once the disease is quiescent.

- Disease modifying antirheumatic drugs: Patients with rheumatoid arthritis should be treated with DMARDs soon after diagnosis, as these have been shown to improve prognosis. They act to ameliorate symptoms and slow progression of structural damage. Methotrexate is normally used as first line, other agents include sulphasalazine, gold and hydroxychloroquine. Combinations of DMARDs are increasingly used. Onset is slow, 10–20 weeks, and all have some degree of toxicity.

- Tumour necrosis factor alpha (TNF-α) inhibitors (etanercept and infliximab) are used in patients with persistently active rheumatoid arthritis that has not responded adequately to at least two DMARDs, including methotrexate.

- Anti-cytokines including anti-IL-1 and anti-IL-6 are undergoing evaluation.

- Because of immobility and steroid therapy patients with rheumatoid arthritis are at high risk for development of osteoporosis. Most patients should be treated with calcium and vitamin D supplementation. Bisphosphonate therapy should be considered in high-risk patients.

- Surgical management aims to help with symptom control and maximise joint function. Procedures include the following:
  1 Synovectomy, which is the removal of excessive synovial swelling from joints and tendons, may help to reduce pain and stiffness in early disease.
  2 Tendon repair and transfer is used particularly in the wrist and hand.
  3 Excision arthroplasty (limited joint excision) or arthrodesis (joint fusion) may be performed for intractable pain at the elbow or wrist; however, there is an inevitable loss of function. Atlantoaxial subluxation may require surgical stabilisation.
  4 Joint replacement has significant postoperative morbidity but can be an effective longer term treatment.

Prognosis

The disease generally progresses insidiously in the majority of cases although most patients experience periods of exacerbation and quiescence.

Seronegative arthritides (spondyloarthropathies)

Ankylosing spondylitis

Definition

Ankylosing spondylitis is a chronic inflammatory arthritis predominantly affecting the axial skeleton, causing pain and progressive stiffness.

Prevalence

0.2% of the population.

Age

Usual onset at 16–40 years.

Sex

5M : 1F, overt disease.

Aetiology

HLA B27 is present in over 90% of Caucasians with ankylosing spondylitis. Environmental factors are implicated due to discordance in identical twins. Suggested agents include bacterial infection (such as *Klebsiella*).

Pathophysiology

There is an inflammatory reaction at the site of ligament to bone attachment (enthesopathy), which then progresses to ligamentous ossification. Microscopically, there is oedema and inflammation, especially in the adjacent bone marrow. Synovitis of the spine and large joints may occur, and there is both synovitis and enthesopathy at the sacroiliac joints. The outer layer of the intervertebral disc becomes calcified and forms a bony bridge between vertebral bodies (syndesmophytes). As these extend up the spine, calcification causes rigidity and a typical 'bamboo' appearance on X-ray.

Clinical features

Patients develop a gradual onset of episodic low-back pain and morning stiffness. There is a loss of normal lumbar lordosis due to muscle spasm and sacroiliac joint tenderness. Movement of the spine is restricted in all planes and a limitation of chest expansion may occur. Late in the disease there is a severe kyphosis (see Fig. 8.2) with marked limitation of movement or complete rigidity of the spine. Acute anterior uveitis, aortic regurgitation and apical lung fibrosis are known extra-articular features.

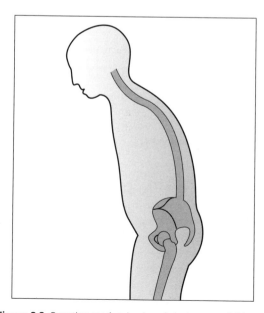

Figure 8.2 Question mark spine in ankylosing spondylitis.

Complications
Spinal fractures may occur with minimal trauma due to localised osteoporosis (secondary to immobility and inflammation). Atlantoaxial subluxation and cauda equina syndrome may occur.

Investigations
- Inflammatory markers (particularly CRP) are often elevated in active phases of the disease, although may be normal even with severe disease.
- X-rays may be normal in early stages.
  1 Early signs on bilateral AP views of sacroiliac joints are of sclerosis and erosions in the sacroiliac joints,
  2 Lateral views of lumbar spine show erosions of edges of vertebral bodies, squaring of the vertebrae, syndesmophyte formation and 'bamboo' spine.

Management
Major objectives are to relieve the pain and stiffness.
- Patients should be encouraged to remain active, avoid prolonged bed rest and avoid lumbar supports. Physiotherapy involvement is important.
- Pain and morning stiffness are treated with non-steroidal anti-inflammatory drugs.
- Large joint involvement may also respond to drugs such as sulphasalazine. Anti-TNF-α antibodies have been shown to be effective in severe disease.
- Surgery may be indicated for disease in large joints (including arthroplasty). A lumbar or cervical spinal osteotomy may be helpful in patients with severe curvature.

Prognosis
There is a wide range of severity: In over 85% there is minimal disability, 50% of patient's children will inherit HLA B27 and of these, 33% will develop the condition.

Psoriatic arthritis

Definition
A chronic inflammatory arthritis occurring with psoriasis.

Prevalence
1% of population have psoriasis of which 5% will get arthritis.

Age
Peak incidence age: 30–50 years.

Sex
1:1

Aetiology
- Genetic factors: Psoriasis and psoriatic arthritis have a familial tendency particularly in first-degree relatives. There are some twin studies suggesting increased monozygotic concordance. A number of HLA antigens are related to the development of psoriasis and psoriatic arthritis especially B27, and there are genetic linkage studies to a number of loci.
- Environmental factors include bacterial and viral infections and trauma. Trauma may be implicated as psoriatic skin lesions exhibit the Koebner phenomenon (lesion develop at sites of trauma).

Pathophysiology
Synovitis is histologically the same as that of rheumatoid arthritis, although bone resorption is sometimes prominent. It is likely that both the skin lesions and the arthritis are immunologically mediated.

Clinical features
There are usually psoriatic lesions of the skin but the severity is unrelated to the development of arthritis (see page 387). Psoriatic nail involvement is related to an increased risk of psoriatic arthritis. Five patterns of arthritis are seen:
1 Distal interphalangeal joint synovitis, which is often asymmetrical.
2 Asymmetric oligo/monoarthritis.
3 Symmetrical rheumatoid-like polyarthritis.
4 Arthritis mutilans is a rare deforming – destructive arthritis with marked bone resorption.
5 Spondyloarthropathy similar to ankylosing spondylitis affects the spine and sacroiliac joints.

Investigations
- Blood tests may show raised inflammatory markers, anaemia of chronic disease and presence of autoantibodies (ANA and RhF).
- X-ray: There is a combination of erosions and new bone formation in distal joints. Other features include periostitis, bone resorption, sacroiliitis and spondylitis.

Management

Pain and inflammation is treated with nonsteroidal anti-inflammatory drugs. Specific Cox II inhibitors may be of value (see indications given in section on Rheumatoid Arthritis). Second line agents include methotrexate and ciclosporin. Anti-TNF-α monoclonal antibodies have been shown to be effective in reducing the progression of psoriatic arthritis. Surgical intervention may prove necessary.

Prognosis

It is not clear whether any medical intervention has disease-modifying potential.

Reactive arthritis

Definition

Acute or chronic synovitis that occurs less than 6 weeks following infections with various organisms, including *Chlamydia*, *Yersinia*, *Salmonella*, *Shigella* and *Campylobacter* species. Reiter's syndrome is a form of reactive arthritis with the triad of arthritis, uveitis, and urethritis.

Incidence

Unknown but not rare.

Age

Peak at 16–35 years.

Sex

M > F

Aetiology

As with other spondylo-arthritides there is a strong association with HLA B27 (60–80% of patients). Inflammatory arthritis is precipitated by an environmental agent, e.g. sexually acquired non-specific urethritis caused by *Chlamydia trachomatis* or *Ureaplasma urealyticum* or enteric infections particularly *Shigella*, *Yersinia* or *Salmonella*.

Pathophysiology

In early synovitis there is intense hyperaemia with inflammatory infiltration. The arthritis is said to be sterile as bacteria cannot be cultured from joints; however, bacterial DNA and RNA and bacterial macromolecules can be detected in the joints.

Clinical features

Typically there is an abrupt onset of asymmetrical lower limb arthritis, sacroiliitis and spondylitis. Achilles tendinitis and plantar fasciitis may also occur. This may have been preceded by a clinical urethritis, prostatitis, cystitis or diarrhoeal disease. Bilateral conjunctivitis and uveitis may also occur.

Investigations

High ESR, anaemia of chronic disease and leucocytosis occur. The synovial fluid white cell count is high. X-rays are initially normal but may show erosions and features similar to ankylosing spondylitis.

Management

Although unlikely to affect the course of arthritis, antibiotics are given for ongoing urethritis. Ophthalmology referral is essential for uveitis and the arthritis is usually managed with nonsteroidal anti-inflammatory drugs. The few patients who develop a chronic arthritis are treated as for rheumatoid arthritis.

Inflammatory bowel disease related arthritis

Definition

An enteropathic arthritis, sacroiliitis, ankylosing spondylitis or rarely hypertrophic osteoarthritis in association with ulcerative colitis or Crohn's disease.

Prevalence

10% of ulcerative colitis patients and 15–20% of Crohn's patients.

Age

Commonest at 20–45 years.

Sex

1:1

Aetiology

The aetiology is unknown but the synovitis may occur in response to bacterial antigens that have passed through the damaged gut wall. Enteropathic arthritis is a seronegative non-erosive synovitis. Sacroiliitis is related to the presence of HLA B27

Clinical features
An acute, self-limiting, asymmetrical non-deforming arthritis usually affecting knees or ankles. Treatment of the inflammatory bowel disease leads to resolution of arthritis.

Management
Inflammatory bowel disease is treated as normal. Use of nonsteroidal anti-inflammatory drugs for treatment of joint pain may make diarrhoea worse. Intra-articular steroid injections may be of value.

Connective tissue disorders

Systemic lupus erythematosus

Definition
Systemic lupus erythematosus (SLE) is a multisystem disorder characterised by inflammation and profound immunological disturbance.

Prevalence
40 per 100,000 in United Kingdom, wide geographic variation (1:250 American black women).

Age
Usually 16–55 years with a peak in early twenties.

Sex
9F : 1M

Geography
Commoner in West Indies, Singapore and Far East.

Aetiology
- Genetics: Up to 60% concordance in monozygotic twins. 5–10% risk in first-degree relatives. HLA-B8, DR2 and DR3 are associated with increased incidence of SLE as are deficiencies in complement factors such as C1q, C2 and C4. Currently studies are underway into a number of chromosomal loci in relation to SLE.
- Hormonal: There is evidence that females are predominantly affected and there are commonly premenstrual and puerperium exacerbations. It is suggested that oestrogen may be involved in the aetiology of SLE.
- Immunological factors: Significant disturbance of normal immunology is seen in patients with SLE; however, it is unclear if these are aetiological factors for, or the consequence of the disorder:
  1 Polyclonal activation of B cells in the early stages of the disease resulting in hypergammaglobulinaemia. B cells also have an increased life span.
  2 T-cell regulation is also affected resulting in decreased cytotoxic T-cell reactions, increased helper T cells and abnormalities in the cytokine balance.
  3 There are also abnormalities in cell-to-cell signaling and in apoptosis within the immune system.
  It is thought that these defects may trigger a cascade of events resulting in the production of autoantibodies. Over time these antibodies undergo maturation of affinity resulting in high affinity antibodies to DNA, Smooth muscle (Sm), RNP, Ro, La, nucleosomes and other nuclear antigens.
- Environmental factors: Suggested factors include viruses, ultraviolet light and reactions to medication.

Pathophysiology
The mechanism by which the aetiological factors interact to cause the disease is still unclear; however, many of the clinical manifestions are the result of the formation of immune complexes and subsequent complement activation (e.g. lupus nephritis).

Clinical features
Systemic lupus erythematosus is a multisystem disorder affecting skin, joints, kidneys, lungs, nervous system, mucous membranes and other organs. The presentation is very variable between individuals. The clinical course is characterised by relapses, which may be prolonged, and remissions. Systemic symptoms include general malaise, fever (sometimes high and swinging) and depression (see Fig. 8.3).

Microscopy
Fibrinoid necrosis around blood vessels (usually arterioles, venules and capillaries) pleura and joint capsules.

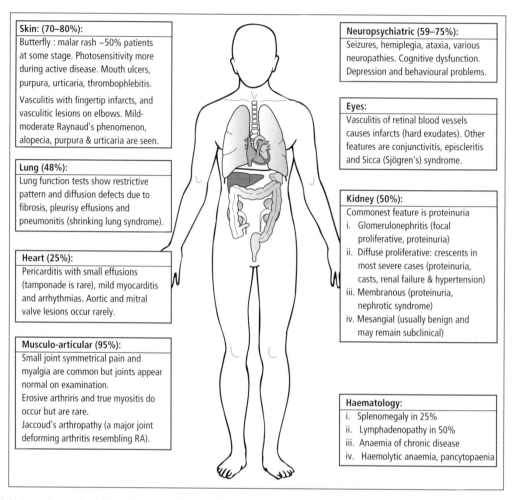

Skin: (70–80%):
Butterfly : malar rash ~50% patients at some stage. Photosensitivity more during active disease. Mouth ulcers, purpura, urticaria, thrombophlebitis.

Vasculitis with fingertip infarcts, and vasculitic lesions on elbows. Mild-moderate Raynaud's phenomenon, alopecia, purpura & urticaria are seen.

Lung (48%):
Lung function tests show restrictive pattern and diffusion defects due to fibrosis, pleurisy effusions and pneumonitis (shrinking lung syndrome).

Heart (25%):
Pericarditis with small effusions (tamponade is rare), mild myocarditis and arrhythmias. Aortic and mitral valve lesions occur rarely.

Musculo-articular (95%):
Small joint symmetrical pain and myalgia are common but joints appear normal on examination.
Erosive arthriris and true myositis do occur but are rare.
Jaccoud's arthropathy (a major joint deforming arthritis resembling RA).

Neuropsychiatric (59–75%):
Seizures, hemiplegia, ataxia, various neuropathies. Cognitive dysfunction. Depression and behavioural problems.

Eyes:
Vasculitis of retinal blood vessels causes infarcts (hard exudates). Other features are conjunctivitis, episcleritis and Sicca (Sjögren's) syndrome.

Kidney (50%):
Commonest feature is proteinuria
i. Glomerulonephritis (focal proliferative, proteinuria)
ii. Diffuse proliferative: crescents in most severe cases (proteinuria, casts, renal failure & hypertension)
iii. Membranous (proteinuria, nephrotic syndrome)
iv. Mesangial (usually benign and may remain subclinical)

Haematology:
i. Splenomegaly in 25%
ii. Lymphadenopathy in 50%
iii. Anaemia of chronic disease
iv. Haemolytic anaemia, pancytopaenia

Figure 8.3 Systemic manifestations of systemic lupus erythematosus.

Immune complex deposition in skin at the dermal–epidermal junction, kidney and blood vessels.

Investigations

- ANAs seen in 95–99% of SLE. Anti-double stranded DNA antibodies are relatively specific but only 50% sensitive. Other autoantibodies seen include anti-RNP, anti-smooth muscle, anti-Ro (SSa) and anti-La (SSb). Rheumatoid factor is seen in 50%.
- Complement is low during active disease suggesting complement activation and consumption by immune complexes.
- False positive tests for syphilis are found in approximately 10% of patients (positive WR or VDRL because cardiolipin is a component of the antigenic mixture used in these assays). The fluorescent *Treponema pallidum* antibody test is negative.
- ESR is raised in active disease, with normal CRP levels.
- Immunoglobulins usually polyclonal increase in gammaglobulins.
- Haematological abnormalities:
  1 Normochromic, normocytic anaemia in 75%.
  2 Direct antiglobulin test positive haemolytic anaemia in 10–20%.
  3 Leucopenia and mild thrombocytopaenia.
  4 Antibodies to clotting factors especially lupus anticoagulant directed against prothrombin activator (see below).

Management

- Most patients with mild disease are treated conservatively.
- Nonsteroidal anti-inflammatory drugs are first-line treatment for articular disease.
- Antimalarials are used for systemic symptoms, refractory arthritis and skin disease.
    Hydroxychloroquine for skin and joint problems.
    Mepacrine causes yellow pigmentation but is useful.
    Six monthly eye-checks are recommended.
- Corticosteroids:
    High dose for widespread vasculitis, acute nephritis, severe CNS vasculitis.
    Moderate dose for pleural effusions or moderate thrombocytopenia.
- Immunosuppressive agents:
    Azathioprine is used as a steroid-sparing agent. Cyclophosphamide is more toxic but may be used in severe diffuse proliferative nephritis or severe neuropsychiatric lupus.

Prognosis

Generally a good prognosis, chronic forms of the disease are seen. Patients with renal or neuropsychiatric involvement have a worse prognosis.

Antiphospholipid syndrome

Definition

A disorder characterised by the presence of autoantibodies directed against phospholipids or plasma proteins bound to phospholipids.

Aetiology/pathophysiology

Antiphospholipid syndrome may be primary/idiopathic or may occur secondary to SLE or other autoimmune disorders. The condition causes a thrombotic tendency due to loss of phospholipid dependent coagulation co-factors. Pro-thrombotic stimuli such as pregnancy, surgery, cigarette smoking, hypertension and the use of oral contraceptives further exacerbate this tendency. Antibodies include the lupus anti-coagulant (anti-coagulant in vitro but procoagulant in vivo), anti $\beta 2$ glycoprotein-I antibodies and anticardiolipin antibodies.

Clinical features

- Thrombosis: Venous thromboses are more common than arterial thromboses. These occur mainly in the deep veins of the calf. Other sites include renal, hepatic, subclavian and retinal veins. Arterial thrombosis in the cerebral vessels, coronary, renal and mesenteric arteries thromboses may also occur. Clinically patients may present with strokes, migraine, pulmonary embolism and infarction, thrombocytopenia, variable degrees of renal failure and amaurosis fugax.
- Pregnancy: Some women suffer recurrent miscarriage especially during the late second and third trimester.
- Non-thrombotic neurological manifestations include epilepsy, transverse myelitis, Guillain–Barré syndrome and chorea.
- Cutaneous manifestations include livedo reticularis (a purplish mottled discolouration of the skin).

Investigations

Diagnosed by presence of anticardiolipin antibodies.

Management

Anticoagulation with aspirin for mild cases and warfarin in more severe cases reduces the risk of thrombosis. During the first and third trimester of pregnancy low-molecular-weight heparin is used due to the teratogenicity of warfarin and risks of bleeding in labour.

Systemic sclerosis and scleroderma

Definition

Sclerosis (hardening due to excessive production of connective tissue) of collagen affecting the skin (scleroderma) and the internal organs (systemic sclerosis).

Incidence

Rare, 3 per million.

Age

Any age, mean onset at 40 years.

Sex

9F : 1M

Aetiology

- Genetic factors are suggested by variations in incidence between ethnic groups and familial clustering.
- Infectious and non-infectious environmental agents have also been implicated. A scleroderma like disorder is seen following exposure to silica, vinyl chloride, petroleum-based solvents, rape seed oil and bleomycin.

Pathophysiology

Immune system activation with the production of autoantibodies including antiendothelial cell antibodies and upregulation of cell adhesion molecules causes damage to blood vessels. This results in the release of activating factors, changes in vascular permeability and the proliferation of active fibroblasts, which produce excessive collagen.

Clinical features

A number of patterns of scleroderma and systemic sclerosis are recognised:

Localised scleroderma

- Morphoea are patches of sclerotic skin on the trunk and limbs, which may be localised or more generalised.
- Linear scleroderma describes a dermatomal distribution of skin and subcutaneous sclerosis.

Systemic sclerosis

- Limited cutaneous systemic sclerosis begins with Raynaud's phenomenon prior to the development of skin sclerosis restricted to the hands (digital ulcers, ischaemia and necrosis), face (beaked nose, small mouth), feet and forearms. Previously this form of systemic sclerosis was referred to as CREST syndrome (calcinosis, Raynaud's disease, esophageal dysmotility, sclerodactyly and telangiectasia).
- Diffuse cutaneous systemic sclerosis refers to extensive skin sclerosis along with multisystem involvement (see Fig. 8.4).
- Systemic sclerosis sine scleroderma is a rare form of the illness in which there is systemic disease in the absence of skin sclerosis.
- Overlap syndromes have combinations of the features of systemic sclerosis, systemic lupus erythematosus, dermatomyositis or rheumatoid arthritis.

Microscopy

Extensive deposition of collagen is seen in the skin, viscera, small and medium-sized arteries, arterioles and capillaries. In the wall of blood vessels concentric proliferation and thickening of the intima and fibrosis of the adventitia is seen.

Investigations

- As with systemic lupus erythematosus the ESR is raised with a normal CRP.
- Autoantibodies include anticentromere, antitopoisomerase-1 (Scl-70), anti-RNA polymerase, and rheumatoid factor is positive in 30%.
- Full blood count may show anaemia of chronic disease or haemolytic anaemia.
- X-ray changes: In the hands there is a loss of the tufts of the terminal phalanges and soft tissue calcification. There is basal fibrosis in the lungs with reticulonodular shadowing. Contrast imaging of the GI tract may demonstrate oesophageal dilation, poor motility and diverticulae of large bowel.

Management

There is no curative treatment, education is essential and symptomatic treatments initiated.

- Raynaud's phenomenon is treated by avoiding cold, and vasodilators such as nifedipine, ACE inhibitors or in severe cases prostaglandin infusions.
- Oesophageal symptoms are treated with H_2 antagonists or proton pump inhibitors, and oesophageal strictures may require repeated dilatation. Malabsorption may require changes in diet.
- Hypertension resulting from renal involvement needs control with ACE inhibitors or calcium channel antagonists.
- The role of immunosuppressive drugs remains unclear.
- Bosentan (an endothelin receptor antagonist) is used in the treatment of pulmonary hypertension secondary to systemic sclerosis and has been shown to reduce the formation of multiple digital ulcers.

Prognosis

Localised forms are milder and do not progress to systemic involvement. No treatment has been shown to alter the long-term progression of scleroderma. Diffuse disease with severe visceral involvement carries the worst prognosis.

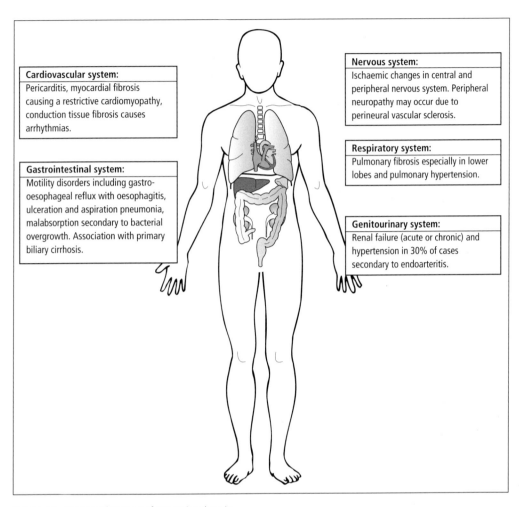

Figure 8.4 Multisystem involvement of systemic sclerosis.

Sjögren's syndrome

Definition
A chronic inflammatory disorder of the lacrimal and salivary glands.

Sex
9F : 1M

Aetiology
Sjögren's syndrome may be primary, or secondary to rheumatoid arthritis, systemic lupus erythematosus, progressive systemic sclerosis or polymyositis. There is an association with non-Hogkin B cell lymphoma.

Pathophysiology
There is lymphocytic infiltration of salivary glands and other exocrine glands in the respiratory and gastrointestinal tract, the skin and the vagina. There is glandular enlargement, with atrophy of the acini and proliferation of the duct lining.

Clinical features
- Ocular manifestations: Sensation of persistent grittiness, photosensitivity, tiredness and an inability to produce tears (keratoconjunctivitis sicca).
- Gastrointestinal system: Lack of saliva (xerostomia) causes difficulty in chewing and swallowing. There

may be oral ulcers, dental caries and firm non-tender enlargement of the parotid gland.

- Other manifestations include arthralgia, Raynaud's phenomenon and an association with other organ specific autoimmune disorders in primary Sjögren's syndrome, e.g. thyroid disease. Occasionally there are systemic features including vasculitis and renal tubular defects.

Investigations

- Anaemia of chronic disease, leucopenia and high ESR
- Rheumatoid factor (RhF) is positive in 80–100%, ANA positive in 60–80%, anti-Ro (SSa) antibodies are seen in primary Sjögren's syndrome and may cause neonatal heart block in offspring of affected women.
- Schirmer's test for keratoconjunctivitis sicca measures tear production. An edge of a strip of filter paper is placed in the lower eyelid and the length that becomes wet is measured.

Management

Artificial tears and saliva replacement solutions provide symptomatic relief.

Polymyositis and dermatomyositis

Definition

Myositis is an inflammatory disorder of striated muscle. When associated with skin manifestations it is termed dermatomyositis.

Prevalence

1 per 100,000 population.

Age

Any, peaks 40–50 years.

Sex

2F: 1M

Aetiology/pathophysiology

Lymphocytic infiltration, autoantibody production and HLA-DR3 association suggests an immune-mediated pathogenesis. There may be environmental trigger factors. Dermatomyositis is associated with malignancy (e.g. lung, stomach carcinoma) predominantly over the age of 40 years. The inflammation within muscle causes necrosis and patchy regeneration with fibrosis and atrophy in later stages. The skin shows collagenous thickening of the dermis with chronic inflammatory cell infiltrates.

Clinical features

Gradual onset of non-specific systemic features followed by symmetrical, progressive, proximal muscle weakness. In more chronic presentations there is muscle atrophy, contractures and calcinosis. Skin manifestations include a purple rash on the eyelids often with oedema (heliotrope rash) and scaly vasculitic patches on the knuckles (Gottron's papules). There may be skin ulceration and Raynaud's phenomenon. Occasionally there is cardiac involvement leading to heart failure, respiratory involvement, including nonspecific interstitial pneumonia, and oesophageal involvement, which may be sufficiently severe so as to require gastrostomy feeding.

Investigations

- Inflammatory markers: The ESR is raised.
- Autoantibodies: Anti-histidyl-tRNA synthetase (anti-Jo1) are seen in 30%, and rheumatoid factor is positive in 30%.
- CK-MB fraction and troponin I can be used to assess cardiac involvement.
- Raised muscle enzymes such as creatine kinase (prior to biopsy).
- EMG: Spontaneous fibrillations at rest, abnormal low-amplitude, short-duration polyphasic motor potentials on voluntary contraction and high-frequency discharges.
- Muscle biopsy is definitive.
- MRI of thighs is routinely performed.

Management

Acute phases are treated with corticosteroids, which should be reduced gradually to a low-maintenance dose. Methotrexate, azathioprine or cyclophosphamide are used in resistant cases.

Prognosis

The condition may last several years. The disease is of variable severity, and spontaneous remissions can occur.

Marfan's syndrome

Definition
Inherited condition resulting in abnormalities of connective tissue causing anomalies in the musculoskeletal, cardiovascular and ocular systems.

Incidence
1 in 15,000.

Aetiology/pathophysiology
Inherited in an autosomal dominant fashion. Mutations occur in the FBN1 gene that codes for the extracellular matrix glycoprotein fibrillin and is on the long arm of chromosome 15. FBN1 mutations also occur in milder phenotypes with features overlapping Marfan's phenotype. Twenty-five per cent of cases represent new mutations.

Clinical features
The phenotype is variable and unrelated to the FBN1 mutation.
- Musculoskeletal: Patients have elongated and asymmetrical faces with a high arched palate. There is a reduced upper to lower body segment ratio and an arm span that exceeds the patient's height. Long thin fingers and toes are termed arachnodactyly. Scoliosis is common along with pectus excavatum (funnel chest).
- Cardiovascular system: There is degeneration of the media of blood vessel walls:
  1 Dilation of the aortic valve ring producing regurgitation.
  2 Mitral valve prolapse and associated mitral valve regurgitation.
  3 Aneurysm formation may occur, usually in the ascending aorta, which may be followed by dissection and/or rupture.
- Ocular: Weakness of the suspensory ligament of the lens may cause an upward lens dislocation (ectopia lentis).

Investigations
The diagnosis is clinical and can be based on clinical criteria scoring. Once diagnosed patients require periodic aortic imaging to detect early dilation.

Management
- β-blockers have been shown to slow aortic dilation, and lifelong therapy is recommended by the European Society of Cardiology.
- At least annual echocardiograms are required with consideration of prophylactic aortic root replacement prior to the development of critical dilatation.
- Dislocated lenses are not removed unless conventional visual correcting aids are ineffective.
- Orthopaedic intervention may be required.
- Genetic counselling should be offered where appropriate.

Ehlers–Danlos syndrome

Definition
An inherited group of conditions resulting from a weakness in collagen.

Aetiology/pathophysiology
At least 10 variants of this condition have been described inherited in a variety of fashions (autosomal dominant, autosomal recessive and X-linked recessive). The underlying pathology is an abnormality in skin, joint and blood vessel collagen resulting in tissue weakness. Some of the subtypes have been mapped to mutations in the collagen genes.

Clinical features
There is hyperextensible skin with normal elastic recoil, hypermobile joints, and fragility of blood vessels causing bruising and occasionally aortic dissection and rupture. Hypermobility can lead to early osteoarthritic changes and damage to the joints. Genetic counselling should be offered where appropriate.

Crystal arthropathies

Crystal-induced arthropathy may result in various disease patterns:
- Monosodium urate crystals cause acute gout and chronic tophaceous gout.
- Calcium pyrophosphate causes pseudogout.
- Crystallised injected corticosteroids may result in iatrogenic acute synovitis.

- Calcium hydroxyapatite crystals are involved in the pathogenesis of osteoarthritis.

The crystals deposited in the joint are phagocytosed by neutrophils. Typically pyrophosphate crystals are seen within a phagolysosomal sac, whereas urate crystals are not confined. Phagolysosomal lysis results in the release of enzymes into the cell cytoplasm. Phagocytosis induces cytokine release leading to chemotaxis and further inflammation.

Gout

Definition

An acute inflammatory arthritis resulting from urate crystal deposition secondary to hyperuricaemia.

Prevalence/incidence

Hyperuricaemia occurs in 5%, gout affects 1–20 per 1000 males.

Age

Peak incidence at the age of 40–50 years.

Sex

10M : 1F

Geography

Mainly a disease of developed countries.

Aetiology

High levels of uric acid cause gout but not all individuals with hyperuricaemia will develop gout. Hyperuricaemia is associated with increasing age, male sex and obesity, and in females urate levels rise after the menopause. Uric acid is formed from the breakdown of purines (see Fig. 8.5). Hyperuricaemia may occur due to increased rates of uric acid production or decreased uric acid excretion.

- Increased uric acid production may be idiopathic or secondary to excessive intake or high turnover as seen in malignancy (especially with chemotherapy).
- Decreased salvage of purines may occur; in Lesch–Nyhan syndrome a defect in HGPRT results in impaired salvage and hence high uric acid levels.

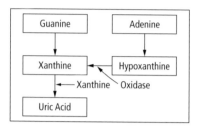

Figure 8.5 Uric acid formation.

- Decreased renal excretion may be idiopathic or secondary to renal failure or drugs such as thiazides or low-dose aspirin.

An acute episode of gout may be precipitated by a sudden increase or decrease in urate concentration. Risk factors include surgery, infection, dehydration, severe illness, starvation, diuretics and alcohol.

Pathophysiology

- In joints an acute synovitis may occur when urate crystals have been phagocytosed. The crystals cause disruption of lysosomal membranes and hence release of inflammatory mediators.
- If chronic, the crystals accumulate in the synovium and sites such as the ear cartilage forming lumps termed tophi.
- In the kidney, urate crystals may precipitate in the collecting ducts or cause stone formation. The result of urate damage is either tubulointerstitial disease (urate nephropathy) or acute tubular necrosis.

Clinical features

In 70–90% the initial attack of gout affects the big toe. It is known as podagra if it first affects the metatarsophalangeal joint. The joint is red, hot, swollen and very tender. There may be an associated fever. These features make it difficult to distinguish from a septic arthritis. Other joints affected include ankles, knees, fingers, elbows and wrists. Chronic gout is unusual but may cause a chronic polyarthritis with destructive joint damage with large erosions on X-ray and deformity. Tophi (smooth white skin and joint deposits) occur at cartilagenous sites particularly in the Achilles tendon and the helix of the ear. This usually reflects severe untreated gout.

Investigations

Urate levels are often high, although they may fall during an acute attack. Inflammatory markers (CRP, ESR) may be raised. Aspiration of joint fluid will demonstrate the negatively birefringent crystals.

Management

Acute gout is managed with high dose nonsteroidal anti-inflammatory drugs. Hyperuricaemia is treated only if associated with recurrent gout attacks.

- Non-pharmacological: Weight loss, high-fluid intake, low alcohol, low-purine diet, avoid thiazides and aspirin.
- Pharmacological: Allopurinol, which inhibits xanthine oxidase. Excess purines are excreted as xanthine rather than uric acid, and the therapy is lifelong. Steroids can be injected into troublesome joints.

Pseudogout

Definition

A crystal arthropathy resulting from calcium pyrophosphate dihydrate (CPPD) deposition in the joints.

Aetiology/pathophysiology

CPPD crystal formation occurs in cartilage located near chondrocytes. It is suggested that excessive cartilage pyrophosphate production leads to local crystal formation. Crystals are thought to enter the joint cavity after being shed from the cartilage in which they have formed.

Clinical features

Chondrocalcinosis may be detected on X-ray in cartilage without joint disease. Acute joint inflammation resembles gout most commonly affecting the knee and other large joints.

Investigation

Examination of the joint fluid will demonstrate positively birefringent crystals.

Management

The pain of pseudogout is relieved by nonsteroidal anti-inflammatory drugs, aspiration of synovial fluid and intra-articular steroid injection.

Metabolic bone disorders

Osteoporosis

Definition

A disease characterised by low bone mass and microarchitectural disruption. It is diagnosed if the race/sex matched bone density falls below 2.5 standard deviations from the average young bone density (WHO).

Incidence

Overall 30% of individuals will have a pathological fracture due to osteoporosis.

Age

Females over 50 and males over 55 years.

Sex

2F : 1M

Aetiology

Bone is continually being remodelled involving reabsorption and synthesis. It is thought that osteoporosis results from a long-term slight imbalance between the two processes. The risk of fractures increases with bone loss and hence with age. Factors that can affect the remodelling balance are as follows:

- Sex: Females have a lower bone mass and a high rate of bone loss in the decade following the menopause. This is largely oestrogen-dependent, early menopause and ovariectomy without hormone replacement therapy predisposes. Gonadal failure and androgen insensitivity are risk factors for osteoporosis in men.
- Age: Age-related bone loss is seen in both sexes; although worse in females, this may be due to decreased calcium absorption.
- Genetic factors implicated include the vitamin D receptors and collagen genes.

- Diseases such as Cushing's syndrome, type I diabetes mellitus, thyrotoxicosis, acromegaly, hyperparathyroidism, rheumatoid arthritis and chronic renal failure.
- Drugs can worsen/cause osteoporosis including systemic corticosteroids, ciclosporin and cytotoxic drugs.
- Smoking increases the risk of osteoporosis.

Pathophysiology

Although there is low bone mass it is normally mineralised. There is disruption of the normal architecture, with fewer and thinner bony spicules and non-supporting horizontal 'struts' that do not join up to any other structure. The structural integrity of the bone is reduced, causing skeletal fragility.

Clinical features

Osteoporosis is not itself painful; however, the fractures that result are. Typical sites include the vertebrae, distal radius (Colles' fracture) and the neck of the femur. Other symptoms of vertebral involvement are loss of height and increasing kyphosis.

Investigations

- Bone density scanning (dual X-ray absorptiometry, i.e. DEXA scan) is the gold standard for diagnosis.
- X-ray investigation shows fractures, a bone scan can be used to demonstrate recent fractures. The generalised bone density is difficult to assess as the appearance is dependent on the X-ray penetration.
- Serum calcium, phosphate and alkaline phosphatase are normal.
- Bone biopsy can be performed to confirm the diagnosis.

Management

- Non-pharmacological interventions include adequate nutrition (calories, calcium and vitamin D), exercise and quitting smoking.
- Bisphosphonates inhibit bone reabsorption and are increasingly being used for the prevention and treatment of osteoporosis.
- Oestrogen therapy in postmenopausal women is protective; however, because of the increased risk of breast cancer and thromboembolic disease it is not recommended for the prevention of osteoporosis. Males with gonadal failure benefit from androgens.

Osteomalacia

Definition

Inadequate mineralisation of growing bone. In adults decreased mineralisation causes osteomalacia, and in children it results in rickets.

Aetiology

Osteomalacia is usually due to a lack of vitamin D or its active metabolites, but it may be caused by severe calcium deficiency or by hypophosphataemia.

Pathophysiology

During bone remodelling vitamin D deficiency results in a failure of calcification of new bone. This causes weakness of the bone and an increased risk of fractures.

Clinical features

Onset is insidious with bone pain, backache and weakness that may be present for years before the diagnosis is made. Vertebral compression and pathological fractures may occur; a biochemical diagnosis may be made prior to onset of clinical disease.

Investigations

- X-ray investigation shows generalised bone rarefaction and possible evidence of fractures. Looser's zones may be seen in which there is a band of severe rarefaction surrounded by sclerosis due to failed healing of a fracture.
- Serum calcium and phosphate levels are generally low with raised alkaline phosphatase. Serum 25-hydroxy vitamin D_3 levels are low.
- Investigation for an underlying cause such as malabsorption or renal disease should be performed.

Management

Treatment is aimed at the underlying disorder but often involves oral calcium and vitamin D replacement.

Paget's disease

Definition

A disorder of bone remodelling with accelerated rate of bone turnover.

Prevalence
Common with 10% of adults affected by age 90.

Age
Rare before 40 years.

Sex
M = F

Aetiology
There may be a genetic component as there is a familial tendency. There are families with an autosomal dominant inheritance of Paget's disease. Viral infections may also be involved in the aetiology, including canine distemper virus and measles. Paget's disease may be due to a latent infection in a genetically susceptible individual.

Pathophysiology
Osteoclastic overactivity causes excessive bone resorption. There follows osteoblast activation in an attempt to repair the lesion. The resultant bone is larger than normal, but abnormal architecture predisposes to fractures.

Clinical features
Most patients are asymptomatic and the disease is discovered incidentally on routine X-ray. Patients may complain of a dull pain, which is worse at night. On examination the bone may be bent and thickened, most obvious if the tibia is affected (sabre tibia). With widespread bone involvement there may be a bowing of the legs and considerable kyphosis.

Complications
Nerve compression may cause pain. Skull involvement may lead to compression of the VIIIth nerve resulting in deafness. High output cardiac failure may occur due to shunting of blood through the vascular bone. Fractures are common especially in the weight-bearing long bones. Osteogenic sarcoma may occur due to Paget's disease and carries a poor prognosis. It may cause a marked increase in bone pain.

Investigations
Characteristically there is a very high serum alkaline phosphatase with a normal serum calcium and phosphate reflecting the high bone turnover. However, during periods of immobilisation in active disease the serum calcium level may rise dramatically. Imaging shows enlargement of bone, osteolysis and sclerosis.

Management
Asymptomatic Paget's disease requires no treatment, patients with persistent bone pain, repeated fractures, neurological complications or high cardiac output are treated with calcitonin and/or bisphosphonates, which suppress bone turnover. Surgical intervention may be required.

Genetic musculoskeletal disorders

Achondroplasia

Definition
Achondroplasia is a form of osteochondroplasia in which the arms and legs are abnormally short.

Incidence
Commonest form of true dwarfism.

Age
Congenital, usually obvious by age 1.

Sex
M = F

Aetiology/pathophysiology
Inherited in an autosomal dominant fashion, most cases however are sporadic. The genetic mutation is within the fibroblast growth factor receptor −3 gene.

Clinical features
Disproportionate shortening of the long bones of the limbs with a normal trunk length. The head is large with a prominent forehead and a depressed bridge of the nose causing a saddle shaped nose. Intelligence is normal. There is a large lumbar lordosis, which causes prominent buttocks, flexed hips and bowed legs. A trident deformity of the hands may be present.

Investigations

Skeletal survey allows accurate measurement of the long bones.

Management

Patients may develop neurological problems due to stenosis of the spinal canal; this may require surgical intervention. Leg lengthening procedures and genu varum correction may be considered.

Osteogenesis imperfecta

Definition

A heterogenous disorder with brittle bones and involvement of other collagen containing connective tissue.

Incidence

1 in 20,000 live births.

Aetiology

Most of the observed phenotypes result from mutations in one of two genes that code for type I collagen precursor proteins (COL1A1 and COL1A2). Blue sclera result from a thinning of the sclera, which allows the colour of the underlying pigmented tissue to be seen.

Clinical features

Features and classification are given in Table 8.4.

Complications

Hearing loss due to otosclerosis. The triad of otosclerosis, blue sclera and brittle bones is termed van der Hoeve's syndrome.

Management

Multidisciplinary approach involving physiotherapy, occupational therapy and orthopaedic surgery.

- Gentle nursing of infant to avoid fractures.
- Prompt splinting of fractures to prevent deformity.
- Mobilisation to prevent further osteopenia.
- Correction of deformities if necessary by surgical intervention.
- New therapies under evaluation include bisphosphonates, growth hormone and bone marrow transplant.
- Genetic counselling should be offered where appropriate.

Bone tumours

Metastatic bone tumours

Definition

Metastatic cancer is much more common than primary bone cancer.

Aetiology/pathophysiology

Two thirds of bone secondaries arise from adenocarcinomas of the breast or prostate. The remainder arise from carcinoma of the bronchus, adenocarcinoma of the kidney and thyroid. Metastases usually appear in the marrow cavity, damaging bone both directly through expansion and indirectly through bone reabsorption.

Clinical features

Patients may present with bone pain or a pathological fracture. Bone metastases may be the first sign of the primary tumour. There may be a leucoerythroblastic

Table 8.4 Features and classification of osteogenesis imperfecta

Type	Inheritance	Features
Type I Tarda (mild)	Autosomal dominant	Fractures are common, sclera are blue and joints are hypermobile; however deformity is uncommon. Heart valve disorders may occur
Type II (lethal)	Recessive disorder	Infants may be still born, or have multiple fractures and deformities of the long bones
Type III (severe deforming)		Normally diagnosed at birth, by 5 yrs of age the child has had multiple fractures and has developed severe deformity. Few children survive into adult life and those who do have severe growth restriction
Type IV (moderately severe)	Autosomal dominant	Similar to type I without the blue sclera

Table 8.5 Primary bone tumours

Tumour	Nature	Epidemiology	Clinical features	X-ray findings	Treatment
Osteoid osteoma	Benign tumour originating from osteoblasts	Adolescents M > F	Localised pain	Radiolucent area surrounded by dense sclerosis	Surgical excision
Non-ossifying fibroma	Benign tumour	Child/adolescent M > F	Coincidental finding	Apparent cystic lesion in cortex of a long bone metaphysis	Resolves spontaneously
Giant cell tumour	Benign, invasive or metastatic tumour of osteoclasts	20–40 years M > F	Pain, swelling and pathological fractures	Asymmetrically positioned low-density area extending to the joint margin	Excision, which may be extensive. Radiotherapy
Osteosarcoma	Malignant tumour of osteoblasts	10–25 yrs/over 65 yrs M > F	Severe pain worse at night, often humerus or knee. May arise in Paget's disease	Bone destruction, & subperiosteal new bone growth, streaks of soft tissue calcification (sun-ray appearance)	Surgery or chemotherapy, metastasises early
Ewing's tumour	Malignant tumour arising from the vascular endothelium	Child/adolescent M > F	Pain and swelling with warm tender lump with ill defined edges	Bone destruction with overlying 'onion skin' layers of periosteal new bone	Surgery often requires amputation followed by chemotherapy
Chondroma	Benign tumour of cartilage	40+ age M > F	Pain, swelling or a fracture often in hands	Low density area in medulla of the bone often with specks of calcification	Excised and replaced with bone graft
Chondrosarcoma	Malignant tumour arising from chondrocytes	30–60 yrs M > F	Pain, fracture or growing exostosis	Destructive medullary tumour containing flecks of calcification	Surgery or chemotherapy, metastasises early

anaemia due to marrow replacement, hypercalcaemia and nerve or spinal cord compression.

Investigations
The X-ray typically demonstrates a destructive lytic bone lesion, although some metastases appear sclerotic (e.g. prostate). Isotope bone scans are used to assess the extent of the lesions and to detect lesions that are not evident on X-ray.

Management
Symptomatic treatments include analgesia, local radiotherapy and chemotherapy, internal fixation of any fractures and spinal decompression in vertebral collapse with spinal cord compression. Hypercalcaemia may require treatment (see page 11).

Primary bone tumours

See Table 8.5.

Vasculitis

Vasculitis is an inflammatory infiltration of the wall of blood vessels with associated tissue damage. The affected

Table 8.6 Classification of vasculitis

Vessel size	Disease	Arteries/organs affected
Large vessels	Giant cell (temporal) arteritis	Temporal arteries
	Takayasu's disease	Aorta and arch branches
Medium vessels	Polyarteritis nodosa	Multiorgan
	Kawasaki's disease	Coronary arteries
Small vessels	Wegner's granulomatosis	Nasal, lung and renal
	Churg–Strauss syndrome	Lung, kidney, heart and skin
	Buerger's disease	Leg arteries and veins
	Hypersensitivity vasculitis	Skin, kidney
	Secondary vasculitis	Multisystems disorders

vessels vary in size, type and location. The underlying mechanisms of the disorders are not fully understood. Vasculitis may be primary or associated with another disorder such as systemic lupus erythematosus, rheumatoid arthritis, scleroderma, malignancy, infection and drugs. Vasculitides may be considered according to the size of vessel affected (see Table 8.6).

Polymyalgia rheumatica

Definition
A clinical syndrome characterised by pain and stiffness in the muscles of the pelvic and shoulder girdle associated with the development of giant cell (temporal) arteritis.

Prevalence
Common, affecting up to 1 in 150.

Age
Rare under 50 years.

Sex
2F : 1M

Aetiology
A history of polymyalgia rheumatica is present in 50% of patients with giant cell arteritis, 15% of patients with polymyalgia rheumatica will develop giant cell arteritis. The conditions may occur separately.

Clinical features
Gradual onset of pain, stiffness and perceived symmetrical weakness in shoulder neck and pelvic girdle. Systemic malaise, anorexia and weight loss may occur. Although fevers occur they are not as severe or swinging as seen in giant cell (temporal arteritis).

Investigations
The diagnosis is made clinically. There are very high inflammatory markers including ESR and CRP. There may be anaemia of chronic disease.

Management
Moderate dose prednisolone is used, and the therapy is monitored and tailored to the response of inflammatory markers. Generally treatment is required for 9–15 months, and prophylaxis against osteoporosis is essential (see page 373).

Temporal (giant cell) arteritis

Definition
Giant cell arteritis (GCA) is a granulomatous arteritis affecting large and medium-sized vessels.

Aetiology
GCA occurs in patients over 50 years of age with familial clustering and an association with smoking. Genetic associations include HLA-DR4 and specific isoforms of intercellular adhesion molecule-1 (ICAM-1). Peaks in incidence every 5 years suggest an infective trigger.

Clinical features
There is a history of polymyalgia rheumatica in up to 50% of cases. Patients present with fever, severe headache and scalp tenderness over the inflamed superficial temporal or occipital arteries. On examination the temporal arterial pulsation is progressively lost as the artery becomes thickened and there may be overlying erythematous skin. Facial, jaw and mouth pain occur due to inflammation of the facial, maxillary and lingual branches

of the external carotid arteries resulting in jaw claudication. Visual disturbances such as ptosis, diplopia and visual loss may occur due to inflammation of the ciliary and/or retinal arteries.

Macroscopy/microscopy
Patchy inflammation of the arterial wall interspersed with segments of normal artery; therefore, a negative biopsy does not mean that the diagnosis is excluded. Affected areas show necrosis, loss of elastic fibres and lymphocytic and occasional giant cell infiltration.

Investigations
Inflammatory markers such as the ESR and CRP are very high. Temporal artery biopsy may be diagnostic (see above).

Management
Corticosteroids are used at high doses to prevent progression to irreversible visual loss. These should be commenced immediately the diagnosis is suspected and should not be delayed by the artery biopsy. The biopsy may still be of diagnostic value up to 5 days after commencing steroids. Once the inflammatory markers have settled, the dose is gradually reduced over a period of months.

Takayasu's syndrome

Definition
A chronic inflammatory arteritis of unknown aetiology affecting the aorta and its main branches.

Incidence
1–3 per 1,000,000 per year.

Age
Commonest between 10 and 40 years.

Sex
80–90% females.

Geography
Largest number of cases in Asia and Africa.

Pathophysiology
Initially inflammation occurs in the left subclavian artery progressing to involve the carotids, vertebral, brachiocephalic, aorta and pulmonary arteries. Inflammation may cause vessel wall thickening, and narrowing, occlusion or dilation of affected vessels. T cells and anti-endothelial antibodies have been implicated in the pathogenesis.

Clinical features
After an initial prodromal illness patients present with weight loss, myalgia and synovitis. On examination patients appear unwell, and the blood pressure may be reduced in one or both arms. However, hypertension often develops due to renal artery or aortic narrowing. Arterial pulses in the limbs are often asymmetrically reduced with bruits on auscultation. There may be features of arterial insufficiency with limb claudication, cool extremities and in severe cases ischaemic ulceration or gangrene.

Microscopy
Intimal proliferation with scarring of the media and loss of elastic fibres. There is lymphocytic infiltration and fibrosis.

Investigations
Inflammatory markers (ESR, CRP) are often raised and there may be anaemia of chronic disease. Although arteriography remains the gold standard for diagnosis, it may be superseded by CT or MR angiography.

Management
Corticosteroids are the mainstay of treatment, with methotrexate and azathioprine used in refractory cases. Percutaneous angioplasty or surgical bypass of affected arteries may be required in irreversible vessel stenosis with significant ischaemia.

Prognosis
Most patients survive at least 5 years.

Polyarteritis nodosa

Definition
Polyarteritis nodosa is a rare intense necrotising vasculitis affecting small and medium-sized arteries.

Age
Middle age

Sex
4M : 1F

Aetiology/pathophysiology
Associated with hepatitis B infection in 10–20% because of hepatitis B surface antigen immune complexes. Also associated with hairy cell leukaemia. Transmural neutrophil infiltration of medium-sized arteries occurs, causing degeneration, weakness and microaneurysm formation. Veins are also affected and the condition may result in thrombosis and tissue infarction.

Clinical features
Polyarteritis nodosa is usually an acute illness characterised by calf pain, general malaise, myalgia and weight loss for a few days prior to visceral manifestations:
- Musculocutaneous: Migratory arthralgia or arthritis, purpura and subcutaneous haemorrhage.
- Cardiovascular system: Coronary arteritis leading to cardiac arrhythmias, failure and myocardial infarction.
- Gastrointestinal system: Mesenteric arteritis causing pain, haemorrhage and mucosal ulceration.
- Genitourinary system: Haematuria, proteinuria, hypertension, renal infarction and renal failure.
- Nervous system: Polyneuropathy (mononeuritis multiplex) with motor and sensory deficits.

Investigations
Raised ESR and white blood count. Patients are usually p-ANCA positive. Angiography reveals multiple microaneurysms of the renal or intestinal vessels. Diagnosis may be made on biopsy of affected organs.

Management
Corticosteroids and immunosuppressive agents (e.g. cyclophosphamide) in severe acute cases.

Wegener's granulomatosis

See page 124 in Chapter 3 (Respiratory System).

Churg–Strauss syndrome (allergic granulomatosis)

Definition
Multisystem disorder consisting of asthma and rhinitis, eosinophilia, eosinophilic infiltration, small vessel vasculitis and extravascular granulomas.

Age
Peak incidence 30–40 years.

Sex
M = F

Aetiology/pathophysiology
It is thought to be an autoimmune disorder.

Clinical features
- Prodromal disorder of allergic rhinitis and asthma.
- Peripheral blood eosinophilia and eosinophilic infiltration of the lung and gastrointestinal tract.
- Systemic vasculitis of the medium and small vessels with vascular and extravascular granulomatosis. Affected organs include the skin with subcutaneous nodules, purpura and haemorrhages; heart with pericarditis, cardiac failure and myocardial infarction; neurological system with a mononeuritis multiplex; kidney with a focal segmental glomerulonephritis; gastrointestinal system with an eosinophilic gastroenteritis and musculoskeletal system causing myalgia and migratory polyarthritis.

Investigations
Chest X-ray may show patchy pneumonia-like shadowing, which can be fleeting. The ESR is raised and there are raised levels of immunoglobulins. Anti-myeloperoxidase anti-neutrophil cytoplasmic antibodies (pANCA) is positive in 70%. The diagnosis can be confirmed on biopsy of affected organs.

Management
Treatment involves steroids and azathioprine.

Buerger's disease

Definition
Buerger's disease or thrombangitis obliterans is an inflammatory occlusion of small and medium-sized peripheral arteries and veins of the upper and lower limbs.

Aetiology/pathophysiology
It occurs almost exclusively in heavy cigarette smokers and is therefore seen more in countries with high levels of smoking. There is segmental chronic inflammatory infiltration of the vessel walls with resultant obliteration of the lumen and secondary thrombosis.

Clinical features
The condition starts with digital ischaemia, ulceration preceded by claudication in the feet, or rest pain in the fingers or toes. The condition is progressive. Wrist and ankle pulses are usually absent but brachial and popliteal pulses are present. There may be a previous history of superficial thrombophlebitis.

Investigations
Arteriography shows narrowing or occlusion of small peripheral arteries with healthy main vessels.

Management
The condition remits with quitting smoking; nicotine replacement therapy cannot be used but bupropion (Zyban) is safe. Prostaglandin infusions, thrombolytic therapy, surgical sympathectomy and revascularistion procedures have been tried.

Henoch–Schönlein Purpura

Definition
A syndrome resulting from a vasculitis of small blood vessels.

Age
Peak 2–8 years, young adults.

Sex
2M : 1F

Aetiology
The aetiology is unknown but several factors have been implicated including upper respiratory tract infection especially by *Streptococcus*. Serum concentrations of IgA are raised in approximately half of patients and IgA-containing immune complexes have been identified. Clusters of cases have been noted with no obvious precipitant.

Pathophysiology
The condition results from inflammation within the walls of small blood vessels, predominantly capillaries but small arterioles and venules are also affected. The inflammation is thought to be the result of a hypersensitivity reaction (type III immune complex mediated). The inflammation of the vessels increases permeability resulting in a leaking of fluid and cells from the circulation into the surrounding tissue. IgA deposition within the glomeruli of the kidney causes a focal segmental pattern of glomerulonephritis with a resultant proliferation of mesangial cells and a nephritic syndrome.

Clinical features
This multisystem disorder may occur with simultaneous or sequential manifestations:
- The characteristic presentation is with the skin lesion. It is unclear whether other lesions can occur without the rash. The rash characteristically affects the lower limbs and buttocks, but is not always confined to these areas. The rash is initially blanching but becomes purpuric and then goes through the classic colour changes of a bruise, lesions of varying ages are present at one time. Oedema of the face, dorsum of the hands and feet, perineum or foreskin may occur especially in young children
- A self-limiting acute arthritis of large distal joints occurs without articular damage with the patient complaining of swollen, tender painful joints exacerbated with movement.
- The gastrointestinal manifestations present with colicky pain, which may be severe, and associated with vomiting. Bleeding from the affected vessels may cause melaena or haematemesis.
- Renal involvement is common with haematuria and proteinuria detectable but is generally not severe in children.

- Rarely there may be CNS involvement with convulsions, paresis and coma.

Microscopy

There is an inflammatory infiltrate in the upper dermis, joint lining and GI mucosa and glomerular mesangium with neutrophils and extravasated red blood cells.

Complications

Gastrointestinal complications include infarction and intussusception as a result of oedema. Renal failure may occur in the acute phase, or may progress over many years.

Investigations

The diagnosis is clinical; erythrocyte sedimentation rate, white cell count and eosinophils may be raised. Urine microscopy should be performed looking for red and white blood cells, casts and protein. Faecal occult blood may be positive without overt bleeding.

Management

No specific treatment is used. Symptomatic relief of joint pain and rash may be achieved with nonsteroidal anti-inflammatory drugs. Gastrointestinal bleeding and CNS manifestations may be improved with the prompt use of steroids. Complications such as acute renal failure and intussusception should be managed promptly.

Prognosis

In most cases the overall prognosis is excellent, the course is variable with cases lasting between a few days and a few weeks. Rarely it may continue for up to a year and there may be a course of relapse and remission. Severe renal involvement and CNS involvement may be life-threatening.

Raynaud's disease and phenomenon

Definition

An exaggerated vascular response to cold, causing a spasm of the arteries supplying the fingers and toes.

Prevalence

Five to ten per cent of young women in temperate climates.

Age

Most common in 15–30 years.

Sex

F > M

Clinical features

Symptoms are symmetrical with fingers affected more than toes, it usually begins in a single digit and then becomes more generalised. There is initial skin pallor due to vasoconstriction progressing through cyanosis to hyperaemia (white to blue to red). There may be tingling or pain in the affected digits especially with restoration of blood supply during rewarming.

Investigations

Primary Raynaud's phenomenon must be distinguished from Raynaud's syndrome occurring with connective tissue disorders such as systemic sclerosis.

Management

Often avoidance of cold is all that is required. In more severe cases calcium channel blockers such as nifedipine are used. In severe cases prostacyclin infusions may be required.

Behçet's syndrome

Definition

A chronic, relapsing multisystem vasculitis characterised by oral ulceration.

Incidence

Rare.

Age

Commonest in 20–40 years.

Sex

M > F

Geography

Much more common in Turkey, Iran, China, Korea and Japan.

Aetiology/pathophysiology

It is thought to be the result of an environmentally triggered autoimmune reaction in a genetically susceptible individual.

Clinical features

Patients have recurrent oral aphthous or herpetiform ulcers. Other manifestations include genital ulceration, ocular disease (uveitis), skin lesions (erythema nodosum), arthritis, gastrointestinal upset, renal, lung and neurological involvement. Patients demonstrate pathergy (a papule or pustule forms at sites of skin puncture) – this is a highly specific finding.

Management

Corticosteroids and immunosuppressive agents are used for severe disease. Colchicine may be of benefit for erythema nodosum and arthralgia.

Clinical

Nomenclature and description

The cornerstone of dermatological diagnosis is accurate observation and description of lesions and rashes. Some terms used to describe specific lesions are given in Table 9.1. Many rashes have classical distributions, which may be symmetrical or asymmetrical. Specific rashes and distributions are considered under individual headings.

Dermatological procedures

- *Shave or tangential excision:* This procedure slices a surface growth off using a blade, often to remove a small growth and confirm its nature at the same time.
- *Punch biopsy:* Under local anaesthesia a full thickness cylinder of skin (1–4 mm diameter) is cut out using a biopsy punch. The resultant hole is sutured and leaves minimal scarring.
- *Electrodesiccation and curettage:* Under local anaesthesia lesions including precancers and benign growths are scraped off with a special tool and the area is cauterised to stop bleeding. Repeated treatment may be required. The area heals often leaving a small hypopigmented mark.
- *Cryotherapy:* Liquid nitrogen is used to freeze the cutaneous lesion. Light freezing causes a peeling, moderate freezing a blistering and hard freezing a scabbing.
- *Mohs' surgery:* This is a technique used in the resection of basal cell and squamous cell carcinomas.

Under local anaesthesia palpable tumour is excised with a curette or scalpel. A thin section a few millimetres around and underneath the resulting defect is taken, divided into pieces, and cut as a fresh frozen specimen. If tumour is seen at a particular margin resection is continued at the appropriate margin, and further sections examined until no further tumour is seen. This technique allows the maximal conservation of normal surrounding tissue. If the resultant defect is large, formal reconstructive surgery may be necessary.

Skin grafts

Skin grafts are sections of skin that are completely detached and transferred to cover large areas of skin defect. The recipient site requires a good blood supply, as the graft has no supply of its own.

- Split skin grafts are used in acute trauma, granulating areas and burns. A guarded freehand knife or an electric dermatome is used to remove epidermis and a variable amount of dermis from the donor site, which heals by re-epithelialisation. If a very large defect needs covering, the graft can be meshed. Split skin grafts take up a blood supply more easily than full thickness grafts, but tend to shrink and have abnormal pigmentation and contour.
- Full thickness grafts, involving epidermis and entire dermis, are used mainly in reconstructive surgery. They leave a donor site, which requires closure by sutures, limiting the size of the graft. They require a very good vascular bed at the recipient site to survive.

Table 9.1 Nomenclature of skin lesions

Bulla	A large fluid-filled blister, may be a primary bullous disorder such as pemphigus or pemphigoid.
Erythroderma	Intense and widespread reddening of the skin due to dilation of blood vessels, often with exfoliation. Normally the most extreme form of an underlying skin pathology.
Excoriation	Stripping of the skin usually by scratching as a result of intense itching of the skin.
Lichenification	A thickening of the skin due to increased keratin production. May be a primary lichenoid disease or a secondary lichenification due to repeated excoriation as seen in chronic eczema.
Macule	Describes a skin lesion that is flat, often well circumscribed with alteration of colour.
Nodule	A lump or swelling within the skin, >1 cm in diameter.
Papule	A small lump or swelling within the skin, <1 cm in diameter.
Plaque	A palpable disc shaped lesion.
Pustule	A visible collection of pus.
Scale	Thick hyperkeratosis overlying normal or abnormal skin.
Vesicle	A small fluid-filled blister below the epidermis.
Weal	A swelling of the skin caused by dermal oedema.

Skin flaps

Skin flaps differ from skin grafts in that they are taken with their own blood supply. The coverage can thus be thicker and stronger than grafts, and can be applied to avascular areas such as exposed bone, tendons and joints. Flaps may be transferred whilst maintaining their original vascular attachments (pedicle flaps), or may be re-anastamosed to local blood supply (free flaps).

Scaly lesions

Eczema

Atopic eczema

Definition
A chronic inflammatory skin disorder associated with atopy, causing dry, scaly, itchy lesions.

Prevalence
Atopic tendency in up to 10–25% worldwide. Atopic eczema in 5%.

Age
More common in children with peak onset usually 2–18 months.

Sex
M = F

Geography
May occur anywhere, but higher incidence in urban areas.

Aetiology/pathophysiology
The term atopy is a disease resulting from allergic sensitisation to normal environmental constituents manifesting as asthma, eczema or hayfever. The underlying cause and mechanisms in eczema have yet to be fully elucidated; however, dry skin (xerosis) is an important contributor. There appear to be genetic and immunological components to allergic sensitisation (see also page 498).

- Genetic: Close concordance in monozygotic twins. Offspring of one atopic parent have a 30% risk of being atopic, which rises to 60% if both parents are atopic.
- Chromosome studies suggest that atopic tendency may be inherited in part on maternal 11q13, which codes for the β subunit of mast cell IgE receptors.
- Exacerbating factors include excessive bathing, drying, emotional stress and detergents. Occasionally, in children less than 1-year old milk allergy may be causative.

Serum IgE is elevated in 85% of individuals and higher values are seen when eczema and asthma are present together. It is thought that the high frequency of secondary infection is a combination of the loss of skin integrity and deficiency of local antimicrobial proteins.

Clinical features

Patients have generalised dry skin (xerosis) along with typical eczematous lesions. These are erythematous and scaly, and intense itching results in superficial abrasions (excoriation). Chronic inflammation of the skin causes thickening termed lichenification. Lesions may weep and have tender tiny blisters termed vesicles especially when superinfection occurs. The distribution is age dependent:

- Babies develop eczema predominantly on the face and head; this may resolve or progress by 18 months to the childhood/adult pattern.
- Children and older patients tend to have lesions in the flexures, such as the antecubital and popliteal fossae, neck, wrists and ankles.

Complications

Staphylococcus aureus is found on the skin of 90%, which may result in acute infection (impetiginised eczema). Primary infection with herpes simplex may give a very severe reaction known as eczema herpeticum, which in the young may cause dehydration and is life-threatening.

Investigations

Patients show high levels of serum IgE; suspected allergic triggers may be identified using skin prick or RAST testing.

Management

There is no curative treatment.

- Avoidance of exacerbating factors is essential. In babies it may be appropriate to either test for cow's milk allergy or to perform a therapeutic trial with a cow's milk protein free formula.
- Generalised dry skin (xerosis) requires regular frequent use of emollient moisturisers especially after bathing/showering. Cream preparations are water based with emulsifiers and preservatives and they tend to dry the skin. Greasier preparations such as white soft paraffin achieve better moisturisation. A balance has to be struck between application of sufficient grease and cosmetic satisfaction. Greasier preparations are usually better tolerated prior to going to bed.
- Topical steroids remain the mainstay of treatment. If used appropriately they are both safe and effective. The lowest potency that is effective should be used and higher potency reserved for resistant cases. It is

also important to use only low-potency steroids on thin areas of skin such as the face.

- Antibiotics are used for secondary bacterial infection. In young children these may be parenteral; aciclovir is used to treat eczema herpeticum.
- Wet wraps consist of the application of topical agents under bandages to facilitate absorption. Emollients may be administered in this way or coal tar may be used as a keratolytic in lichenified skin. If steroids are applied under wet wraps the dose/potency must be decreased as increased absorption may result in systemic side effects.
- Antihistamines have not been shown to be effective in reducing itching. Sedating antihistamines are used at night to improve sleep, reduce nocturnal scratching and hence break the 'itch-scratch-itch' cycle.
- Topical tacrolimus, an immunosuppressant, is being increasingly used in children prior to the use of high-potency steroids. It appears safe and effective; however, the long-term risks are unknown, as it is a relatively new preparation. Pimecrolimus is under study as a similar agent without systemic immunological effects.
- PUVA or combination UVA and UVB are used in very resistant eczema; however, therapy is expensive and increases the risks of skin cancer.

Prognosis

Eczema has a fluctuating course with approximately 50% resolving by 18 months, and few have problems beyond childhood.

Contact dermatitis

Definition

Contact dermatitis is an allergic or irritant-induced dermatitis arising from direct skin exposure to a substance.

Age

Most common in children and adult women.

Sex

F > M

Geography

Exposure is most common in the home or industrially related.

Aetiology/pathophysiology

- Irritant contact dermatitis (80%) is caused by over-exposure to substances that cause damage to the skin. Once the epidermal barrier is damaged a secondary inflammatory response occurs. Irritants include soapy water, detergents, acid and alkaline solutions.
- Allergic contact dermatitis (20%) occurs in sensitised individuals exposed to a specific low-molecular-weight chemical, such as nickel in jewellery, and components of hair dyes and perming solutions, perfumes, topical medicines and plants. Allergens are processed and presented by Langerhans' cells in the skin causing a Th1 mediated type IV hypersensitivity response.

Clinical features

Contact dermatitis often affects the hands or face. Lesions may also affect the legs of patients with chronic venous insufficiency, when sensitivity to dressings is thought to be the cause. Lesions are erythematous itchy papules or blisters occasionally with oedema and fissures. Allergic contact dermatitis may be acute or chronic.

Management

The allergens can be identified by patch testing (see page 467) and avoided. Where contact is unavoidable appropriate protection for the skin such as gloves should be used. For irritant contact dermatitis, topical steroids can be used. Use of aqueous cream instead of soap helps to reduce itching.

Seborrhoeic dermatitis

Definition

Seborrhea means excessive oily secretions. Seborrhoeic dermatitis is a chronic scaly inflammatory eruption affecting areas rich in sebaceous glands.

Aetiology/pathophysiology

Evidence suggests a role of *Malasezia furfur/Pityrosporum ovale*, a yeast that colonises the skin of patients with seborrhoeic dermatitis; however, it is unclear if this is the cause or effect of the condition. Seborrheic dermatitis is common in patients with HIV infection and may be a presenting feature.

Clinical features

The lesions appear pinkish due to mild erythema and scaly due to increased epidermal proliferation. The commonest areas affected are the eyebrows and around the eyes extending into the scalp. The areas around the nose and upper lip are also affected. In babies a widespread lesion of the scalp (cradle cap) is seen, and in the elderly lesions are often more diffuse.

Management

Seborrhoeic dermatitis is treated with a combination of low-potency steroids and topical antifungal creams/shampoos.

Psoriasis

Definition

Psoriasis is a chronic, non-infectious, inflammatory condition of the skin, characterised by well-demarcated erythematous patches and silvery scaly plaques.

Prevalence

It affects 3% of the population worldwide.

Age

Peak of onset in teens and early 20s and late onset 55–60 years.

Sex

M = F

Geography

Less common in Africa and Japan.

Aetiology

The aetiology is not fully understood but genetic environmental and immunological components are suggested.

- Psoriasis has a familial tendency with 40% of patients having a first-degree relative affected. There is concordance in monozygotic twins and a suggestion of genes located within the major histocompatibility complex close to the class I HLA locus.
- Immunological mechanisms include inflammatory infiltrates within the dermis, activation of growth factors (TGF-α and -β) and expression of various cytokines.
- There is a suggestion of environmental components. Group A streptococcal sore throat can lead to guttate

psoriasis, psoriatic lesions occur at sites of trauma and damage (the Köebner phenomenon) and certain drugs may exacerbate psoriasis (β blockers, lithium, antimalarials).

Pathophysiology

The epidermis is thickened with increased epidermal stem cells and keratinocytes. There is increased cellular DNA synthesis, shortened cell cycle and rapid epidermal turnover (turnover time is reduced from 28 to 4 days).

Clinical features

Psoriasis varies in severity. Typical lesions are clearly demarcated erythematous patches 1–10 cm in diameter. There is a thick silvery scale, which when lifted off characteristically reveals small areas of punctate bleeding. Different distribution patterns are recognised.

- Plaque psoriasis is the most common form. It usually affects extensor surfaces especially the elbows and knees, scalp and hair margin or sacrum.
- Guttate (drop-like) psoriasis is an acute onset of multiple small psoriatic lesions on the trunk often in a child or young adult with no previous history of psoriasis. It often follows a streptococcal pharyngitis. It is usually self-limiting.
- Pustular psoriasis is the most severe form and can be life-threatening. There is acute onset of diffuse erythema and scaling with sheets of superficial non-infected pustules. If the entire skin is affected, it is termed erythrodermic (the von Zumbusch variant). This may be associated with systemic upset (malaise, fever, diarrhoea) and is potentially life-threatening. Localised forms of pustular psoriasis also occur, such as palmoplantar pustulosis.
- Flexural or inverse psoriasis affects the inguinal region, axillae and submammary areas. There may not be scales visible due to moisture, the plaques therefore appear erythematous and smooth.
- Nail involvement includes pitting, ridging and onycholysis. Nail involvement is specifically associated · with psoriatic arthropathy.
- Psoriatic arthritis occurs in 5% of patients (see page 363).

Microscopy

There is infiltration of the strium corneum with neutrophils, epidermal hyperplasia with hyperkeratosis and a thin or absent granular layer. Dilated capillaries are seen in the oedematous papillary dermis.

Management

Psoriasis is a chronic disorder that is managed rather than cured. Treatments are chosen on the basis of disease pattern and severity, patient preference and clinical response.

- Emollients both topical and in the bath help reduce the scaling and dryness.
- Keratolytic agents (e.g. coal tar) are used both in the form of topical applications and shampoos to remove the scales before applying other treatments.
- Topical corticosteroids are often used; however, there is a risk of rebound psoriasis on stopping treatment.
- Calcipotriol, a vitamin D analogue, is increasingly used either as single therapy or in combination with topical steroids.
- Phototherapy with ultraviolet B (UVB), or with UVA light and an oral psoralen (PUVA), is used in patients with extensive refractory disease. These treatments are expensive and increase the risk of skin cancer. An alternative may be the use of a high-energy laser that treats only the affected skin.
- Systemic therapy is used in life-threatening or refractory psoriasis including methotrexate, ciclosporin and retinoids all of which have systemic toxicity requiring monitoring.

Prognosis

Psoriasis is a lifelong disease with variability in severity over time.

Pityriases

Pityriasis rosea

Definition

Pityron is Greek word for bran. The pityriases are skin diseases characterised by fine, bran-like scales. Pityriasis rosea is an acute, self-limiting condition with scaly oval papules and plaques mainly occurring on the trunk.

Aetiology

The cause is unknown, human herpes virus 7 has been suggested; however, the virus is not always detectable in patients with pityriasis rosea.

Clinical features

Most cases commence with a herald patch, a single salmon pink lesion 2–5 cm in diameter with central clearing and peripheral scaling. Days later crops of similar smaller oval plaques appear and proximal extremities. The lesions distribute along dermatomal lines, which is most evident on the back appearing in a 'Christmas tree' pattern.

Management

Steroids and phototherapy may be of value for associated itching.

Prognosis

Self-limiting. The condition fades in 1–2 months.

Pityriasis versicolor

Definition

Pityriasis (bran-like) versicolour (varying in colour) is a chronic infection characterised by multiple macular patches varying in size and degree of brown pigmentation occurring on the trunk.

Aetiology

Caused by infection by the commensal yeast *Pityrosporum orbiculare* (also known as *Malessezia furfur*, *Pityrosporum ovale* and *Malassezia ovalis*). Infection results from conversion of the yeast to the mycelial or hyphal form, which may be triggered by heat and humidity and immunosuppression. The yeast releases carboxylic acids, which inhibit melanin production.

Clinical features

Lesions are superficial hypopigmented macules appearing light brown or salmon coloured with a fine scale. They are most seen commonly on the upper trunk and proximal limbs.

Management

Treated with topical antifungal agents for 2 weeks. Oral antifungals may be used for extensive disease. Recurrence is common, and frequent relapses may require prophylaxis with topical selenium sulfide or an oral conazole. The loss of colour in the skin may persist for several months after treatment.

Ichthyoses

Definition

The ichthyoses are disorders of keratinisation, which may be congenital or acquired characterised by a generalised scaling of the skin due to hyperkeratosis (see Table 9.2).

Management

Topical emollients and bath additives are used to help avoid the dryness. Oral retinoids are used in the more severe forms.

Erythematous lesions

Erythema multiforme

Definition

A self-limiting hypersensitivity reaction affecting the skin and occasionally mucous membranes.

Table 9.2 Forms of ichthyosis

Condition	Inheritance	Clinical features
Ichthyosis vulgaris	Autosomal dominant	1 in 300, onset 1–4 yr, small bran-like scales are seen, often mild
Sex-linked ichthyosis	X-linked recessive	1 in 6000 males, generalised involvement with large dark scales, onset before 1 year.
Lamellar ichthyosis	Autosomal recessive	1 in 60,000, may at birth cause the collodion baby with red scaly skin and ectropion, may resolve or progress to other forms
Acquired ichthyosis	Non-inherited	Associated with inflammatory disorders, endocrine anomalies, and neoplasia especially Hodgkin's disease

Aetiology
50% of cases have no obvious underlying cause. Aetiological agents include:
- Herpes simplex in 33% of cases; may cause recurrent attacks.
- *Mycoplasma pneumoniae.*
- Other infections, e.g. vaccinia, orf, streptococci, tuberculosis, histoplasmosis.
- Drugs, e.g. sulphonamides, penicillin, phenytoin, barbiturates and carbamazepines.
- Connective tissue disorders, such as systemic lupus erythematosus.

Clinical features
Lesions are pinkish red erythematous papules/plaques with central clearing or concentric rings (target lesions). Distribution is usually symmetrical affecting the backs of limbs, hands and feet. Disseminated rash with mucosal involvement with conjunctivitis and necrotic mucosal ulcers is termed Stevens–Johnson syndrome. This is often associated with systemic symptoms.

Management
The withdrawal of any causative drug and treatment of any associated infection is essential. Short courses of oral steroids are sometimes used but their efficacy and safety are unclear. Patients with recurrent erythema multiforme resulting from herpes simplex can be prevented with prophylactic aciclovir.

Prognosis
Disease is usually self-limiting clearing in 2–3 weeks but death can occur with Stevens–Johnson syndrome.

Erythema nodosum

Definition
Erythema nodosum is an immune-mediated disorder resulting in red tender pretibial subcutaneous nodules.

Incidence
1–5 per 100,000 per year.

Age
Peak incidence 15–40 years.

Sex
F > M

Aetiology
- Streptococcal pharyngitis is the most common associated condition.
- Many cases are idiopathic but this is a diagnosis of exclusion.
- Drugs: Penicillin, oral contraceptive pill.
- Pregnancy.
- Conditions with hilar lymphadenopathy: Sarcoidosis, tuberculosis, coccidioidomycosis, histoplasmosis, Hodgkin's lymphoma and *Chlamydophila pneumoniae.*
- Gastrointestinal disorders: Inflammatory bowel disease, Behçet's syndrome and bacterial gastroenteritides.

Clinical features
Painful bluish-red nodules up to 5 cm in diameter appear in crops over 2 weeks on the anterior surface of both lower legs. They slowly fade leaving bruising and scarring of skin. Malaise, fever and arthralgia may accompany the rash.

Management
Symptomatic treatment and management of any underlying cause is essential. Recovery may take weeks, and there may be recurrence.

Urticaria

Definition
Urticaria is an itchy erythematous eruption ranging from nettle rash to large weals/plaques with palpable skin oedema. Most cases of urticaria are acute and self-limiting within a few hours, occasionally with recurrent episodes for up to 6 weeks. Acute urticaria often has an identifiable trigger. Chronic urticaria lasts from 6 weeks and up to 10 years. There is often no identifiable trigger in chronic urticaria.

Prevalence
Affects up to 25% of the population.

Age
Most common in children and young adults.

Table 9.3 Aetiology of urticaria

Mechanism	Example
IgE mediated	Food allergy (egg, milk, peanut)
	Drug reaction (penicillin, cephalosporin)
	Insect stings (bees, wasps)
	Contact allergy (latex)
Complement mediated	Hereditary angio-oedema
	Serum sickness
	Transfusion reactions
Direct mast cell degranulation	Opiates (morphine, codeine)
	Neuromuscular blocking agents (atracurium, vecuronium)
	Vancomycin
	Radiological contrast agents
Infections	Coxsackie A and B
	Hepatitis A, B and C
	HIV infection
Prostaglandin inhibitors	Aspirin
	Nonsteroidal anti-inflammatory drugs
Physical	Dermatographism
	Cold

Sex

M = F

Aetiology

Aetiological agents for urticaria are given in Table 9.3. Rarely urticaria may bepart of a systemic disease, such as systemic lupus erythematosus, or autoimmune thyroid disease and may be the presenting feature.

Pathophysiology

Urticaria results from the degranulation of cutaneous mast cells causing dilation of local capillaries and leakage of fluid into the skin. Mediators include histamine.

Clinical features

Rapid onset of itchy erythematous swellings or weals anywhere on the body. The accompanying soft tissue oedema (angio-oedema) often occurs around the face including the tongue and larynx causing potentially life-threatening upper airways obstruction, presenting as stridor.

Management

The management of anaphylaxis is discussed on page 499. Any trigger factor should be identified and avoided wherever possible. Medical treatment is used for symptom relief in acute urticaria and chronic urticaria where triggers are not identifiable.

1 Antihistamines
   - H_1 receptor blockers such as loratadine are the mainstay of treatment.
   - H_2 receptor blockers such as ranitidine may be useful in conjunction with an H_1 blocker in refractory cases.
2 Corticosteroids may be useful in individuals in whom antihistamines are ineffective. Prolonged courses in chronic urticaria are associated with significant side effects and adrenal suppression.

Lichenoid lesions

Lichen planus

Definition

Lichen planus is pruritic skin disorder causing bluish purple papules involving flexor surfaces, mucous membranes and genitalia symmetrically.

Age

Most common between 30–60 years. Uncommon in very young and very old.

Sex

M = F

Aetiology/pathophysiology

The exact cause is unknown but it is thought that there is a T cell autoimmune reaction to keratinocytes. There is also some evidence of an association with HLA DR1. There is a lichen planus like eruption, associated with many drugs (see Table 9.4).

Clinical features
- Patients develop small, flat, polygonal, bluish purple papules often affecting the wrists, shins and lower back. On close inspection there are white, lacy patterns on the surface of the papules; these are termed

Table 9.4 Drugs causing a lichen planus like eruption

Anti-rheumatoid agents, e.g. gold, penicillamine
Antibiotics, e.g. streptomycin, tetracycline
Antimalarial drugs, e.g. choroquine, quinine
Antituberculosis drugs, e.g. isoniazid
Diuretics, e.g. chlorothiazide
Antipsychotic drugs, e.g. phenothiazines

Wickham's striae. Patients often describe severe pruritus, and healing results in hyperpigmentation. Hypertrophic lichen planus is a variant with hyperkeratotic plaques seen on the legs.

- Lichen planus of the scalp is termed lichen planopilaris, which can cause a scarring alopecia.
- Nail involvement ranges from mild dystrophy to nail loss.
- Mucous membrane involvement may be Wickham's striae in the mouth, or plaques or erosive ulceration.
- Anogenital lichen planus results in bluish purple papules on the glans penis or vulva. An erosive lichen planus affecting the orogenital regions is seen in women termed vulvovaginal-gingival syndrome.

Management
High potency topical steroids are the mainstay of treatment. Refractory cases may respond to systemic steroids, oral retinoids, ciclosporin or azathioprine.

Prognosis
Most lesions clear within 2 years leaving hyperpigmented patches. Hypertrophic, anogenital and mucosal involvement is more persistent and more refractory to treatment.

Lichen sclerosus

Definition
Lichen sclerosus (previously lichen sclerosus et atrophicus) is an uncommon chronic progressive disorder of the skin characterised by inflammation and epithelial thinning.

Age
Most common in postmenopausal women, but can occur at any age.

Sex
F > M

Aetiology/pathophysiology
The cause is unknown; however, there is a familial tendency possibly with an HLA association. There is also an association with autoimmune conditions such as thyroid disorders. Trauma may play a role as lesions occur at sites of skin trauma (Köebner phenomenon).

Clinical features
Lichen sclerosis is most commonly seen in the anogenital region. Patients may complain of itching, dysuria and dyspareunia. On examination there are atrophic, white macules on vulva or penis, occasionally extending to involve the perineum. There may be fissures, excoriation and secondary lichenification with loss of architecture (phymosis in males). Extragenital white plaques due to hyperkeratosis may occur on other areas of skin or rarely, the oral cavity.

Complications
Longstanding disease predisposes to squamous cell carcinoma.

Investigations
A biopsy may be required if the diagnosis is not clear. The epidermis may show areas of thinning and hyperkeratosis. A lymphocytic infiltrate is seen in the lower dermis, and immunofluorescence may be required to exclude cicatricial pemphigoid.

Management
Genital lesions may be treated with potent topical steroid ointments. Hydroxychloroquine is used in refractory cases. Maintenance therapy may be required to prevent recurrence. Surgery is avoided due to the Köebner phenomenon but may be required for adhesions, phymosis or introital stenosis. Long-term follow-up with biopsy of any area suspicious of squamous cell carcinoma is recommended.

Prognosis
The condition responds well to potent topical steroids. Spontaneous remission may occur in childhood cases around puberty.

Lichen simplex chronicus (neurodermatitis)

Definition
Lichen simplex chronicus or nodular prurigo refers to a cutaneous response to rubbing or scratching normal skin.

Aetiology
More common in Asian, African and Oriental patients and is associated with atopic tendency.

Clinical features
Following intense itching and recurrent scratching of a patch of skin, lichen simplex chronicus presents as a single plaque often on the lower leg, neck or the perineum. Nodular prurigo presents as multiple itchy nodules, which are more diffusely distributed.

Management
Lesions are often refractory to treatment although topical steroids, tar bandages and phototherapy are tried.

Bullous disorders

Pemphigus

Definition
Pemphigus is a group of severe, chronic, autoimmune, superficial blistering diseases of the mucous membranes and skin. The commonest form is pemphigus vulgaris. Two other forms have been described: pemphigus foliaceus and paraneoplastic pemphigus.

Incidence
Uncommon

Age
Peaks in the middle-aged and elderly.

Sex
M = F

Geography
Increased incidence in Ashkenazi Jews.

Aetiology/pathophysiology
Patients have IgG autoantibodies against desmoglein (dsg), which are adhesion molecules that hold epidermal cells together. The absence of epidermal adhesion results in intraepidermal blisters. The genetic predisposition to develop these autoantibodies may be HLA related. Paraneoplastic pemphigus is associated with lymphoreticular malignancies such as non-Hodgkin's lymphoma, chronic lymphocytic leukaemia and Waldenström's macroglobulinaemia. Drugs such as penicillamine, penicillin or captopril may induce pemphigus or unmask latent disease.

Clinical features
- Pemphigus vulgaris presents with flaccid painful blisters and erosions often initially in the oropharynx and then the scalp, face, groin and chest. The blisters rupture easily, so often only erosions are seen. Sliding pressure easily dislodges the epidermis at the edge of blister (Nikolsky sign).
- Pemphigus foliaceus causes a more superficial epidermal weakness causing erosions rather than blisters. Patients present with erythema, and crusting on the face and scalp, chest and back without involvement of the mucous membrane.
- Paraneoplastic pemphigus causes severe disease involving both the skin and mucosal membranes.

Complications
There may be extensive fluid and protein loss and secondary infection particularly due to the immunosuppressive nature of medications.

Investigations
Diagnosed by biopsy of an early, small blister or the edge of new erosion. Light microscopy and direct immunofluorescence for IgG deposition at epidermal cell junctions. Identification of anti-dsg autoantibodies may be useful.

Management
High-dose systemic corticosteroids tailored dependent on clinical response. If control cannot be maintained on low-dose steroids, immunosuppressive agents are used as steroid sparing agents including azathioprine, cyclophosphamide and methotrexate. Plasmapheresis and intravenous immunoglobulin have been used in refractory cases.

Prognosis

Without treatment pemphigus carries a high risk of mortality. With combination therapy the mortality rate is around 5%, mainly due to sepsis and other drug complications. Most patients require long-term immunosuppressive treatment with maintenance therapy to remain in remission.

Pemphigoid

Definition

Pemphigoid is a chronic, blistering autoimmune disease of the skin.

Incidence

Twice as common as pemphigus.

Age

Mainly affects patients over 60 years.

Sex

M = F

Aetiology/pathophysiology

Linear polyclonal IgG autoantibodies and complement are found at the junction of the dermis and epidermis causing the release of proteolytic enzymes, which damage the basement membrane. Circulatory autoantibodies against basement membrane glycoproteins BP230 and BP180 can be demonstrated in the serum of most patients. These may however result from keratinocyte damage rather than be the cause. Individual's HLA haloptype may make them susceptible to production of these autoantibodies. Drugs including penicillamine and furosemide may cause an acute pemphigoid, which resolves on stopping the medication or they may unmask latent pemphigoid that persists and behaves like non-drug-induced illness.

Clinical features

Patients present with widespread blisters and erosions typically in the flexures, groin and axillae, which are often itchy. Cicatricial pemphigoid predominantly involves the mucous membranes, especially the oropharynx and genital region with scarring.

Investigations

Biopsy of an intact blister for light microscopy and direct immunofluorescence for IgG and complement seen in a linear pattern along the basement membrane of the blister.

Management

Patients have traditionally been treated with systemic corticosteroids, with azathioprine, cyclophosphamide and methotrexate used as steroid-sparing agents. Recent data however suggests that topical corticosteroid therapy is effective in both moderate and severe pemphigoid.

Prognosis

Often self-limiting with remission allowing cessation of treatment after 1–2 years.

Dermatitis herpetiformis

Definition

Dermatitis herpetiformis is a primary blistering disorder associated with coeliac disease and other autoimmune disorders.

Prevalence

1 in 350–400 patients with coeliac disease.

Age

Teenagers and young adults.

Sex

M > F

Aetiology

Eighty-five per cent of individuals with dermatitis herpetiformis have small bowel mucosal changes with variable villous atrophy on small bowel biopsy even if they do not have the clinical features of coeliac disease. Both disorders have similar HLA haplotypes and autoantibodies to endomysial, gliadin and reticulin antigens. Dermatitis herpetiformis is also associated with other organ specific autoimmune conditions.

Clinical features

Erythematous itchy papules and vesicles over the extensor surface of the extremities and on the trunk.

Investigations

It is a clinical diagnosis; however, biopsy of affected skin shows a subepidermal blister with neutrophil infiltration. Immunofluorescence staining of skin biopsy taken from an unaffected area shows granular IgA deposits along the basement membrane. Serological testing and small bowel biopsy may be required to identify gluten sensitivity (see page 165).

Management

Even without clinical coeliac disease patients often respond to a gluten-free diet. The rash responds dramatically to dapsone (this has been used as a diagnostic test). The concomitant use of cimetidine (which inhibits cytochrome p450 enzymes) helps to reduce side effects caused by the metabolic products of dapsone.

Prognosis

Condition often shows relapses and remissions.

Facial dermatoses

Acne vulgaris

Definition

Acne is a chronic inflammatory disease of the pilosebaceous units, which may result in comedones (black- or white-headed spots), papules, pustules, cysts and scars.

Prevalence

Acne will affect approximately 85% of individuals at some time.

Age

Generally confined to adolescence but may persist.

Sex

M = F (females affected earlier).

Aetiology/pathophysiology

- The process of acne begins in the keratinocytes within the follicles of the pilosebaceous glands. Increased proliferation and reduced loss of keratinocytes increases their number and blocks the follicles with a hyperkeratotic plug (microcomedo).

- Increased androgens around puberty and an increased sensitivity to androgens causes hyperplasia of the sebaceous glands and increase sebum production. Accumulation of the sebum in a follicle obstructed by hyperkeratosis creates a closed comedo or white-headed spot. Reopening of the follicle due to distension causes the formation of an open comedo, which appears as a blackhead.

- *Propionibacterium acnes*, an anaerobic commensal of the skin, is able to grow in the anaerobic environment produced by the combination of increased sebum production and blockage of the follicular canals.

- Rupture of a follicle into the dermis and/or the hydrolysis of lipids in the sebum by *P. acnes* results in an inflammatory reaction that may cause cysts, pustules, papules, and scarring.

- Exacerbating factors include excess androgen production, oily creams and cosmetics, humidity and heavy sweating. Mechanical trauma such as excessive scrubbing increases inflammation and scarring. Diet does not affect sebum production or acne. Excess steroids, either endogenous or exogenous, can induce a pustular form of acne mainly affecting the back and shoulders. Infantile acne is a self-limiting condition seen in babies due to the effect of maternal androgens.

Clinical features

Lesions occur at sites where there are many sebaceous glands such as face, shoulders, back and upper chest. Scars may follow healing particularly when cysts have formed, leaving skin depressions, and may result in keloid formation.

Management

- Local treatments include topical retinoids, which normalise keratinisation and prevent follicular blockage, benzoyl peroxide, a keratolytic agent, and topical antibiotics, such as tetracycline. These may be used in combination in more severe acne.

- Systemic treatments are used for refractory acne or if scarring occurs:
  Low-dose oral antibiotics such as erythromycin, tetracycline or trimethoprim may be used but need to be continued for up to 6 months.
  Cyproterone acetate and ethinyl oestradiol, a combined oral contraceptive, also has an antiandrogen

effect. It can be used in women eligible for oral contraceptives.

Oral retinoids are derivatives of vitamin A. They have an anti-inflammatory action and reduce sebum production for up to a year, this in turn causes a decrease in *P. acnes* due to reduced sebum. These are very effective with 80% of patients achieving long-term remission after a single course of treatment. However, retinoids are highly teratogenic causing spontaneous abortions and severe life-threatening congenital malformations. Women require a pregnancy test prior to starting therapy and should ideally use both an oral contraceptive and a barrier contraceptive during and for 1 month after treatment. Retinoids may rarely cause hepatitis, jaundice and pancreatitis. Patients require regular liver function tests and lipid profile measurement during treatment.

Rosacea

Definition
A chronic inflammatory facial dermatosis affecting the central face characterised by vascular dilation, erythema and pustules.

Age
Generally affects patients aged 30–60 years.

Sex
F > M

Aetiology/pathophysiology
There is dilation of dermal blood vessels, hyperplasia of sebaceous glands but normal excretion of sebum. The cause is unknown but it is more common in individuals with fair skin, light hair and light eye colour. Some evidence suggests a role for hair follicle mites.

Clinical features
Symptoms begin with recurrent flushing of the face, which worsens on exposure to hot drinks, alcohol, stress and sunlight. This may precede, by years, erythema of the nose and cheeks. Telangiectasia are seen on the cheeks and sebaceous gland hyperplasia results in the formation of papules and pustules. There may be a sensation of a foreign body in the eye, telangiectasia and inflammation of lid margins (blepharitis), conjunctivitis and keratitis.

Hypertrophy of the sebaceous glands and connective tissue around the nose, most commonly in middle-aged men, causes rhinophyma.

Management
- Topical treatments using antibiotic gels, such as metronidazole, are used for at least 4–6 weeks.
- Systemic treatments are used in refractory cases and in patients with ocular symptoms. Prolonged courses of metronidazole, tetracycline, oxytetracycline or erythromycin are generally used, which is changed to a retinoid if symptoms remain. See section Acne Vulgaris for details regarding the use and safety of retinoids.
- Rhinophyma may require electrosurgical resection.

Prognosis
Rosacea is a chronic condition, and topical metronidazole may be required to maintain remission.

Hair and nail disorders

Alopecia

Definition
Alopecia is defined as hair loss; it is classified into diffuse and localised, scarring and non-scarring.

Aetiology/pathophysiology
The growth of hair from follicles passes through a cycle (see Fig. 9.1). Causes of alopecia are given in Table 9.5.

Clinical features and management
- Androgenic alopecia has a genetic tendency and is androgen-dependent. Males are affected more than females, starting from late teens increasing in incidence throughout life. In males the hairline recedes initially in the temporal regions before hair loss at the

Table 9.5 Causes of alopecia

Diffuse non-scarring	Androgenic alopecia, metabolic, drug induced, telogen effluvium.
Localised non-scarring	Alopecia areata, ringworm, traumatic, traction.
Scarring	Discoid lupus, burns, radiation, lichen planus.

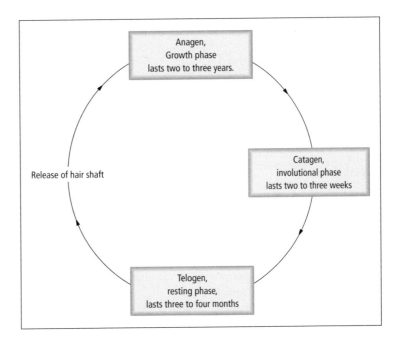

Figure 9.1 Normal hair growth.

crown. In women there is more diffuse thinning of the hair. Topical minoxidil produces some response in up to 30% of cases. Finasteride is also used in androgenic alopecia in males.

- Telogen effluvium occurs when the normally asynchronous cycles in follicles synchronises after childbirth, surgery or severe illness. The hair loss typically occurs 3 months after the precipitating event. It is self-limiting.
- Alopecia areata is associated with autoimmune conditions in which anagen is prematurely arrested. Patients develop well-demarcated circular patches of hair loss, which may coalesce causing alopecia totalis. Pathognomonic is the presence of exclamation mark hairs, narrower at the scalp. Alopecia areata is refractory to treatment.
- Metabolic disorders may present with hair loss: hypo/hyperthyroidism, hypopituitarism or hypoadrenalism, iron deficiency and malnutrition.

Hirsutism

Definition
Hirsutism is the androgen-dependent growth of hair in a woman, which is in the same distribution as in males.

Table 9.6 Causes of hirsutism

Idiopathic	Possible steroidogenic abnormality
Iatrogenic	Danzol, some oral contraceptive pills
Pituitary	Hyperprolacinaemia
Adrenal	Congenital adrenal hyperplasia, Cushing's syndrome
Ovarian	Polycystic ovaries, hyperthecosis, some tumours

Aetiology/pathophysiology
There is a wide geographical variation in the 'normal' body hair independent of androgen production. Hirsutism is caused by increased androgen production or, more rarely, increased sensitivity of hair follicles to androgens (see Table 9.6). There may be associated menstrual problems.

Clinical features
Patients present with male pattern hair growth on the lip, chin, chest, abdomen, back, arms and legs more than that expected for a woman of the same ethnic background. Women with a normal menstrual cycle are unlikely to have an endocrine cause. Other features may include acne, seborrhoea, androgenic alopecia, deepening of the voice and clitoromegaly. The abdomen should be examined for masses.

Table 9.7 Causes of hypertrichosis

Drugs	Phenytoin, penicillamine, minoxidil, ciclosporin
Systemic illness	Hypothyroidism, anorexia nervosa, malnutrition, porphyria cutanea tarda
Paraneoplastic syndrome	

Investigations

Dependent on the level of virilisation and menstrual anomalies found; hormone profile and abdominal imaging may be required.

Management

- Any underlying cause for excess androgen production should be identified and treated.
- Physical methods of hair removal include shaving, chemical depilatories, bleaching, electrolysis and laser treatments.
- Combined oral contraceptives may slow hair growth; antiandrogens may also be effective.

Hypertrichosis

Definition
Hypertrichosis is excessive hair in a non-androgenic distribution. Causes of hypertrichosis are given in Table 9.7.

Clinical features
Patients present with fine terminal hair diffusely on the face, limbs and trunk. As there is often an underlying cause, thorough investigation is indicated.

Infections of the skin and soft tissue

Bacterial infections

Impetigo

Definition
Impetigo is a contagious superficial skin infection occurring on exposed skin predominantly in children.

Aetiology/pathophysiology
The commonest cause of impetigo is *Staph. aureus*; group A *Streptococci* also cause impetigo. Increased incidence of impetigo is seen in conditions damaging the integrity of skin such as eczema, and its spread is facilitated by overcrowding and poor hygiene.

Clinical features
Impetigo appears as erythematous erosions with a characteristic golden brown crusting. There may be associated localised lymphadenopathy. Bullous impetigo describes punched-out blistering lesions with crusting due to Staphylococcal toxin production.

Management
Swabs should be taken. Localised disease may be treated with topical agents such as fucidin cream. Often the condition requires treatment with oral penicillin (*Streptococcus*) and flucloxacillin (*Staphylococcus*). Erythromycin is an alternative for penicillin-sensitive individuals.

Cellulitis

Definition
Cellulitis is an acute diffuse spreading infection of the skin extending into the soft tissues. Erysipelas is an acute infection of the skin not extending into the soft tissues.

Aetiology/pathophysiology
The main causative organisms are β-haemolytic *Streptococci* and *Staph. aureus*. Risk factors for development of cellulitis include damage to skin integrity (leg ulcer, traumatic wounds), venous insufficiency, leg oedema, diabetes and obesity. The mechanisms of infection are not clearly understood but may involve bacterial exotoxins and cytokine release.

Clinical features
Patients have a well-demarcated patch of erythema with swelling of the underlying soft tissues. There is warmth and tenderness to touch, often with local lymphadenopathy. If untreated, there is spreading of the erythema, abscess formation and secondary septicaemia. Systemic symptoms may include fever, fatigue and myalgia.

Complications

Abscess formation, septicaemia, toxic shock-like syndrome.

Investigations

The diagnosis is clinical; blood cultures should be taken but are usually negative.

Management

Initial management with penicillin (*Streptococcus*) and flucloxacillin (*Staphylococcus*); erythromycin is useful for patients who are penicillin allergic. If the cellulitis is advanced or if it fails to respond to oral therapy, parenteral penicillin and flucloxacillin are used, and clindamycin, if penicillin allergic. It is useful to outline the erythema to allow the condition to be followed. Abscesses may require surgical drainage.

Clostridial myonecrosis (gas gangrene)

Definition

Gangrene refers to death of tissue, and myonecrosis refers specifically to muscle. Clostridial infection of wounds may result in significant infection of muscle, which develops rapidly and is potentially life-threatening.

Aetiology/pathophysiology

The most common cause is *Clostridium perfringens* found in soil and in the faeces of animals and humans. Infection occurs after deep penetrating trauma. Compromise of the blood supply as a result of the traumatic damage or as a result of longstanding vascular disease, creates an acidic anaerobic environment and facilitates bacterial proliferation. It is thought that τ-toxin produced by *Clostridium* prevents the normal inflammatory cell infiltration and therefore allows the infection to spread rapidly causing extensive necrosis. α-toxin has a direct negative inotropic effect on the heart and may lead to shock.

Clinical features

Patients develop severe pain due to myonecrosis at a site of trauma with induration, blistering and oedema. In a limb distal pulses may be lost and crepitus is felt in the muscle late in the disease process. Systemic signs include pyrexia, tachycardia, progressing to multiorgan failure.

Investigations

- Imaging may allow detection of gas in muscle too deep for palpation (crepitus on palpation is as sensitive in superficial muscle).
- Diagnosis is confirmed by identifying clostridia in the wound.

Management

Prevention of clostridial infections involves adequate wound care at the time of original trauma including excision and debridement of necrotic tissue. Wounds that may be infected should not undergo primary closure. In established cases penicillin is the drug of choice. Aggressive surgical intervention with wide excision, opening of fascial compartments, and meticulous debridement of all necrotic tissue is essential. This may require subsequent reconstruction and skin grafting. The use of hyperbaric oxygen (HBO) to reduce anaerobic conditions is controversial.

Leprosy

Definition

Leprosy is a chronic indolent mycobacterial infection mainly of the skin.

Incidence

Rare since WHO eradication programmes.

Geography

Leprosy is found primarily in Africa and Asia.

Aetiology

Leprosy is caused by an intracellular acid-fast bacillus, *Mycobacterium leprae*. The mode of transmission is uncertain and the incubation may be many years.

Clinical features

Five patterns of disease are recognised that are dependent on the immunological response of the individual (see Table 9.8).

There are two immunological reactions that may occur in borderline or lepromatous leprosy.

- Reversal reaction (lepra type I) is seen following treatment of borderline leprosy. It is a type IV hypersensitivity reaction resulting in acute inflammation

Table 9.8 Patterns of leprosy

Type	Skin Lesions	Nerve Involvement
Tuberculoid (TT)	Single hypopigmented erythematous macule with a well-defined, raised margin and central healing	The nerve supplying the patch is thickened with loss of sensation and muscle atrophy
Borderline tuberculoid (BT)	Skin lesions as for tuberculoid but multiple, smaller lesions	Peripheral nerves are thickened causing deformity of hands and feet.
Borderline (BB)	Skin lesions are numerous, vary in size characteristic annular rimmed, punched out lesion	Widespread nerve involvement causing deformity of limbs
Borderline lepromatous (BL)	Large number of florid variable asymmetrical skin lesions	
Lepromatous (LL)	Erythematous macules, papules and/or nodules, or occasionally diffuse disease without distinct lesions. Infiltration at ear lobes and face results in typical leonine facies	Glove and stocking neuropathy

characterised by erythema and oedema of skin lesions, accompanied by neuritis.

- Erythema nodosum leprosum (lepra type II) is a type III hypersensitivity reaction seen in boderline and lepromatous leprosy. It is characterised by fever and multiple erythematous tender nodules.

Investigations

The diagnosis is clinical but can be confirmed with demonstration of acid-fast bacilli in skin scrapings. PCR can be used.

Management

Patients are treated with dapsone and rifampicin. Clofazimine is added in BB, BL and LL types. Patients may require surgery and physiotherapy for deformities. Reversal reaction is treated with prednisolone. Erythema nodosum leprosum is treated with analgesia, chloroquine, clofazimine and antipyretics (thalidomide has also been used).

Viral skin infections

Herpes simplex

Definition

Herpes simplex virus (HSV) can cause a variety of clinical presentations.

Aetiology/pathophysiology

There are two subtypes:

- HSV type 1 is usually the cause of perioral lesions, ocular infections, non-genital skin lesions and encephalitis. It spreads by direct contact with oral secretions and via droplet spread; infection is very common and most individuals are seropositive by adult life. Genital infections may occur due to orogenital contact. Immunocompromised patients are at particular risk for recurrent and disseminated infection.
- HSV type 2 is transmitted by direct contact; it usually causes genital herpes and is therefore a sexually transmitted disease.

After primary infection, the latent non-replicating virus resides within the dorsal root ganglion, shielding the virus from the immune system. Reactivation may follow exposure to sunlight, fever, trauma or emotional stress.

Clinical features

- HSV type 1 primary infection usually occurs during childhood and is often asymptomatic. Symptomatic infection usually manifests as acute gingivostomatitis with vesicles on the lips and painful ulcers within the mouth accompanied by fever and malaise. Local herpes inoculation into a site of injury may present as a herpetic whitlow – a painful vesicle or pustule on a digit. Ocular infections and encephalitis (see page 304) may occur with or without kin lesions.
- HSV type 2 primary infection is often asymptomatic, but may cause acute vulvovaginitis, penile or perianal lesions.

Latent infection occurs and recurrence is often heralded by a burning or tingling sensation. It usually occurs at the site of the primary infection and in adjacent areas. Hours or days later vesicles reappear.

Complications
Patients with atopic eczema may develop eczema herpeticum (see page 385). Disseminated herpes may occur in the newborn or immunosuppressed. HSV is the most common cause of recurrent erythema multiforme.

Management
Aciclovir is of value if used early enough. Topical treatment at the onset of tingling may prevent a recurrence. As aciclovir works to prevent reactivation it is of limited value in established disease. However, immunosuppressed patients should be treated aggressively with parenteral aciclovir to prevent dissemination.

Herpes zoster (shingles)

Definition
Herpes zoster or shingles is an acute self-limiting dermatomal vesicular eruption occurring in a dermatomal distribution.

Incidence
Affects 10–20% of the population at some time in their lives.

Age
Incidence increases progressively with age.

Sex
M = F

Aetiology/pathophysiology
Primary infection with the varicella-zoster virus (VZV) causes chickenpox. Like other herpes virus infections, it then remains as a latent infection in the sensory dorsal root ganglia. It is thought that gradual loss of immunity underlies reactivation explaining the increased incidence with age and the association with immunocompromise including HIV.

Clinical features
Pain, tenderness or paraesthesia develops in the distribution of a single dermatome 3–5 days prior to the onset of the rash. Erythema and crops of vesicles then develop in the same dermatomal distribution. Additional discrete non-dermatomal lesions are also commonly found. The vesicles become pustular and then form crusts. They heal over 2–3 weeks leaving scars.

Complications
Corneal ulcers and corneal scarring may result from trigeminal infection with ocular involvement. Dissemination is seen in immunosuppressed individuals. Postherpetic neuralgia is found in 5–10% of patients presenting as a continued burning pain.

Investigations
The virus can be isolated from vesicular fluid and identified on electron microscopy.

Management
Adequate analgesia is essential. Aciclovir is effective in shortening the duration of pain when started within 48 hours of the onset of the rash. It should be given parenterally in the immunocompromised.

Human papillomavirus (viral warts)

Definition
Human papillomavirus (HPV) infections affecting epithelial tissues and mucous membranes.

Aetiology
Human papillomaviruses are double-stranded DNA viruses. Over 70 subtypes are identifiable and different subtypes cause infections at different sites of the body: HPV type 2 causes hand warts, type 1 and 2 cause plantar warts, and various subtypes cause genital warts and anogenital intraepithelial neoplasia. HPV types 16–18 are high-risk subtypes for neoplasia and are associated with cervical and oral cancer. The virus is spread direct by direct contact, anogenital warts, and HPV infection of the cervix may be sexually transmitted.

Clinical features
1 Common warts are well-demarcated dome shaped papules or nodules with an irregular papilliferous surface. Commonly occur on the back of hands, between fingers and around the nail edge.

2 Plantar warts (often called verrucae) are seen on the soles of feet particularly in children. They appear as thickened plaques with overlying callous, which may reveal underlying black dots if removed.

3 Flat warts are smooth-topped papules often multiple and refractory to treatment.

Microscopy

The epidermis is hyperkeratotic and thickened. Infection of keratinocytes in the granular layer results in a vacuolated appearance.

Management

No treatment is universally successful, and as there is a high spontaneous resolution, management may be expectant. Available treatments include topical keratolytics such as salicylic acid, cryotherapy, surgical excision and laser treatments.

Prognosis

Most warts spontaneously resolve over 2 years.

Fungal skin infections

Candida albicans

Definition

Candida albicans, a commensal yeast of the gastrointestinal tract, may cause opportunistic infections such as mucocutaneous candidiasis.

Aetiology/pathophysiology

Candida is a dimorphic fungus occurring as a yeast on mucosal surfaces. In immunocompetent patients most infections result from disruption of the normal body flora. Patients with cell-mediated immune deficiency tend towards more extensive persistent mucous membrane infections. Neutropenic patients are at risk of widespread disseminated illness. Predisposing factors to opportunistic infection include moist and opposing skin folds, obesity, diabetes mellitus, pregnancy, poor hygiene and the use of broad-spectrum antibiotics.

Clinical features

1 Oral candidiasis is commonly seen in babies and patients treated with antibiotics or chemotherapy. Patients develop white plaques on the oral mucosa, palate and tongue.

2 Candidal oesophagitis causes painful swallowing most commonly seen in patients with human immunodeficiency virus (HIV) infection. The diagnosis requires direct visualisation on endoscopy.

3 Vulvovaginal candidiasis is the most common form of mucosal candidiasis associated with increased oestrogens, systemic steroids, antibiotics, diabetes mellitus and HIV infection. Women develop itching and discharge occasionally with dysuria or dyspareunia. There is erythema and a white vaginal discharge.

4 Candidal balanitis may occur in uncircumcised men. Patients present with an inflamed glans and prepuce.

5 Systemic infections may occur in the immunosuppressed.

Management

Topical antifungals are used in the form of creams, lozenges or pessaries. Resistant, recurrent or severe infections may require systemic antifungal medication.

Dermatophyte (ring worm) fungi

Definition

Dermatophytes or ringworm fungi invade keratin and cause skin and nail infections.

- Tinea Capitis: Tinea capitis is a ringworm infection of the scalp, which occurs in small children especially of African origin. Infection is spread by close contact. Lesions are single or multiple erythematous, scaly, well-demarcated patches on the scalp that gradually spread. Hairs within the patch break off giving a patch of alopecia. A kerion is a boggy swollen mass containing pus and exudate. It is a form of immune response to the fungus. Prolonged courses of oral terbinafine, itraconazole or griseofulvin are effective even in kerion.

- Tinea Pedis: Tinea pedis or athlete's foot is the most common dermatophyte infection. Infection is spread by contact with shed spores. Patients develop itchy or painful, erythematous scaling lesions between the toes. It may be acute self-limiting or a persistent chronic infection. Topical antifungal agents are usually effective if applied regularly.

- Tinea Unguium: Nail infection with ringworm is common especially in the elderly. Patients develop asymmetrical discoloured (white/yellowish black) thickened nails with crumbling white material under the nail plate. This condition may respond to a prolonged course of systemic antifungals as for tinea capitis.
- Tinea Cruris: Tinea cruris affects the groin with erythema and scaling is surrounded by a well-defined edge. Infection may extend over the perianal region. If mild, treatment is with topical antifungals. Severe or refractory cases require oral antifungals as for tinea capitis.

Parasitic skin infections

Head lice

Definition
Infestation with the head louse *Pediculosis capitis.*

Incidence
Common

Age
Occurs mainly in school children.

Sex
F > M (due to longer hair).

Aetiology/pathophysiology
Pediculosis capitis or head louse is a grey-white insect that grasps on to hair and sucks blood. Eggs laid by the female are closely adherent to hair. Insects are spread by contact but as insects can survive for hours away from the host, transfer on clothing, shared combs, towels and beds may occur.

Clinical features
Infestations are often asymptomatic although allergy may result in itching and lymphadenopathy. The head louse is difficult to find but eggs (nits) may be seen along the hair shaft. A fine-toothed nit comb is often used to detect lice and nits.

Management
Topical shampoo containing insecticides such as malathion and permethrin may be used, although there is some evidence of increasing resistance. Treatment should be repeated after 7 days. Mechanical removal of lice nit combs from wet hair is an alternative strategy. Household members should be examined and treated if infested.

Scabies

Definition
Skin infestation by the mite *Sarcoptes scabiei*, causing itching.

Aetiology/pathophysiology
Transmission of the mite occurs by skin–skin contact with an infested individual or contaminated clothing or bedding. The mite burrows down into the stratum corneum of the skin and then the female lays eggs.

Clinical features
- There is often a widespread, erythematous urticating rash all over the body as a result of a hypersensitivity reaction to the mite. Patients present with severe itching usually worse at night.
- On examination small papules and linear tracks, caused by burrowing mites, are seen around the wrists, finger webs and ankles (and scrotum in the male).
- In immunosuppressed patients, Norwegian/crusted scabies may occur with diffuse scaly erythematous patches especially on the scalp, hands and feet.

Investigations
The burrows and distribution pattern is very suggestive of the diagnosis. The mite can be visualised using a dermatoscope.

Management
Patients are extremely infectious and require barrier nursing. The entire skin except the face should be treated with malathion or permethrin. All close contacts require treatment, and clothing and bed linen should be thoroughly machine-washed. Norwegian/crusted scabies may require repeated treatments.

Skin and soft tissue lumps

Seborrhoeic keratoses

Definition
Seborrhoeic keratoses are a benign localised proliferation of the basal layer of the epidermis. They are sometimes termed basal cell papillomas; however, they are not neoplastic and are not premalignant.

Incidence
Common; by age 40 approximately 10% of individuals have one seborrhoeic keratosis.

Age
Increase in incidence with increasing age.

Sex
M = F

Aetiology/pathophysiology
The cause of seborrhoeic keratoses is unclear, although they occur more commonly on sun-exposed skin.

Clinical features
Lesions occur most commonly on the trunk. They are flat, raised or pedunculated with a yellow brown appearance of the overlying skin. With time the surface becomes irregular and wart-like. Lesions may cause concern due to bleeding, itching or surrounding inflammation.

Management
If treatment is required, cryotherapy or currettage are usually effective.

Solar keratoses

Definition
Solar keratoses or actinic keratoses are single, small scaly plaques occuring as a result of sun damage to the skin.

Incidence
Common.

Age
Occurs in the middle-aged and elderly.

Aetiology/pathophysiology
Solar keratoses are seen in fair-skinned patients associated with sun exposure. They are most common in patients who burn easily and tan poorly. There is debate as to whether solar keratoses leads to squamous cell carcinoma, or whether squamous cell carcinomas arise in the same areas due to the sun damage.

Clinical features
Lesions initially appear as a small, well-demarcated, red brown plaque that progress to become more erythematous and hyperkeratotic. Solar keratoses bleed easily with minor trauma.

Management
Treatment includes cryotherapy, curettage or topical 5-fluorouracil.

Dermatofibromas

Definition
A dermatofibroma is a cutaneous nodule containing macrophages or histiocytes.

Incidence
Common.

Age
Can occur at any age, more common in adults.

Sex
4F : 1M

Aetiology/pathophysiology
Historically dermatofibromas have been associated with trauma or insect bites, although the cause is unknown.

Clinical features
Lesions occur most commonly on the lower limbs. They are solitary firm elevated nodules with pigmentation of the overlying skin. Although classically asymptomatic they may cause itching or pain.

Management
Dermatofibromas are removed only if troublesome or if there is diagnostic uncertainty.

Benign naevi

Definition
A naevus is a hamartoma of the skin (a benign overgrowth of normal tissue). A melanocytic naevus is a proliferation of pigmented melanocytes.
- Melanocytic naevi occurring only in the dermal–epidermal junction are referred to as junctional naevi.
- Melanocytic naevi occurring only in the dermis are referred to as dermal naevi. Blue naevi are acquired naevi occurring in the mid dermis.
- Melanocytic naevi in the dermal–epidermal junction and the dermis are referred to as compound naevi.

Aetiology/pathophysiology
Almost all naevi are benign, but malignant change may occur with junctional naevi at greatest risk. There is a familial dysplastic naevus syndrome (autosomal dominant, gene on the short arm of chromosome 1).

Clinical features
All individuals have one or more benign naevi, they appear as small hyperpigmented flat or slightly raised areas of skin. Atypical features and those suggestive of malignancy are described later in section Malignant Melanoma (see page 407).

Management
Benign naevi do not require any treatment. If there is any diagnostic uncertainty an elliptical excision biopsy and histopathological evaluation should be performed.

Haemangiomas

Definition
A haemangioma is an arteriovenous malformation or proliferation of abnormal blood vessels.
- A strawberry naevus or capillary cavernous haemangioma is a raised nodular patch of strawberry-coloured skin, which can appear anywhere on the body. They usually develop in the first few weeks of life, grow to a maximum in the first year and then gradually resolve. Treatment is not required unless they involve the eye, bleed or become recurrently infected. Treatments include laser therapy and courses of steroids.
- Cavernous haemangioma are larger and deeper vascular lesions, which may be covered by normal skin.

Large haemangiomas can trap platelets leading to thrombocytopenia (Kasabach–Merritt syndrome).
- Port-wine stains are irregular reddish-purple macules caused by permanent vascular dilatation, which may darken and become irregular with age. They are treated with laser therapy. A port-wine stain in the ophthalmic division of the trigeminal nerve may have an associated vascular malformation in the brain or meninges leading to epilepsy, hemiplegia and developmental delay (Sturge–Weber syndrome).
- Pyogenic granuloma is an acquired haemangioma consisting of a bright red or blood-crusted nodule, which often follows trauma. Surgical curettage is possible but they occasionally recur.

Lipoma

Definition
A lipoma is a lobulated slow growing benign tumour of fatty tissue encased by a thin fibrous capsule.

Clinical features
Lipomas typically present as soft, fluctuant mass separate from the overlying skin. Lipomas that occur in the fat of intramuscular septa become more prominent when the muscle is contracted. Soft tissue X-ray confirms a radiolucent mass.

Management
Lipoma may require surgical removal.

Epidermoid cysts

Definition
An epidermoid cyst is an epithelium-lined cavity within the dermis filled with oily or fatty semisolid material.

Aetiology/pathophysiology
Epidermoid cysts are common in the hair-bearing areas and are thought to arise from the blockage of a hair follicle. The commonest scalp cysts are pilar cysts, which may be inherited.

Clinical features
Patients present with a lump in the skin, so the skin cannot be moved over it. A characteristic surface punctum

is often visible. If there is a superimposed infection the lump may become red, hot and tender.

Management
- Uninfected cysts are excised under local anaesthesia, if required using an elliptical incision.
- Infected cysts are first incised and drained. Excision is performed if still necessary once the infection has been treated.

Dermoid cysts

Definition
A cyst arising from deep implanted epidermal cells.

Aetiology/pathophysiology
Dermoid cysts arise from epidermal cells, which have been implanted into the dermis either during embryonic development or following trauma. They are lined with squamous epithelium and contain sebum, cells and occasionally hair.

Clinical features
Cysts present as soft rubbery swellings deep to the skin. There may be fixation to the deep tissues.
- Congenital dermoid cysts are found at sites of embryonic fusion. The commonest congenital dermoid cyst occurs at the junction between the frontal bone and the maxilla at the lateral border of the orbit (external angular dermoid).
- Implantation cysts occur following traumatic implantation of epidermal cells. The surrounding skin and subcutaneous tissue may be erythematous and swollen.

Management
Dermoid cysts are surgically removed. Congenital dermoid cysts require general anaesthesia due to the deep extension.

Ganglion

Definition
A benign cystic swelling occurring over a joint or tendon sheath.

Aetiology
It is thought that there is herniation of synovial tissue from a joint capsule or tendon sheath. The ganglion has a fibrous capsule and contains mucoid material.

Clinical features
A ganglion may present as a swelling or pain commonly around the wrist or the dorsum of the hand. On examination the swelling transilluminates.

Management
Ganglia may resolve or may be recurrent. Aspiration and injection of a crystalline steroid may be useful, and injection of hyaluronidase into the lesion prior to aspiration may improve results. Surgical removal is effective, although recurrence may still occur.

Skin tumours

Basal cell carcinoma

Definition
Basal cell carcinoma (BCC) is a locally invasive skin cancer arising from the basal layer of epidermis.

Incidence
Approximately 75% of all skin tumours.

Age
Increases in incidence with age.

Sex
M > F

Geography
Most common in Caucasians, and uncommon in dark-skinned populations.

Aetiology
Basal cell carcinomas are predisposed to by light and ionising radiation. Sun exposure is the most important aetiological factor particularly in individuals with fair skin, pale eyes and red hair. Childhood sun exposure appears to be important, especially if there is repeated intermittent intense exposure.

Pathophysiology

Mutations in the tumour suppressor gene and patched (PTCH) on chromosome 9 have been identified in both sporadic basal cell carcinoma and familial basal cell nevus syndrome. As with other tumour suppressor genes both copies need to be damaged before tumours develop. With the familial form, patients inherit one inactive gene and are therefore susceptible to tumour development. Only a minority of basal cell carcinomas become locally aggressive or metastasise.

Clinical features

Most basal cell carcinomas occur on the face. And three patterns are recognised:
- Nodular basal cell carcinoma is the most common type (60%) appearing as a firm pink-coloured raised nodule, often with telangiectatic vessels within the nodule. Central ulceration is common (rodent ulcer).
- Superficial basal cell carcinoma (30%) occurs on the trunk as a flat scaly red plaque, often with an irregular micropapular edge.
- Morphoeic basal cell carcinoma (10%) is typically flat smooth, flesh-coloured, or a plaque with indistinct edges.

Investigations

Suspicious lesions are investigated by excision biopsy.

Management

Complete excision is curative, local recurrence may occur especially with morphoeic and superficial types. Radiotherapy can be used for large superficial carcinomas especially in older patients.

Prognosis

Excision achieves a 95% cure with a recurrence rate of 5% at 5 years.

Squamous cell carcinoma

Definition

A malignant tumour originating from squamous cells on the outer layer of the skin.

Aetiology/pathophysiology

Sunlight and ionising radiation predispose to the development epidermal dysplastic lesions:

- Keratoacanthoma (KA) is a rapidly growing hyperkeratotic nodule with a central keratin plug. This is probably a low-grade malignancy that originates in the pilosebaceous glands. It is considered by some to be a variant of invasive squamous cell carcinoma. Most resolve spontaneously but they may rarely progress to invasive or metastatic carcinoma. Surgical excision is often advocated.
- Bowen's disease is squamous carcinoma in situ. It appears as a red patch or plaque with variable scaling on sun damaged skin. Such areas require 5-fluorouracil cream, cryotherapy or curettage.

Clinical features

Most squamous cell carcinomas present with a locally invasive and well-differentiated papule, nodule or plaque, which frequently ulcerate if left untreated. Sometimes they have a rolled everted edge. Squamous cell carcinoma metastasise initially to regional lymph nodes which should be examined.

Management

Surgical excision is the treatment of choice; this may necessitate reconstruction and skin grafting. Lymph nodes should be examined and removed if involved. Radiotherapy is an alternative in patients unfit for surgery.

Malignant melanoma

Definition

Malignant skin tumour, which arises from melanocytes usually in the epidermis.

Incidence

Commonest skin cancer, rising in incidence.

Age

Median age 50–55 years, rare in children.

Geography

Particular problem in Caucasians.

Aetiology

Around 30% of melanomas arise from the junctional component of a pre-existing naevus, which has become dysplastic. Excess sun exposure, particularly a history of childhood sunburn, is the major risk factor. Highest incidence in Caucasians with fair skin. Melanomas have a familial tendency and there is recent evidence for the role of tumour suppressor genes.

Clinical features

Most lesions are new lesions not arising in a pre-existing benign naevus. Features suggestive of malignancy include asymmetry, irregular borders, variations in colour in a single lesion and large size. Bleeding, crusting or changes in sensation may also indicate malignant change in a pre-existing lesion.

- Superficial spreading malignant melanoma (70%) occurs anywhere on the body. Lesions are flat with radial growth and microinvasion of the dermis.
- Nodular malignant melanoma (20%) presents as a raised brown-black nodule, although occasionally amelanotic lesions are seen. Tumours grow by vertical extension, the skin lesion may therefore not increase in size.
- Lentigo maligna melanoma (5%) arises from lentigo maligna (a form of intra-epithelial neoplasia). The malignant change is heralded by the appearance of a nodule in lentigo maligna.

- Acral lentiginous malignant melanoma (5%) is confined to hands and nail beds.

American Joint Committee on Cancer (AJCC) staging system:

Stage I: Primary lesions are subdivided according to the thickness of the lesion.

Stage II: Regional nodal spread or satellite lesions within 2 cm of the primary lesion.

Stage III: Fixed metastatic regional lymph nodes or more distal node spread.

Stage IV: Distant metastases.

Management

Primary therapy is wide surgical excision. Lymph node dissection is required if there is evidence of lymph node involvement. Radiotherapy, immunotherapy and chemotherapy are used in metastatic disease.

Prognosis

Prognosis is worse with increasing thickness and stage, and with increasing age and male sex.

Clinical

Symptoms

Breast lumps

Breast tissue is normally lumpy and women commonly have premenstrual breast changes including generalised tenderness, lumpiness and nodularity, which recedes after menstruation. Nodularity may be generalised or localised and it may be difficult to differentiate a localised area of nodularity from a discrete breast lump. It should however be noted that particularly in younger women, breast cancer may present as an area of localised nodularity. Further assessment is required for any new discrete lump, a new lump within pre-existing nodularity or asymmetrical nodularity that persists after menstruation.

Many women develop one or more breast lumps during their lifetime. Whilst the finding of a lump is very distressing, the majority are due to benign breast disorders (see page 412) and only a minority are due to carcinoma of the breast. A lump larger than 1 cm in size is usually palpable, although some are missed until they are much larger.

The clinical approach to breast lump assessment uses a triple approach combining clinical examination, imaging and fine needle aspiration cytology (FNAC) and/or needle core biopsy (see page 412). This combined approach gives a diagnostic accuracy exceeding 99%.

Clinical features

The history should include when and how the lump was discovered, whether it has grown and whether there have been any previous lumps. Other important aspects include a family history of breast cancer (including the number of first- and second-degree relatives affected and their age at diagnosis), history of oestrogen usage, including the combined oral contraceptive pill or hormone replacement therapy, pregnancy history and history of breast feeding. A menstrual history including the date of last menstrual period should also be documented.

Inspection of the breasts starts with the woman sitting upright with her arms to the side and then raised above her head. The symmetry of the breasts and evidence of any skin changes (see Table 10.1) should be noted. The breasts should be palpated (normal breast first) examining each quadrant in turn. Both axillae should be palpated for lymph nodes.

- A firm discrete lump with no associated skin features in a younger woman is most likely to be a fibroadenoma.
- A cyst may be soft, firm or tense and hard. It is generally spherical.
- Signs suggestive of a malignant lump include hard texture, poorly defined edges and fixation to skin or underlying tissues. There may be associated

Table 10.1 Skin changes suggestive of malignancy

Nipple retraction
Asymmetry of the breast contour
Skin tethering (dimpling or flattening of the skin, best elicited by asking the patient to raise their arms above their head or when she pushes her hands against her hips)
Paget's disease – a dry, scaling or red weeping appearance of the nipple
Peau d'orange is a late sign due to oedema of the skin due to obstruction of the lymphatics and has the appearance of orange peel
Ulceration of the skin is a very late sign seen in women who have neglected the lump

lymphadenopathy or bloody nipple discharge. Skin changes suggestive of malignancy are given in Table 10.1.

Breast pain (mastalgia)

Mastalgia is any pain felt in the breast. A thorough history of the pain (documenting the site, onset and relationship to the menstrual cycle) should be taken. Mastalgia may occur premenstrually (cyclical mastalgia) or may be unrelated to the menstrual cycle. The history should also include any previous or family history of breast disease including carcinoma. A thorough breast examination including examination of the regional lymph nodes may reveal a cyst, an abscess or localised inflammation secondary to mastitis. In non-cyclical mastalgia the chest wall should also be palpated.

- Cyclical mastalgia: Most premenopausal women get some breast discomfort premenstrually. Symptoms including heaviness, tenderness and increased nodularity of the breast tend to gradually increase during the premenstrual period. The symptoms tend to subside as menstruation starts and generally resolve within a few days. If no other abnormalities are detected imaging is not normally required for cyclical mastalgia.
- Non-cyclical mastalgia may arise from the breast or from non-mammary causes. True breast pain may be caused by acute mastitis, a breast abscess, fat necrosis or benign breast disorders. Focal mastalgia may rarely be a presentation of breast cancer therefore mammography must be considered for women over the age of 35 years with non-cyclical focal mastalgia.
- Non-mammary causes include Tietze's disease (chostochondritis) in which patients present with a sharp pain exacerbated by movement and reproduced by pressure on the costochondral junctions. It usually

resolves with rest and nonsteroidal anti-inflammatory drugs. Pain arising from the chest wall may require infiltration of local anaesthetic agents and steroids in severe cases. Breast pain may also be referred pain from conditions such as angina, pleural inflammation, pneumonia and oesophageal inflammation.

Once underlying pathology has been excluded the majority of patients can be effectively managed with reassurance. Lifestyle changes have been suggested including the use of a well-fitting sports bra, reduction of stress, relaxation therapy and dietary manipulation. Various drug therapies have been shown to be effective including danazol (a synthetic testosterone), tamoxifen and bromocriptine although all have significant side effects limiting their clinical use. Recent advances include lisuride (a dopamine agonist with fewer side effects than bromocriptine) for cyclical mastalgia and the use of topical nonsteroidal anti-inflammatory preparations for all types of mastalgia.

Nipple discharge

Nipple discharge may arise from single or multiple ducts and be unilateral or bilateral. Causes are given in Table 10.2.

Clinical features

There may be a mass palpable, which when pressed produces the discharge. Even if no mass is palpable, the discharge may come from one duct when one segment of the breast is pressed. Lymph nodes should be looked for.

Investigations

Any associated breast lump should be investigated (see page 412). Unilateral blood-stained discharge is suggestive of an intraductal papilloma and also requires a triple

Table 10.2 Causes of nipple discharge

Serous, milky	Physiological (lactation, during pregnancy)
	Drug induced
	Hyperprolactinaemia
Blood stained	Duct papilloma
	Intraduct carcinoma Invasive carcinoma (very rare)
Yellowish, green or brown	Perimenopausal
	Multiple/bilateral in duct ectasia
Pus	Breast abscess, periductal mastitis

assessment. Copious bilateral milky discharge (galatorrhoea) may indicate a prolactinoma (see page 421) hence a serum prolactin level should be sent.

Management

If there is no mass, a non-bloody discharge and the investigations have proved negative, management is conservative. Surgical intervention is indicated if the discharge is profuse and embarrassing or if malignancy cannot be excluded. For management of specific causes see relevant conditions.

Investigations/procedures

Imaging in breast disease

There are two main modalities of imaging used in assessment of breast disease depending on the age of the patient:

- Ultrasound is the imaging method of choice for establishing the nature of a breast mass in younger women (less than 35 years). Mammograms can be difficult to interpret in young women because of increased breast tissue density.
- Mammography is more useful in older women to confirm the morphology and site of any mass. Cysts are seen as well demarcated masses with a surrounding halo. Carcinomas are often less well defined and have spiculation, distortion of the normal breast architecture or microcalcification. Mammography alone has a 10% false negative rate, hence it is used as part of the triple assessment (clinical examination, imaging, breast tissue sampling).

Breast tissue sampling

Needle core biopsy and fine needle aspiration are both effective methods for taking tissue samples from breasts, but as needle core biopsy is more likely to give an unequivocal result and inadequate sampling is less common, most centres in the United Kingdom now perform needle core biopsy. However, needle core biopsy false negative rates are higher than fine needle aspiration and fine needle aspiration allows aspiration of cystic lesions. Fine needle aspiration may also provide cytology results on the same day (one stop clinic) helping to alleviate anxiety at a particularly stressful time for the patient.

- Fine needle aspiration: The lesion is fixed between the index finger and thumb and a fine needle attached to a syringe (often in a holder) is inserted into the lesion through the stretched skin and subcutaneous tissue. Aspiration is performed by exerting gentle negative pressure through the syringe. A number of passes are made through the lesion at differing angles whilst negative pressure is maintained.
- Needle core biopsy: Local anaesthetic is infiltrated into the area. A small skin incision is made to allow insertion of the core biopsy needle. Under ultrasound guidance the needle is advanced to the edge of the lesion and the biopsy gun is fired. Ultrasound is used to confirm that the needle passes through the lesion. One or two passes are usually sufficient to obtain diagnostic material.

Cytology from either procedure is graded into five categories (see Table 10.3).

Breast reconstruction

Following a mastectomy breast reconstruction can be performed at the same time or as a delayed procedure. Reconstruction may need to be delayed to allow effective

Table 10.3 Grading of FNAC and needle core biopsy

FNAC	Core biopsy	Definition
C1	B1	Inadequate sample (FNAC), normal core biopsy
C2	B2	Benign
C3	B3	Probably benign
C4	B4	Probably malignant
C5	B5	Malignant

local therapies such as radiotherapy to the chest wall. Other factors to be taken into consideration when deciding on breast reconstruction include the following:

- Patient preference.
- The risk of recurrence. If there is a high risk of recurrence reconstruction may be delayed.
- Previous irradiation does not rule out breast reconstruction but may affect the choice of surgical techniques.

Reconstruction of the breast involves either the use of a breast prosthesis or an autologous myocutaneous flap:

- Breast prostheses such as silicone gel implants are usually inserted under the muscles of the chest wall. The skin may need to be gradually stretched first using a tissue expander. Expansion to form a cavity slightly larger than the implant allows the reconstructed breast to hang naturally (ptosis). Previously irradiated skin may be too rigid to allow stretching. Complications include capsular contracture, infection and pain.
- Myocutaneous flap reconstruction involves taking a piece of muscle with its overlying skin to create a breast mound. A pedicle flap retains its original blood supply and is tunnelled under skin to the breast. A free flap requires its blood vessels to be surgically re-anastomosed such as a latissimus dorsi flap. A TRAM (transverse rectus abdominus myocutaneous) flap is an ellipsoid piece of skin, fat and muscle taken from across the whole width of the abdomen. It may be used as a pedicle or free flap. Complications of myocutaneous flaps include necrosis of the flap and scarring of the donor site.

Nipple reconstruction may be achieved by shaping of the reconstructed breast tissue and tattooing to achieve the correct colour. Nipple prostheses offer an alternative to further surgical treatment.

Sufficient counselling on the advantages and disadvantages, the problems and complications of the techniques must be given to all patients.

Benign disorders of the breast

Benign breast disease

Definition

Abnormalities that occur during the normal cycle of breast proliferation and involution. Previously known

Table 10.4 Aberrations of normal development and involution

Normal process	Aberration of normal development and involution
Breast development	Fibroadenoma, juvenile hypertrophy
Cyclical activity	Cyclical mastalgia, cyclical nodularity
Involution	Breast cysts, duct ectasia

under various names (fibroadenosis, fibrocystic change, mammary dysplasia) these have now been classified as aberrations of normal development and involution (ANDI) (see Table 10.4).

Incidence

Common, affecting most women to some extent.

Age

From puberty onwards, peaks in later reproductive life, declines after menopause.

Aetiology

Benign breast disease is thought to occur due to an abnormal tissue response to hormones.

Clinical features and investigations

Some women develop generalised breast nodularity and others present with more localised nodularity (see also section Breast Lumps, page 409). If excised most areas of nodularity show either no abnormality or aberrations of the normal involutional process such as focal areas of fibrosis or sclerosis. Triple assessment (clinical examination, imaging and tissue sampling) is required for any new discrete lump, a new lump within pre-existing nodularity or asymmetrical nodularity that persists after menstruation.

Management

For management of specific forms of ANDI see individual conditions.

Fibroadenoma

Definition

Previously fibroadenomas were considered to be benign neoplasms of the breast. However, as they do not develop from a single cell and are under normal hormonal control they are best considered as an aberration of normal breast development (ANDI).

Incidence
Most common cause of a discrete breast lump in young women.

Age
Peak 25–35 years, but can occur any time from menarche to menopause.

Pathophysiology
Fibroadenomas are usually solitary lesions that result from a hyperplastic or proliferative process in a single terminal ductal unit. Fibroadenomas are under hormonal control, they may enlarge during pregnancy and involute at menopause.

Clinical features
Patients (normally young women) present with a smooth, firm, painless nodule that is well-demarcated and freely mobile (breast mouse). Fibroadenomas may be multiple in 10–15%.

Juvenile fibroadenoma is a rare subtype that occurs in female adolescents and grows rapidly. Histologically they resemble common fibroadenomas and are benign. However, local recurrence can only be prevented by complete excision.

Macroscopy/microscopy
An encapsulated rubbery white lesion with a glistening cut surface. It consists of a fibrous connective tissue component and abnormally proliferated ducts and acini (adenoma) in varying proportions.

Investigations
Investigation of any breast lump involves a triple assessment consisting of clinical examination (see page 409), imaging normally by ultrasound as patients are young and sampling by core biopsy or fine needle aspiration (see page 412).

Management
If confirmed as a fibroadenoma on triple assessment, small lesions may be left unless the patient requests excision. Larger lesions and those with equivocal histology should be excised.

Prognosis
Untreated only 10% of fibroademonas increase in size over a 2-year period most of which occur in teenage women. It is thought that most fibroadenomas involute if left untreated.

Breast cysts

Definition
A common fluid filled epithelial lined space in the breast presenting as a mass.

Incidence
Palpable cysts occur in 7% of women in Western countries and account for 15% of all discrete breast masses.

Aetiology/pathophysiology
Breast cysts are a very common finding in the years leading up to the menopause and are thought to arise due to an anomaly of breast involution.

Clinical features
Patients present with a solitary or multiple lump(s). These are typically well-demarcated, soft or firm and not fixed to underlying tissue. There should not be any associated lymphadenopathy.

Investigations
Patients require a triple assessment consisting of clinical examination (see page 409), imaging using ultrasound or mammography (see page 412) and in the case of a cyst fine needle aspiration (see page 412).

Management
Patients with a single cyst do not need to be reviewed following an otherwise normal ultrasound and successful fine needle aspiration. Patients with multiple cysts do not need all their cysts aspirated and therefore should remain under regular review. Indications for surgical biopsy include bloody fluid detected on fine needle aspiration, a residual mass following aspiration, or multiple recurrence at the same site.

Duct ectasia

Definition
A benign breast disorder with dilation (ectasia) of the subareolar ducts as part of breast involution with accumulation of cellular debris and inflammation.

Age
Most common in women approaching the menopause.

Aetiology/Pathophysiology
The dilated ducts are filled with inspissated secretions with a chronic inflammatory response in the surrounding breast tissue. The cause is unknown.

Clinical features
Duct ectasia may be asymptomatic or may cause nipple discharge (often green) and localised tenderness around the areola. Duct fibrosis and shortening can cause nipple retraction without a lump.

Macroscopy/microsopy
The ducts may be dilated as much as 1 cm in diameter and are filled with proteinaceous secretions, lipid-laden macrophages and epithelial cells. There is periductal chronic inflammation and fibrosis.

Investigations
Any lump should be investigated using the triple assessment (see page 409). Although ductography or ductoscopy are possible, they are not routine investigations.

Management
Once the diagnosis is confirmed surgery may be required to exclude malignancy, if the discharge causes distress or to evert the nipple. Treatment is by subareolar excision of the affected ducts.

Duct papilloma

Definition
A benign proliferation of the epithelium within large mammary or lactiferous ducts.

Aetiology pathophysiology
Papillomas usually arise less than 1 cm from the nipple and obstruct the natural secretions from the gland. In younger women multiple smaller peripheral ducts may be involved, termed peripheral papillomatosis. This is associated with an increased risk of developing breast cancer.

Clinical features
Most patients present with a bloody or serous nipple discharge. It is often possible to identify the discharge as arising from a single point on the nipple, where a dilated slit-like orifice may be visible. There may be a small swelling at the areolar margin (30%), which if pressed may produce discharge.

Macroscopy/microscopy
One to two centimetres sized papilloma within a dilated duct with secretions collected behind it. The lesion usually consists of fronds of vascular tissue covered by a double layer of cells resembling ductal epithelium. Malignant change is rare.

Investigations
Mammography and/or ductography show the dilated duct and filling defect.

Management
A wire is often passed into the responsible duct, which is excised as a microdochectomy with the breast segment that drains into it.

Fat necrosis

Definition
An uncommon condition in which there is death of fat cells within the breast.

Aetiology/pathophysiology
The aetiology is unclear, it is suggested that the death of fat cells may result from trauma. There is an acute inflammatory response, which in some cases progresses to chronic inflammation and organisation with fibrous tissue. The result may be a hard, irregular mass, which can mimic carcinoma.

Clinical features
Patients present with a hard mass, which may also have skin tethering; often in an obese patient with large breasts. Although the patient may recall trauma, this is

not helpful in diagnosis, as many cases of breast carcinoma are discovered after incidental trauma.

Microscopy

Plasma cells predominate. Lipid-laden macrophages (foam cells/lipophages) may form multinucleate giant cells.

Investigation/management

As for breast lump (see page 409), using a triple assessment to exclude malignancy.

Infections of the breast

Acute mastitis

Definition

Acute bacterial inflammation of the breast is related to lactation in most cases.

Aetiology/pathophysiology

- Breast-feeding predisposes to infection by the development of cracks and fissures in the nipple and areola. The infectious agents are most commonly *Staph. aureus*; other causes include *Staph. epidermidis* and *Strep. pyogenes*.
- Periductal non-lactating mastitis is associated with smoking in 90%. It has been suggested that smoking may damage the subareolar ducts, predisposing to infection. Peripheral non-lactating mastitis is uncommon, but is associated with diabetes, rheumatoid arthritis, steroid treatment and trauma. Infections include *Bacteroides*, *Staph. aureus*, *Enterococci* and anaerobic *Streptococci*.

Clinical features

Patients present with painful tender enlargement of the breast, often with a history of a cracked nipple. If left untreated an abscess may form after a few days.

Investigations

Swab any pus and send breast milk (where appropriate) for culture and sensitivities.

Management

- In lactating mastitis, flucloxacillin is usually sufficient. Breast-feeding should be encouraged as this aids drainage of the affected segment of the breast. There is no evidence of harm to the baby. If pain prevents breast-feeding, the baby should be fed from the non-infected breast and expression of milk used to drain the affected breast.
- In non-lactating mastitis, co-amoxiclav is used, with a combination of erythromycin and metronidazole in those who are penicillin-sensitive.
- Surgical drainage is rarely required but may be needed once an abscess has formed. An alternative is daily ultrasound-guided aspiration with antibiotics until the infection has resolved.

Breast cancer

Definition

Breast cancer is the most common malignancy of females in the developed world.

Incidence

Approximately 2/1000 p.a. 1 in 12 women (lifetime risk); 20% of all cancers.

Age

Adults. Peak 50–60 years

Sex

99% in females, and 1% in males.

Geography

More common in North America (1 in 10) and Northern Europe. It is associated with higher social class. Migrants from low-risk to high-risk areas have increased incidence.

Aetiology

In most cases it appears to be multifactorial with a strong environmental influence.

- Exposure to oestrogen is important. Increased risk with early menarche, late menopause, nulliparity, low parity and late first pregnancy.
- Family history of breast cancer.

- History of previous breast disease especially atypical hyperplasia.
- Current evidence indicates a slightly increased risk from the oral contraceptive pill from 2/1000 to 3/1000.
- Hormone replacement therapy postmenopause increases risk.
- Dietary factors (obesity and high alcohol intake) have been implicated.
- Genetic: Two genes have been identified, autosomal dominant with variable penetrance:
  1 BRCA-1 on the long arm of chromosome 17 accounts for <5% of cases of breast cancer, but possessing the gene gives an 80% lifetime risk of developing breast cancer and increased risk of ovarian cancer.
  2 BRCA-2 on chromosome 13 is less common. There is increased breast and prostate cancer in the family. This gene is particularly associated with male breast cancer.
  3 Mutations in the p53 tumour suppressor gene are also associated with an increased risk of developing breast cancer.

Pathophysiology

Most tumours of the breast are adenocarcinomas, which develop from the epithelial cells of the terminal duct/lobular unit. They may either take a lobular or ductal histological appearance on the basis of cell differentiation and architecture. Lobular and ductal carcinoma behave differently in terms of spread.

1 If the atypical cells have not penetrated the basement membrane, it is termed carcinoma in situ. These tumours form approximately 20% of carcinomas of the breast.
  - Ductal carcinoma in situ is now classified according to histological characteristics (including nuclear grade and the presence or absence of necrosis), which helps to predict the potential of the lesion to recur within the breast or to progress to invasive breast cancer. This grading helps to guide management allowing conservative surgery with or without radiotherapy, whereas previously all patients underwent mastectomy.
  - Lobular carcinoma in situ is not palpable and has no characteristic findings on mammography. It is identified as a coexistent finding during microscopic examination of breast tissue samples taken for other reasons (e.g. fibrocystic change). Lobular carcinoma in situ is thought to represent a non-obligate precursor of invasive carcinoma, which may occur at sites other than that of the original biopsy. Management is by close surveillance.

2 Once cells invade the basement membrane, they spread locally and may metastasise and are said to be 'infiltrating' or invasive carcinoma of the breast:
  - Invasive ductal carcinoma is the most common primary malignant tumour (approximately 80%).
  - Invasive lobular breast cancer accounts for approximately 10%.
  - Lobular carcinoma is not a feature in males.

Clinical features

The woman (or rarely, a man) usually presents with a painless lump in the breast or after routine mammographic screening. It most often occurs in the upper outer quadrant of the breast. Occasionally the lump aches or has an unpleasant prickling sensation. Signs of malignancy on examination include the following:

- A firm non-tender irregular lump with ill-defined edges, which is tethered or fixed to skin or underlying muscle.
- Palpable lymph nodes in the axilla, hard in texture, which may be discrete or matted together or to overlying skin or subcutaneous tissue.
- Arm oedema is a late sign, because of involvement of axillary lymph nodes.
- Skin changes suggestive of malignancy are given in Table 10.1.

Some patients present with metastatic disease and a hidden primary. Back pain due to vertebral collapse, shortness of breath or pleuritic chest pain due to spread to the lungs and jaundice due to liver involvement are signs of disseminated disease. Weight loss and malaise are also late symptoms.

Macroscopy/microscopy

The macroscopy of invasive tumours is largely determined by the stromal reaction around the cells. Most tumours excite a lot of reaction forming gritty nodules. If they excite little reaction, they are soft and fleshy.

- Invasive ductal carcinoma: The majority of these have no special histological features, reflecting their lack of differentiation. Approximately 50% of invasive tumours are pure ductal carcinoma, a further 25% have ductal mixed with another type (usually lobular).

- Invasive lobular carcinoma: Characteristically consists of small, bland, homogeneous cells that invade the stroma in 'Indian file' pattern. It is often multifocal and may be bilateral in up to 15% of cases.
- Other forms of invasive breast cancer exist, which have certain well-differentiated features and so are described as medullary, papillary, mucinous or tubular. These (particularly the tubular and mucinous types) have a better prognosis than invasive ductal or lobular carcinoma.
- Tumours can be stained for oestrogen receptors, which affects response to treatment.
- In Paget's disease of the nipple, the skin of the nipple and areola is reddened and thickened, mimicking eczema. It is a form of ductal carcinoma arising from the large excretory ducts. The epidermidis is infiltrated by large pale vacuolated epithelial cells, and there is almost always an in situ or invasive ductal carcinoma in the underlying breast tissue.

Complications

Lymphatic and haematogenous spread. Ninety to ninety-five per cent of the breast drains to the axillary nodes, the remainder drains to the internal mammary nodes. Haematogenous spread may occur before or after lymphatic spread. The most common organs affected are bone, liver, lung and pleura, brain, ovaries (Krukenberg tumour is an enlarged ovary due to 2° tumour cells) and adrenal glands.

Investigation

Investigation of a breast lump involves a triple assessment:

1 Clinical history and examination (see page 409).
2 Imaging using mammography or ultrasound in younger women (see page 412).
3 Breast tissue sampling using needle core biopsy or fine needle aspiration (see page 412). This also allows staining for hormone receptors, which guides management.

If a malignancy is confirmed patients may undergo a chest X-ray, full blood count and liver function tests for staging. Isotope bone scan, liver ultrasound and CT brain scan may also be required if clinically indicated (see Table 10.5).

Management

Early or operable breast cancer (Up to T2, N1, M0 breast cancer with or without mobile lymph nodes on the same

Table 10.5 The TNM classification of breast cancer

Primary tumour	
Tis	Carcinoma in situ
	Paget's disease (no tumour)
T0	No evidence of primary tumour
T1	Tumour <2cm
	(T1a <5mm, T1b 5–10mm, T1c 10–20mm)
T2	Tumour 2–5 cm
T3	Tumour >5cm
T4	Any size with direct extension to chest wall or skin
Regional lymph nodes	
N0	No regional node metastases
N1	Metastases to movable ipsilateral axillary nodes (histologically <3 nodes)
N2	Fixed ipsilateral nodes
N3	Metastases to ipsilateral internal mammary nodes
Distant metastases	
M0	No evidence of distant metastases
M1	Distant metastases (including metastases to supraclavicular LN's)
MX	Metastases suspected but unproven

side and no evidence of metastases) is potentially curable. The decision between differing combinations of therapy is complex and involves factors such as breast size, patient choice, multifocality, tumour site, tumour type, recurrence of previously treated tumours and where radiotherapy is contraindicated.

Local treatment:

- Breast conservation surgery involves a wide local excision of the lesion. Conservative breast surgery with radiotherapy has been shown to be as effective as mastectomy in terms of long-term survival.
- Simple mastectomy describes the removal of breast parenchyma including nipple and areolar.

Lymph node treatment:

- Assessment of the presence of spread to the lymph nodes may be achieved by axillary lymph node sampling or dissection (the latter is also therapeutic). Sentinel node biopsy involves sampling the first 2–4 axillary lymph nodes draining the breast. These sentinel nodes may be identified by intraoperative injection of a tracer around the tumour site. If the sentinel nodes are free from metastases, this indicates that there has been no spread to the remainder of the axilla (5% false negative rate) and no further treatment is required.
- If axillary node sampling or sentinel biopsy have demonstrated nodal metastases, axillary clearance or radiotherapy is required.

Locally advanced disease: Patients are treated with preoperative systemic therapy and then if they become operable they undergo surgery. In more than 65% of women, the tumour shrinks by more than 50%, which makes it more likely that the whole tumour is excised at surgery and in some patients allows breast conservation. This form of treatment may also be used in patients with stage T2 tumours to facilitate breast-conserving surgery. Radiotherapy and further systemic therapy may be used with or without surgery.

Metastatic breast cancer: The aim of treatment is palliation of symptoms and improving quality of life as currently most of these patients die from breast cancer. Treatments include radiotherapy, systemic treatment and surgery to debulk the primary tumour, which may be ulcerating through the skin and alleviate symptoms such as bone pain, pleural and pericardial effusions.

Systemic therapy: The choice of which therapies are used depends on whether patients are pre- or post-menopausal, if they have oestrogen-receptor positive

disease, their risk of recurrence and the stage of their disease.

- Hormonal therapy should be used in all patients with oestrogen-receptor positive tumours. Premenopausal women are given LHRH analogues and tamoxifen. Postmenopausal women receive either tamoxifen or an aromatase inhibitor, which reduces the peripheral conversion of androgens to oestrogen. Aromatase inhibitors appear to be as effective as tamoxifen with fewer side effects.
- Adjuvant combination chemotherapy has been shown to be more effective than a single agent. Most regimens are administered 3–4 weekly for 4–6 cycles. A new class of chemotherapeutic agents called taxanes has resulted from yew tree-derived products, e.g. paclitaxel and docetaxel.
- Recent advances have occurred in monoclonal antibodies directed against HER2, which is overexpressed in 15–20% of breast cancers. Trastuzumab (Herceptin) has been shown to prolong survival in patients with metastatic breast cancer that overexpresses HER2.

Prognosis

The important prognostic indicator is the TNM staging (see Table 10.5):

T: Increasing size of tumour indicates worse prognosis.

N: Nodal involvement reduces 5-year survival from 80 to 60%.

M: Haematogenous spread has a much poorer prognosis (5-year survival is only 10%). Average survival is 14–18 months with chemotherapy.

Well-differentiated cells also improve the prognosis.

Breast cancer screening

UK programme

Females aged 50–69 years are invited every 3 years for screening by a craniocaudal and a mediolateral oblique mammogram (see also page 412). Screening aims to detect tumours of <1 cm size before they become palpable. If identified, a stereotactic needle core biopsy can be performed to obtain tissue for histology. A hooked wire can be inserted under radiological guidance into the lesion prior to surgery. The lump can then be identified and either undergo excision biopsy or wide local excision with the removal of a margin of surrounding normal tissue. If the histology demonstrates malignancy further treatments for breast cancer may be required (see page 417).

The evidence of the breast cancer screening programme is difficult to assess. Trials have investigated the effect of screening on mortality, but as the range of mortality rates exceed the reduction of mortality by screening it is difficult to demonstrate a statistical benefit. Overall it appears that one woman in every 1000 who undergoes breast screening may be prevented from dying from breast cancer. This must be balanced against false positive screening results and unnecessary biopsies, which are the cause of significant patient morbidity.

Endocrine system

Clinical

Principles of endocrine testing

The endocrine system is the mechanism by which information is communicated around the body using chemical messengers (hormones). These messengers are secreted by glands and may be transported through the bloodstream to a distant target organ (endocrine activity) or may act directly on local tissue (paracrine activity). Hormones are of various types including peptides, glycoproteins, steroids or amines such as catecholamines.

- Peptide, glycoprotein and amine hormones act by binding to cell surface receptors, which initiate a cascade of intracellular signalling molecules. These hormones may be synthesised and stored as inactive precursors (prohormones).
- Steroid hormones and thyroid hormones circulate freely and bound to plasma proteins. It is only the unbound (free) hormone that is biologically active. The bound hormone acts as a buffer against rapid changes in hormone levels. Steroid hormones act via intracellular receptors, which travel to the cell nucleus and regulate DNA transcription and hence protein synthesis.

The sensitivity of target organs to a hormone is dependent on the level of receptor expression. Prolonged exposure to a hormone often results in receptor downregulation, whereas absent or minimal hormone exposure leads to receptor upregulation.

Hormones may act on glands to cause the secretion of other hormones and may also act to downregulate their own production (negative feedback), for example the action of thyroid hormones on the anterior pituitary (see Fig. 11.1).

Endocrine dysfunction generally results in over or under functioning of a gland. Reduced function may result from a number of mechanisms. For example, hypothyroidism may result from a failure of the anterior pituitary gland or a failure of the thyroid gland. Endocrine testing is used to both identify the lack of hormone and to elucidate the underlying cause. For example,

- measurement of thyroid hormones is used to detect hypothyroidism
- measurement of thyroid stimulating hormone (TSH) helps to identify the cause. A low TSH signifies failure of the anterior pituitary (secondary hypothyroidism). A high TSH signifies failure of the thyroid gland (primary hypothyroidism).

Clinical features of apparent hormone deficiency may also result from a failure of response at the target organs.

Some hormones have cyclical or pulsatile secretion. In these cases a single random hormone sample will not determine whether the level is high or low. In such instances either testing at specific times of day (e.g. early morning cortisol levels) or dynamic endocrine testing is required. Dynamic endocrine testing uses techniques to stimulate or suppress hormone secretion. For example, cortisol is secreted from the adrenal glands in response to adrenocorticotrophin hormone (ACTH). Administering a synthetic ACTH (Synacthen) allows the response of the adrenal glands to be assessed.

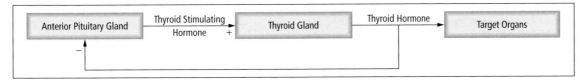

Figure 11.1 An example of negative feedback control.

The hypothalamus and pituitary

Introduction to the hypothalamus and pituitary

The pituitary gland lies in the sella turcica, which is a tightly enclosed bony space at the base of the cranium, roofed by a reflection of the dura. The optic chiasm lies just above the pituitary fossa and the cavernous sinuses run lateral to it. These structures may be affected by expansion of the pituitary gland. It consists of two lobes:

- The posterior lobe is a physical and functional extension of the ventral hypothalamus. The nerve endings within the posterior pituitary contain and secrete oxytocin and vasopression (antidiuretic hormone).
- The anterior lobe originates from Rathke's pouch. Although the anterior lobe is of separate origin to the hypothalamus, it is under its close control. Hypothalamic hormones reach the anterior pituitary in high concentrations via hypophyseal–pituitary portal veins.

The hypothalamus lies just above the pituitary, and has centres for appetite (the satiety centre), thirst, temperature control and the sleep–wake cycle. The hypothalamus secretes polypeptide hormones that regulate anterior pituitary hormone secretion, mostly by stimulation. They are secreted episodically and some, e.g.

corticotrophin-releasing hormone and thyrotrophin–releasing hormone have an important circadian (*circa*-about, *dia* - day) rhythm.

The hypothalamus and pituitary form the basis of the central control of various endocrine axes, which are vital to everyday function (see Fig. 11.2). Disorders of the hypothalamus itself are very rare; however, disorders of the pituitary are common.

Pituitary adenomas

Definition
Pituitary adenomas are benign slow growing tumours arising from the anterior pituitary.

Aetiology
The cause of most pituitary adenomas is unknown. Gene mutations have been characterised in some pituitary adenomas, for example in the condition multiple endocrine neoplasia (MEN) type 1 tumours including pituitary adenomas occur due to the loss of tumour suppressor genes.

Pathophysiology
Seventy per cent of pituitary adenomas are functioning, i.e. hormone secreting. These tend to present earlier than the other 30% non-functioning tumours.

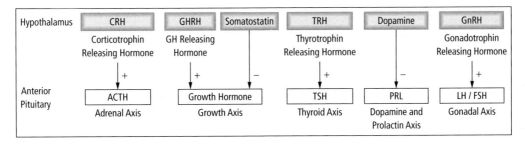

Figure 11.2 Hypothalamic and pituitary secretion.

Table 11.1 Common hormone secreting pituitary adenomas

Hormone producing pituitary adenoma	Clinical syndrome
Prolactin (60%)	Hyperprolactinaemia (e.g. amenorrhoea and subfertility in women)
Growth hormone (20%)	Acromegaly Gigantism
Adrenocorticotrophic hormone (10%)	Cushing's disease

Clinical features

Pituitary adenomas produce symptoms through local pressure such as headache, and visual loss due to pressure on the optic chiasm (bilateral temporal heminanopia). Continuing growth disrupts other hormone secretion and can result in hypopituitarism. Symptoms may also result from the effects of hormone excess (see Table 11.1).

Macroscopy

- Tumours less than 1 cm in diameter without enlargement of, or extension outside the pituitary fossa are defined as microadenomas.
- Tumours larger than 1 cm in diameter are called macroadenomas and may cause pituitary fossa enlargement.
- Tumours ≥1–2 cm may extend outside the fossa towards the hypothalamus and optic chiasm, laterally into the cavernous sinus or downwards into the sphenoid sinus.

Investigations

- A mass within the sella turcica (pituitary fossa) may be identified on plain skull X-ray.
- MRI scanning using gadolinium contrast is the imaging modality of choice. Microadenomas take up less contrast and macroadenomas take up more contrast.
- If a pituitary mass is identified, hormone assays should be undertaken to identify functioning adenomas. Testing also helps identify any associated hypopituitarism, with stimulation or suppression testing where appropriate.

Management

- For prolactinomas medical treatment with a dopaminergic drug is the treatment of choice (see section on Hyperprolactinaemia, page 424).

- For other pituitary adenomas, transsphenoidal resection is the treatment of choice, with postoperative radiotherapy for patients where complete resection has not been possible. Major postoperative complications include CSF leakage, meningitis or visual impairment, which are most frequent in patients undergoing large resections. Transient diabetes insipidus or syndrome of inappropriate anti-diuretic hormone (SIADH) may also occur. Increasingly asymptomatic pituitary adenomas are found at incidental imaging. In elderly or infirm patients surgery may not be appropriate.
- All patients require regular assessment for hormone deficiencies with replacement therapy used as necessary.

Hypopituitarism

Definition

Hypopituitarism is a clinical term referring to underfunction of the pituitary gland. This may imply a deficiency of single or multiple hormones.

Aetiology

The commonest causes are pituitary or hypothalamic tumours, or secondary to pituitary surgery or cranial radiotherapy (see Table 11.2).

Pathophysiology

Hypopituitarism may be primary due to destruction of the anterior pituitary gland or secondary to a deficiency of hypothalamic stimulation (or excess of inhibition).

Clinical features

Symptoms and signs are related to the deficiency of hormones (see Table 11.3). General symptoms of panhypopituitarism include dry, pale skin with sparse body hair. On examination postural hypotension and bradycardia may be found with decreased muscle power and delayed deep tendon reflexes.

Investigations

All functions of the pituitary should be assessed using basal levels, stimulation tests and suppression testing where appropriate.

Table 11.2 Causes of hypopituitarism

Type	Causes
Invasive	Large pituitary adenoma
	Craniopharyngioma or primary CNS tumour
	Metastasic tumour (esp. breast)
Infarction	Postpartum necrosis (Sheehan's syndrome)
	Pituitary apoplexy (haemorrhagic infarction of pituitary tumour)
Infiltration	Sarcoidosis, haemochromatosis, histiocytosis X
Injury	Head trauma
Immunologic	Organ-specific autoimmune disease
Iatrogenic	Surgery, irradiation
Infectious	Mycoses, TB, syphilis
Idiopathic	Familial
Isolated	
GH	Dwarfism, emotional deprivation
LH, FSH	Kallmann's syndrome, weight loss, sickle cell anaemia
TSH	Chronic renal failure, pseudohypoparathyroidism
ACTH-LPH	Lymphocytic hypophysitis, familial
PRL	Pseudohypoparathyroidism

Management

Treatment of the underlying cause may be required. Hormone replacement depends on the results of pituitary function testing:

- In ACTH deficiency, lifelong glucocorticoid replacement is essential.
- In TSH deficiency, oral thyroxine is given and titrated according to free T_4. Thyroxine replacement may aggravate any partial adrenal insufficiency, if present, by increasing cortisol clearance.
- Gonadotrophin deficiency in women may be treated with cyclical oestrogen replacement to maintain secondary sexual characteristics and prevent osteoporosis. Progestagen is used to induce bleeding and prevent endometrial hyperplasia. In men testosterone replacement restores libido and potency, maintains beard growth and muscle power, prevents osteoporosis and improves sense of well-being. In adolescent males testosterone induces epiphyseal closure, so replacement therapy should be delayed as long as possible. Treatment of associated infertility requires complex hormone replacement to stimulate ovulation/spermatogenesis.
- Growth hormone deficiency is treated with recombinant human growth hormone.

Dopamine and prolactin axis

Dopamine from the hypothalamus acts to inhibit prolactin secretion from the pituitary (see Fig. 11.3).

- If the hypothalamic pituitary connection is disrupted, e.g. by stalk section or hypothalamic lesions then pituitary prolactin (PRL) secretion is uncontrolled.
- PRL release is stimulated by drugs that block dopamine receptors (e.g. metoclopramide) or cause a reduction in hypothalamic dopamine (e.g. methyldopa). Stress, sleep and nipple stimulation increase PRL.
- Oestrogens during pregnancy increase PRL secretion but also suppress milk production. As oestrogens fall postpartum, milk production accelerates.
- Administration of dopamine or levodopa inhibits PRL release. Pituitary haemorrhage causing death of the lactotrophs results in failure of lactation (Sheehan's syndrome).

Table 11.3 Features of pituitary hormone deficiency in order of frequency

Hormone	Clinical features
Growth hormone deficiency	Changes in body composition, osteopenia and insulin resistance
	Reduced growth in childhood
Gonadotrophins (LH, FSH) deficiency	Amenorrhoea in women
	Decreased libido, impotence in men
Thyroid stimulating hormone deficiency	Hypothyroidism
Adrenocorticotrophic hormone deficiency	Adrenocortical insufficiency, but less severe than primary adrenal failure. The zona glomerulosa and aldosterone secretion usually remains relatively intact, so Addisonian crisis is rare. Symptoms are more common at times of stress, such as illness.
	Reduced adrenal androgens causes loss of body hair
Prolactin deficiency	Failure to lactate after giving birth

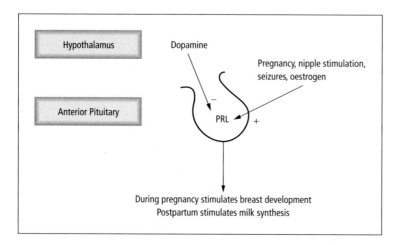

During pregnancy stimulates breast development
Postpartum stimulates milk synthesis

Figure 11.3 Factors affecting prolactin secretion.

Table 11.4 Factors affecting prolactin secretion

Increased prolactin (hyperprolactinaemia)	Decreased prolactin
PRL-secreting pituitary adenoma (prolactinoma)	Any cause of panhypopituitarism (see page 422)
Other pituitary tumours (reduces dopamine concentration)	Sheehan's syndrome
Hypothalamus/pituitary stalk damage	Dopamine agonists (bromocriptine/ cabergoline)
Drugs: opioids, monoamine oxidase inhibitors, cimetidine, verapamil	
Hypothyroidism (direct effect of raised TRH and TSH)	
Renal failure	
Polycystic ovarian syndrome	

- Other factors affecting PRL secretion are shown in Table 11.4.

Hyperprolactinaemia

Definition
Hyperprolactinaemia is a raised serum prolactin level causing galactorrhoea and gondadal dysfunction.

Incidence
Most common endocrine abnormality of the hypothalamic–pituitary axis.

Aetiology
Prolactin (PRL) is under the inhibitory control of dopamine released from the hypothalamus. Causes of hyperprolactinaemia are shown in Fig. 11.4 and Table 11.4.

Pathophysiology
Hyperprolactinaemia causes disturbance of the hypothalamic–pituitary–gonadal axis in both men and women, probably by a local hormonal interaction between prolactin and hypothalamic gonadotrophin-releasing hormone (GnRH) secretion.
- Gonadotrophin (luteinising hormone and follicle stimulating hormone (LH and FSH) secretion is abnormal and the mid-cycle surge in LH in women is suppressed.
- Hyperprolactinaemia in women is commonly physiological, and in men it is almost always of pathological significance.

Clinical features
In women hyperprolactinaemia causes primary or secondary amenorrhoea, oligomenorrhoea with anovulation or infertility. Galactorrhoea is variably present. Oestrogen deficiency can cause vaginal dryness and osteopenia. Hirsutism can occur, with weight gain and anxiety depression and hot flushes. In men galactorrhoea occurs occasionally, but the most common early features are decreased libido and sexual dysfunction, sometimes with impotence and infertility.

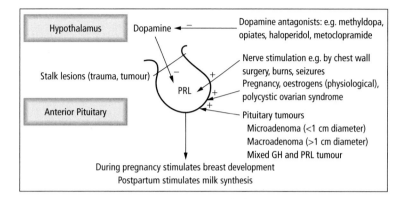

Figure 11.4 Causes of hyperprolactinaemia.

Complications
Headache, visual impairment and hypopituitarism due to local effects of the adenoma.

Investigations
Raised PRL in the absence of another cause of hyperprolactinaemia is the feature of a functioning pituitary adenoma. The serum prolactin level is in proportion to tumour size. All the pituitary hormone axes have to be tested to look for associated hypopituitarism. Plain skull X-ray is usually normal, whereas MRI will demonstrate the lesion, usually <1 cm in size.

Management
Prolactinomas are treated with dopaminergic drugs such as cabergoline. The minority of tumours that do not respond to medical treatment and hyperprolactinaemia due to stalk compression are treated surgically.

Growth axis

Growth hormone releasing hormone (GHRH or GRH) secreted from the hypothalamus in a pulsatile manner. Growth hormone (GH also called somatotrophin) promotes linear growth mainly through insulin-like growth factor (IGF-I previously known as somatomedin C), see Fig. 11.5.

Conditions that affect levels of growth hormone are shown in Table 11.5.

Acromegaly

Definition
Acromegaly is a clinical syndrome caused by growth hormone (GH)-secreting pituitary adenomas in adults.

Incidence
GH-secreting pituitary adenomas are second in frequency to prolactinomas.

Age
Can occur at any age but mean onset 40 years.

Sex
M = F

Aetiology
- 95% of cases result from growth-hormone-secreting pituitary adenoma (somatotroph). A mutation in the G_s protein leading to excessive cAMP production has been found in 40% of GH-secreting adenomas. Acromegaly may occur as part of multiple endocrine neoplasia (MEN) type I.
- In around 5% of cases there is ectopic GHRH secretion from a carcinoid tumour, GH from a pancreatic islet cell tumour, or inappropriate hypothalamic production of GRH.

Pathophysiology
Excess production of GH leads to the release of high levels of IGF-I (insulin-like growth factor) from the liver.

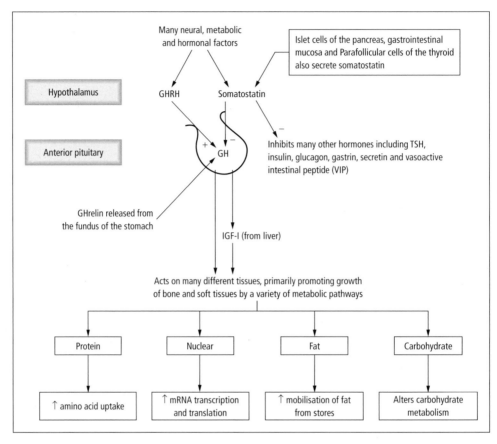

Figure 11.5 The growth axis.

Table 11.5 Causes of growth hormone excess and deficiency

Increase	Decrease
Sleep, exercise, stress	
Hypoglycaemia	Postprandial hyperglycaemia/ free fatty acids
	Glucocorticoids (hence short stature in children on long-term oral steroids)
Acromegaly	Hypopituitarism
(GH secreting tumour)	

The combination of high levels of GH and IGF-I leads to following:

- Overgrowth of bone and soft tissue, particularly the face and skull.
- These hormones are lipolytic, diabetogenic and cause sodium and water retention. Other endocrine and

metabolic abnormalities may occur, due to the local mechanical effect of the adenoma on normal pituitary tissue.

Clinical features

The course of the disease is slowly progressive. Soft tissue overgrowth is the characteristic early feature, causing enlargement of hands and feet, coarse facial features.

- Face and skull: Thickened calvarium, prominent supraorbital ridges, enlarged nose, prognathic mandible, widely spaced teeth and puffiness of the face due to soft tissue overgrowth.
- Hands and feet are bulky, with blunt, spade-like fingers.
- Bones and joints: Arthralgia and degenerative arthritis of the spine, hips and knees due to bone and cartilage overgrowth. Carpal tunnel syndrome is common.

- Skin is thickened, oily and sweaty. Acne, sebaceous cysts and skin tags are common. Acanthosis nigricans of the axillae and neck may occur. Hypertrichosis in women.
- Cardiovascular: Hypertension in 25% of patients, and left ventricular hypertrophy and cardiomyopathy leading to cardiac failure in about 15%.
- Organomegaly: Thyroid and salivary gland enlargement, hepatomegaly.
- Diabetes in 40% of patients.

Macroscopy/microscopy
The tumour is solid and trabecular, often 1 cm in diameter by the time of diagnosis. Immunohistochemistry can be used to stain for GH.

Complications
- Renal calculi occur in 10% as a result of the hypercalciuria induced by GH excess.
- Local effects of a pituitary tumour include headache, and pressure effects such as bitemporal hemianopia. Panhypopituitarism may occur.
- Increased risk of uterine tumours and possibly of colonic polyps.

Investigations
- IGF-I and GH levels are raised, but GH levels are unreliable due to episodic secretion. An oral glucose suppression test is performed – a glucose load will fail to suppress growth hormone production.
- Imaging of the pituitary fossa by X-ray, CT or MRI.
- If there is no evidence of a pituitary adenoma GHRH may be assayed.

Management
- Wherever possible transphenoidal resection of the adenoma is the treatment of choice. Large tumours may be resected by transfrontal craniotomy. Prior to surgery hypopituitarism must be treated using cortisol and thyroxine.
- Octreotide or lanreotide, a long-acting somatostatin analogue, may be used prior to surgery, following incomplete resection or in elderly patients not fit for surgery. Dopamine agonists may be added in refractory cases.
- Irradiation may be used as an adjuvant to other therapies.

- Accompanying hypopituitarism is treated as appropriate with corticosteroids, thyroxine and gonadal steroids or gonadotrophins.

Prognosis
Follow-up is required for recurrence or loss of pituitary function. Acromegaly causes increased morbidity and mortality mainly due to diabetes and cardiovascular disease.

Thyroid axis

The thyroid axis
Thyrotrophin-releasing hormone (TRH) is released from the hypothalamus episodically and with a circadian rhythm. It stimulates the production of thyroid stimulating hormone (TSH) from the anterior pituitary gland. TSH is a glycoprotein, which binds to high-affinity receptors (TSH-R) in the thyroid gland. This in turn stimulates iodide uptake by the thyroid gland, and the synthesis and release of thyroxine (T_4) and triiodothyronine (T_3) through activation of adenylate cyclase (see Fig. 11.6).

Somatostatin and dopamine agonists decrease TSH secretion conversely dopamine antagonists increase TSH secretion. Other hormones affecting the thyroid axis include glucocorticoids, which in excess can impair the sensitivity of the pituitary to TRH and hence reduce TSH secretion. Oestrogens conversely increase the sensitivity of the pituitary to TRH.

Production and action of the thyroid hormones (T_3 and T_4)
The epithelial cells of the thyroid gland produce thyroglobulin, which can be seen in the centre of thyroid follicles and stains as pink 'colloid'. TSH stimulates the re-absorption of colloid by the cells and the production of T_3 and T_4. These hormones circulate in the blood bound to thyroxine binding globulin (TBG) and albumin. The majority of T_3 is converted from the less active T_4 by peripheral tissues. Disorders of the thyroid axis are shown in Table 11.6 and Fig. 11.7.

Goitre
A goitre is a visible or palpable enlarged thyroid. The enlargement may be generalised enlargement or diffuse

Table 11.6 Disorders of thyroid axis

	Increased hormone	Decreased hormone
TSH	Hypothyroidism (thyroid failure and lack of feedback) TSH secreting pituitary adenoma (rare) Thyroid hormone resistance	Primary thyrotoxicosis, e.g. Graves' disease, toxic multinodular goitre (due to increased thyroid hormone negative feedback)
T$_3$ and T$_4$	Graves' disease Toxic multinodular goitre Early Hashimoto's disease	Hashimoto's disease Iatrogenic: following thyroidectomy or radioiodine treatment Iodine deficiency

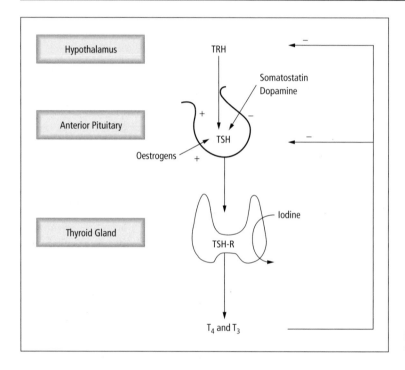

Figure 11.6 Production and action of the thyroid hormones.

goitre; or may consist of single or multiple nodules. Further classification is based on whether the patient is hyperthyroid, euthyroid or hypothyroid (see Table 11.7) and below.

Multinodular goitre

Definition
Irregular multinodular enlargement of the thyroid gland, which may be hyperthyroid (toxic) or is commonly euthyroid (nontoxic).

Incidence/prevalence
25% of cases of thyrotoxicosis are due to multinodular goitre.

Age
Increases with age.

Sex
F > M

Aetiology
Unknown. May be due to varying response of the thyroid tissue to TSH over many years.

Clinical features
Patients may present for cosmetic reasons, with thyrotoxic symptoms, or because of complications. Multinodular goitre can present with a particularly prominent thyroid nodule or a diffusely nodular gland. Most

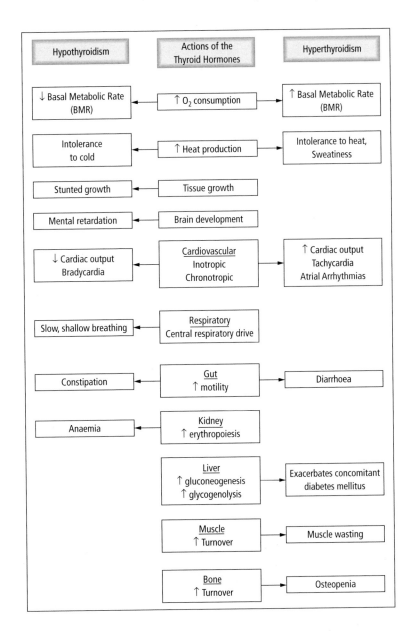

Figure 11.7 Actions of thyroid hormones in thyroid dysfunction.

Table 11.7 Causes of goitre

Hyperthyroid (toxic goitre)	Euthyroid (nontoxic goitre)	Hypothyroid
Graves' disease (thyrotoxicosis)	Pregnancy, puberty	De Quervain's thyroiditis
Toxic multinodular goitre	Endemic goitre (iodine deficiency)	Iodine deficiency
Solitary toxic nodule	Nontoxic multinodular goitre	Hashimoto's (autoimmune) thyroiditis
	Solitary thyroid nodule or cyst	

patients are euthyroid with a goitre, occasionally one or more nodules develop, which are TSH-independent and so cause thyrotoxicosis.

Macroscopy/microscopy

The thyroid is enlarged with irregular nodules of varying sizes. Nodules may be cystic, haemorrhagic and fibrosed. Microscopy reveals hyperplastic acini, with varying amounts of colloid.

Complications

Enlargement of the gland can cause tracheal compression leading to shortness of breath and choking. This is more common with retrosternal goitre, when the nodule(s) are in the isthmus. Toxic multinodular goitre has a particularly high incidence of cardiac arrhythmias and other cardiac complications.

Investigations

Thyroid function tests (TSH and thyroid hormone levels) are used to assess thyroid status. A chest X-ray can demonstrate any retrosternal mass or tracheal deviation. Ultrasound scanning of the thyroid may be useful to examine the structure of the thyroid and nature of lesions. Isotope scans are used to demonstrate areas of increased uptake in toxic multinodular goitres. Cysts and nodules may be aspirated by fine needle aspiration for cytology.

Management

Subtotal thyroidectomy may be required for cosmetic reasons or due to compression symptoms or thyrotoxicosis. Patients must be medically treated and euthyroid before surgery.

Solitary thyroid nodule

Definition

A solitary mass within the thyroid gland that may be solid or cystic.

Incidence

5% of population have a palpable solitary thyroid nodule. Up to 50% of population have a solitary nodule at postmortem.

Aetiology/pathophysiology

Solitary thyroid nodules are most commonly benign (over 90%). Causes include the following:

- Benign follicular adenoma: Single lesions with well-developed fibrous capsules. Adenomas are not under the control of TSH and continue to secrete thyroid hormones, which may result in hyperthyroidism. There are low levels of circulating TSH and hence suppression of the remainder of the thyroid gland.
- Colloid nodule that may be a dominant nodule in a multinodular goitre (see page 428).
- Malignant tumours of the thyroid follicle cells.
- Thyroid cyst (15–25%): These may be simple cysts or bleeding into a colloid nodule or adenoma. About 15% are necrotic papillary tumours.

Clinical features

Patients may present with a palpable lump or may be diagnosed on incidental imaging. Features suggestive of malignancy:

- Rapid painless growth.
- Family history of thyroid tumours or MEN 2 syndrome (see page 450).
- History of neck irradiation exposure.
- Hoarseness and vocal cord paralysis suggesting recurrent laryngeal nerve palsy.
- Malignancy is more common in children and patients over 60 years.

Investigations

- Thyroid function tests are used to determine thyroid status. Isotope scans may also be used to demonstrate either a cold nodule, a hyperactive gland (toxic multinodular goitre) or a 'cold' gland containing a 'hot' nodule (toxic adenoma). Cold nodules suggest malignancy.
- Ultrasound scan may be used to determine the anatomy of the lesion and distinguish solid from cystic nodules.
- Fine needle aspiration for cytology is used to differentiate benign cells, suspicious cells or malignant cells.

Management

Benign lesions only require treatment if they cause hyperthyroidism or for cosmetic reasons. Treatment options include surgical excision and radioactive iodine.

If suspicious cells are identified on cytology a thyroid lobectomy should be performed.

Graves' disease (primary thyrotoxicosis)

Definition
Graves' disease is an autoimmune thyroid disease.

Age
Any. Peak 20–40 years.

Sex
F > M

Aetiology
Graves' disease results from production of an autoantibody that binds to the TSH receptor and causes continuous gland stimulation.

- Fifteen per cent of patients have a close relative with Graves', and 50% of relatives have circulating thyroid autoantibodies.
- Associated with HLA-B8 and DR3 in Caucasians, and with HLA-B17 in Blacks.
- Environmental 'triggers' suggested: Pregnancy, iodide excess, infection.

Pathophysiology
Breakdown of self-tolerance results in the formation of stimulating autoantibody acting at the TSH receptor. This causes a generalised, uncontrolled stimulation of the thyroid gland initially causing hyperthyroidism. After many years the gland becomes non-functional and the patient becomes hypothyroid.

- The thyroid antigen shares epitopes with antigens on the orbital muscles, so that cytotoxic T-cells attack these tissues causing them to swell. Other complications of Graves' disease may also be due to similar epitopes being present in other tissues, e.g. skin and nail beds. These complications do not resolve on treatment to reduce the overactivity of the thyroid.
- Some symptoms of Graves' disease relate to apparent catecholamine (noradrenaline and adrenaline) excess, for example tachycardia, tremor and sweating. Thyroid hormones induce cardiac catecholamine receptors.

- The autoantibody can cross the placenta, causing neonatal hyperthyroidism.

Clinical features
Hyperthyroidism produces palpitations, nervousness, fatigue, diarrhoea, sweatiness, tremor and intolerance of heat. Weight loss with increased or normal appetite and hyperactivity are common. There is often muscle weakness, which can be severe.

The patient may have noticed the neck swelling, which is usually soft, diffusely and symmetrically enlarged. Proptosis (exophthalmos) with lid retraction, stare and lid lag are prominent features, and in its most severe form it may cause sight loss due to damage to the optic nerve. Involvement of the orbital muscles may also cause diplopia.

Less common symptoms and signs include atrial fibrillation and heart failure, depression (see also Fig. 11.7). Thyroid dermopathy (also called pretibial myxoedema) is a thickening or 'orange-peel appearance' of the skin, most often affecting the lower leg. Onycholysis (weakening, thinning and broken nails) may occur. Thyroid acropachy (osteopathy), which is a form of clubbing, is rare and may be complicated by hypercalcaemia.

Microscopy
The thyroid epithelial cells are increased in number and size with large nuclei. The colloid in the centre of the follicle shows scalloped edges, which although an artefact of processing does seem to indicate increased removal of colloid for production of thyroxine. Focal lymphocyte infiltration may also be seen.

Investigations
Thyroid function tests generally show high free tri-iodothyronine (T_3) and usually thyroxine (T_4), with a low thyroid-stimulating hormone (TSH). The diagnosis is made by a combination of clinical features and detection of thyroid autoantibodies.

Management
Antithyroid drugs (usually carbimazole) are given to suppress the gland. Graves' disease commonly enters remission after 12–18 months, so a trial of withdrawal is appropriate. Patients who are severely symptomatic with hyperthyroidism also benefit from β-blockers. Relapse is common (50%); treatment options include a

second course of antithyroid drugs, radioiodine therapy or surgery. Subtotal thyroidectomy results in normalisation of thyroid function in 70%. Recurrence can be treated by further surgery. The patient must be made euthyroid before surgery with antithyroid drugs and β-blockers (see page 436).

Prognosis

Thirty to fifty per cent of patients used to undergo spontaneous remission without treatment. Recurrence after treatment may be more likely in those with HLA association. Approximately 20% become hypothyroid with all types of treatment.

Thyrotoxic crisis (storm)

Definition

A rare syndrome of severe acute thyrotoxicosis, which may be life-threatening.

Aetiology

Surgery or radioactive iodine therapy in a patient with inadequately controlled thyrotoxicosis may precipitate a thyrotoxic storm. Other causes include severe illness or accident, uncontrolled diabetes, acute infection, severe drug reaction or myocardial infarction.

Pathophysiology

Levels of thyroid-binding protein in the serum fall and catecholamines are released. This results in increased free T3 and T4, coupled to increased sensitivity of the heart and nerves due to the presence of catecholamines.

Clinical features

The symptoms include life-threatening coma, heart failure and cardiogenic shock. There is a high fever (38–41°C), flushing and sweating, tachycardia, often with atrial fibrillation and heart failure. Central nervous symptoms include agitation, restlessness, delirium and coma. Nausea, vomiting, diarrhoea and jaundice occur.

Management

Concomitant use of propranolol, potassium iodide, antithyroid drugs and corticosteroids.

Table 11.8 Causes of hypothyroidism

Primary	Idiopathic/autoimmune thyroid atrophy
	Hashimoto's thyroiditis
	Iatrogenic: radioactive iodine, surgery, drugs
	Iodine deficiency (common in Nepal, Bangladesh)
	Inborn errors of hormone synthesis
Secondary	Panhypopituitarism due to pituitary adenoma
	Iatrogenic: pituitary ablative therapy/surgery
Tertiary	Hypothalamic dysfunction (rare)
	Peripheral resistance to thyroid hormone (rare)

Prognosis
Mortality of 10%.

Hypothyroidism (myxoedema)

Definition
Hypothyroidism is a clinical syndrome resulting from a deficiency of thyroid hormones.

Aetiology
Hypothyroidism may be divided into primary thyroid failure, secondary hypothyroidism due to lack of pituitary TSH and tertiary hypothyroidism due to lack of hypothalamic thyrotrophin releasing hormone (TRH) (see Table 11.8).

Pathophysiology
Congenital hypothyroidism causes permanent developmental retardation. In children it causes reversible delayed growth and puberty, and developmental delay. Precocious puberty may occur in juveniles, due to pituitary hypertrophy. In adults it causes decreased removal of glycosaminoglycans and hence deposition in the extracellular space, especially skin, heart and skeletal muscle. There is also increased capillary permeability to albumin.

Clinical features
Usually insidious onset. Common symptoms are increasing lethargy, forgetfulness, intolerance to cold, weight gain, constipation and depression (see also Fig. 11.7).
- Cardiovascular system: The heart is less contractile causing bradycardia and reduced cardiac output. Hypercholesterolaemia increases the incidence of atherosclerosis.

- Respiratory system: Respiration may be slow and shallow. Respiratory failure occurs in myxoedema coma.
- Gastrointestinal system: Reduced peristalsis, leading to chronic constipation. Ileus may occur.
- Genitourinary system: Impaired ability to excrete water predisposes to water overload. Women may have menstrual irregularities, particularly heavy periods.
- Haematological: Anaemia (normally normochromic/ normocytic).
- Other signs include a cool rough dry skin, hair loss, puffy face and hands, a hoarse husky voice and slowed reflexes. The skin may be yellowish (due to reduced conversion of carotene to vitamin A).

Complications
Pericardial and pleural effusions. Carpal tunnel syndrome. Deafness due to fluid in the middle ear.

Investigations
- Hypothyroidism is confirmed by a low T_3 and T_4 (except in end organ resistance) with a raised TSH in primary hypothyroidism. Thyroid autoantibodies are present in patients with autoimmune disease.
- Other investigations are aimed at diagnosing the underlying cause and are indicated according to the history and clinical suspicion.

Management
Thyroxine replacement starting with a low dose is required for life. Treatment of elderly patients should be undertaken with care, as any subclinical ischaemic heart disease may be unmasked. Thyroxine dosing is titrated according to thyroid function tests.

Hashimoto's disease (autoimmune thyroiditis)

Definition
Organ-specific autoimmune disease causing thyroiditis and later hypothyroidism.

Age
Peak in middle age.

Sex
F > M (10:1)

Aetiology
Patients have detectable anti-microsomal antibody and antithyroglobulin antibodies in most cases. Other autoantibodies include anti-thyroid cell cytosol and anti-microsomes associated with HLA-DR5 and other autoimmune diseases such as vitiligo and SLE.

Clinical features
The patient, typically a postmenopausal female, presents with a diffuse goitre. Although most patients are euthyroid, thyrotoxicosis can occur and if presentation is late, hypothyroidism may be present. On examination, the thyroid is firm and symmetrically enlarged with a bosselated surface.

Macroscopy/microscopy
The thyroid is diffusely enlarged and has a fleshy white cut surface due to lymphocytic infiltration, which is seen on microscopy around the destroyed follicles.

Investigations
High titres of circulating antithyroid antibodies, associated with a goitre on examination.

Management
Thyroxine may cause regression of small goitres. Large goitres require subtotal thyroidectomy if causing compression of local structures such as the oesophagus or trachea. Surgical complications include damage to the recurrent laryngeal nerves or parathyroids. Post-surgery or following significant thyroid destruction patients become hypothyroid requiring treatment with thyroxine for life.

Myxoedema coma

Definition
This is the end-stage of untreated hypothyroidism, leading to progressive weakness, hypothermia, respiratory failure, shock and death.

Incidence/prevalence
Rare

Age
Mainly in elderly.

Sex

F > M

Aetiology

May occur in any patient with hypothyroidism (see page 432). Myxoedema coma may be precipitated by inter-current illness or disorder, such as heart failure, perhaps following a myocardial infarction, stroke, pneumonia; iatrogenic causes include water overload and sedative or opiate drugs.

Pathophysiology

Thyroid hormones maintain many metabolic processes in the body. Severe and chronic lack of these hormones without adequate exogenous replacement leads to

- respiratory failure with CO_2 retention and hypoxia,
- water intoxication due to the syndrome of inappropriate antidiuretic hormone (SIADH) and hypothermia and
- adrenal insufficiency.

Clinical features

There may be a history of previous thyroid disease, followed by gradual onset of symptoms from lethargy through stupor to coma. The patient appears obese with hypothermia, yellowish dry skin, thinned hair, puffy eyes and has a slow pulse, respiration and reduced reflexes.

Investigations

Diagnosis may be made clinically, but is supported by a low free thyroxine (T_4) and a high TSH. Thyroid autoantibodies, blood gases, blood sugar, ECG, CXR are also required.

Management

Myxoedema coma requires admission to intensive care.

- Respiratory failure requires support and may necessitate ventilation.
- Thyroxine replacement is essential either orally or intravenously.
- Corticosteroids must be given if adrenal insufficiency is present.
- Patients also require gradual re-warming and dextrose support to prevent hypoglycaemia.

Prognosis

Myxoedema coma has a poor prognosis, particularly as it tends to occur in elderly patients who have little respiratory and cardiological functional reserve.

Malignant tumours of the thyroid
Papillary adenocarcinoma

Definition

A slow-growing, well-differentiated primary thyroid tumour arising from the thyroid epithelium.

Incidence/prevalence

50% of malignant tumours of the thyroid.

Age

Rare after the age of 40 years. Occurs in young adults.

Sex

F > M

Clinical features

Presents as a solitary or multifocal swelling of the thyroid. Lymph nodes are palpable in one-third of patients, and may be the only sign when there is a microscopic primary. Papillary tumours spread via lymphatics within the thyroid resulting in multifocal lesions and to neck nodes. Widespread metastases are rare.

Macroscopy/microscopy

Non-encapsulated mass in contrast to adenomas, which have a capsule. There is often infiltration into the surrounding tissue with associated fibrosis.

Investigations

Patients may be identified during investigation for a solitary thyroid nodule (see page 430). Definitive diagnosis is by histology, although cytology from fine needle aspiration may indicate malignancy.

Management

Total thyroidectomy with excision of involved neck lymph nodes and preservation of the parathyroid glands. Radical neck dissection is not necessary. Metastases may be treated by resection. Radioactive iodine therapy may be used prophylactically or as treatment for metastases. Thyroxine replacement is necessary after surgery as replacement and to suppress TSH (in order to reduce the risk of recurrence).

Prognosis

Ten year survival rates of almost 90%. Cervical lymph nodes do not make the prognosis significantly worse, but if the tumour has spread from the thyroid into adjacent structures it has a poor prognosis.

Follicular adenocarcinoma

Definition

A primary malignancy of the thyroid gland arising from the thyroid epithelium.

Incidence/prevalence

Approximately 20% of cases of thyroid malignancies.

Age

Middle age

Sex

F > M

Clinical features

Typically presents as a solitary thyroid nodule in middle-aged patients.

Investigations

Patients are investigated as for a solitary thyroid nodule (see page 430). Isotope scanning of the nodule reveals it to be non-functioning or 'cold'. Definitive diagnosis requires tissue from fine needle aspiration.

Complications

Predominantly haematogenous spread. Twenty per cent of patients have metastases in the lungs, bone or liver.

Macroscopy/microscopy

Resembles a benign solitary thyroid nodule, a round encapsulated mass, but less colloid and more solid in appearance. Histology reveals invasion of the capsule, blood vessels and surrounding gland.

Management

Total thyroidectomy with preservation of the parathyroids is required. All palpable lymph nodes are removed. If these contain tumour, a modified radical neck dissection is required. A postoperative radioisotope scan of the skeleton and neck detects metastases as 'hot spots', and further treatment is with radioiodine. Thyroxine is given to suppress TSH secretion, as well as for replacement.

Prognosis

Follicular carcinoma is more aggressive than papillary carcinoma. Ten year survival is 50%. Plasma thyroglobulin levels can be monitored for recurrence.

Medullary carcinoma

Definition

Tumour of the thyroid that arises from the parafollicular C-cells, which secrete calcitonin.

Aetiology

Approximately one-third are seen in children and young adults as part of MEN (multiple endocrine neoplasia) type II syndrome (see page 450). The other two-thirds are sporadic cases.

Pathophysiology

The parafollicular cells originate from neural crest tissue during embryonic life, but merge with the embryonic thyroid and are dispersed amongst the follicular cells. Parafollicular cells normally secrete calcitonin, a polypeptide, in response to small increases in calcium. The tumour cells secrete calcitonin and carcinoembryonic antigen (CEA) and are also capable of secreting prostaglandins and serotonin.

Clinical features

One or both thyroid lobes are enlarged and firm. Cervical lymph nodes are palpable in about half of cases, but the tumour is generally slow growing and tends only to metastasise to local lymph nodes. Those associated with MEN syndrome tend to be more aggressive.

Microscopy

The tumour is composed of sheets of small cells containing neuroendocrine granules with a hyaline stroma between them. Spread is mainly to local lymph nodes.

Investigations
Calcitonin levels are raised, although serum calcium levels are normal. Calcitonin is also used for follow-up and for screening of relatives.

Management
Total thyroidectomy and dissection of lymph nodes in the central neck compartment.

Anaplastic carcinoma

Definition
This is a highly malignant tumour of the thyroid.

Incidence/prevalence
10–15% of cases of malignant tumours of the thyroid.

Pathophysiology
There is evidence that these are poorly differentiated adenocarcinomas derived from thyroid epithelium. They often arise in elderly patients with a long history of goitre in whom the gland suddenly enlarges.

Clinical features
These tumours are rapidly growing and invade local structures early, most patients present with a rapidly enlarging neck swelling and complications such as hoarseness, dyspnoea and stridor, dysphagia and Horner's syndrome (miosis, partial ptosis and anhydrosis).

Macroscopy/microscopy
Diffusely infiltrative mass, often invading neighbouring tissues. Composed of various undifferentiated cells.

Management
Resection is rarely possible, but may be carried out for palliative relief of tracheal compression. Radioactive iodine and radiotherapy are ineffective.

Prognosis
Poor: 1-year survival is ~30%.

Thyroidectomy

Hyperthyroid patients must be made euthyroid before thyroid surgery using antithyroid drugs and β-blockers to reduce complications such as cardiac arrhythmias, excessive sympathetic activity and bleeding.

The thyroid is exposed via a transverse skin-crease incision above the sternal notch. The lobes of the thyroid are supplied by the superior and inferior artery, and drained by the middle and inferior veins. These are dissected out, ligated and divided removing the desired amount of thyroid tissue. Surrounding structures that require identification and protection include the parathyroid glands and the recurrent laryngeal nerves.

- Complications include haemorrhage, leading to tracheal compression; damage to the superior or recurrent laryngeal nerve; damage or excision of parathyroid glands; and scarring. Neuropraxia (temporary damage) of the recurrent laryngeal nerve occurs in 5% of operations. The ipsilateral vocal cord becomes paralysed and fixed midway between closed and open. Bilateral nerve injury is rare but causes stridor and may subsequently require laryngoplasty or permanent tracheostomy.
- Postoperative calcium levels should be monitored to look for hypocalcaemia, which is usually transient, due to damage to the parathyroid glands. Subsequent hypothyroidism is treated with lifelong thyroxine supplements.

Adrenal axis

Corticotrophin releasing hormone (CRH) is secreted from the hypothalamus in a diurnal pattern. Adrenocorticotrophic hormone (ACTH) is secreted by the pituitary in response to CRH that in turn activates the enzyme desmolase in the adrenal glands converting cholesterol to pregnenolone. This is the rate-limiting step for the production of all the adrenocortical hormones. Cortisol is mainly controlled in this way, aldosterone is mainly controlled by the renin-angiotensin system, and androgens

Table 11.9 Abnormalities of the adrenal axis

	Increased hormone	Decreased hormone
CRH	Cushing's disease	
	CRH-secreting tumour (very rare)	
ACTH	Cushing's disease	Hypopituitarism
	(ACTH-secreting pituitary tumour)	
	Addison's disease	
	Nelson's syndrome	
Mineralocortic oids	Primary hyperaldosteronism (adenoma or hyperplasia)	Adrenocortical insufficiency
	Secondary hyperaldosteronism	
Glucocorticoids	Cushing's syndrome	Adrenocortical insufficiency
	Causes include nodular hyperplasia, adrenal cortex tumour	
Androgens	Congenital adrenal hyperplasia	Adrenocortical insufficiency
	Also hyperplasia and tumours	

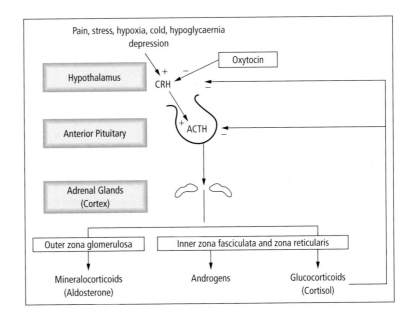

Figure 11.8 The adrenal axis.

are also secreted by the gonads (see Fig. 11.8 and Table 11.9).

Aldosterone

Aldosterone is the corticosteroid with the most mineralocorticoid activity, so-called because it controls sodium, potassium and water balance. Its production is stimulated mainly by the renin–angiotensin system. Renin is secreted from the juxtaglomerular apparatus in the kidney in response to reduced renal blood flow, for example due to hypotension. In response aldosterone acts on the kidney and vasculature (see Fig. 11.9).

When aldosterone levels are high this may be due to high renin levels (secondary hyperaldosteronism) or it may be independent of renin production (primary hyperaldosteronism).

Cortisol

Cortisol is the major glucocorticoid, although aldosterone and corticosterone also have some effect. The glucocorticoids control glucose metabolism, for example gluconeogenesis, and mobilisation of fat stores (lipolysis) amongst other actions. Cortisol exerts a negative feedback on ACTH and CRH secretion. Glucocorticoids

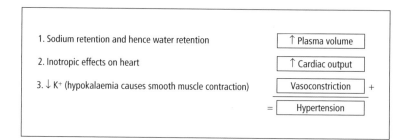

Figure 11.9 Effects of aldosterone.

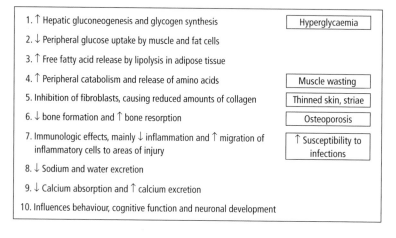

Figure 11.10 Effects of cortisol.

are most important during fasting, illness or surgery (see Fig. 11.10).

Androgens

Androstenedione is produced by the adrenal cortex and is converted to testosterone and dihydrotesterone. In males, 95% of active testosterone is derived from the testis, so adrenal androgen excess or deficiency is relatively insignificant. In females 50% of the peripheral production of testosterone is from adrenal androgens. Female neonates with congenital adrenal hyperplasia have ambiguous genitalia (clitoromegaly). Adults with Cushing's syndrome and adrenal tumours with hypersecretion of adrenal androgens have acne, hirsutism and virilisation.

Cushing's syndrome

Definition

Cushing's syndrome is the clinical syndrome resulting from excess circulating glucocorticoids.

Aetiology

The excess of glucocorticoid may be endogenous or exogenous. Endogenous glucocorticoids may result from high ACTH causing excessive adrenal stimulation or may result from a primary adrenal disease in which case ACTH levels will be low (see Table 11.10).

Pathophysiology

Cortisol opposes insulin, with a catabolic effect. Adrenal mineralocorticoid secretion is mildly raised, but the glucocorticoids also have some mineralocorticoid effect. Excess androgens can cause mild hirsutism, menstrual irregularities in women, and can inhibit LH and testosterone secretion in men, reducing libido.

Clinical features

Common features include centripetal obesity (moon face, buffalo hump), plethora, osteoporosis, proximal myopathy, easy bruising, striae, acne, hirsutism, poor wound healing and glucose intolerance. Gonadal dysfunction leads to oligo- or amenorrhoea or impotence.

Table 11.10 Causes of Cushing's syndrome

ACTH-dependent (83%)	
Pituitary-dependent (~80%)	Pituitary hyperplasia
	Pituitary adenoma (Cushing's disease)
	Pituitary carcinoma
Ectopic ACTH secretion (<20%)	Neuroendocrine tumours: oat cell carcinoma, bronchial carcinoid tumour, medullary thyroid carcinoma, pancreatic carcinoma, phaeochromocytoma
Non-ACTH dependent (16%)	
Primary adrenal disorder	Adrenal adenoma (58%)
	Adrenal carcinoma (42%)
Unknown/mixed aetiology (1%)	Multinodular hyperplasia of the adrenals
Cushingoid appearance	
Iatrogenic	Glucocorticoid therapy
	ACTH therapy (rare)
Pseudo-Cushing's syndrome	Alcoholics
	Severe depression

Hypertension, hypokalaemia and metabolic alkalosis may be present. Euphoria, mania and depression may also be features.

Patients with ectopic ACTH syndrome may have profound hypokalaemia, weight loss (therefore lack of obesity) and anaemia. Hyperpigmentation in an Addisonian distribution (skin creases, pressure points, in the mouth) suggests ACTH excess, and thus an ACTH-dependent cause.

Investigations

Initial diagnosis is confirmed by demonstrating high cortisol levels. As there is a diurnal rhythm and variable cortisol secretion a 24-hour urine collection or low-dose dexamethasone suppression test is used (see Fig. 11.11).

Management

Adrenal adenomas and carcinomas should be resected if possible. Pituitary tumours may also be resected. If surgery is not possible, drugs that block cortisol synthesis such as metyrapone, which inhibits 11-hydroxylase, are used, but these cause a rise in ACTH, which overcomes the inhibition. Radiotherapy is used in treatment of unresectable pituitary adenomas.

Prognosis

Patients require lifelong steroid replacement therapy after bilateral adrenalectomy, but may only need it for 1–2 years after unilateral removal.

Cushing's disease

Definition

In 1932, Harvey Cushing described pituitary adenomas as a cause of adrenocortical excess.

Incidence/prevalence

80% of Cushing's syndrome are due to a pituitary cause.

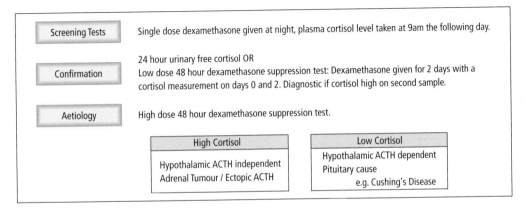

Figure 11.11 Tests used in the screening for and diagnosis of Cushing's syndrome.

Age
Any age, peak 20–40 years.

Sex
8F : 1M

Aetiology
In virtually all patients, an ACTH-secreting pituitary adenoma is found, occasionally the cause is hypothalamic oversecretion of corticotrophin releasing hormone (CRH).

Pathophysiology/clinical features
As for Cushing's syndrome. Unlike patients with ectopic ACTH syndrome, patients with pituitary adenomas rarely have hypokalaemia, weight loss, anaemia or hyperpigmentation.

Macroscopy
Bilateral adrenocortical hyperplasia twice the size of normal, with thickening of zona reticularis and the zona fasciculata. The zona glomerulosa appears normal, because mineralocorticoid production is controlled primarily by the renin–angiotensin system.

Microscopy
The pituitary tumour is normally a microadenoma. The cells contain ACTH and its related peptides.

Investigations
As for Cushing's syndrome (see page 438).

Management
The treatment of choice is transsphenoidal hypophysectomy. Irradiation is used post-surgery, for patients where complete resection was not possible. Drugs which inhibit adrenal cortisol synthesis are often used as adjunctive therapy, e.g. ketoconazole, metyrapone and aminoglutethimide. Their disadvantage is that they increase ACTH secretion so this enzyme inhibition is overcome and the clinical effect is short-lived.

Bilateral adrenalectomy is still used if the adrenals have become semi-autonomous, however it must be followed by pituitary treatment (e.g. irradiation) as otherwise the pituitary adenoma can progress to cause hyperpigmentation, local pressure effects and Nelson's syndrome (an ACTH-secreting tumour of the pituitary which enlarges post-bilateral adrenalectomy).

Addison's disease

Definition
First described by Thomas Addison in 1857, Addison's disease is primary adrenal insufficiency.

Aetiology
In Western countries autoimmune disease is the commonest cause (80%). It is familial, and associated with other organ specific autoimmune diseases, especially thyroid failure (Schmidt syndrome), autoimmune gastritis, pernicious anaemia and vitiligo. Presence of HLA-B8 association carries a x12 risk of developing disease. Worldwide, tuberculosis is still a very important cause (see Table 11.11).

Pathophysiology
- The mineralocorticoids (90% activity by aldosterone, some by cortisol) act on the kidneys to conserve sodium by increasing Na^+/K^+ exchange in the distal tubules and collecting ducts. In Addison's disease, gradual loss of these hormones causes increased sodium and water loss with a consequent decrease in

Table 11.11 Causes of adrenal insufficiency

Primary
  Congenital/familial
    Adrenal enzyme defects
    Congenital adrenal hypoplasia
  Acquired
    Infectious – TB, histoplasmosis, HIV associated
      cytomegalovirus
    Autoimmune
    Vascular – haemorrhage (associated with meningococcal
      septicaemia – Waterhouse-Friderichsen syndrome),
      thrombosis
    Neoplastic – secondary carcinoma (e.g. lung)
    Degenerative – amyloid
Secondary
  Hypopituitarism
  Isolated ACTH deficiency
  Following glucocorticoid therapy
Drug-induced glucocorticoid metabolism
  Rifampicin, carbamazepine

extracellular fluid volume. Failure to exchange Na^+ for H^+ ions can lead to a mild acidosis.

- The glucocorticoids (cortisol) allow gluconeogenesis to maintain glucose concentrations between meals, and mediate protein and fat mobilisation from the tissues. Reduced cortisol may lead to symptomatic hypoglycaemia.
- Lack of cortisol feedback leads to increased ACTH (adrenocorticotrophin) secretion from the anterior pituitary. When ACTH is secreted by the anterior pituitary, other hormones are also secreted such as β-endorphin and melanocyte-stimulating hormone (MSH) causing skin pigmentation.
- Once mineralocorticoid secretion ceases completely, the patient will die within 2 weeks if not treated, from progressive weakness and eventual shock.

Clinical features
Patients present with gradual onset of weakness, tiredness and fatigue. There are often gastrointestinal complaints such as anorexia, nausea, vomiting, abdominal pain, constipation or diarrhoea. The patient may report salt craving.

Examination reveals weight loss, hyperpigmentation especially in mouth, skin creases and pressure areas. Chronic dehydration leads to general and especially postural hypotension.

Complications
Renal failure due to decreased perfusion. Sudden cardiac arrest or arrhythmias due to electrolyte imbalance.

Investigations
- Hyponatremia, hyperkalemia and a hyperchloraemic acidosis due to mineralocorticoid deficiency. Glucose should be measured to detect hypoglycaemia.
- Screening can be performed by measurement of early morning cortisol and 24 hour urinary cortisol.
- Primary adrenal insufficiency is confirmed by use of the short Synacthen (ACTH analogue) test. Cortisol levels are measured before and 30 mins after administration of synacthen and show a low base line and a lack of rise in Addison's Disease. Adrenal insufficiency that results from ACTH deficiency (secondary and tertiary adrenal insufficiency) will result in an appropriate rise in cortisol following Synacthen. A long Synacthen test using a depot injection and repeated cortisol

samples over a 24-hour period is used to distinguish between Addison's disease (primary adrenal failure) and adrenal suppression.

Management
Chronic adrenal insufficiency is treated with glucocorticoids and mineralocorticoids. Patients require significant education about the illness and how to manage co-existing illness or stress, such as at the time of operations when increased steroids may be required. Parenteral steroids are needed if vomiting occurs. All patients requiring replacement steroids should carry a steroid (blue) card.

Addisonian crisis

Definition
Acute presentation of complete adrenal failure.

Aetiology
Patients may already be diagnosed with Addison's Disease or may present in crisis for the first time. Precipitating factors include trauma, illness or surgery. It may also be caused acutely by bilateral adrenal haemorrhage, due to meningococcal septicaemia (Waterhouse-Friderichsen syndrome) or anti-coagulant therapy. An Addisonian crisis may also occur on cessation of glucocorticoid treatment including inhaled glucocorticoids in children.

Pathophysiology
In adrenal failure, there is no glucocorticoid response to stress. If exogenous high-dose steroids are not provided the condition is fatal.

Clinical features
The patient is ill with anorexia, vomiting and abdominal pain. This may suggest an acute abdomen. Signs include pyrexia and dehydration with tachycardia, hypotension (postural drop) decreased skin turgor and sunken eyes. Increased pigmentation may be noticed, especially in mouth, skin creases and pressure areas.

Investigations
- Urgent cortisol and ACTH if possible.
- U&Es (hyponatraemia, hyperkalaemia and hyperchloraemia).

- Blood sugar monitoring to detect hypoglycaemia.
- Definitive investigations should not delay treatment, steroids will not interfere with test results in the short-term.

Management

Immediate fluid resuscitation with 0.9% saline (and 5% dextrose if hypoglycaemia is present). Intravenous hydrocortisone and broad-spectrum antibiotics are given. Any underlying causes need to be identified and appropriately managed.

Prognosis

Has a high mortality.

Conn's syndrome

Definition

Conn's syndrome is a condition of primary hyperaldosteronism.

Incidence/prevalence

Rare. Accounts for 1% patients with hypertension.

Aetiology

Eighty per cent of cases are due to an adrenal adenoma. In the remainder, there is diffuse hyperplasia of the zona glomerulosa. Very rarely it is caused by an adrenal carcinoma. Raised aldosterone is much more commonly a physiological response to reduced renal perfusion as in renal artery stenosis or congestive cardiac failure.

Pathophysiology

Aldosterone is the most important mineralocorticoid produced by the zona glomerulosa. It acts on the Na^+/K^+ pump in renal tubular epithelial cells in the collecting tubules, distal tubule and collecting duct increasing the absorption of sodium and hence water with increased loss of potassium. The rise in blood volume increases renal perfusion and arterial blood pressure. However there is a significant loss of K^+ leading to hypokalaemia and resistance to antidiuretic hormone. This causes increased urinary volumes and hence increased thirst.

Clinical features

Hypertension and symptoms resulting from the hypokalaemia such as cardiac arrhythmias, muscle weakness, cramps, latent tetany and paraesthesiae. The muscle weakness may present with paralysis. Polydipsia and polyuria may be a feature.

Macroscopy/microscopy

Adrenal cortical adenomas are well-circumscribed, yellow lipid laden tumours within the adrenal cortex. Adrenal cortical carcinomas are larger, with local invasion and metastatic spread. In hyperplasia, the glands are enlarged, with increased number, size and secretory activity of the cells within the zona glomerulosa.

Investigations

- Urea and electrolytes demonstrate the hypokalaemia and may show a mild rise in sodium. Hypokalaemia may lead to a mild metabolic alkalosis (H^+/K^+ exchange in the kidney). However, the use of diuretics to treat hypertension may mimic or mask these features. A high urinary K^+ (>30 mmol/24 h) suggests primary aldosteronism.
- The definitive test is to measure aldosterone and renin baselines after a night's rest (low in 1° aldosteronism, high in 2° aldosteronism) and after being upright (stimulates renin in normal individuals, but aldosteronism suppresses renin).
- CT scan of the adrenal glands. If negative, selective blood sampling may be required to find the source of aldosterone.

Management

Bilateral adrenal hyperplasia is usually treated with spironalactone (inhibits the Na^+/K^+ pump, i.e. antagonises aldosterone) to control the blood pressure. Adenomas and carcinomas should be removed surgically. Spironalactone may be used prior to surgery.

Prognosis

30% have persistent hypertension after treatment, thought to be due to irreversible renal damage.

Phaeochromocytoma

Definition

An APUD (amine precursor uptake and decarboxylation) tumour of the adrenal medulla which produces adrenaline and noradrenaline.

Incidence

Uncommon. The cause of 0.2–0.5% of cases of adult hypertension.

Age

Peak age 40–60 years.

Sex

M = F

Aetiology

Associated with the Multiple Endocrine Neoplasia (MEN) type II (see page 450). Also may be associated with von Hippel-Lindau syndrome, neurofibromatosis, tuberose sclerosis and the Sturge-Weber syndrome.

Pathophysiology

10% of cases are malignant, 10% are extra-adrenal and 10% are bilateral. The adrenal medulla is functionally related to the sympathetic nervous system, secreting adrenaline and noradrenaline in response to sympathetic stimulation. High levels of sympathetic stimulation result in increased heart rate, blood pressure, and sweating. There is decreased blood supply to the gut, increased sphincter activity and metabolic effects, such as diabetes and thyrotoxicosis.

Clinical features

Patients normally present with episodic headache, sweating, and palpitations. They are found to be hypertensive which may be paroxysmal or continuous. Other signs include pallor, dilated pupils and tachycardia. There may be a postural hypotension secondary to volume depletion. Phaeochromocytoma may present in pregnancy, or with sudden death following trauma or surgery.

Macroscopy

Usually up to 5 cm spherical tumour with a pale cut surface that oxidises to brown when exposed to air. Extramedullary tumours are usually found in the sympathetic chain, alongside the abdominal aorta.

Complications

Cardiovascular disease or cerebral haemorrhage. Persistent hypertension causes hypertensive retinopathy.

Investigations

Diagnosis is by measuring plasma levels of noradrenaline, and urinary adrenaline and noradrenaline or their metabolites vanillylmandelic acid (VMA) and homovanilyic acid (HVA). The paroxysmal secretion of the hormones may mean repeated measurements are needed. Adrenal CT scan is used to locate the tumour, scanning with a radiolabelled catecholamine precursor (MIBG) can identify extra-adrenal tumours.

Management

- Surgical excision where possible is the treatment of choice. Surgery has a high peri-operative risk and requires expert anaesthetic supervision. The blood pressure must be carefully monitored and any rise countered with i.v. phentolamine (α-receptor antagonist) or nitroprusside. Intensive care postoperatively is preferred.
- Adrenergic blockade is necessary to oppose the catecholamine effects before surgery. Phenoxybenzamine (an α-receptor antagonist) is used initially, followed by β-blockade with propanolol.
- In cases where surgery is not possible combined long term α- and β-blockers are used.

Prognosis

10% of phaechromocytomas are malignant these have a 5 year survival of less than 50%. Overall recurrence rate of 10–15%.

Adrenalectomy

Surgical removal of the adrenal glands may be necessary for a number of conditions (see Table 11.12). Large tumours, which may be malignant, are removed via a

Table 11.12 Indications for adrenalectomy

Unilateral adrenal adenomas	Cushing's syndrome Conn's syndrome Phaeochromocytoma Secondary metastases, e.g. renal cell carcinoma

Bilateral adrenalectomy	Bilateral tumours
	Nodular hyperplasia
	   (causing Cushing's or
	   Conn's syndrome)
	Cushing's syndrome if
	   pituitary treatment fails

flank incision following removal of a rib. The diaphragm, pleura and peritoneum are left intact wherever possible. A posterior approach through the bed of the 11th or 12 rib is more difficult, but has a lower morbidity. Lifelong corticosteroid (both glucocorticoid and mineralocorticoid with hydrocortisone and fludocortisone) replacement therapy is needed following bilateral adrenalectomy. Laparoscopic adrenalectomy is increasingly being used.

Replacement is monitored by blood pressure measurement, serum electrolytes and patient well-being. Stress, infection and surgery may all increase corticosteroid requirements, and may precipitate an Addisonian crisis (see page 441). Patients need to be advised of the signs and symptoms and management of such events.

Thirst axis

Syndrome of inappropriate anti-diuretic hormone secretion (SIADH)

Definition
SIADH is characterised by the persistence of ADH secretion despite decreased plasma osmolality and normal or increased extracellular fluid volume.

Aetiology
See Table 11.13.

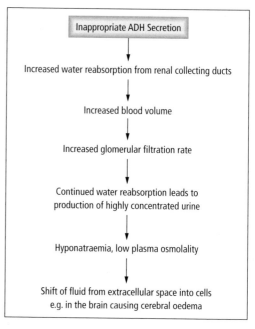

Figure 11.12 Pathophysiology of SIADH.

Pathophysiology
ADH is a peptide hormone similar to oxytocin which is normally secreted from the posterior pituitary, in response to an increase in plasma osmolality. It acts on the collecting tubules in the kidney to make them more permeable to water molecules. Hence its secretion causes water retention (see Fig. 11.12).

Table 11.13 Causes of syndrome of inappropriate anti-diuretic hormone secretion (SIADH)

Ectopic secretion	Small-cell bronchial carcinoma
	Rarely carcinoma of the thymus, prostate, pancreas, duodenum, adrenal, ureter or nasopharynx
	Lymphoma, leukaemia
Inappropriate secretion (hypothalamus)	
Lung disease	Pneumonia, tuberculosis, aspergillosis
	Positive pressure mechanical ventilation (stretch receptors)
Neurological	Trauma (including neurosurgery or major surgery)
	Encephalitis, post-meningitis
	Ischaemia (stroke, vasculitis)
	Tumours
Drugs	Carbamazepine, chlorpropamide, tricyclics, phenothiazines, syntocinon, narcotics and cytotoxic drugs (vinca alkaloids – cyclophosphamide, vincristine)
Other	Pain, intermittent acute porphyria, Guillain–Barré syndrome, hypothyroidism, symptomatic HIV infection or AIDS

Clinical features

Patients present with headache, confusion, behavioural changes, convulsions and coma. On examination there is no peripheral oedema. There may be muscle twitching with an extensor plantar reflex.

Investigations

Electrolyte analysis will reveal hyponatraemia with reduced plasma osmolality, and high urinary osmolality and sodium. Plasma osmolality can be estimated from the sodium, urea and glucose concentrations ($\sim$2x [Na] + [Urea] + [glucose]).

Management

Fluid restriction is the mainstay of treatment, although this is unpleasant for the patient and often difficult to enforce. It is also a useful diagnostic test. Demeclocycline, an ADH antagonist at the renal collecting ducts can be used, but is nephrotoxic, especially in the elderly. If water intoxication is severe, diuretics with hypertonic saline infusion is used. Any underlying cause should be identified and treated.

Prognosis

In many cases the syndrome is temporary.

Diabetes insipidus

Definition

Polyuria, thirst & polydipsia resulting from deficiency of or resistance to antidiuretic hormone (vasopressin).

Aetiology

Diabetes insipidus results from either a deficiency in anti diuretic hormone (central or cranial diabetes insipidus, see Table 11.14) or from renal resistance to ADH (nephrogenic diabetes insipidus, see Table 11.15).

Pathophysiology

Normally ADH acts on the renal collecting ducts to increase water reabsorption preventing plasma osmolality from rising. Lack of vasopressin, or renal resistance to vasopressin leads to loss of water (water depletion), leading to polyuria. Unless the thirst centre is also impaired, rising osmolality stimulates thirst and the person drinks water in increased quantities. The urine is dilute.

Table 11.14 Causes of cranial diabetes insipidus

Cranial causes (more common)	Examples
Infective	Meningitis, encephalitis
Inflammatory	Granulomatous (TB, sarcoidosis, etc)
Vascular	Ischaemia (CVA)
Trauma	Head injury
Neoplastic	Craniopharyngioma, secondary tumours, pituitary tumours with suprasellar extension
Iatrogenic	Intracranial surgery (often transient)
Idiopathic	DIDMOAD (diabetes insipidus, diabetes mellitus, optic atrophy and nerve deafness)

Table 11.15 Causes of nephrogenic diabetes insipidous

Nephrogenic causes	
Congenital	X-linked recessive genetic
Metabolic	Hypokalaemia, hypercalcaemia
Drugs	Lithium, demeclocycline
Kidney disease	Post-obstructive uropathy
Chronic kidney diseases	Pyelonephritis, polycystic kidneys, amyloid, Sickle cell disease

Clinical features

Polyuria, polydipsia. Daily urine output may be >10 L a day.

Complications

Hypernatraemia if patient is denied access to water or is unconscious. If left untreated there is progression to severe irreversible brain damage and cerebral vessels may tear causing intracranial haemorrhage (see page 3). Rapid rehydration can cause a similar problem.

Investigations

Plasma osmolality is normal to high (>295 mmol/kg) with associated hypernatraemia, The urine osmolality is low. In the water deprivation test the patient is weighed, plasma and urine osmolality measured, then they are deprived of fluid for 8 hours under constant supervision.

- Diabetes insipidus is diagnosed if body weight falls by >3%, if plasma osmolality exceeds 300 mmol/kg, or if the urine:plasma osmolality ratio remains <1.9 (provided plasma osmolality exceeds 285 mmol/kg).

After 8 hours, the patient is allowed to drink freely and desmopressin (DDAVP – desamino-D-arginine vasopressin, a long-acting vasopressin analogue) is given intranasally or i.v. Urine output is monitored.

- If the kidneys are then able to produce concentrated urine the diabetes insipidus is due to ADH deficiency, i.e. central diabetes insipidus. If the urine remains dilute the kidneys are insensitive to ADH, i.e. nephrogenic diabetes insipidus.

Management

Any underlying cause should be sought and treated if possible. DDAVP intranasally is used in cranial diabetes insipidus. There is no specific treatment for nephrogenic diabetes insipidus.

Disorders of the parathyroids

Hyperparathyroidism

Definition

Increased secretion of parathyroid hormone (PTH) from the parathyroid glands located on the posterior surface of the thyroid gland.

Aetiology

Hyperparathyroidism may be primary, secondary or tertiary (see Table 11.16). Secretion of PTH like peptide is seen in squamous cell bronchial carcinoma (see page 134).

Pathophysiology

PTH is an 84 amino acid polypeptide, which controls normal calcium homeostasis (see Fig. 11.13).

Primary hyperparathyroidism

Definition

Primary oversecretion of parathyroid hormone (PTH) by the parathyroid glands.

Incidence/prevalence

Common amongst middle-aged and elderly. In patients over the age of 40, incidence may be as high as 1 in 1000 to 1 in 2000.

Age

Increases with age.

Sex

2–4F : 1M

Aetiology

Neoplasia of the parathyroid gland(s). There are thought to be genetic and environmental predisposing factors including a family history of Multiple Endocrine Neoplasia (see page 450) and neck irradiation.

- Single benign adenoma 75%
- Multiple adenomata or hyperplasia 24%
- Parathyroid carcinoma 1%

Pathophysiology

Autonomous hypersecretion from one or more glands result in hyperparathyroidism, with hypercalcaemia, hypophosphataemia and osteoporosis.

Clinical features

Presentation ranges from asymptomatic (diagnosed incidentally on a calcium measurement) to severe and life-threatening hypercalcaemia. Patients commonly remain asymptomatic for many years, then develop insidious

Table 11.16 Causes of hyperparathyroidisim

Type	Causes
Primary hyperparathyroidism	Primary tumour or hyperplasia of the parathyroid gland(s)
Secondary hyperparathyroidism	Appropriate increased PTH in response to prolonged hypocalcaemia or vitamin D deficiency especially in chronic renal failure
Tertiary hyperparathyroidism	Prolonged secondary hyperparathyroidism, causing autonomous secretion of PTH and hypercalcaemia
Pseudohypoparathyroidism	End-organ resistance to PTH leads to hypocalcaemia and therefore increased PTH occurs

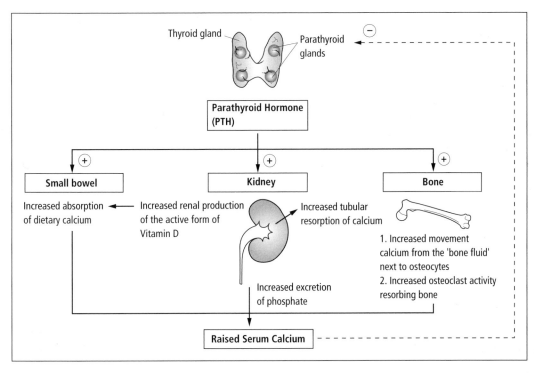

Figure 11.13 Effects of parathyroid hormone.

weakness, fatigue, anorexia, thirst, constipation and confusion.

- Bones: Increased calcium resorption, classically causes bone cysts (osteitis fibrosa cystica) which may present with diffuse pain or rarely fractures.
- Stones: Urinary stones and nephrocalcinosis (calcification of the kidney), due to hypercalciuria. Hypertension is common, possibly due to renal damage.
- Groans: Abdominal symptoms such as nausea, vomiting, pain and constipation.
- Moans: Psychosis, confusion and drowsiness.

Complications
Fractures, complications of urinary stones, seizures, coma, sudden death due to cardiac arrest. Dehydration occurs secondary to hypercalcaemia, which can cause a nephrogenic diabetes insipidus.

Investigations
- Serum calcium, PTH and albumin levels (for corrected calcium) should be measured. If hypercalcaemia is found, and PTH is detectable the likely diagnosis is primary or tertiary hyperparathyroidism. In other causes of hypercalcaemia, PTH is suppressed to below detectable values.
- Ultrasound of the neck may be able to differentiate between parathyroid adenoma or hyperplasia. The tumour(s) may be located by technetium-thallium subtraction scanning or selective venous catheterisation to assay PTH and find the source.

Management
- Surgery is the only curative option. The parathyroids are exposed by a transverse neck incision. Each lobe of the thyroid is mobilised and the parathyroids identified. Abnormal glands are removed and frozen sections examined. If all four glands are enlarged, all but a portion of one gland is removed.
- If symptomatic, treatment should be directed at correcting the hypercalcaemia with fluids. If Ca >3.5 mmol/L, the patient is vomiting, pyrexial or there

are severe symptoms or signs such as confusion, intravenous saline together with iv furosemide are used. Potassium and magnesium often fall and need supplements. Bisphosphonates may also be used, although they can take some time to act.

- If surgery is not possible, oral phosphates or bisphosphonates reduce bone resorption and osteoclast activity.

Secondary hyperparathyroidism

Definition
This is a syndrome of appropriately raised parathyroid hormone (PTH) in response to hypocalcaemia.

Incidence/prevalence
Increasing because of survival of renal patients on dialysis.

Aetiology
Common causes of chronic hypocalcaemia are chronic renal failure and vitamin D deficiency.

Pathophysiology
1 Chronic renal failure leads to reduced hydroxylation of inactive vitamin D (25-hydroxycholecalciferol 25(OH)D$_3$) to the active vitamin D (calcitriol or 1,25(OH)$_2$D$_3$) in the kidney, and hence a functional vitamin D deficiency.
2 Chronic hypocalcaemia caused by vitamin D deficiency stimulates chronically increased parathyroid hormone secretion, which may cause some restoration of serum calcium. The failing kidney also retains phosphate which binds calcium, reducing serum levels further.
3 The pathological effects are due to raised PTH levels which cause loss of calcium from the skeleton.

Clinical features
This condition is usually asymptomatic and chronic, although hyperparathyroidism may cause vague bone pains. Hypocalcaemia is rarely severe.

Complications
Tertiary hyperparathyroidism (hypercalcaemia due to autonomous parathyroids).

Investigations
Low or normal serum calcium, with a raised PTH. Phosphate is high. Skeletal X-ray classically shows subperiosteal erosions, 'brown tumours' which are areas of radiolucency which mimic lytic bone lesions and a ground-glass appearance of the skull.

Management
Dietary calcium and Vitamin D supplements. For renal patients alfacalcidol and calcitriol are suitable forms of vitamin D, as they do not require hydroxylation by the kidney to become active.

Tertiary hyperparathyroidism

Definition
Development of parathyroid hyperplasia or adenomas and autonomous parathyroid hormone (PTH) secretion following chronically low calcium levels.

Aetiology
Any cause of chronic secondary hyperparathyroidism, in particular chronic renal failure. Often becomes apparent post-renal transplantation.

Pathophysiology
During secondary hyperparathyroidism, the glands may become autonomous, either developing an adenoma or hyperplasia which secretes excessive PTH resulting in hypercalcaemia. In a patient with renal failure and secondary hyperparathyroidism who undergoes renal transplantation, PTH secretion may fall as the glands recover normal activity.

Clinical features
History of previous secondary hyperparathyroidism. Clinical features are those of hypercalcaemia (bones, stones, groans and moans).

Complications
Acute severe hypercalcaemia may cause seizures, abdominal pain, nausea and vomiting, confusion and pyschosis.

Investigations
Hypercalcaemia with markedly raised PTH.

Management

Total parathyroidectomy possibly with autotransplantation of parathyroid tissue equivalent to a normal gland into the arm, where it can be readily accessed for further treatment. Calcium replacement, phosphate binders and alfacalcidol (1-alpha hydroxyvitamin D_3) to increase calcium absorption and serum levels may be effective by negative feedback on the parathyroids.

Hypoparathyroidism

Definition

A deficiency of parathyroid hormone (PTH) characterised by hypocalcaemia and hyperphosphataemia, with normal renal function.

Aetiology

Most commonly occurs following surgery with removal of abnormal parathyroid glands or removal of neck malignancies. Gland failure may be caused by direct damage to the glands or their blood supply.

Idiopathic hypoparathyroidism:

- Genetic abnormalities are usually autosomal recessive and manifest at an early age. Associated with autoantibodies specific for parathyroid and adrenal tissue.
- Associated autoimmune syndromes include pernicious anaemia, ovarian failure, autoimmune thyroiditis, and diabetes mellitus.
- Late onset idiopathic hypoparathyroidism occurs without circulating autoantibodies.

Functional hypoparathyroidism occurs in patients with chronic hypomagnesaemia which results in a failure of PTH release.

Pathophysiology

PTH is normally released in response to hypocalcaemia, to restore calcium levels. The consequences of reduced PTH are decreased calcium levels, increased phosphate levels, decreased $1,25(OH)_2D_3$ and alkalosis (due to decreased bicarbonate excretion).

- In chronic cases of hypoparathyroidism, calcification of the basal ganglia causing extrapyramidal signs and calcification of cornea may occur.
- Cardiovascular problems with prolongation of the QT interval in ECGs associated with hypocalcaemia, hypotension and refractory congestive heart failure.

Clinical features

Hypocalcaemia and alkalosis cause increased neuromuscular excitability: paraesthesias of the fingertips and toes, tetany (spasms of muscles of extremities and face)

- Trousseau's sign: Inflating a blood pressure cuff to above systolic BP for at least 2 minutes causes carpal spasm, which does not relax for a few seconds after deflation.
- Chvostek's sign: Tapping the facial nerve anterior to the ear lobe causes twitching of the facial muscles.
- Convulsions occur more commonly in young people.

Investigations

Low calcium with normal or high phosphate with no detectable PTH on immunoassay. Alkaline phosphatase is normal. U&Es should be normal, or a renal cause is suspected.

Management

Replacement therapy with $1,25(OH)_2D_3$ (calcitriol, vitamin D_2) or $1(OH)D_3$. Serum and urinary calcium must be measured, as hypercalcaemia and hypercalciuria can occur. Vitamin D intoxication causes irreversible renal damage. Thiazide diuretics which increase renal tubular reabsorption of calcium may be useful in treating hypercalciuria.

Prognosis

Lifelong treatment and follow-up.

Pseudohypoparathyroidism

Definition

This is a rare condition in which there is impaired response to circulating parathyroid hormone, and hence hypocalcaemia and hyperphosphataemia.

Aetiology

Failure of the target cell response to parathyroid hormone, thought to be due to a PTH receptor defect or its coupling to the second messenger system, adenylate cyclase.

Clinical features

Round face, short stature with short fourth and fifth metacarpals and metatarsals. Other features are the same as those of hypoparathyroidism. Some patients have the somatic manifestations, but without the biochemical abnormalities and clinical signs of hypocalcaemia and hyperphosphataemia. This is called 'pseudopseudoparathyroidism'.

Investigations
Low calcium with normal or high phosphate, unlike primary hypoparathyroidism or high PTH and alkaline phosphatase.

Management
Lifelong replacement therapy with $1,25(OH)_2D_3$ or $1(OH)D_3$.

Multiple endocrine neoplasia syndrome

Multiple endocrine neoplasia (MEN)

Definition
Multiple endocrine neoplasia is a group of inherited syndromes characterised by multiple tumours of endocrine glands.

Multiple endocrine neoplasia type I
- Inherited in an autosomal dominant pattern. The function of the gene products are unknown but it is suggested that susceptible individuals inherit a gene defect from one parent, tumour growth occurs when the remaining copy of the gene is inactivated by somatic mutation.
- Tumours occur within the parathyroids in 90% (resulting in primary hyperparathyroidism), anterior pituitary (pituitary adenomas see page 421) and pancreatic islet cells (see page 222). MEN I is defined as the presence of at least two of the three main tumour types.

Multiple endocrine neoplasia type II
- Inherited in an autosomal dominant pattern with high penetrance. Mutations occur in the RET protooncogene.
- Tumours include medullary carcinoma of the thyroid, phaeochromocytomas (may be bilateral or multiple) and parathyroid tumours.

- Type IIb MEN may also have numerous mucosal neuromas, intestinal ganglioneuromas and a Marfanoid appearance.

Management
Tumours are surgically removed wherever possible, however recurrence is common. When an index case has been identified family members require screening either using genetic probes (when the mutation is known) or with endocrine testing for glandular dysfunction.

Diabetes mellitus

Diabetes mellitus type 1

Definition
Type 1 diabetes mellitus is a chronic disorder of carbohydrate, fat and protein metabolism with hyperglycaemia resulting in most cases from autoimmune destruction of pancreatic β cells.

Incidence/prevalence
Rare in infancy but rises to 2 per 1000 at age 16. Approximately 10% of all diabetic patients in the UK have Type 1 diabetes.

Age
Any age. Most present aged less than 20 years (peaks at 3–4 years and around puberty).

Geography
Wide variation between countries. High in Northern Europe, low in Japan.

Aetiology
Environmentally triggered autoimmune destruction of the pancreatic islet β-cells in a genetically susceptible individual. There is a concordance of 20–40% in monozygotic twins.
- Patients have autoantibodies directed against pancreatic islet constituents which may precede the clinical diagnosis by many years.
- Polygenic inheritance with Class II MHC associated genes. The IDDM1 major susceptibility gene is involved in familial clustering.

- There are specific high risk MHC II haplotypes including HLA-DR3 and -DR4. Having both HLA-DR3 and -DR4 gives an even greater risk than having one or the other. The MHC class II encoded for by these high risk haplotypes is able to present the auto-antigen causing lymphocyte activation and hence autoimmune destruction of islet β-cells. The target autoantigens include glutamate decarboxylase, and insulin. β-cells may be induced to express MHC Class II by viral infection, which makes the β-cell present one of its components as an auto-antigen on the cell surface.
- Non-MHC related genes are also of importance.
- The autoimmune destruction of islet β-cells is probably triggered by an environmental agent. Type 1 diabetes presents most commonly in autumn and winter, with suggestion of a role for both coxsackie and enteroviruses. Type 1 diabetes is the culmination of an occult process of β-cell destruction. The autoimmune activity begins up to 10 years before the presentation, which occurs when >95% of the β-cells have died.

Pathophysiology
The actions of insulin are anabolic (see Fig. 11.14).

In type 1 diabetes, there is hyperglycaemia due to failure of glucose uptake and uncontrolled gluconeogenesis, glycogenolysis, lipolysis and proteolysis:
- Osmotic diuresis – there is a renal threshold for glucose reabsorption, once the levels in the blood rise above 10 mmol/L the kidney is no longer able to completely reabsorb it from the proximal tubule resulting in glycosuria and an osmotic diuresis.

- Polydipsia is secondary to the hyperosmolarity and water depletion.
- Increased appetite occurs.

Clinical features
Patients may present with a history of polyuria, polydipsia and weight loss often despite increased appetite. Young patient often present acutely in diabetic ketoacidosis (see page 460).

Complications
Acute complications include insulin-induced hypoglycaemia and diabetic ketoacidosis.

Chronic complications can be considered as microvascular or macrovascular.
- Microvascular (microangiopathic) disease includes diabetic retinopathy, diabetic nephropathy and the neuropathies seen in diabetes.
- Macrovascular (large vessel) disease due to atherosclerosis which leads to complications such as myocardial infarction, strokes, gangrene of the legs and mesenteric artery occlusion.

Investigations
Diagnosis is made on finding symptoms of diabetes (i.e. polyuria, polydipsia and unexplained weight loss) plus one of:
- A random venous plasma glucose concentration ≥11.1 mmol/L or
- A fasting plasma glucose concentration ≥ 7.0 mmol/L or

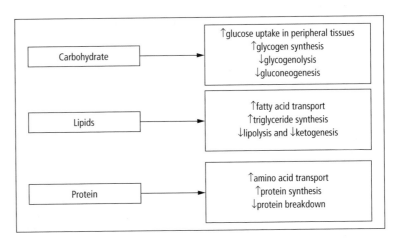

Figure 11.14 The anabolic actions of insulin.

- A plasma glucose concentration ≥ 11.1 mmol/L 2 hours after 75 g anhydrous glucose in an oral glucose tolerance test (OGTT).

If there are no symptoms diagnosis should not be based on a single glucose determination. Impaired Fasting Glucose (IFG) is defined as a fasting plasma glucose above the normal range but below those diagnostic of diabetes (≥ 6.1 mmol/L but <7.0 mmol/L). These patients require an oral glucose tolerance test to exclude diabetes. This is also a risk factor for the future development of diabetes.

Impaired Glucose Tolerance (IGT) is a state of impaired glucose regulation defined as a fasting plasma glucose < 7.0 mmol/L and OGTT two hour value ≥ 7.8 mmol/L but <11.1 mmol/L). This is a risk factor for the development of diabetes and cardiovascular disease.

Other investigations that may be of value include C-peptide measurement (the cleavage product when pro-insulin is converted to insulin) and detection of autoantibodies. These tests are useful in distinguishing patients with type 1 from type 2 diabetes.

Management

Diabetes requires a combination of education, dietary advice, insulin regimens and careful monitoring and follow-up.

Diet: Good nutrition based on a normal proportion of carbohydrate particularly high fibre evenly divided between three main meals. In addition, snacks between meals and at bedtime may be required.

Insulin: It is difficult for subcutaneous insulin therapy to mimic the normal pancreatic secretion into the portal system. Normally the liver immediately takes up 50% of insulin output of the pancreas. Most patients are managed on a twice-daily regimen or basal bolus regimen (see page 454).

Good control of blood glucose reduces small vessel disease. The Diabetes Control and Complications Trial has shown that only 12% of intensively monitored and treated patients developed retinopathy after 9 years, compared to >50% of the conventionally treated patients.

Monitoring:
- Regular capillary blood glucose measurement often pre-meals, two hours post meals and during the night when changing doses, or at times of instability. Once a patient is stabilised on a particular regimen monitoring may be less frequent.

- Glycosylated Hb (HbA1c) is used to assess long-term glycaemic control. It gives an estimate of the average blood glucose over the previous 1–2 months.
- Patients should be regularly assessed for the development of long-term complications such as nephropathy, neuropathy and retinopathy.

Research is continuing into pancreatic and islet-cell transplantation. Immunosuppression itself may prevent autoimmune destruction of islet β-cells and can prevent the development of diabetes in animal models. However there are severe side effects to this treatment.

Diabetes mellitus type 2

Definition

Type 2 diabetes mellitus is a chronic disorder of carbohydrate, fat and protein metabolism with hyperglycaemia as its principal feature. It is characterised by impaired insulin secretion and insulin resistance.

- Type 2 diabetes used to be called non-insulin dependent diabetes (NIDDM) but this term is confusing, as many patients require insulin for good diabetic control.

Incidence/prevalence

Approximately 2% prevalence in UK; 75% of UK diabetic patients.

Age

Increases with age.

Sex

M = F

Geography

Wide geographic variation. More common in Asian immigrants to UK than indigenous population.

Aetiology

A combination of genetic and environmental factors both in the development of insulin resistance and impaired insulin secretion. The overall concordance in monozygotic twins is up to 90%. Environmental factors include diet both in relation to obesity, lack of exercise and the epidemiological evidence that once 'westernised' ethnic migrants have significantly increased prevalence.

Maturity onset diabetes of the young (MODY) occurs in a small subgroup of patients who present under the age of 25. MODY results from specific mono-genetic disorders which are inherited in an autosomal dominant fashion.

Pathophysiology
- Insulin resistance in the liver, skeletal muscle and adipose tissue (by about 40%) secondary to a decrease in the number of insulin receptors, decreased receptor tyrosine kinase activity and post-receptor defects causing impaired glucose transport.
- Defective insulin secretion due to islet cell dysfunction with increased secretion of proinsulin and cleavage products. Amylin, an amyloid protein, is found in increased amounts in the islets cells. It may disrupt the normal insulin secretion.
- Reduced effective insulin causes increased gluconeogenesis by the liver and reduced peripheral uptake, leading to hyperglycaemia. However, there is sufficient insulin to suppress lipolysis and ketogenesis, so that ketosis and ketoacidosis do not occur.

Clinical features
Type 2 diabetes may be diagnosed on routine blood testing (this may follow detection of glycosuria). Symptomatic patients have an insidious onset of polyuria, polydipsia and are usually obese. Diabetes causes an increased predisposition to infections, such as abscesses, pyelonephritis and candidiasis.

Complications
- Acute complications: Hyperglycaemic coma which is usually hyperosmolar non-ketotic coma and complications of therapy such as hypoglycaemia due to insulin or sulphonylureas, metformin-induced lactic acidosis.
- Chronic complications include:
  Microvascular (microangiopathic) disease: Includes diabetic maculopathy and retinopathy, nephropathy and neuropathy.
Macrovascular (large vessel) disease: Atherosclerosis which leads to complications such as myocardial infarction, strokes, gangrene of the legs and mesenteric artery occlusion.

Investigations
The diagnostic criteria are as for type 1 diabetes.

Management
Involves changing the diet, lifestyle (exercise, losing weight) and using oral hypoglycaemic drugs if the former are not effective. Some patients require insulin for adequate glycaemic control.

Loss of weight by an obese patient can lead to normalisation of blood glucose levels and resolution of symptoms. It also reduces insulin resistance. Dietary recommendations include:
- Increase complex carbohydrates (CHO) i.e. bread, cereal, pasta.
- Decrease refined sugars i.e. cakes and sweets.
- Decrease fats, particularly saturated fat.
- Decrease alcohol if excessive, and dry wine is better than beer (less CHO).

Oral hypoglycaemic drugs:
- Biguanides (metformin) reduce insulin resistance, but may cause lactic acidosis with a mortality rate of up to 50%. It may be prevented by avoiding the use of biguanides in patients with moderate renal or hepatic failure.
- Sulphonylureas (glicazide and glibenclamide) increase insulin secretion by the β-cells. These increase levels of plasma insulin and may result in more weight gain, insulin resistance and a higher risk of complications, they are often avoided in the early treatment, unless symptoms are severe.
- Thiazolidinediones (glitazones) increase peripheral insulin sensitivity. They take 3–4 months to achieve maximal effect. They can be used as monotherapy or combined with other drugs.
- α-glucosidase inhibitors (acarbose) which reduce the activity of the enzyme responsible for digesting carbohydrates in the intestine, thus delaying and reducing postprandial blood glucose peaks.

Management also requires careful monitoring for and treatment of complications.

Prognosis
75% of patients die from vascular and related disease.

Secondary diabetes mellitus

Definition
Chronic hyperglycaemia and other metabolic abnormalities seen in diabetes mellitus due to another identifiable cause.

Pancreatic disease: At least two thirds of the pancreas must be lost to cause a type 1 diabetes like syndrome. Causes include chronic pancreatitis, post-pancreatectomy, pancreatic cancer, cystic fibrosis or haemochromatosis.

Insulin counter-regulatory hormones inhibit insulin secretion or cause insulin resistance. This includes drugs and results in a type 2 diabetes like syndrome.

- Growth hormone (acromegaly)
- Glucocorticoids (Cushing's syndrome or disease, iatrogenic)
- Glucagon (glucagonoma)
- Catecholamines (phaeochromocytoma)
- Somatostatin (pancreatic somatostatinoma)
- Oral contraceptives and pregnancy probably due to the oestrogens (and also increased cortisol seen in pregnancy).

Drugs may inhibit insulin secretion or cause damage to the pancreatic islets.

- Thiazides and phenytoin inhibit insulin secretion.
- Pentamidine damages the β-cells.

Insulin receptor defects. These are rare disorders and include:

- DIDMOAD (diabetes insipidus, diabetes mellitus, optic atrophy and deafness)

- Insulin-resistant diabetes with acanthosis nigricans
  i. Young women who have polycystic ovaries and reduced numbers of insulin receptors due to mutations in the allele for the receptor gene.
  ii. Older patients with antibodies to insulin receptors reducing their affinity for insulin.

Insulin therapy

Synthetic insulin is administered subcutaneously in a variety of regimens. Various insulins have been 'designed' with different pharmacokinetic effects (see Table 11.17).

Two common regimens are used (see Fig. 11.15):

- A twice daily adminstration of biphasic insulin, with two thirds of the total daily dose given before breakfast and one third given before the evening meal.
- A bolus of short or immediate acting insulin given three times a day at meal times and a medium or long-acting insulin given at night. The advantage of this regimen is that meal times and quantities can be varied. If immediate acting insulin is used it is taken at or immediately after the meal, if short acting is used then this is administered 30 minutes before the meal.

Table 11.17 Insulin regimens

Type of Insulin (length of action)	No. of injections per day (usual)	Description	Name
Immediate Onset Immediate Duration 4 h	2 or 3 (plus once daily medium or long acting)		Lispro Novorapid
Short Onset 0.5 h Peak 2–4 h Duration 4–6 h	2–4 (plus once daily medium or long acting)	Soluble	Actrapid Velosulin Humulin S
Medium Onset 3 h Peak 6–10 h Duration 12–24 h	2	Isophane (insulin zinc and protamine (a protein) suspension) Insulin detemir (soluble insulin analogue)	Insulatard Protaphane Humulin I Levemir
Long Onset 3–4 h Peak 12–18 h Duration ~24 h	1	Insulin zinc suspension (protein and zinc crystals) Insulin glargine (forms slowly absorbed subcutaneous crystals)	Human ultratard Lantus
Biphasic Onset 0.5 h Peak 2–10 h Duration 12–18 h	1–2	Mixture of soluble and isophane	Human mixtard Humulin M5

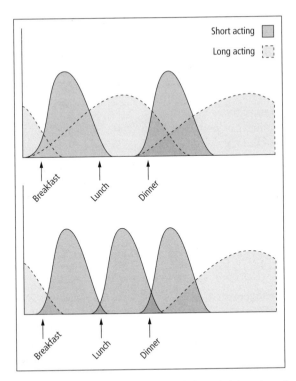

Figure 11.15 Twice daily and basal bolus administration of insulin.

A continuous subcutaneous insulin infusion or continuous intravenous infusion via a tunelled line may also be used. An infusion pump controls the rate and preprandial boosts can be given simply and easily. They are expensive and if they fail, they can cause diabetic ketoacidosis, as there is no longer-acting reserve.

The site of injection also affects the absorption rate:
- The abdominal wall is quickest (use before mealtimes).
- The arms are intermediate.
- The legs are the slowest (night-time).

Temperature and exercise affect absorption. Exercise also increases the use of glucose and hence reduces the amount of insulin needed. Patients must be educated about the problems with insulin therapy. For example, common sites of injection may develop fat hypertrophy or fat atrophy. These sites then release insulin poorly. Rotating the sites prevents these problems. Hypoglycaemia may result from having too much insulin and not eating enough, or exercising. If a patient is not eating, e.g. with vomiting due to gastroenteritis, then insulin

treatment should not be omitted, as the body still requires insulin to utilise glucose. Instead, lower amounts should be used with careful monitoring, or the patient will need to be admitted for intravenous glucose and insulin to avoid either diabetic ketoacidosis or hyperosmolar non-ketotic coma.

Complications of diabetes

Diabetic microvascular disease

Definition
Microvascular diabetic complications includes diabetic retinopathy, nephropathy and the neuropathies.

Aetiology
It is thought that microvascular complications are secondary to the metabolic derangements of diabetes, in particular hyperglycaemia. Good glycaemic control of diabetes and control of hypertension can reduce the incidence of complications.

Pathophysiology
- Hyperglycaemia leads to glycosylation of proteins including haemoglobin, collagen and proteins of blood vessels by non-enzymatic means. This may impair the function of the proteins.
- Intracellular hyperglycaemia in nerves, kidney, blood vessels and the lens which do not require insulin for glucose uptake. The excess intracellular glucose is metabolised to sorbitol and fructose increasing the osmolarity so that water is drawn into cells, causing cell injury.
- Increased blood flow in the capillaries of the retina, kidney and other microcirculations could cause increased damage to the capillary wall. Other factors include smoking (at least as common in diabetics as non-diabetics) and hypertension.
- An inherited factor has been postulated as some patients do not develop microvascular disease.

Diabetic retinopathy

Definition
Diabetes can affect almost all the structures of the eye but the retina and the lens are most commonly affected.

Incidence

Leading cause of blindness under the age of 65 in the developed world. After 20 years of diabetes almost all patients have some retinopathy. Around 40% of type 1 and 20% of type 2 diabetics have proliferative retinopathy.

Aetiology

Control of blood sugars and concomitant hypertension has been shown to reduce risk of retinopathy and other microvascular complications.

Pathophysiology

There is a thickening of the capillary basement membrane and hyaline arteriosclerosis. Microaneurysms (dot haemorrhages) occur in some vessels while others become occluded. The weakening of the vessel walls leads to blot haemorrhages, and transudates of fluid and lipid (hard exudates). The obliteration of capillaries causes retinal ischaemia (cotton wool spots) which in turn stimulates the formation of new vessels at the surface of the retina and iris.

Clinical features

All patients with diabetes should be screened regularly for diabetic retinopathy.
- Background diabetic retinopathy is the earliest sign of diabetic retinopathy. Initially there are microaneurysms later accompanied by blot haemorrhages and scattered hard exudates. Vision is generally unaffected.
- Diabetic maculopathy causes gradual loss of vision due to:
  i. Capillary leakage causing macular oedema
  ii. Lipid deposition
  iii. Extensive obliteration of macular capillaries
- Pre-proliferative retinopathy is seen most commonly in young patients on insulin for about 10 years. Retinal ischaemia is seen as 'soft exudates' or cotton wool spots. Fifty per cent of patients with pre-proliferative changes develop proliferative retinopathy within a year.
- Proliferative retinopathy: New vessels develop most commonly at the optic disc on the venous side adjacent to the temporal vessels. They grow into the vitreous and round to the front of the eye when they are visible on the iris. These vessels may bleed either as vitreous (blue-grey opacity) or pre-retinal haemorrhages (usually flat upper surface), which may cause obscuring of

vision for months or years. Scar formation leads to a traction retinal detachment. New vessels forming at the iris are accompanied by obstruction at the drainage angle causing a neovascular or thrombotic glaucoma (a type of secondary closed angle glaucoma).

Complications

Proliferative retinopathy may cause sudden loss of vision from extensive haemorrhage or retinal detachment. Thrombotic glaucoma may also occur.

Investigations

Screening is by fundoscopic or retinal camera examination. Patients require dilation of the pupils. Fluorescein angiography can be used to show very early disease. Acuity testing should be performed to detect early macular disease.

Management

- No specific treatment is required for background retinopathy except to maximise diabetic control and manage any coexisting hypertension.
- Maculopathy is treated by laser to the centre of a hard exudate.
- Proliferative retinopathy is treated by panretinal photocoagulation (PRP), widespread pinpoint laser treatment to the periphery of the retina, destroying the ischaemic retina. There is then reduction in the growth factors which promote neovascularisation and hence regression of new vessels. Laser treatment also helps prevent neovascular glaucoma.
- Surgery may be required to remove vitreous haemorrhage and fibrous tissue or to repair a detached or torn retina.

Prognosis

Prevention is the best management, by regular screening and good control of blood sugar.

Diabetic nephropathy

Definition

Diabetic nephropathy is a microvascular disease of type 1 and 2 diabetes.

Incidence

Patient individual risk is falling however due to increasing rates of diabetes the overall prevalence of diabetic nephropathy is rising.

Age
Increases with age.

Aetiology
Associated with hypertension, smoking and poor glycaemic control.

Pathophysiology
In addition to the other microvascular mechanisms hypertension can accelerate nephropathy by causing further thickening of the capillary walls and reduced glomerular filtration rate. This further increases hypertension.

Glomerular basement membrane (GBM) thickening and glomerulosclerosis due to an increase in the mesangial matrix. It leads to diffuse sclerosis of the glomerulus, which later condenses into nodular lesions, called Kimmelstiel-Wilson lesions. The thickening of the basement membrane increases its permeability to albumin. As the disease progresses, the amount of protein lost increases.

The glomerular filtration rate is initially normal, but falls with progressive renal damage and chronic renal failure occurs around 5–7 years after macroalbuminuria occurs.

Clinical features
The condition is asymptomatic until chronic renal failure or nephrotic syndrome develops. Patients should be screened annually for all diabetic complications and hypertension.

Microscopy
The GBM is thickened (can be seen on electron microscopy). There are exudative lesions on the surface of the glomerulus, which are masses of red-staining fibrin protein. The mesangial matrix is expanded and there are round hyaline areas in the glomeruli (Kimmelstiel-Wilson nodules).

Investigations
Annual screening of urine for microalbuminuria. Amount of albumin lost per 24 hours:

30–300 mg/24 hours	Microalbuminuria
>300 mg/24 hours	Proteinuria
>3.6 g/24 hours	Hypoalbuminaemia and Nephrotic syndrome

Diabetic patients may have other causes for proteinuria and renal failure, so particularly if there are atypical features such as haematuria, rapid onset or absent retinopathy further investigation must be carried out to look for another cause.

Management
- Microalbuminuria and proteinuria require aggressive treatment of hypertension (<130/75), better glycaemic control and cessation of smoking. ACE inhibitors and angiotensin II blockers appear to be most effective in reducing protein loss and delaying progression.
- End-stage renal failure is treated as for non-diabetics. Haemodialysis may be more complicated because of increased cardiovascular disease and autonomic neuropathy which exacerbates postural hypotension. Hypoglycaemia may occur because insulin and sulphonylureas accumulate in renal failure.
- Renal transplantation is the preferred option in younger patients, and pancreatic-renal transplants may be of value in reducing diabetic complications.

Diabetic neuropathy

Definition
Nerve damage is one of the microvascular complications of diabetes mellitus.

Incidence/prevalence
Diabetes is the most common metabolic disorder causing neuropathy: 10% of diabetics have significant symptoms and 30% have evidence on testing.

Aetiology
It is thought to be secondary to hyperglycaemia and microvascular disease.
There are three main types of diabetic neuropathy:
- Symmetrical peripheral neuropathy: Affecting sensory and motor function diffusely, particularly in the lower limbs. This can be a painful neuropathy.
- Focal and multifocal neuropathy: Affecting one or more cranial or peripheral nerves.
- Autonomic neuropathy: Affecting the sympathetic and parasympathetic nerves.

Pathophysiology
- Hyperglycaemia may damage nerves through non-enzymatic glycosylation of proteins or through the

accumulation of sorbitol in nerve cells, which can take up glucose without the aid of insulin.

- Microvascular damage (which itself is thought to be secondary to hyperglycaemia and other factors) to the capillaries which supply nerves probably cause ischaemic nerve damage. Focal nerve palsies may be due to sudden occlusion of a larger vessel causing infarction.

Symmetrical peripheral neuropathy

A diffuse symmetrical pattern of damage to the nerves, most commonly the sensory nerves, which has a glove and stocking distribution. There is Schwann cell injury, myelin degeneration and axonal damage.

Clinical features

Sensory neuropathy:

- Sensory symptoms in the feet and legs are most common and may be insidious or sudden in onset. In the case of the latter it may follow an episode of severe hyperglycaemia. Paraesthesia (pins and needles, burning, shooting pains) which may be precipitated by normal sensations such as contact with bedclothes, this is called allodynia. The pain is worse at night and keeps the patient awake.
- Chronic loss of sensation, most importantly of pain. The patient completely loses the sense of pain, so that severe damage such as burns, cuts, ulcers, infection and gangrene can occur without being noticed by the patient (the neuropathic foot).
- On examination, there is reduced sensation, often in a glove and stocking distribution, and tendon reflexes may be reduced or absent. Vibration sense is often lost early in the course of peripheral neuropathy. Motor nerve damage causes muscle wasting. The feet and ankles in particular may be damaged.

Motor neuropathy:

- This may be asymptomatic, accompanying the sensory neuropathy.
- Painful neuropathy: It may also cause intense pain in a glove and stocking distribution.

Investigations

A careful neurological examination should be carried out, including joint position sense, vibration, pinprick and light touch, tendon reflexes and muscle power. Most cases do not require further investigation as the cause is clear, however, occasionally it is appropriate to exclude other causes of the neuropathy e.g. by checking vitamin B_{12} level.

Management

Improving glycaemic control may be of benefit. Pain can be treated by a step-wise approach using aspirin and codeine, tricyclic antidepressants, carbamazepine or gabapentin. Feet should be inspected and examined at each review including sensation to a 10 g monofilament or vibration and palpation of foot pulses. Examination may need to be repeated 1–3 monthly in high-risk patients. New ulceration, swelling, discolouration is a foot care emergency and requires multidisciplinary assessment within 24 hours.

Prognosis

The acute form may resolve with time and better glycaemic control. The chronic form is persistent and irreversible. Symptoms may be intractable in some patients.

Focal and multifocal neuropathy

Pathophysiology

A focal nerve lesion, either of a cranial or peripheral nerve, which is thought to be due to occlusion of a larger vessel supplying the nerve, or pressure damage, when it may be seen in the context of impaired sensation of pain. Several nerves may be affected.

- The cranial nerves most affected are III, IV and VI.
- The peripheral nerves most affected are the median, ulnar and lateral popliteal nerves.
- If a large nerve trunk or root is affected, such as the femoral nerve, radiculopathy results, causing proximal pain and wasting, for example in the thigh, with weakness and wasting of quadriceps (diabetic amyotrophy).

Clinical features

Any nerve(s) can be involved.

- Third nerve palsy typically presents with pain, diplopia and ptosis. It may resolve spontaneously.
- Peripheral nerve palsies recover only slowly and often incompletely.

- Diabetic amyotrophy present with sudden onset of pain and weakness with an absent tendon jerk (usually the knee). The important differential diagnosis is a spinal or cauda equina cause of the radiculopathy.

Investigations

In most cases, this is not necessary, as the cause is clear. Occasionally, it may be useful to exclude other causes, particularly in cranial nerve palsies when a space-occupying lesion may be excluded with CT or MRI.

Management

Management is as for diffuse symmetrical neuropathies.

Autonomic neuropathy

Incidence

About 40% of diabetic patients have autonomic neuropathy on screening. It increases with the duration of the disease.

Pathophysiology

This probably has similar pathogenesis to the diffuse, symmetrical neuropathy. The autonomic nervous system is involved, causing disturbance of functions such as postural vasoconstriction, gastrointestinal motility, bladder emptying, sexual function (erection and ejaculation). Life-threatening disturbances include reduced awareness of hypoglycaemia and cardiorespiratory arrest. Sudden unexplained death is more common.

Clinical features

- Postural hypotension, causing dizziness, faints and falls.
- Nausea, vomiting and diarrhoea or constipation due to abnormal gastrointestinal motility.
- Bladder problems include incomplete emptying, chronic urinary retention and this predisposes to more severe urinary tract infections, such as pyelonephritis.
- Failure of erection is due to reduced parasympathetic activity (may also result from depression or atheroma in the pudendal arteries). Failure of ejaculation due to impaired sympathetic activity.
- Increased sweating.

Examination shows a >20 mmHg fall in systolic BP on standing, loss of normal sinus arrhythmia on breathing and lack of reflex bradycardia on the Valsalva maneouvre. The bladder may be palpable.

Complications

Pyelonephritis, overgrowth of bowel bacteria causing diarrhoea.

Management

Treatment depends on the symptoms and complications. Postural hypotension is treatable with fludrocortisone (a mineralocorticoid), but this may cause hypertension to be worse. Impotence is treatable with sildenafil.

Prognosis

Symptomatic autonomic neuropathy is associated with a reduced life expectancy.

Diabetic ketoacidosis (DKA)

Definition

The hyperglycaemic and metabolic acidotic state which occurs in Type I diabetes due to excess ketone production as a result of insulin deficiency.

Aetiology

Precipitating factors include infection, trauma, surgery, burns and myocardial infarction. It is associated with poor diabetic control.

Pathophysiology

- Patients may omit or reduce their insulin when ill, because they are eating less and therefore believe they require less insulin. In fact, stresses such as an intercurrent infection increase the secretion of glucagon and other counter-regulatory hormones which oppose insulin, so that insulin requirements increase during illness.
- The result of this is a severe catabolic state: there is uncontrolled glycolysis, lipolysis and protelolysis. This causes hyperglycaemia and a rise in free fatty acids which are the substrates for ketone body formation (ketogenesis) within the liver. Normally insulin opposes ketogenesis, but in conditions of insulin deficiency, glucagon and catecholamines increase ketogenesis. The ketone bodies produced are acetoacetic acid, acetone and hydroxybutyrate which result in a metabolic acidosis.

- As the production rate exceeds the body's capacity to utilise ketone bodies, both ketone body and glucose concentrations rise, causing hyperosmolarity of the extracellular fluid. The renal threshold for glucose reabsorption (~10 mmol/L) is exceeded, and an osmotic diuresis occurs so that water and electrolytes, especially sodium and potassium, are rapidly lost. This causes a severe dehydration, hypovolaemia and this compounds the problem by reducing renal perfusion, thereby reducing glucose clearance.
- Dehydration is exacerbated by vomiting, which is due to central effects of ketosis.
- Death is usually due to cardiac arrest.

Clinical features
Nausea, vomiting, abdominal pain, hyperventilation, shock, coma, signs of dehydration and ketotic smelling breath. Normally this occurs in a known diabetic, but it may occur as the presenting feature, particularly in young patients.

Complications
Shock and acute renal failure, cerebral oedema may occur during rehydration, adult respiratory distress syndrome, acute gastric dilatation, aspiration, hypothermia, and coma.

Investigations
The diagnosis requires the demonstration of diabetes, ketosis and a metabolic acidosis. Blood glucose should be checked on capillary bedside testing and confirmed with a laboratory sample. Ketones may be detected in the urine on urinalysis. Some bedside blood glucose monitors can also detect ketones. An arterial blood gas sample is also required to demonstrate and assess the severity of metabolic acidosis.
- U&Es and osmolality should be sent urgently.
- Full blood count, amylase, blood cultures, urine culture, CXR and ECG are checked to identify underlying causes and complications. Consider cardiac enzymes in older patients. Serum amylase greater than threefold normal is suggestive of acute pancreatitis, which may be the cause of DKA in up to 10% of cases.

Management
DKA is a medical emergency. The initial management is rehydration and correction of electrolyte imbalances.

Insulin replacement is also needed to correct the hyperglycaemia and prevent further osmotic diuresis. Any underlying illness must be treated as appropriate. Patients require a nasogastric tube for gastric decompression and emptying as there is a high risk of aspiration. Fluid and electrolytes: Patients can be as much as 10 L fluid depleted, with a K^+ and Na^+ deficit. Monitor fluid balance (urine output etc.) during treatment. A central venous catheter may be placed to measure central venous pressure to guide fluid management. Care must be taken not to change the osmolality too rapidly, as this can lead to cerebral oedema. The osmolality will drop as glucose levels fall, and so sodium and potassium need to be given to counter this. For this reason, normal saline is always used initially:
- 1st hour   1.5 L
- 2nd hour   1.0 L
- 3rd to 4th hour   1.0 L over 2 hours
- > 5th hour   2.0 L every 8 hours
- Change to 5% or 10% dextrose, 1 L every 8 hours once the patient is rehydrated and blood glucose is back down to 12 mmol/L. Replacement should be faster if patients are shocked and slower if there are signs of cardiac failure, fluid overload or cerebral oedema.

There is always a depletion of total body potassium, but serum K^+ may be normal, high or low. Supplementation is always needed, because potassium follows glucose into the cells. However, there is a danger of hyperkalaemia, causing cardiac arrhythmias, so if K^+ levels are >5 mmol/l withhold K^+ and recheck after 30 minutes.

Normal K^+	20 mmol per litre of fluid
<3.5 (hypo)	40 mmol per litre

Insulin: Soluble insulin is administered intravenously by an infusion pump – start with 10 units per hour and then titrate to response. Therapy should aim to produce a gradual reduction to a glucose level of 10–15 mmol/L over a period of several hours. Hourly blood sugar and 1–2 hourly U&E's, plasma osmolality monitoring are required. If intravenous access is not possible then subcutaneous or intramuscular insulin can reverse the ketoacidosis.

Bicarbonate: The use of bicarbonate is contentious. It is unlikely to improve the acidosis and has the potential of doing harm including making cerebral oedema more likely. It therefore should not normally be used in the treatment of diabetic ketoacidosis.

Prognosis

Overall mortality is ~10% and as high as 50% in older patients with severe intercurrent illness. It is the most common cause of death in diabetic patients under 20 years old.

Hyperosmolar, non-ketotic coma (HONK)

Definition

This occurs in people who have type 2 diabetes mellitus and is characterised by hyperglycaemia without severe hyperketonaemia or metabolic acidosis.

Age

More common in the elderly.

Sex

M = F

Aetiology

Precipitating factors include infection, myocardial infarction and stroke, or diabetogenic drugs such as glucocorticoids and thiazide diuretics.

Pathophysiology

The pathophysiology is essentially the same as for diabetic ketoacidosis (DKA), except that because the person has enough insulin to suppress lipolysis and ketogenesis, uncontrolled ketogenesis does not occur. There is insufficient insulin to prevent increased glucose production and reduced glucose uptake by cells and so hyperglycaemia occurs. The hyperglycaemia is often much more extreme than in DKA and causes severe hyperosmolarity with an osmotic diuresis which unless compensated for by water intake leads to progressive severe dehydration. This compounds the hyperosmolarity caused by the hyperglycaemia, which increases blood viscosity, predisposing to thromboembolic disorders. If untreated, it leads to confusion and eventually coma.

Clinical features

Often occurs in elderly undiagnosed patients, who present with polyuria, intense thirst, weight loss and blurred vision. The symptoms and signs of ketoacidosis are absent (hyperventilation, ketotic breath) but confusion, drowsiness and coma are more common.

Complications

Thromboembolic disease, such as stroke, mesenteric artery thrombosis, deep vein thrombosis and pulmonary embolism.

Investigations

- Blood and urinary ketones are absent or only slightly raised.
- Blood glucose is raised and can be as high as 100 mmol/L.
- U&Es: Markedly raised sodium (often over 155 mmol/L) and urea due to dehydration.
- Very high plasma osmolality (>350 mosmol/kg) but anion gap is normal, as is pH on arterial blood gas.
- Full blood count, blood cultures, urine culture, CXR and ECG are checked to identify underlying causes and complications. Consider cardiac enzymes in older patients.

Management

Patients require emergency fluid resuscitation with normal saline and potassium replacement (as for diabetic ketoacidosis). Low-dose intravenous insulin is used to reduce the hyperglycaemia but patients are often very sensitive and rapid reductions in glucose should be avoided. Prophylactic low-dose heparin to prevent thromboembolic complications. Any underlying cause should be identified and treated.

Prognosis

Mortality is higher overall (~30%) than DKA, because these patients are more elderly.

Hypoglycaemia

Definition

Low serum glucose caused by insufficient hepatic glucose production for peripheral requirements.

Aetiology

Insulin overdose (accidental or deliberate self harm), sulphonylurea overdose, malnutrition, fasting, exercise or severe liver disease. Alcohol impairs gluconeogenesis and can cause hypoglycaemia in diabetic patients. Rare causes include insulinomas (see page 222) and Addison's disease (see page 440).

Clinical features

Patients become irritable, pale, weak and sweaty. In patients who have regular hypoglycaemic episodes and in autonomic neuropathy the awareness of symptoms is reduced. Untreated the condition progresses to confusion, seizures and coma. Prolonged or severe hypoglycaemia risks permanent neurological damage and death.

Investigations

The diagnosis can be confirmed on bedside blood sugar testing, a formal laboratory glucose sample should be sent but treatment should not be delayed. Other tests may be required to identify the underlying cause.

Management

This is a medical emergency and requires immediate treatment.

- In conscious patients the blood sugar can be raised by oral administration of a sugary drink. This should be followed by a more complex carbohydrate to prevent a further rebound hypoglycaemia.
- In unconscious patients or those unable to tolerate oral fluids blood sugar can be raised by administration of glucose gel to the gums (e.g. Hypostop), intravenous dextrose or intramuscular glucagon.
- Further management depends on severity and the underlying cause.

Haematology and clinical immunology

Clinical

Signs

Lymphadenopathy

The usual function of lymph nodes is to allow antigen recognition, proliferation and affinity maturation of mature lymphocytes. They usually become enlarged when active/reactive because of infection. Enlargement of lymph nodes can be localised or generalised (see Table 12.1).

Table 12.1 Causes of lymphadenopathy

Localised lymphadenopathy
    Infection, e.g. cervical lymphadenopathy in tonsillitis,
        lymphadenitis
    Carcinoma, e.g. lymph node enlargement in the axilla
        with breast carcinoma
    Hodgkin's disease (can also be generalised)
    Non-Hodgkin's lymphoma (can also be generalised)
    Tuberculosis can present as a single enlarged painless
        lymph node
    Sarcoidosis often begins with bilateral hilar
        lymphadenopathy
Generalised lymphadenopathy
    Infectious mononucleosis
    Toxoplasmosis
    Human immunodeficiency virus can cause a
        persistent generalised lymphadenopathy
    Chronic lymphocytic leukaemia
    Lymphoma

Splenomegaly

The spleen is not normally palpable on clinical examination. The spleen may by moderately or massively enlarged see Table 12.2.

Hypersplenism occurs when the spleen is functionally overactive and can result from any cause of splenomegaly. It causes pancytopenia and haemolysis.

Bleeding tendency

Characterisation of a bleeding tendency requires multiple tests; however, a number of important factors can be elucidated clinically.

- Differentiating between an inherited or acquired disorder may be suggested by the age. A full family history is also essential to establish any affected relatives.
- Generalised haemostatic defects are suggested by bleeding from multiple sites, spontaneous bleeding and bleeding into the skin.

Table 12.2 Causes of splenomegaly

Moderate splenomegaly	Massive Splenomegaly
Infectious mononucleosis	Chronic myeloid leukaemia
Septicaemia, infective endocarditis	Myelofibrosis
Hodgkin's disease, non-Hodgkin's lymphoma	Storage disorders such as Gaucher's disease
Leukaemia	
Haemoglobinopathies	
Cirrhosis with portal hypertension	

- Bleeding disorders may result from abnormalities of blood vessels platelets and coagulation:
  1 Vascular/platelet disorders are suggested by bruising, purpura and petechiae.
  2 Inherited coagulation disorders are associated with haemarthroses (bleeding into the joints) and muscle haematomas.

Investigations

- Full blood count and blood film to examine the number and morphology of platelets.
- Platelet aggregation times (spontaneous and stimulated) can be used to assess the function of platelets.
- A full coagulation screen is performed comprising a prothrombin time (PT), thrombin time (TT) and activated partial thromboplastin time (APTT), see page 465.
- Bleeding time is a measure of platelet function. A blood pressure cuff is applied and inflated to 40 mmHg. An incision is made that is 1-cm long and 1-mm deep. The time taken for bleeding to stop is measured. The bleeding time is prolonged in quantitative and qualitative platelet disorders.
- Factor assays can be used to measure the levels of any components of the coagulation cascade.

Investigations and procedures

Full blood count

The full blood count is the most commonly performed investigation in medicine. It measures the five types of white blood cell (neutrophil, lymphocyte, monocyte, eosinophil and basophil), the red blood cells and the platelets. The mean cell volume (MCV), packed cell volume (PCV), mean cell haemoglobin content (MCH) and the mean cell haemoglobin concentration (MCHC) are also either measured or calculated. Further details about cellular morphology can be obtained by examining the blood film.

Neutrophils

A neutrophilia is seen in bacterial infections, tissue necrosis, inflammation, myeloproliferative diseases and corticosteroid therapy. A leukaemoid reaction is when overproduction of white cells leads to the release of immature cells. It occurs in severe infections, tuberculosis or malignant infiltration of the bone marrow. A leucoerythroblastic anaemia occurs when nucleated red cells and immature white cells are released into the circulation. This may result from marrow infiltration or myelofibrosis.

A neutropenia may occur in viral infections and severe bacterial infections. It occurs with any cause of pancytopenia, in association with rheumatoid arthritis (Felty's syndrome). There is a recognised racial neutropaenia in Afro-Carribbeans.

Lymphocytes

A lymphocytosis is seen in viral infections particularly Epstein Barr virus and cytomegalovirus. Chronic inflammation including tuberculosis and toxoplasma may cause a rise in lymphocytes. Malignant proliferation may result from leukaemias and lymphomas.

Monocytes

Monocytes are the blood and bone marrow located precursors of tissue macrophages (including liver Kupffer cells, pulmonary alveolar macrophages and Langerhan cells in the skin) and dendritic antigen presenting cells. They are phagocytic and are involved in antigen processing and presentation.

A monocytosis may be seen in viral infections such as glandular fever and in chronic bacterial infections such as endocarditis, tuberculosis and myelodysplasia. In cyclical neutropenia the monocytes rise as the neutrophil count falls.

Eosinophils

Eosinophils are phagocytic, with a particular affinity for antigen–antibody complexes and are involved in allergic reactions and parasitic infections.

An eosinophilia may arise in parasitic infections, allergic disorders (hay fever, hypersensitivity), skin disorders (urticaria, eczema), pulmonary disorders (asthma, allergic aspergillosis, Churg Strauss syndrome) and in hyper eosinophilic syndrome.

Basophils

Basophils are thought to be the circulating equivalent of tissue mast cells, the granules contain proteoglycans, heparin, histamine. They have surface IgE receptors and are increased in myeloproliferative disorders particularly chronic myelogenous leukaemia (see page 482).

Red blood cells

Polycythaemia (increased red cell count) may result from reduced plasma volume (diarrhoea, vomiting, diuretics). True polycythaemia may be primary (see page 483) or secondary. Secondary polycythaemia may be due to

- Hypoxia, which may be physiological (neonates, altitude), or due to respiratory disease (smoking, COAD) or cyanotic heart disease.
- Inappropriate erythropoetin production: Renal cell carcinoma, renal cysts or following renal transplant.
- Tumour secretion: Hepatoma, cellular haemangioma.

Severe polycythaemia may result in hyperviscosity of the blood, which prediposes to thrombosis, haemorrhage and cardiac failure.

Platelets

Thrombocytopenia (reduced platelet count) may be due to failure of bone marrow production or excess destruction of platelets. Bone marrow platelet production may fail due to aplasia, marrow infiltration or the effects of drugs. Peripheral platelet destruction may result from immune mechanisms (see page 495), from excess coagulation in disseminated intravascular coagulation (see page 494) or thrombotic thrombocytopenic purpura (see page 258).

Coagulation screening tests

The basic coagulation cascade (excluding co factors) is outlined below; the cascade style of reaction allows a small stimulus of negative charge contact (such as collagen) or the release of thromboplastin from the tissues to create a large amount of fibrin product (see Fig. 12.1).

Factors II (prothrombin), VII, IX and X require vitamin K for their synthesis. The coagulation screen is made up of a combination of tests:

- The thrombin time (TT) is initiated by adding thrombin to a sample and thus assesses deficiencies/dysfunctions in fibrinogen. Fibrinogen levels and fibrin degradation (D-dimers) products can also be measured as a measure of intravascular clot breakdown, e.g. disseminated intravascular coagulation or pulmonary embolism.
- The prothrombin (PT) time is initiated by the addition of thromboplastin and thus measures the extrinsic and final common pathway. It is prolonged in deficiencies

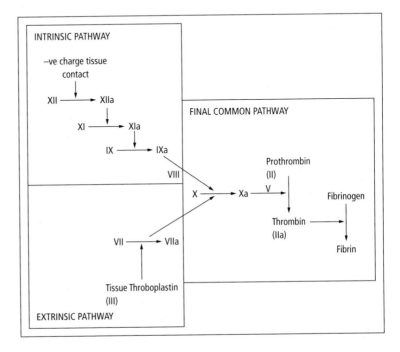

Figure 12.1 The coagulation cascade.

of factors VII, V, X or II. It is also prolonged in liver disease and in patients taking warfarin.

- The activated partial thromboplastin time (APTT) or partial thromboplastin time with kaolin (PTTK) is initiated by adding an activator such as kaolin and thus measures the intrinsic and final common pathway. It is prolonged in deficiencies of factors XII, XI, IX, VIII, X or V.
- If the coagulation times are prolonged, a 50:50 mix of patients and normal plasma is made. If such a mixture does not correct the time then the result is suggestive of the presence of an inhibitor of coagulation rather than a factor deficiency. If heparin is suspected as the cause of a prolonged TT then reptilase or protamine is added to the sample, which reverses the effects of heparin.

Bone marrow sampling

Bone marrow sampling is often essential in diagnosing haematological conditions. There are two sampling techniques available:

- Bone marrow aspiration: Sampling normally occurs from the iliac crest. Following skin preparation local anaesthetic is infiltrated into the skin and down to the periosteum. The aspiration needle is inserted through the skin and advanced rotating clockwise and counterclockwise until the marrow cavity is entered. The stylet is then removed and 2–3 mL of marrow is aspirated using a syringe. The sample is spread onto glass slides and stained as required.
- Bone marrow trephine: Following skin preparation, anaesthetic and incision the biopsy needle (e.g. Jamshidi needle) is inserted and advanced until it makes contact with the bone. The stylet is then removed and the needle advanced using alternating clockwise-counterclockwise motion into the bone marrow cavity. The sample is removed from the needle, fixed, decalcified and stained as required.

Haemopoeitic progenitor cell transplantation

Haemopoetic progenitor cell transplantation is used in an attempt to cure various haematological and immunological conditions. Treatment begins with ablation of the existing diseased marrow using cytotoxic drugs and/or total body irradiation. This induces pancytope-

nia and severe immunodeficiency risking bacterial infection, bleeding and anaemia. Total body irradiation has a number of potential late complications including thyroid underactivity, gonad underactivity, cataract formation, diarrhoea, sun burn and nausea.

During this pancytopaenic period support includes the following:

- Blood transfusion, if haemoglobin falls below 10.0 g/dL, (CMV negative if patient and donor have not had CMV). Blood is irradiated to prevent graft versus host disease.
- Platelet transfusions may be used.
- Patients are maintained in a filtered air environment.
- Prophylactic antibiotics and antivirals can be used.

The pancytopaenia is reversed by haemopoetic progenitor cell transplantation (infusion into a peripheral vein of haemopoetic progenitors, which finds its own way to the marrow cavity and regenerates it). Grafts may be allografts (HLA matched sibling or unrelated donors) or autologous (from self) either bone marrow or more recently peripheral blood stem cell transplants and cord blood.

Allografts risk the negative effect of graft versus host disease (GVHD) where mature T cells in the transplant recognise the rest of the body as 'non-self' and therefore attempt to reject it. Coupled to this is a positive phenomenon known as the graft versus leukaemia effect (GVL) where the donor marrow recognises any remaining leukaemic cells and mounts an immunological attack. Acute GVHD may occur within the first 3 months and subsequently chronic GVHD may develop. Acute GVHD affects HLA-rich tissue with desquamation of the skin, impairment of liver function and diarrhoea. Lymphocyte-depleted marrow reduces the risk of GVHD, but also eliminates the graft versus leukaemia effect and may thus increases the risk of relapse.

Chronic GVHD, which occurs after 3 months may be an extension of acute GVHD or may occur in patients who never showed clinical evidence of acute GVHD.

- Ocular manifestations: Irritation, photophobia, and SICCA syndrome (see page 369).
- Gastrointestinal system: Abdominal pain dysphagia, odynophagia, weight loss, malabsorption and liver disease.
- Respiratory system: Obstructive lung disease usually nonresponsive to bronchodilator therapy.
- Neuromuscular system: Weakness, neuropathic pain, muscle cramps.

Autografts (frozen haemopoetic progenitors from the patient) is not associated with GVHD or GVL and may involve re-infusion of leukaemic cells. However, they have the advantage of availability. Peripheral stem cell transplants are now used more frequently than autologous bone marrow transplantation. They have the advantage that more progenitor cells are collected and thus rescue from pancytopenia occurs more rapidly.

Allergy testing

Allergy testing most commonly involves skin prick tests and may include the radioallergosorbent test (RAST) and rarely diagnostic allergen challenge. The choice of test is dependent on the suspected allergen and the nature of any previous allergic reaction. Testing of patients with a history of anaphylaxis may be confined to RAST and should only be undertaken by an allergy specialist.

- Skin prick tests allow the testing of multiple allergens simultaneously. Small amounts of a specific suspected allergen or a panel of common allergens is applied to the skin, which is then pricked to allow the allergens to penetrate the skin. An erythematous reaction followed by a weal occurs within minutes when positive. The test is read at 15 minutes and a weal diameter of ≥ 3 mm is normally considered positive. Skin tests are useful in detection of respiratory allergies, food allergies and allergies to penicillin and insect bites. Patients should not be taking antihistamine medication at the time of the test.
- RAST measures specific IgE antibodies in the blood to individual allergens.
- Food allergies can normally be diagnosed on a good clinical history. If doubt exists skin prick tests or RAST tests (usually if there is a history of anaphylaxis) can be helpful. True identification may require food challenges with the patient blinded to the food being tested, as there may be a psychological component to presumed food allergies.
- Other tests include immunoglobulin and complement measurements and blood eosinophil counts.

Haemoglobin disorders and anaemia

Anaemia

Definition
A fall in the concentration of haemoglobin below the reference level for the age and sex of the individual.

Aetiology
Anaemia is usually due to a fall in haemoglobin; rarely it may result from a rise in plasma volume, e.g. in fluid overload or during pregnancy. Anaemia is usually classified according to the size of the red blood cells (see Fig. 12.2).

Clinical features
Symptoms suggestive of anaemia include fatigue, faintness, headaches, breathlessness, angina of effort, intermittent claudication and palpitations. On examination there may be pallor, tachycardia, a systolic flow murmur and/or cardiac failure.

Investigations
The cause of anaemia must always be found. Initial investigations must include a full blood count and blood film.

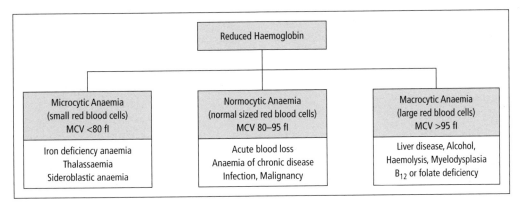

Figure 12.2 Important causes of anaemia.

These provide information on the degree of anaemia, whether the disorder is confined to haemoglobin or whether it includes abnormalities of white blood cells and/or platelets. The full blood count also provides information on the mean corpuscular volume (MCV) to guide further investigations. The blood film demonstrates the morphology of red blood cells, white blood cells and platelets.

- In microcytic anaemia, a serum iron and ferritin, and total iron binding capacity (TIBC) are measured to assess iron stores.
- In macrocytic anaemia with normal vitamin B_{12} and folate levels, or in suspected haematological malignancy, a bone marrow aspiration and trephine is usually performed (see page 466).

Microcytic hypchromic anaemia

Iron deficiency anaemia

Definition
A fall in haemoglobin concentration secondary to depleted iron stores.

Aetiology
Causes of iron deficiency:
- Inadequate supply due to poor dietary intake (normal requirements 0.5–1 mg per day).
- Inadequate absorption, e.g. in coeliac disease or post-gastrectomy.
- Increased demand such as during growth or pregnancy.
- Increased loss from bleeding including occult gastrointestinal bleeding or menstruation.

Pathophysiology
Most of the iron within the body is circulating as haemoglobin. The remainder is stored in the bone marrow, hepatocytes and skeletal muscle cells. As an individual becomes iron deficient the bone marrow stores are depleted prior to the development of a microcytic anaemia.

Clinical features
Symptoms of anaemia include fatigue, faintness, headaches and breathlessness. In patients with known iron deficiency anaemia, it is important to enquire about dietary iron intake, history of blood in faeces, menorrhagia and a history of taking nonsteroidal anti-inflammatory drugs, aspirin or warfarin. On examination there may be pallor, tachycardia, cardiac failure and specific features of iron deficiency including glossitis, angular stomatitis and brittle spoon shaped nails (koilonychia). A rectal examination should be performed.

Investigations
- Full blood count demonstrates a microcytic (low MCV) hypochromic (low MCH, MCHC) anaemia. Blood film confirms small, pale staining (hypochromic) cells, variable shaped red blood cells (poikilocytosis) and variable sized red blood cells (anisocytosis). The white blood cells and platelets should be normal.
- A low serum ferritin is the normal diagnostic investigation; however, it is falsely raised in liver disease and renal failure.
- Other tests include a low serum iron and raised total iron binding capacity. Bone marrow aspiration is not usually required, but shows erythroid hyperplasia and a lack of iron stores on Perl's staining.
- Investigation of established iron deficiency may require faecal occult blood testing and upper or lower gastrointestinal endoscopy.

Management
The underlying cause must be identified and treated where possible. Iron deficiency is treated with oral iron supplements, which should result in a rise of 1 g/dL of haemoglobin per week. Supplements are usually required for at least 6 months to replenish iron stores. Failure of response may be due to poor compliance, severe malabsorption, continued significant blood loss or another cause of anaemia. Rarely parenteral iron treatment may be required. In severely symptomatic anaemia, blood transfusion may be required; however, this may interfere with subsequent investigations.

Sideroblastic anaemia

Definition
Disordered haem synthesis resulting in abnormal accumulation of iron within red blood cells.

Aetiology/pathophysiology

Haem synthesis is abnormal with a failure of iron incorporation. There is accumulation of iron in the mitochondria of erythroblasts, which stain as a ring around the nucleus (ring sideroblasts). Sideroblastic anaemia may be congenital or acquired:

- Congenital X-linked disease.
- Primary acquired sideroblastic anaemia is one of the myelodysplastic syndromes.
- Secondary acquired sideroblastic anaemia may be caused by drugs (e.g. isoniazid) or toxins such as lead or alcohol.

Clinical features

Patients initially present with symptoms and signs of anaemia. As sideroblastic anaemia results in a microcytic hypochromic anaemia, it may be misdiagnosed as iron deficiency. The anaemia is however refractory to iron supplementation.

Investigations

- The full blood count and film may reveal diamorphic red cells, i.e. there are two populations of cells – one normal sized and a population of microcytic hypochromic cells.
- Serum iron and ferritin are normal or raised.
- Perl's staining of bone marrow samples shows a ring of iron around the nucleus in erythrocyte precursors. The presence of these ring sideroblasts are diagnostic.

Management

Congenital sideroblastic anaemia may respond to pyridoxine. Primary acquired sideroblastic anaemia is treated as for myelodysplastic syndrome (see page 481). In secondary acquired sideroblastic anaemia any causative agent should be removed where possible.

Normocytic anaemia

Anaemia of chronic disease

Definition

Anaemia of chronic disease is a condition of impaired iron use where haemoglobin is reduced but iron stores are normal or high.

Table 12.3 Conditions that may cause anaemia of chronic disease

Infections	Subacute infective endocarditis, tuberculosis, osteomyelitis
Inflammation	Rheumatoid arthritis, systemic lupus, erythematosus, connective tissue disease
Chronic renal failure	
Malignancy	

Aetiology/pathophysiology

Anaemia may result from any chronic disease, see Table 12.3. The exact mechanisms are unknown but may include the following:

- Bone marrow iron stores are not incorporated into developing erythrocytes.
- There is a relative resistance to erythropoetin.
- Circulating red cells have a reduced life span.
- These changes may be mediated by cytokines such as IL-1, TNF and interferon.

Clinical features

Symptoms and signs of anaemia (see page 467).

Investigations

The anaemia is usually normocytic but may be slightly microcytic. Serum iron is low but ferritin is normal or high. The total iron binding capacity is low. The ESR is usually raised.

Management

Treating the underlying cause may result in a resolution of the anaemia. Erythropoeitin may be of benefit.

Macrocytic anaemia

Macrocytic normoblastic anaemia

Definition

Macrocytosis (large circulating red blood cells) are seen with normal erythrocyte progenitor cells in the bone marrow (normoblasts).

Aetiology/pathophysiology

Macrocytic normoblastic anaemia may be physiological (in pregnancy and in neonates), pathological, e.g.

alcohol, liver disease, hypothyroidism or drug induced, e.g. azathioprine. The exact mechanism is not understood, but there is often an increased lipid deposition in the membrane of the red cells.

Clinical features
Symptoms and signs of anaemia (see page 467).

Investigations
Full blood count shows anaemia with large cells (raised MCV). Serum vitamin B_{12} and red cell folate are normal. Thyroid function tests and liver function tests (including γGT) should be performed.

Management
Any underlying cause should be treated where appropriate.

Megaloblastic anaemia

Definition
Megaloblastic anaemia is characterised by the presence in the bone marrow of megaloblasts and macrocytic red blood cells.

Aetiology
The causes of megaloblastic are shown in Fig. 12.3.

Pathophysiology
Defective DNA synthesis (see Fig. 12.4) causes delayed nuclear maturation in red cell precursors (erythroblasts), which are enlarged (megaloblasts) and develop into enlarged red blood cells (macrocytes). There is also abnormal neutrophil development.

Clinical features
Symptoms and signs of anaemia (see page 467).

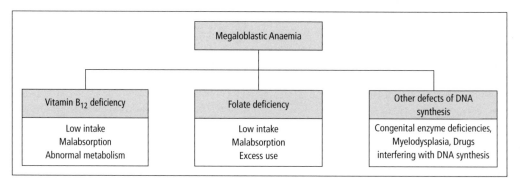

Figure 12.3 Causes of megaloblastic anaemia.

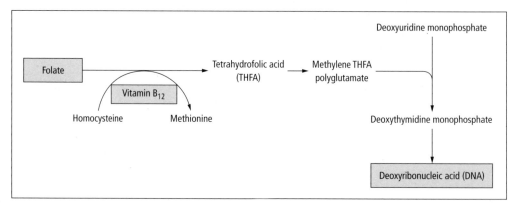

Figure 12.4 Simplified pathway of DNA synthesis and the role of vitamin B_{12} and folate.

Investigations

Full blood count demonstrates anaemia with macrocytosis (raised MCV). Blood film also reveals neutrophils with a hypersegmented nucleus. Serum vitamin B_{12} and red cell folate levels should be measured. For further investigations and management see below.

Vitamin B_{12} deficiency

Definition

Deficiency of vitamin B_{12} (cobalamins) causes macrocytic megaloblastic anaemia.

Aetiology

- Low intake occurs in vegans and chronic alcoholics. Vitamin B_{12} is found in animal products such as liver, kidney, fish, red meats, eggs and cheese. Increased requirements occur in pregnancy and haemolysis.
- Malabsorption may occur in pernicious anaemia (see below), terminal ileal disease (e.g. Crohn's disease), pancreatic failure and following gastrectomy or small bowel resection.

Pathophysiology

Vitamin B_{12} is absorbed mainly in the terminal ileum, by binding to intrinsic factor (IF) secreted by gastric parietal cells. There is 3–4 years supply stored in the liver. Vitamin B_{12} is involved in nucleic acid synthesis (see Fig. 12.4). It also controls fatty acid synthesis in myelin sheaths of nerves.

Clinical features

In addition to symptoms of anaemia, patients with vitamin B_{12} deficiency may have neurological complications such as peripheral neuropathy, optic atrophy, subacute combined cord degeneration and dementia.

Investigations

The diagnosis is made by serum B_{12} levels. The Schilling test is used to identify the cause of the deficiency (see Table 12.4). Gastrointestinal endoscopy can be used to demonstrates gastric atrophy and achlorydia. Intrinsic factor antibodies can be detected in the serum of 50% of patients with pernicious anaemia as the cause.

Management

Treatment is by vitamin B_{12} replacement, which may be given orally if due to dietary insufficiency or

Table 12.4 Schilling test

Part I
- A loading dose of parenteral vitamin B_{12} is given to the fasting patient to saturate plasma and liver binding sites. Oral radioactive vitamin B_{12} is then given.
- Urinary excretion of labelled vitamin B_{12} is then measured.
- A high urinary excretion indicates a primary deficiency of B_{12} intake, whereas a low urinary excretion indicates malabsorption of B_{12}, which should be further investigated.

Part II
- Oral radioactive B_{12} complexed to intrinsic factor is given.
- If excretion is increased, this indicates that lack of IF is responsible for the malabsorption. If not, there is malabsorption due to some other cause.

intramuscularly if due to malabsorption. Complications of treatment include hypokalaemia, gout and the unmasking of iron deficiency.

Pernicious anaemia

Definition

In pernicious anaemia, atrophy of the gastric mucosa causes failure of intrinsic factor production, vitamin B_{12} deficiency and megaloblastic anaemia.

Incidence

1 in 8000 over 60 years.

Age

More common in the elderly.

Sex

F > M

Aetiology/pathophysiology

The gastric parietal cells normally produce intrinsic factor (IF) that binds to vitamin B_{12} allowing it to be absorbed in the terminal ileum.

- 90% of patients with pernicious anaemia have autoantibodies to the gastric parietal cells; however, autoantibodies may occur in association with gastric atrophy without pernicious anaemia.
- 50% of patients have antibodies to intrinsic factor, which are specific for this diagnosis and may be

blocking antibodies (bind to intrinsic factor and prevents binding to B_{12}) or binding antibodies (bind to the IF:B_{12} complex preventing absorption).

Atrophic gastritis is present with plasma cell and lymphoid infiltration affecting the fundus and body of the stomach. There is achlorydia and absent secretion of intrinsic factor.

Clinical features

The onset of pernicious anaemia is usually insidious with worsening symptoms of anaemia (see page 467). Patients may also have neurological complications of vitamin B_{12} deficiency (see page 471).

Investigations

Full blood count will demonstrate a macrocytic anaemia (raised MCV). Vitamin B_{12} is low. The Schilling test is used to differentiate the causes of vitamin B_{12} deficiency (see Table 12.4).

Management

Parenteral vitamin B_{12} replacement is required for life. Clinical improvement can be seen in 48 hours and a reticulocytosis can be demonstrated 2–3 days after commencing therapy.

Folate deficiency

Definition

Deficiency of folate causes a megaloblastic anaemia due to abnormal DNA synthesis.

Aetiology/pathophysiology

Folic acid is the precursor to the folates, which are involved in the synthesis of DNA (see Fig. 12.4). Causes of folic acid deficiency:

- Low intake is most common in elderly, people living in poor social conditions and chronic alcoholics. Folic acid is found in fresh vegetables and meat, but may be destoyed by overcooking.
- Malapsorption occurs due to small bowel disease (especially if affecting the jejunum) such as coeliac disease.
- Increased requirements occur in haemolytic conditions, myeloproliferative disorders, other rapidly growing tumours and severe inflammatory disease. In pregnancy there are increased requirements and

deficiency is associated with neural tube defects in the fetus.
- Antifolate drugs include methotrexate, trimethoprim, anticonvulsants and alcohol.

Clinical features

Symptoms and signs of anaemia (see page 467). Patients may also complain of a sore mouth and tongue (glossitis).

Investigations

Red cell folate level are low. In many cases the cause is not obvious and further investigations may have to be undertaken including barium follow through or upper gastrointestinal endoscopy and biopsy.

Management

The underlying cause should be identified and treated where possible. Prior to treatment with oral folic acid supplements, concurrent vitamin B_{12} deficiency must be identified and treated to avoid the neurological complications of B_{12} deficiency. Prophylaxis is advised in pregnancy, haemolytic anaemias, premature babies, dialysis patients and those taking methotrexate.

Haemolytic anaemia

Definition

Haemolytic anaemia is defined as an anaemia resulting from increased breakdown of red cells and shortened red blood cell life span (normal 120 days).

Aetiology

The causes of haemolytic anaemia are shown in Table 12.5.

Pathophysiology

Shortening of the life span of red cells does not always cause anaemia. If the increased loss can be compensated for by an up-regulation of the bone marrow (which can increase output between six and eight times) then a compensated haemolytic state will arise. In addition to bone marrow up-regulation, reticulocytes (red cell precursors) may be released prematurely. Haemolysis can be divided into two categories:

Table 12.5 Causes of haemolytic anaemia

Type	Mechanism	Examples
Inherited	Red cell membrane defects	Hereditary spherocytosis
		Hereditary elliptocytosis
	Haemoglobin abnormalities	Thalassaemia
		Sickle cell disease
	Metabolic defects	Glucose-6-phosphate dehydrogenase deficiency
		Pyruvate kinase deficiency
Acquired	Immune	
	Autoimmune	Warm autoimmune disease
		Cold autoimmune disease
	Alloimmune	Haemolytic transfusion reactions
		Haemolytic disease of the newborn
		Post allogeneic bone marrow/organ transplant
		Drug induced
	Non-immune	
	Membrane	Paroxysmal nocturnal haemoglobinuria
	Mechanical	Micro angiopathic haemolytic anaemia
		Valve prosthesis
	Systemic	Secondary to renal and liver failure
	Miscellaneous	Infections, e.g. malaria
		Drugs and chemicals causing membrane damage
		Hypersplenism
		Burns

- Extravascular haemolysis: This is the more common type in which the red cells are removed predominantly in the spleen by macrophages.
- Intravascular haemolysis: Red blood cells are broken down within the circulation releasing haemoglobin, which is scavenged by haptoglobin.

Complications

A chronically high serum bilirubin predisposes to the formation of pigment gallstones. Chronic haemolysis predisposes to folate deficiency and thus levels should be monitored and replacement given as required. Parvovirus infections that cause a temporary bone marrow failure may result in an aplastic crisis.

Investigations

- Haemolysis is suggested by a rise in bilirubin, high urinary urobilinogen (due to bilirubin breakdown in the intestine) and reduced plasma haptoglobin. In intravascular haemolysis, red cell fragments are seen in the blood film, whereas spherocytes may be present in extravascular haemolysis. The reduced red cell life span can be demonstrated using labelled red cells.

- Haemolysis results in an increase in red cell production by the bone marrow, which is detected by a peripheral blood reticulocytosis.
- There may be evidence of abnormal red cells depending on the underlying cause.

Inherited haemolytic anaemia

Hereditary spherocytosis

Definition

An autosomal dominant condition in which the red cells are spherical. Hereditary elliptocytosis is an autosomal dominant condition similar but clinically milder than hereditary spherocytosis.

Incidence

Commonest inherited haemolytic anaemia; 1 in 5000.

Aetiology/pathophysiology

There is a high new mutation rate with 25% of patients not having an affected parent. The underlying cause is a weakness in the link between the cytoskeleton and the red cell membrane. This may be a quantitative or functional abnormality of any of the membrane proteins (spectrin, ankyrin, protein 4.1). Part of the abnormally weak cell membrane is removed as the cells pass through the spleen, changing the cell shape from a biconcave disc to a sphere. These cells are more rigid than normal and are subject to further damage in the microcirculation.

Clinical features

Spherocytosis may present as neonatal jaundice or anaemia with chronic malaise and splenomegaly. Normal infections cause a relative increase in haemolysis and may result in jaundice. Complications as for haemolytic anaemia may occur (see page 473).

Investigations

Anaemia is usually mild. A blood film will demonstrate the spherocytes, but this cell morphology is not diagnostic. The diagnosis can be confirmed by demonstrating the osmotic fragility of the red blood cells.

Management

Splenectomy is often required but should be delayed to adulthood if possible to prevent overwhelming septicaemia from encapsulated organisms. Patients are given pneumococcal vaccinations and prophylactic antibiotics post splenectomy.

Haemoglobinopathies

Haemoglobinopathies are abnormalities in the normal structure of the haemoglobin molecule. Normal haemoglobin is made up of four polypeptide chains each containing a haem group. HbA is the main adult form comprising two α chains and two β chains. Adults also have a minor haemoglobin HbA$_2$, which makes up around 2% of the circulating haemoglobin and consists of two α chains and two δ chains. Abnormal haemoglobins result from:
- Abnormal globin chain production such as thalassaemia.
- Abnormal structure of the globin chain in sickle cell disease.

Sickle cell anaemia

Definition

Autosomal recessive condition in which there is abnormal structure of the globin chain.

Incidence

Most common haemoglobinopathy.

Age

As HbF synthesis is normal, it presents at 6 months.

Sex

M = F

Geography

Occurs most frequently in Africa, Middle East, India and the Mediterranean.

Aetiology

A point mutation on chromosome 11 results in a substitution valine for glutamine at the sixth codon on the β globin chain to form haemoglobin (Hb)S. Infection, dehydration, hypoxia and cold may precipitate a sickle crisis. Classical sickle cell anaemia is a result of the presence of two mutations, i.e. HbSS, other combinations that produce sickle cell anaemia include Sβ thal, SD, SE and SC variants.

Pathophysiology

HbS molecules, when deoxygenated tend to aggregate into rigid polymers. The red blood cells become inflexible and sickle shaped and become trapped in the microcirculation, especially within bones, resulting in microvessel occlusion.

Clinical features

Sickle cell trait (the carrier state) is asymptomatic, but offers protection against falciparum malaria. Sickle cell anaemia is a clinical spectrum ranging from asymptomatic to severe haemolytic anaemia and recurrent sickle crises. Painful vascular occlusive crises typically produce symptoms of bone pain and pleuritic chest pain with a low-grade fever. Severe occlusive crises may result in seizures and hemiparesis due to cerebral vessel occlusion, haematuria due to occlusion of the renal microcirculation, priapism, splenic infarcts and liver damage. Other patterns of crisis:
- Acute sequestration (pooling of blood in liver and spleen) requires transfusion for apparent hypovolaemia.
- Pulmonary infarction may occur in association with pneumonitis termed acute chest syndrome.

Complications

Patients have a susceptibility to infections including streptococcal infections and osteomyelitis often due to salmonella. Avascular necrosis particularly of the femoral head may occur. Patients may develop renal failure due to recurrent renal damage and papillary necrosis. Retinal detachment and proliferative retinopathy may result in blindness. See also complications of haemolytic anaemia (page 473).

Investigations

- Full blood count shows anaemia. Blood film shows a high reticulocyte count and sickle shaped red blood cells.
- Sickle screening tests use a reducing solution, which causes HbS to precipitate. They are used as a first line test and for screening preoperatively.
- Haemoglobin electrophoresis is used to diagnose both sickle cell trait and sickle cell disease (see Fig. 12.5).
- X-ray of the tubular bones may show destruction and medullary sclerosis together with periosteal bone formation.

Management

Treatment is largely symptomatic with prophylactic antibiotics, folic acid and pneumococcal vaccination. Management of a painful crisis includes oxygenation, adequate hydration and analgesia. Any associated bacterial infection should be treated with antibiotics. Acute sequestration requires blood transfusion, as patients become shocked. Severe crises such as priapism, acute chest syndrome or cerebral infarction require exchange blood transfusions to remove sickle cells. Transfusions may also be indicated in patients with regular severe crises and preoperatively.

Prognosis

There is marked variation in the severity of the condition, some patients have a relatively normal life span with few complications. In the most severe cases patients die from severe infarctions or sequestration.

α-Thalassaemia

Definition

Inherited haemoglobinopathy with defective synthesis of the α-globulin genes. It is mainly found in the Far East, Middle East and Africa.

Aetiology

α-Thalassaemia is caused by gene deletions. There are four copies of the α gene, two on each chromosome 16. Deletion may be of one or both α chain genes on each of the chromosomes.

Clinical features

- Deletion of all four copies of the α gene ($-/-$) prevents production of any viable haemoglobin. This disorder is also termed haemoglobin Bart's (γ_4) hydrops syndrome and results in a stillbirth or neonatal death.
- Deletion of three genes ($-/\alpha-$) causes HbH disease (a moderate anaemia with splenomegaly and the production of HbH (β_4) from the excess β chains). Treatment is not usually required.
- Deletion of one ($-\alpha/\alpha\alpha$) or two genes ($-\alpha/-\alpha$ or $-/\alpha\alpha$) causes α-thalassaemia trait in which there are microcytic red blood cells with or without a mild anaemia.

Investigations

Full blood count shows microcytosis with or without anaemia. The diagnosis may be confirmed by quantitative globin chain synthesis.

β-Thalassaemia

Definition

Inherited haemoglobinopathy with defective synthesis of the β-globulin chain.

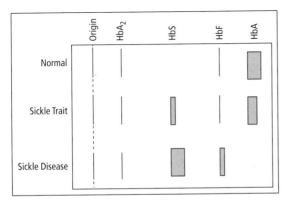

Figure 12.5 Haemoglobin electrophoresis in sickle cell anaemia.

Incidence

In the Mediterranean there is a carrier rate of 10–15%.

Age

Congenital

Sex

No sexual preponderance.

Geography

Most common in Asian and Mediterranean races.

Aetiology/pathophysiology

β-Thalassaemia results from point mutation in the β globin gene; over 100 defects have been characterised. These mutations may result in no β chain production (β^0) or very reduced production (β^+).

- Patients homozygous for β^0 or β^+ have very little or no production of β globin and have the clinical picture of β-thalassaemia major.
- Patients heterozygous for β^0 or β^+ have reduced β chain production and have a milder clinical picture termed β-thalassaemia minor.

Excess α chains precipitate in the red blood cells or combine with δ resulting in increased HbA$_2$, and γ resulting in increased levels of fetal haemoglobin (HbF).

- If there are defects in both β and δ genes, patients have thalassaemia intermedia (homozygous) or thalassaemia minor (heterozygous).
- If there are defects in β, γ and δ, this results neonatal haemolysis and thalassaemia minor in heterozygous patients. Homozygous combined β, γ and δ are incompatible with life.

Clinical features

- Thalassaemia minor/trait is asymptomatic with a mild hypochromic microcytic anaemia.
- Thalassaemia intermedia causes symptomatic moderate anaemia with splenomegaly.
- Thalassaemia major presents in infancy with failure to thrive and recurrent infections. At 6 months the production of fetal haemoglobin ceases and the patient becomes symptomatic with a severe anaemia. Extramedullary haemopoesis causes hepatosplenomegaly, maxillary overgrowth and trabeculation on bone X-rays.

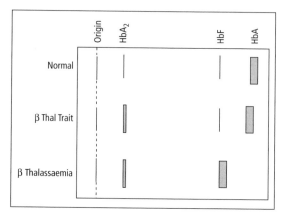

Figure 12.6 Haemoglobin electrophoresis in β-thalassaemia.

Investigations

- Full blood count shows anaemia with a microcytic hypochromic appearance. The reticulocyte count is raised and there are nucleated red cells.
- Haemoglobin electrophoresis with quantification of HbA$_2$ is diagnostic (see Fig. 12.6).

Management

- Thalassaemia minor does not require treatment; however, iron supplements should be avoided unless co-existent iron deficiency has been demonstrated. The partners of women with thalassaemia minor should be screened to allow appropriate genetic counselling.
- Thalassaemia intermedia may require treatment for worsening anaemia or complications of haemolysis or extramedullary haemopoeisis.
- Thalassaemia major and symptomatic thalassaemia intermedia are treated by regular blood transfusions to maintain a haemoglobin above 10 g/dL. This aims to suppress ineffective erythropoesis and prevent bony deformity, while allowing normal growth and development. Iron overload is prevented by the use of the chelating agent desferrioxamine, which is administered intravenously or by subcutaneous infusion. Splenectomy should be considered in patients over 6 years with high transfusion requirements. Bone marrow transplantation has been used successfully in young patients with severe β-thalassaemia major. Other treatments under investigation include gene therapy and drugs to maintain the production of fetal haemoglobin.

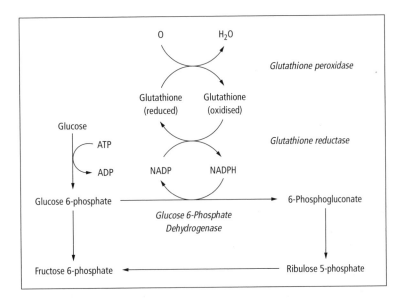

Figure 12.7 The pentose phosphate pathway.

Metabolic defects

Glucose-6-phosphate dehydrogenase (G6PD) deficiency

Definition
An X-linked genetic enzyme deficiency resulting in abnormal metabolism within red cells and haemolysis.

Incidence
Affects 200 million people worldwide.

Age
Congenital

Sex
Males affected, females have 50% of cells affected.

Geography
More common in Africa, Mediterranean, Middle East and South East Asia.

Aetiology
The gene for G6PD is carried on the X chromosome. There are over 400 structural types of the G6PD gene, it can therefore be considered to be a polymorphism rather than a defect. Differing isoforms have differing activity. The incidence of abnormal genes in some countries is so high that females may have two X chromosomes each with an abnormal G6PD coded. Random X inactivation (Lyonisation) means that some heterozygous females may also have symptoms.

Pathophysiology
Normally red cells are protected from the action of free radicals by glutathione. The pentose-phosphate pathway is used to keep glutathione in its reduced form. G6PD is one of the enzymes involved in the pentose phosphate pathway (see Fig. 12.7).

G6PD deficiency leads to haemolysis in times of high oxidative stress and results in

- Membrane oxidation and cross-linking of spectrin, which decreases flexibility and increases permeability of the red cell membrane.
- Oxidation of haemoglobin to methaemoglobin; the globin chains then precipitate as Heinz bodies, which are removed from the red cells in the spleen.

Clinical features
With such a wide variety of genes and enzymatic activity, a spectrum of clinical conditions occur. G6PD deficiency is a cause of prolonged neonatal jaundice. The WHO classifies G6PD deficiency into two categories:

- Class I: Extremely low G6PD activity causing lifelong haemolytic anaemia.
- Class II and III: No chronic haemolysis but susceptibility to haemolytic episodes at times of high

oxidant stress such as with infections or drugs, e.g. primaquine, sulphonamides, nitrofurantoin, ciprofloxacin, dapsone and naphthalene (mothballs). Favism is acute haemolysis following ingestion of fava (broad) beans.

Complications

After an oxidant shock the haemoglobin levels may fall dramatically with death following unless transfused.

Investigations

During an attack the blood film may show irregularly contracted cells, bite cells (indented membrane), blister cells (cells in which haemoglobin appears detached from the cell membrane), Heinz bodies and increased reticulocytes. Between attacks the G6PD level can be measured.

Management

Avoid causative drugs and foods, treat infections and transfuse as required.

Acquired haemolytic anaemia

Autoimmune haemolytic anaemia

Definition

Acquired disorders resulting in haemolysis due to red cell autoantibodies.

Aetiology

Autoimmune haemolytic anaemia is subdivided according to the temperature at which the antibodies bind to the red cells:

- Warm autoimmune haemolytic anaemia: Antibodies bind best at 37°C
- Cold autoimmune haemolytic anaemia: Antibodies bind at lower temperatures, this type is further subdivided into cold haemagglutinin disease (CHAD) and paroxysmal cold haemoglobinuria.

Pathophysiology

IgM or IgG antibodies are produced, which bind to red cells.

- IgM (and IgG which fully activates complement) cause lysis of cells within the vessel (intravascular haemolysis).
- IgG which only partially activate complement cause extravascular haemolysis with opsonised red cells either completely phagocytosed in the spleen or partially phagocytosed leading to the formation of spherocytes.
- The antibody coated red cells characteristic of autoimmune haemolytic anaemias are detected by the direct antiglobulin (Coomb's) test (see Fig. 12.8).

Clinical features

The clinical features, specific investigations and management are summarised in Table 12.6.

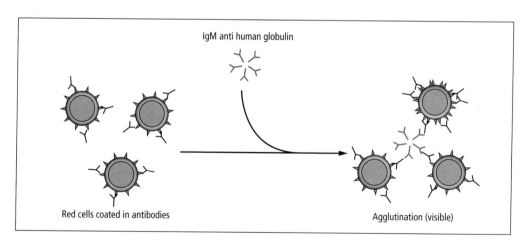

Figure 12.8 The direct antiglobulin test.

Table 12.6 Autoimmune haemolytic anaemia

Disorder	Aetiology	Pathophysiology	Management
Warm antibodies	Primary or secondary to autoimmune disorders, lymphomas, chronic lymphatic leukaemia, carcinoma and drugs such as methyldopa	IgG antibodies often specific for rhesus antigens. Complement fixation is unusual.	Corticosteroids produce a remission in ~80%. Splenectomy may be indicated if haemolysis is severe and refractory. Immunosuppressants such as azathioprine may be of value.
Cold haemagglutinin disease	May be primary or secondary to *Mycoplasma pneumoniae*, infectious mononucleosis and rarely other viral infections	IgM antibodies agglutinate best at 4°C, often against minor red cell antigens. Complement fixing.	Treat any underlying cause and avoid extremes of temperature. Steroids or chlorambucil may be tried.
Paroxysmal cold haemoglobinuria	Usually secondary to childhood viral exanthems or syphilis	Polyclonal IgG antibodies with specificity for the P red cell antigen. Complement fixing.	The haemolysis is usually self-limiting; however, transfusions may be required.

Aplastic anaemia

Definition
A pancytopenia due to a loss of haematopoetic precursors from the bone marrow.

Aetiology/pathophysiology
Aplastic anaemia can be either congenital or much more commonly acquired:

- There are several forms of congenital aplastic anaemia the most common of which is Fanconi's anaemia. This is an autosomal recessive aplastic anaemia with limb deformities.
- Idiopathic acquired aplastic anaemia is the most common form. It is thought to be due to an immune mechanism.
- Secondary acquired aplastic anaemia may result from direct injury to stem cells by external radiation or cytotoxic drugs. Other drugs may cause aplastic anaemia through dose dependent (e.g. gold) or idiosyncratic (e.g. nonsteroidal anti-inflammatory drugs) reactions, or by both mechanisms (e.g. chloramphenicol). Other causes include solvents, pesticides, industrial chemicals and insecticides and viruses (e.g. parvovirus B19 and HIV).

Clinical features
Patients present with the features of pancytopenia:
- Symptoms and signs of anaemia (see page 468).
- Recurrent infections due to leucopenia.
- Bruising and purpura due to thrombocytopenia.

Investigations
Full blood count and blood film will demonstrate a pancytopenia with absence of reticulocytes. A bone marrow aspirate and trephine shows a hypocellular marrow with no increased reticulin (fibrosis).

Management
Treatment should include withdrawal of any causative agents, supportive care (blood and platelet transfusions) and some form of definitive therapy. Blood and platelet transfusions should be used selectively in patients who are candidates for stem cell transplantation to avoid sensitisation.

Stem cell transplantation is the treatment of choice in young patients with acquired severe aplastic anaemia who have an HLA identical sibling.

Immunosuppressive therapy is used as first line treatment in patients over 35–45 years, younger patients without an HLA identical sibling or those with less severe aplastic anaemia. Regimens include anti-thymocyte globulin and cyclosporine. Androgens may be used as additional therapy.

Prognosis
The course is dependent on the severity of the disease and the age of the patient. In young patients who undergo stem cell transplantation the 3-year survival rate

is 75–85%. Immunosuppressive therapy has a similar 3 year survival but there is a significant risk of developing paroxysmal nocturnal haemoglobinuria, myelodysplastic syndrome or acute myeloid leukaemia.

Malaria

Definition
Malaria is an infection caused by one of the four species of the genus *Plasmodium*.

Incidence
Worldwide there are 300–500 million cases of malaria per year with a mortality rate of up to 1%. In the United Kingdom there are 1500–2000 cases per year, most of which are caused by *Plasmodium falciparum*. The incidence in the United Kingdom is rising.

Geography
Endemic malaria is found in parts of Asia, Africa, Central and South America, Oceania and certain Caribbean islands. In the United Kingdom, travellers to these areas who do not take adequate precautions are at greatest risk.

Aetiology
Four species of *Plasmodium* affect humans: *P. falciparum*, *P. malariae*, *P. ovale* and *P. vivax*. Transmission occurs predominantly by the bite of the female *Anopheles* mosquito although transmission may occur by blood transfusion or transplacentally. The life cycle of malaria is shown in Fig. 12.9.

Pathophysiology
Parasites consume red cell proteins, glucose and haemoglobin. They affect the red cell membrane making the cell less deformable and ultimately causing cell lysis. *Falciparum* induces cell surface adhesion molecules on red cells causing adhesion to small vessels and uninfected red cells. This leads to occlusion within the microcirculation and organ dysfunction. Resistance to malaria is conferred by genetic variation:

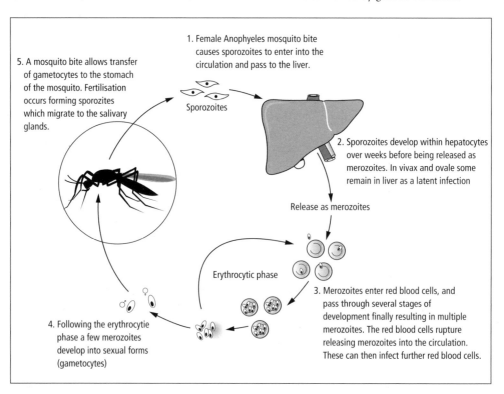

1. Female Anophyeles mosquito bite causes sporozoites to enter into the circulation and pass to the liver.

5. A mosquito bite allows transfer of gametocytes to the stomach of the mosquito. Fertilisation occurs forming sporozites which migrate to the salivary glands.

Sporozoites

2. Sporozoites develop within hepatocytes over weeks before being released as merozoites. In vivax and ovale some remain in liver as a latent infection

Release as merozoites

Erythrocytic phase

3. Merozoites enter red blood cells, and pass through several stages of development finally resulting in multiple merozoites. The red blood cells rupture releasing merozoites into the circulation. These can then infect further red blood cells.

4. Following the erythrocytie phase a few merozoites develop into sexual forms (gametocytes)

Figure 12.9 The life cycle of malaria.

- The Duffy red cell antigen is necessary for invasion by *P. vivax*. Many Africans do not express this antigen and have a relative resistance.
- The sickle cell gene reduces mortality in *P. falciparum* infections.
- *α* thalassaemia increases susceptibility to *P. vivax* reducing subsequent *P. falciparum* infection.
- *β* thalassaemia reduces parasite multiplication due to the persistence of fetal haemoglobin which is resistant to digestion by malaria.

Symptoms are associated with the asexual stages. In the gametocyte stage there is genetic recombination causing antigenic variation.

Clinical features

Most patients have a history of recent travel to an endemic area. Patients develop symptoms including cough, fatigue, malaise, spiking fever and rigors, arthralgia and myalgia. The classical description of paroxysmal chills and shivering followed by a spike of high temperature is only seen in the minority of patients. Other symptoms include anorexia, nausea, vomiting, diarrhoea and headache. Examination may reveal tachycardia, pyrexia, hypotension, pallor and in chronic cases splenomegaly. There should be a high index of suspicion for malaria in any patient presenting with symptoms following travel to endemic areas.

Complications

P. falciparum is potentially life threatening due to cerebral malaria (progressive headache, neck stiffness, convulsions and coma), severe anaemia (red cell lysis and reduced erythropoesis), hypoglycaemia, hepatic and renal failure. It may also lead to severe intravascular haemolysis causing dark brown/black urine (blackwater fever) particularly after treatment with quinine.

Investigations

Diagnosis is by identification of parasites on thick and thin blood films. Although the first specimen is positive in 95% of cases at least three negative samples are required to exclude the diagnosis. The thick film is more sensitive for diagnosis and the thin film is used to differentiate the parasites and quantify the percentage of parasite infected cells. Other diagnostic tests include ELISA antigen detection and polymerase chain reaction (PCR) tests. Other investigations should include a full blood count, U&E, liver function tests, clotting, urine

and blood cultures. If there are signs of neurological involvement a CT scan of the head should be performed but should not delay treatment.

Management

If causative species is not known, or if the infection is mixed, initial treatment should be as for *P. falciparum*.

- *P. falciparum* is treated by oral quinine, mefloquine, Malarone (proguanil and atovaquone), or Riamet (artemether with lumefantrine). If the patient is unable to swallow, is vomiting or has impaired consciousness intravenous quinine is used. Falciparum malaria can progess rapidly in unprotected individuals. Treatment should be considered in patients with features of severe malaria even if the initial blood tests are negative. Other supportive treatments include monitoring for, and correction of hypoglycaemia, blood transfusion for severe anaemia. In severe cases intensive care may be required.
- Benign malaria (*P. vivax P. ovale* or *P. malariae*) is treated with chloroquine although some *P. vivax* is developing resistance. *P. malariae and ovale* require subsequent treatment with primaquine to eradicate latent parasites in the liver (after exclusion of G6PD deficiency).
- Chemoprophylaxis is dependent on the area that is to be visited and specialist advice should be sought. In general where there is no chloroquine resistance weekly chloroquine is used. In areas of chloroquine resistance a combination of chloroquine and proguanil may be used. Alternative regimes include mefloquine, Maloprim (dapsone and pyrimethamine) or doxycycline. Prophylaxis should begin prior to entering an endemic area (in order to detect establish tolerance) and should continue for 4 weeks after leaving the endemic areas. Mosquito repellent nets and sprays, and protective clothing should also be used.

Myelodysplastic and myeloproliferative disorders

Myelodysplastic syndromes

Definition

Myelodysplastic syndrome (MDS) is a pre-malignant condition in which there are abnormal stem cells resulting in production of abnormal cells, anaemia, neutropenia and thrombocytopenia.

Incidence
20 per 100,000 per year over the age of 70 years.

Age
More than 80% of patients are over the age of 60 years.

Sex
M>F

Aetiology
Myelodysplastic syndromes are classified using the WHO classification dependent on the peripheral blood and bone marrow findings into:
- Refractory anaemia (RA).
- Refractory anaemia with ringed sideroblasts (RARS).
- Refractory cytopenia with multilineage dysplasia (RCMD).
- Refractory cytopenia with multilineage dysplasia and ringed sideroblasts (RCMD-RS).
- Refractory anaemia with excess blasts-1 (RAEB-1).
- Refractory anaemia with excess blasts-2 (RAEB-2).
- Myelodysplastic syndrome, unclassified (MDS-U).
- MDS associated with isolated deletion (5q).

Pathophysiology
The disorder arises from a single abnormal stem cell. MDS is initially indolent due to inhibitory cytokines, however over time oncogenes are activated and tumour suppressor genes inactivated resulting in a pro-proliferative aggressive condition which may progress to acute myeloid leukaemia (see page 486). Dysplastic stem cells are refractory to haemopoetic growth factors resulting in a peripheral cytopenia.

Clinical features
Patients with myelodysplastic syndrome typically present with symptoms of anaemia, thrombocytopenia (spontaneous bruising and petechiae or mucosal bleeding) or leucopenia (recurrent infections of the skin, mucosal surfaces or lungs).

Investigations
Bone marrow aspirate examination shows normal or increased cellularity with megaloblastic cells and sometimes ring sideroblasts and abnormal myeloblasts.

Management
Supportive therapy includes red blood cell and platelet transfusions and the use of antibiotics for infections. Allogeneic stem cell transplantation is potentially curative but is only used in the rare cases arising in young patients. In older patients chemotherapy may be used especially in the more aggressive forms of MDS. Patients with less aggressive forms of MDS may benefit from the use of haemopoetic growth factors.

Myeloproliferative diseases

Myeloproliferative diseases are characterised by the clonal proliferation of one or more stem cells in the bone marrow (occasionally additionally in the liver and spleen). The WHO classification includes chronic myelogenous leukaemia (CML), polycythemia vera (PV), myelofibrosis (MF), essential thrombocythemia (ET). These conditions have some common features:
- Extramedullary haemopoesis in the spleen and liver.
- Marrow hyperplasia often extending into the fatty marrow.
- Increased marrow reticulin.
- Platelet dysfunction, clumping or non-adhesion.
- Hyperuricaemia due to high nucleic acid turnover, particularly if cytotoxics are used.

There may be transformation from one condition to another or to acute myeloid leukaemia.

Chronic myelogenous leukaemia

Definition
Chronic myelogenous leukaemia (CML) is a myeloproliferative disorder arising from clonal proliferation of haemopoietic stem cells giving rise to a high peripheral white blood cell count.

Incidence
1 per 100,000 per year.

Age
Most common 40–60 years.

Sex
M>F

Aetiology/pathophysiology

Almost all patients have the Philadelphia chromosome, a balanced reciprocal translocation between the long arms of chromosomes 9 and 22 t(9;22). This results in the *c-abl* proto-oncogene translocating to the *bcr* gene producing a novel *bcr/abl* fusion gene which encodes Bcr-Abl tyrosine kinase.

CML has three phases possibly mediated by further genetic changes. Initially there is a chronic indolent phase lasting 3–5 years, followed by an accelerated phase lasting 6– to 18 months. Finally a blast crisis develops similar to an aggressive acute leukaemia.

Clinical features

Most patients with CML are asymptomatic, the disease is often found from an incidental full blood count. Patients may develop non-specific symptoms of fatigue, anorexia, weight loss, sweats and fever. On examination splenomegaly may be present.

Investigations

- Full blood count and blood film reveal a high neutrophil count with a left shift (immature granulocytic forms). There may also be an increase in other granulocytes (basophils and eosinophils), thrombocytosis and anaemia. In the chronic phase blast cells account for <10% of peripheral white blood cells. The blast count rises in the accelerated phase and blast crisis.
- Bone marrow aspirate shows a hypercellular marrow with an increase in myeloid precursors.
- Cytogenetic studies can be used to demonstrate the Philadelphia chromosome.
- Neutrophils can be stained for alkaline phosphatase, which is low in CML and high in neutrophilia caused by infection.

Management

- Hydroxyurea can induce a haematologic remission and decrease splenomegaly but does not treat the underlying cytogenetic abnormality.
- Interferon-α can achieve both haematologic and cytogenetic remission in up to 35% of patients but has severe flu-like side effects.
- Imatinib, a competitive inhibitor of the Bcr-Abl tyrosine kinase, is recommended for Philadelphia-chromosome-positive CML in the chronic phase in adults who are intolerant of interferon-α therapy or

in whom interferon-α has failed to control the disease. Cytogenetic remission is achieved in 70% of patients. It is also recommended for the treatment of adults with Philadelphia-chromosome-positive CML in accelerated phase or blast crisis provided they have not received it at an earlier stage.

Allogeneic stem-cell transplantation is used in younger patients with HLA-matched donor.

Polycythaemia vera

Definition

Polycythaemia vera (PV) is an overproduction of mature red blood cells due to a clonal proliferation in the bone marrow. Myeloid precursors and megakaryocytes may also be increased.

Prevalence

5 per 1,000,000 population.

Age

Most commonly presents over the age of 50 years.

Sex

M>F

Aetiology

Idiopathic disorder, although genetic and environmental factors have been suggested.

Pathophysiology

There is clonal expansion of a pluripotent stem cell capable of differentiating into red blood cells, granulocytes and platelets. Erythroid precursors in PV are very sensitive to erythropoietin leading to increased red blood cell production. Polycythemia results in increased blood viscosity increasing the risk of arterial or venous thrombosis. Platelet function is often disrupted risking bleeding.

Clinical features

Patients may be asymptomatic and the diagnosis made on incidental full blood count. Patients may complain of pruritus especially after a hot bath or shower. Hyperviscosity may result in headache or blurred vision. On examination patients may appear plethoric and have splenomegaly or hepatomegaly.

Complications

- Thrombosis may result in ulceration or gangrene of extremities, myocardial infarction, deep vein thrombosis, transient ischaemic attacks and stroke.
- Abnormalities in platelet function can lead to epistaxis, bruising and mucosal bleeding (including peptic ulcer disease) although severe bleeding is unusual.
- Increased blood cell turnover can lead to hyperuricemia and gout.

Investigations

Full blood count shows an increased red blood cell count, haemoglobin and packed cell volume. The whole blood viscosity is raised although plasma viscosity is normal. Polycythaemia vera can be distinguished from other causes of polycythaemia by an increase in white cell count, platelets and a high neutrophil alkaline phosphatase.

Management

Treatment is aimed at maintaining a normal blood count (PCV below 45%) and prevention of the associated complications.

- Venesection may be of benefit in treating symptoms but has not been shown to reduce complications. It induces iron deficiency and reduces whole blood viscosity but may increase the platelet count.
- Cytotoxic therapy is avoided if possible due to increased risk of acute myeloid leukaemia. Although hydroxyurea has been considered safe for long-term maintenance it is also associated with increased risk of development of leukaemia in comparison with venesection.
- Newer therapies under evaluation include α interferon, venesection with low doses of aspirin and anagrelide (for treatment of associated thrombocythaemia).

Prognosis

The median survival is 10–20 years with treatment. 10% of patients develop myelofibrosis on average 10 years after diagnosis with polycythaemia vera. 3% of patients treated with venesection only develop acute myeloid leukaemia.

Myelofibrosis

Definition

A myeloproliferative disorder characterised by an increase in reticulin and collagen in the marrow cavity.

Prevalence

2 per 1,000,000 population.

Age

Most commonly diagnosed 60–70 years.

Sex

M = F

Aetiology

Increased risk following exposure to benzene or radiation. Myelofibrosis may develop late in the course of polycythaemia vera or essential polycythaemia.

Pathophysiology

Myelofibrosis is characterised by proliferation of fibroblasts in the marrow as a response to growth factors secreted by abnormally proliferating myeloid cells. As the bone marrow cavity becomes fibrotic, extramedullary haematopoiesis occurs in the liver and spleen causing hepatosplenomegaly.

Clinical features

Patients may present with symptoms of anaemia, anorexia, weight loss, and night sweats. On examination there is massive splenomegaly. Symptoms and signs of marrow failure (anaemia, recurrent infections and bleeding) may be present.

Investigations

A blood film shows a leucoerythroblastic anaemia with teardrop poikilocytes, nucleated red blood cells and immature myeloid elements. Marrow aspiration is normally impossible, the trephine shows dense fibrosis.

Management

- Symptomatic management with red blood cells and platelet transfusions and haemopoetic growth factors. Iron chelation therapy may be required if multiple transfusions are necessary.

- Splenectomy may be required if the enlarged spleen is painful or to reduce transfusion requirements.

Prognosis

The median survival of patients with myelofibrosis is 3–6 years. Ten to twenty per cent of patients develop acute myeloid leukaemia.

Essential thrombocythaemia

Definition

A myeloproliferative disorder characterised by increased platelets due to clonal proliferation of megakaryocytes in the bone marrow.

Pathophysiology

Platelets although increased in number have disrupted function causing them to clump intravascularly leading to thrombosis, and to fail to aggregate causing bleeding.

Clinical features

Essential thrombocythaemia presents with bruising, bleeding and cerebrovascular symptoms. Initially there is splenomegaly but recurrent splenic thromboses lead to a small atrophic spleen.

Investigations

The blood film shows increased numbers of platelets and giant platelets. Bone marrow aspiration demonstrates increased megakaryocytes.

Management

Mild disease may be treated with long term aspirin. Patients with a higher risk of thrombosis are treated with hydroxyurea. Patients with life-threatening haemorrhagic or thrombotic events should be treated with thrombocytopheresis in addition to hydroxyurea. Angrelide is occasionally used.

Prognosis

Essential thrombocythaemia may eventually transform to myelofibrosis or acute leukaemia but the disease may not progress for many years.

Leukaemia and lymphoma

Acute leukaemia

Acute lymphoblastic leukaemia (ALL)

Definition

Clonal proliferation of lymphoid progenitor cells.

Incidence

85% of all childhood leukaemias.

Age

Predominantly seen in childhood with a peak incidence at 5 years. In adults incidence increases with advancing age.

Sex

M = F

Aetiology

ALL is more common in Down's syndrome and in syndromes involving chromosomal instability like Fanconi anaemia. Risk factors include exposure to excessive radiation and benzene.

Pathophysiology

In acute leukaemias there is replacement of the normal bone marrow progenitor cells by blast cells, resulting in marrow failure. Acute lymphoblastic leukaemia arises from the lymphoid side of the haemopoetic system (see Fig. 12.10). It can be subdivided into:
Common ALL arising from the common progenitors.
Pre B/B cell ALL.
Pre T/T cell ALL (50% present with a thymic mass).
The blast cells of ALL tend to form reservoirs within the testes and CNS.

Clinical features

Often there is an insidious onset of anorexia, malaise and lethargy due to anaemia. There is often a history of recurrent infections and/or easy bruising and mucosal bleeding. Other presentations include lymph node enlargement, bone and joint pain and symptoms of raised intra cranial pressure. On examination there may be pallor, bruising, hepatosplenomegaly, lymphadenopathy,

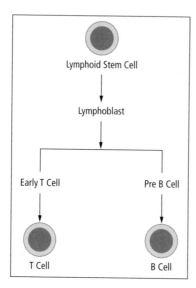

Figure 12.10 Lymphocyte development.

papilloedema, cranial nerve palsies, testicular enlargement and occasionally superior vena caval obstruction.

Microscopy

The normal marrow is replaced by abnormal monotonous leukaemic cells of the lymphoid cell line. The leukaemia is typed by cytochemical staining and monoclonal antibodies to look for cell surface markers. The FAB (French/American/British) classification is based on morphology (FAB L1- homogenous population of small cells, FAB L2 heterogeneous population of cells, FAB L3 rare, cells similar to those in Burkitt's lymphoma).

Investigations

Lymphoblasts are seen in a peripheral blood film. Full blood count shows a low haemoglobin, variable white count, low platelet count. Bone marrow aspiration shows increased cellularity with a high percentage of blast cells. Bone marrow cytogenetics and immunophenotyping is used to type the ALL and look for prognostic indicators.

Management

The current treatment protocol is UKALL-12. Which consists of:

- Induction: Phase 1 involves intravenous chemotherapy (daunorubicin and vincristine) oral prednisolone

and intramuscular L-asparginase. Phase 2 involves intravenous chemotherapy (cyclophosphamide and cytosine) with oral 6-mercaptopurine.

- Intensification: This involves intravenous methotrexate and folinic acid, with intramuscular L-asparginase.
- Consolidation: This involves several cycles of chemotherapy at lower doses.
- Maintenance: Therapy consists of 18 months of oral cytotoxic therapy with intravenous vincristine given every 3 months.

CNS treatment involves a combination of intrathecal methotrexate and cytosine and cranial irradiation.

Supportive treatment: Cytotoxic therapy and the leukaemia itself depresses normal bone marrow function and causes a pancytopenia with resulting infection, anaemia and bleeding. Supportive therapy includes red cell concentrates, platelet transfusions, broad-spectrum antibiotics and prophylaxis for pneumocystic pneumonia.

The role of early bone marrow and haemopoetic stem cell transplantation is currently under investigation.

Prognosis

Prognosis is related to age, subtype and inversely proportional to the peripheral blast count. Over 90% of children respond to treatment, the rarer cases occurring in adults carry a worse prognosis.

Acute myeloid leukaemia

Definition

Malignant expansion of cells from the myeloid cell line.

Age

Most common in the middle aged and elderly

Sex

M = F

Aetiology

Aetiology is largely unknown although previous exposure to radiation, benzene or chemotherapy are known to be precipitating factors.

FAB sub classification (see Fig. 12.11)

M0 Undifferentiated myeloblasts

M1 Myelocytic leukaemia without differentiation

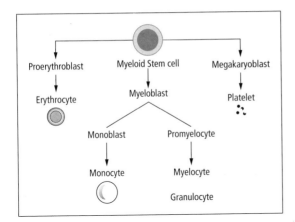

Figure 12.11 Myeloid haemopoesis.

M2 Myelocytic leukaemia with differentiation

M3 Acute promyelocytic leukaemia

M4 Acute myelomonocytic leukaemia

M5 Acute monocytic leukaemia proliferation of mono-
blasts

M6 Acute erythroblastic leukaemia (myeloblasts &
proerythroblasts)

M7 Acute megakaryocytic leukaemia – myeloblasts &
megakaryoblasts (uncommon)

- Patients with M3 (acute promyelocytic leukaemia) are
particularly prone to disseminated intravascular coagulation due to the presence of procoagulants within
the cytoplasmic granules of the promyelocyte. In M3
there is a characteristic chromosomal translocation
t(15:17), the promyelocytic leukaemia (PML) gene
and the retinoic acid receptor come to lie next to
each other and are therefore deregulated. Ninety-five
per cent of patients with M3 are induced into remission by treatment with high dose retinoic acid. This
is not sustained and chemotherapy should also be
used.
- Cells in M5 (acute monocytic leukaemia) secrete
lysozyme (an antibacterial enzyme) which can damage the renal tubules causing hypokalaemia. Gum
hypertrophy and hepatosplenomegaly is common
within this subgroup.

Clinical features

Often there is an insidious onset of anorexia, malaise
and lethargy due to anaemia. There is often a history of
recurrent infections and/or easy bruising and mucosal
bleeding. Other presentations include lymph node enlargement, bone and joint pain. On examination there
may be pallor, bruising, hepatosplenomegaly and lymphadenopathy.

Microscopy

Abnormal leukaemic cells of the myeloid cell line replace
the normal marrow. Morphologically the blast cells in
AML may contain a stick like inclusion – Auer rods.
The leukaemia is typed by cytochemical staining and
monoclonal antibodies to look for cell surface markers.

Investigations

Blasts are seen in a peripheral blood film. Full blood
count shows a low haemoglobin, variable white count,
low platelet count. Bone marrow aspiration shows increased cellularity with a high percentage of the abnormal cells. Bone marrow cytogentic studies allow classification into prognostic groups (e.g. t(8:21) and inv 16
are good prognostic indicators, whereas −7 and −5 and
poor prognostic indicators).

Management

High dose cytotoxic drugs doxorubicine, cytosine,
etoposide are given cyclically. Supportive treatments include red blood cell transfusions, platelet transfusions
and broad-spectrum antibiotics. Bone marrow transplantation may be used.

Prognosis

70% of those under 60 years will achieve remission with
combination chemotherapy although the majority relapse within 3 years.

Chronic leukaemia

Chronic lymphocytic leukaemia

Definition

Chronic lymphocytic leukaemia (CLL) is a leukaemic
proliferation of mature B lymphocytes.

Incidence

1.8–3 per 100,000 per year

Table 12.7 Staging of CLL

Stage 0	Lymphocytosis of blood and marrow
Stage I	Lymphocytosis and lymphadenopathy
Stage II	Lymphocytosis with enlarged liver or spleen
Stag III	Stage 0–II with haemoglobin <11 g/dL
Stage IV	Stage 0–III with platelets <100 × 10^9/L

Age
Peak diagnosis 60–70 years

Sex
M > F

Pathophysiology
Although there is a proliferation in B cells they have abnormal function resulting in hypogammaglobulinaemia. Staging is shown in Table 12.7.

Clinical features
Patients may be asymptomatic. Symptoms result from marrow failure (anaemia, infection and bleeding). On examination there may be lymphadenopathy and hepatosplenomegaly.

Investigations
- Full blood count reveals a low or normal haemoglobin, a white cell count >15 × 10^9/litre of which at least 40% are lymphocytes, platelets are low or normal. Autoimmune haemolytic anaemia/thrombocytopenia are present in 10%.
- Blood film demonstrates a high lymphocyte count and because these are fragile they appear as smear or basket cells.
- Hypogammaglobulinaemia may be present.

Management
CLL frequently requires no treatment other than supportive measures. Symptomatic disease may be treated with intermittent chemotherapy such as chlorambucil or fludarabine.

Prognosis
Prognosis is related to clinical staging.

Chronic myelogenous Leukaemia
See Myeloproliferative disorders page 482.

Lymphoma

Hodgkin's disease

Definition
Hodgkin's disease is a primary neoplastic disease of lymphoid cells characterised by proliferation of an atypical form of lymphoid cell termed Reed-Sternberg (RS) cell.

Incidence
4 per 100,000 per year.

Age
Bimodal distribution with a peak in young adults (15–34 years) and older individuals (>55).

Sex
2M : 1F

Aetiology
Infectious agents particularly Epstein Barr virus have been implicated. There is an increased incidence in patients with HIV. There may be a genetic predisposition.

Pathophysiology
RS cells are a clonal proliferation of B lymphocytes arising from the germinal centres of lymph nodes. They do not produce antibodies. Some of the clinical manifestations are attributed to the production of cytokines. Oncogenes have been implicated in the pathophysiology, upregulation of *bcl2* has been shown to be of prognostic significance.

Clinical features
Patients present with a painless lymphadenopathy most often within the neck. Fatigue, anorexia, pruritus and alcohol induced nodal pain may also occur. Involvement of mediastinal lymph nodes may cause cough, shortness of breath and chest pain. B symptoms may be present (fever >38°C, drenching night sweats, weight loss of more than 10% within 6 months). On examination there is lymph node enlargement, and hepatic or splenic enlargement. The staging of Hodgkin's's disease is according to the Ann Arbor system, which is suffixed by B if B symptoms are present and A if they are absent (see Table 12.8).

Table 12.8 Staging of lymphoma

Stage	Disease
Stage I	Disease confined to one lymph node group
Stage II	Two or more nodes on the same side of the diaphragm
Stage III	Nodes on both sides of the diaphragm
Stage IV	Disseminated involvement of one or more extranodal tissue such as the liver or bone marrow.

Microscopy
Classical Reed-Sternberg cells are large cells with a pale cytoplasm and two nuclei with prominent nucleoli said to resemble owl eyes. There are three main types of Hodgkin's disease:
- Nodular sclerosis which affects predominantly young adults.
- Lymphocyte predominant disease seen mainly in young male adults.
- Mixed cellularity disease which mainly affects older patients.

Investigations
Diagnosis is made by lymph node biopsy. Staging requires chest X-ray, CT chest abdomen and pelvis, and bone marrow aspiration and trephine.

Management
Treatment involves chemotherapy, involved field radiotherapy or a combination depending on the stage of disease, whether the disease is bulky (defined as a mass >5–10 cm or a mediastinal mass larger than one third of the chest diameter) and the presence or absence of B symptoms.

Prognosis
The 5-year mortality from Hodgkin's disease depends on the staging (stage I and II – 10%, stage III – 16% and stage IV – 35%).

Non-Hodgkin's lymphoma

Definition
Non-Hodgkin's lymphoma (NHL) is a tumour originating from lymphoid tissue. NHL includes many subtypes but can be subdivided into indolent and aggressive lymphomas (see Table 12.9).

Incidence
20 per 100,000 per year.

Age
Median age at diagnosis 65 years.

Sex
1.5 M : 1F

Aetiology
Most NHLs are of B-cell origin. Tumours arise due to multiple genetic lesions affecting proto-oncogenes

Table 12.9 WHO classification of NHL

	B-cell lymphoma	T-cell lymphoma
Indolent	**B-cell chronic lymphocytic leukaemia/small lymphocytic lymphoma** B-cell prolymphocytic leukaemia Lymphoplasmacytic lymphoma Hairy cell leukaemia **Plasma cell myeloma/plasmacytoma** **Follicular lymphoma** Marginal zone B-cell lymphoma **Mantle cell lymphoma**	T-cell large granular lymphocyte leukaemia **Mycosis fungoides** T-cell **Mycosis fungoides** prolymphocytic leukaemia Enteropathy associated T cell lymphoma (EATL)
Aggressive	**Diffuse large B-cell lymphoma** **Burkitt lymphoma** **Precursor B lymphoblastic leukaemia/lymphoma**	**Anaplastic large cell lymphoma** Peripheral T-cell lymphoma Adult T-cell lymphoma/leukaemia **Precursor T lymphoblastic leukaemia/lymphoma**

More common conditions are given in bold

or tumour suppressor genes. Multiple chromosomal translocations have been identified. Other factors include viruses (Epstein-Barr virus particularly associated with Burkitt lymphoma), enviromental factors, congenital and acquired immunodeficiency and some autoimmune conditions. *Helicobacter pylori* is associated with primary gastrointestinal lymphomas.

Clinical features

- Indolent: Most patients present with painless slowly progressive lymphadenopathy. Lymph nodes may reduce in size spontaneously making it difficult to distinguish from reactive lymphadenopathy. B symptoms (fever >38°C, drenching night sweats, weight loss of more than 10% within 6 months) are not common at presentation. Bone marrow failure leads to anaemia, recurrent infections and bleeding. On examination there is lymphadenopathy and hepatosplenomegaly.
- Aggressive lymphomas: Most patients present with lymphadenopathy, extranodal involvement (gastrointestinal tract, skin, genitourinary tract, thyroid and central nervous system) and B symptoms. On examination there is bulky lymphadenopathy and hepatosplenomegaly.
- Mycosis fungoides (Sézary's Syndrome) is a rare cutaneous T cell lymphoma. The cells are trophic to the skin particularly the hands and feet, and result in plaques and lumps of associated with generalised lymphadenopathy.
- Extranodal lymphomas can occur at any site of lymphoid tissue (gastrointestinal tract, salivary glands, lung, thyroid, skin, gonads, bone and brain). Gastrointestinal lymphoma is particularly common in the Middle East and is also seen in association with coeliac disease.

The staging of NHL is a measure of its extent and distribution according to the Ann Arbor system, which is suffixed by B if B symptoms are present (see Table 12.8)

Investigations

The diagnosis is made by lymph node biopsy, cytogenetic studies of lymphoma cells may give prognostic information. Full blood count may show anaemia and thrombocytopenia suggestive of marrow involvement. Staging involves CT scan of the abdomen and a chest X-ray or CT.

Management

Treatment is dependent on the nature and distribution of the lymphoma. Available options include chemotherapy, radiotherapy and monoclonal antibody treatment. The role of bone marrow transplantation is under investigation.

Prognosis

Indolent lymphomas have a predicted median survival time of 5–10 years. Aggressive lymphomas are more responsive to chemotherapy but have a predicted median survival 2–5 years.

Paraproteinaemias

Multiple myeloma

Definition

Multiple myeloma is a malignant clonal proliferation of plasma cells.

Incidence

3 per 100,000.

Age

Most commonly diagnosed 60–65 years.

Sex

2M : 1F

Pathophysiology

There is expansion of a single clone of plasma cells that replace normal bone marrow and produce monoclonal immunoglobulins. Cleavage of these immunoglobulins result in the production of Fab and Fc fragments; the Fab fragment is termed the Bence-Jones protein and is found in the urine of patients with myeloma. If the antibody polymerises there may be hyperviscosity of the blood. There is also production of osteoclast stimulation factor causing lytic bone lesions, bone pain and hypercalcaemia. Incomplete immunoglobulins may precipitate in the tissues as amyloid. Renal damage may result from deposition of light chains, amyloid or hypercalcaemia.

Clinical features

- Marrow infiltration results in anaemia, thrombocytopenia and leucopenia.
- Lytic bone lesions most commonly in the axial skeleton may result in pathological fractures and bone pain. Spinal cord compression occurs in approximately 10–20% of patients at some time during the course of disease. Hypercalcaemia causes thirst, polyuria, constipation and abdominal pain.
- Renal failure.

Investigations

The diagnosis of myeloma is made if there are:
- Bone marrow aspirate has at least 10–15% plasma cells.
- Lytic lesions on skeletal survey.
- Monoclonal immunoglobulins in the urine or blood.

Other investigations include:
- FBC may show signs of marrow infiltration anaemia, thrombocytopenia, leucopenia.
- The ESR is raised if there is a serum paraprotein.
- Serum calcium may be raised.
- Hyperuricemia due to increased cell turnover.

Management

Chemotherapy with single alkylating agents improves prognosis. High dose combination chemotherapy with or without haemapoetic progenitor cell transplantation is used in younger patients. Recently, thalidomide has been demonstrated to produce a significant response in 30% of patients whose disease progressed following other therapy. Supportive care includes blood transfusion, radiotherapy for localised bone pain, correction of hypercalcaemia with bisphosphonates and management of renal impairment.

Waldenström macroglobulinaemia

Definition

Lymphoplasmacytoid proliferation resulting in a high level of a macroglobulin (IgM), elevated plasma viscosity and bone marrow infiltration.

Incidence

0.5 per 100,000 per year.

Age

Onset most commonly aged 60 years.

Sex

M > F

Pathophysiology

The abnormal proliferation of lymphoplasmacytoid cells produces high levels of IgM, which polymerises and results in increased plasma viscosity. Marrow infiltration may result in pancytopenia.

Clinical features

Hyperviscosity presents as weakness, tiredness, confusion and coma. Platelet opsonisation results in a functional deficiency and hence an increased risk of bleeding. Patients also often have peripheral lymphadenopathy. Marrow failure may lead to symptoms and signs of anaemia, recurrent infections and bleeding.

Investigations

- Full blood count: Haemoglobin, white cell count and platelets may be low or normal.
- Bone marrow demonstrates lymphoplasmacytoid cell infiltration.
- Protein electrophoresis shows an IgM paraproteinaemia.
- Plasma viscosity is raised.

Management

Chemotherapy produces a variable response. Plasmapheresis is used for symptomatic hyperviscosity.

Monoclonal gammopathy of undetermined significance (MGUS)

Definition

An abnormal clone of plasma cells producing a mildly raised monoclonal immunoglobulin without features of multiple myeloma.

Aetiology/pathophysiology

The immunoglobulin secreted is normally IgM. It polymerises and causes a mild increase in plasma viscosity. Unlike multiple myeloma there are preserved levels of normal immunoglobulins, no lytic bone lesions and no renal failure.

Investigations
Electropheresis of serum protein demonstrates a raised monoclonal band within the immunoglobulin region, without suppression of other proteins.

Management
A proportion of patients will go on to develop multiple myeloma and therefore all patients require followup looking for any increase in monoclonal protein levels or the development of lytic bone lesions.

Bleeding disorders

Clotting disorders

Haemophilia A

Definition
An inherited coagulation disorder resulting from factor VIII deficiency.

Incidence
1–2 in 10,000 two thirds of whom have severe disease.

Age
Inherited, age at presentation depends on severity.

Sex
X linked; males only affected.

Aetiology
Mutations on the X chromosome including deletions, frame shifts and insertions. One third of cases are new mutations.

Pathophysiology
The factor VIII complex is a cofactor in the intrinsic pathway's activation of factor X (see Fig. 12.12). VIII:c is coded for on the X chromosome and it is this part of the complex that is deficient.

Clinical features
As there are various mutations there is a resultant spectrum of clinical severity dependent on the level of normal VIII complex that is formed:
- Factor VIII levels of less than 1% present within the first 2 years of life with recurrent spontaneous bleeding.
- Factor VIII levels of less than 5% result in severe bleeding following injury although spontaneous haemorrhage does occur.

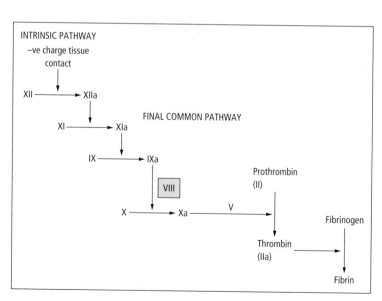

Figure 12.12 Factor VIII in the coagulation cascade.

- Factor VIII levels above 5% causes bleeding only following trauma or surgery, they may not present until later life.

Sites of bleeding include haemarthroses (bleeding into a joint causing pain and restriction of movement), muscle bleeds (often quadriceps, iliopsoas or forearm), intracranial bleeding (presenting as headache, vomiting and lethargy), haematuria and mucosal bleeding.

Complications

There has been significant HIV and Hepatitis C transmitted in factor VIII concentrates during the 1980s, recombinant factor VIII is now the treatment of choice. About 10% of patients develop antibodies to factor VIII:c making them very difficult to treat.

Investigations

- Activated partial thromboplastin time is raised, but correctable with 50% normal serum (ie not due to an inhibitor of coagulation) other coagulation measures are normal.
- Factor VIII:c assay is low, Factor VIII:vwf is normal.

Management

- Bleeding is treated by intravenous administration of factor VIII concentrates. Prophylaxis is the mainstay of treatment for those severely affected to prevent recurrent haemarthroses and permanent joint damage. Patients who develop antibodies to factor VIII concentrates may be successfully treated with recombinant factor VIIa.
- 1-desamino-8-D-arginine vasopressin (DDAVP) releases factor VIII from endothelial cells. The response is proportional to the pre-treated factor VIII levels and thus is useful in mild disease.
- Carrier detection is possible and antenatal diagnosis uses chorionic villus sampling or fetal blood sampling. Genetic counselling should be offered to patients and carriers.

von Willebrand disease

Definition

An inherited coagulation disorder resulting in platelet dysfunction and low levels of circulating factor VIII.

Aetiology/pathophysiology

von Willebrand factor (vWF) is a glycoprotein that has two functions in haemostasis. vWF acts as a bridging molecule between allowing platelet aggregation and adhesion to damaged endothelium. vWF acts as a carrier protein for circulating factor VIII increasing the half-life of factor VIII five-fold.

- Type 1 (autosomal dominant) is the most common type. It causes are reduction in the amount of vWF.
- Type 2 (usually an autosomal dominant) causes functional abnormalities of vWF. There are at least four subtypes.
- Type 3 (autosomal recessive) causes extremely reduced or undetectable levels of vWF.

Clinical features

Type 1 and 2 causes mild disease with bleeding following injury, menorrhagia and epistaxis. Type 3 causes spontaneous bleeding from early life.

Investigations

- Activated partial thromboplastin and prothrombin times are raised, but correctable with 50% normal serum other coagulation measures are normal.
- Factor VIII:vWF and VIII:c assays are low.

Management

Treatment of bleeding and prophylaxis in severe disease uses intermediate purity factor VIII concentrates or VIII:vWF concentrates. 1-desamino-8-D-arginine vasopressin (DDAVP) releases factor VIII from endothelial cells and is of value in mild to moderate disease.

Haemophilia B

Definition

An inherited coagulation disorder resulting from a factor IX deficiency.

Incidence

1 in 30,000.

Age

Inherited

Sex

X linked; males only affected.

Aetiology/pathophysiology

Mutations on the X chromosome including deletions, point mutations and insertions. Factor IX is the last component of the intrinsic pathway (see Fig. 2.12).

Clinical features

Similar to haemophilia A with mild deficiency causing only bleeding post surgery and trauma. Severe deficiency presents in early life with recurrent joint and muscle bleeds.

Investigations

- Activated partial thromboplastin time is raised, but correctable with 50% normal serum (i.e. not due to an inhibitor of coagulation) other coagulation measures are normal.
- Factor XI levels are low.

Management

Treated with factor IX concentrates. Patients who develop antibodies to factor IX concentrates may be successfully treated with recombinant factor VIIa.

Disseminated intravascular coagulation

Definition

Disseminated intravascular coagulation (DIC) is a generalised activation of the coagulation system causing widespread generation of fibrin within blood vessels and consumption of clotting factors.

Aetiology

Causes include Gram −ve and meningococcal septicaemia, disseminated malignant disease, haemolytic transfusion reactions, trauma, burns, surgery and *P. falciparum* malaria.

Pathophysiology

Widespread activation of intrinsic, extrinsic pathways and platelet aggregation causes consumption of platelets and clotting factors (a consumptive coagulopathy) resulting in a severe bleeding risk. Fibrin is deposited in small vessels within the brain, kidney and lungs causing ischaemic damage. Red cells are fragmented during passage through occluded vessels causing a micro angiopathic haemolytic picture.

Clinical features

The first signs may be bleeding into the tissues particularly mouth, nose and at venepuncture sites. Patients are shocked and acutely ill, they develop multi organ ischaemia and dysfunction.

Investigations

- Coagulation studies reveal prolonged clotting times and low fibrinogen levels.
- Fibrinogen degradation products are raised (D-dimer).
- There is thrombocytopenia, blood film reveals fragmented red blood cells.

Management

DIC is managed by treating the underlying cause and blood components using platelets, fresh frozen plasma, cryoprecipitate and red cell concentrates. Patients require supportive care and normally are managed in intensive care units.

Vitamin K deficiency

Definition

Deficiency of vitamin K, a fat-soluble vitamin, leads to a bleeding tendency.

Aetiology

Insufficient vitamin K intake or absorption. Sources of dietary vitamin K include vegetables, peas, beans and liver. Deficiency occurs in obstructive jaundice and certain malabsorption syndromes. Warfarin prevents the reduction of vitamin K to its active form leading to functional vitamin K deficiency.

Pathophysiology

Vitamin K is a co factor in the synthesis of clotting factors II (prothrombin), VII, IX and X. In its absence the factors do not have an active binding site and are therefore functionally deficient. Vitamin K is also involved in producing proteins required for bone calcification.

Clinical features

Patients present with bruising, mucosal bleeding and haematuria.

Investigations

The prothrombin time and the partial thromboplastin time are prolonged.

Management

Vitamin K (phytomenadione) can be given as iv. or im injections. If given orally in malabsorption syndromes it must be in a water-soluble form.

Acute immune thrombocytopenia purpura

Definition

Purpura arising secondary to a fall in platelet count thought to be of immune origin.

Incidence

Commonest cause of thrombocytopenia.

Age

More common in childhood, peak onset 2–10 years.

Sex

M = F

Aetiology

The cause is largely not understood but it may arise 1–4 weeks after a viral infection. Platelet associated IgG antibodies are detectable in the serum of patients.

Pathophysiology

The autoantibody binds to circulating platelets, which are then removed in the spleen. Clinical problems only become apparent when the platelet count falls below 50×10^9 per litre.

Clinical features

Children present with petechiae and superficial bruising, however in severe cases mucosal bleeds occur such as epistaxis and menorrhagia. Cerebral haemorrhages are rare. There may be a history of a viral illness in the previous four weeks.

Investigations

Full blood count shows the level of platelets. Bone marrow aspiration can be used to confirm the diagnosis (normal megakaryocytes) and exclude haematological malignancy.

Management

Treatment is often not necessary. Steroids and intravenous immunoglobulin (acts by saturating the Fc receptors within the spleen) shorten the course of the condition. Prior to using steroids a bone marrow aspirate must be performed to exclude leukaemia. Platelet transfusions are not used unless life threatening bleeds occur. In refractory cases splenectomy can be considered. Previous response to intravenous immunoglobulin is suggestive of a favourable outcome of splenectomy.

Prognosis

In children 80% of cases are acute self limiting with a full recovery within 6 months, most within 8 weeks.

Chronic idiopathic thrombocytopenia purpura

Definition

Chronic idiopathic thrombocytopenia purpura (ITP) is a fall in platelet count thought to be of immune origin.

Age

Chronic ITP is seen predominantly in adults.

Sex

F > M

Aetiology/pathophysiology

Chronic ITP may occur with other autoimmune disorders such as systemic lupus erythematosus and thyroid disease. Platelet associated IgG antibodies are often detectable.

Clinical features

Patients present with easy bruising, purpura, epistaxis and menorrhagia.

Investigations

Full blood count and blood film identify the low platelet count, a bone marrow aspirate demonstrates normal or raised megakaryocytes.

Management

Prednisolone may produce a complete or partial remission. Intravenous immunoglobulin works by blocking the Fc receptors in the spleen. The effect is transient but is useful in severe bleeding and predicts the potential success of splenectomy. Other drugs used include azathioprine, vincristine and danzol. Platelet transfusions are only used in life threatening haemorrhage.

Thrombotic thrombocytopenia purpura

See page 252.

Thrombotic disorders

Thrombophilia

Definition
Thrombophilia is a group of disorders resulting in an increased risk of thrombosis.

- Factor V Leiden (Activated Protein C resistance): This is the commonest form of thrombophilia. It is present in 2–3% of the population and results from a point mutation in the factor V gene. The mutation results in a resistance of factor V to inactivation by Protein C. This failure in the normal control of the coagulation cascade results in a thrombotic tendency. This risk is further increased in homozygotes, in women taking the oral contraceptive pill and in pregnancy.
- Protein C & S deficiency, Antithrombin III deficiency: Deficiency in normal factors that downregulate the coagulation cascade increase clotting tendency. Inheritance of a single mutation for any of these conditions results in recurrent thrombotic episodes in young patients.

For clinical features and management of venous thromboembolism see page 81.

Anti-phospholipid syndrome

See page 367.

Vascular causes of bleeding

See also Henoch Schönlein Purpura (see page 381).

Hereditary haemorrhagic telangiectasia

Definition
Rare autosomal dominant vascular disorder resulting in telangiectasia and recurrent bleeding.

Clinical features
Dilation of small arteries and capillaries result in characteristic small red spots that blanch on pressure (telangiectasia) in the skin and mucous membranes particularly the nose and gastrointestinal tract. Patients suffer from recurrent epistaxis and chronic gastrointestinal bleeds.

Complications
Patients are prone to chronic iron deficiency anaemia.

Transfusion medicine

Transfusion medicine

Blood grouping
Grouping is the process by which the patient's ABO and rhesus D status are determined. The patient's blood sample is separated into cells and serum. These are grouped separately in order to act as a double check.

- The patient's red cells are incubated with commercial antibody preparations against the A, B and D antigens. By examining the pattern of agglutination the blood group can be determined.
- The patients serum is incubated with red cells of known blood group (A, B, AB and O Rh$^+$) and the agglutination patterns are read to check the blood group.

Antibody screening
The patient's serum is also tested for atypical red cell antibodies using at least two Group O donors who express a wide range of antigens. Any IgM antibodies present will automatically agglutinate the donor red cells suspended in saline (see Fig. 12.13). IgG antibodies are detected by the indirect Coomb's test (see Fig 12.14).

Cross matching
A group matched blood unit (antigen matched if patient has atypical antibodies) is cross matched with the patient's serum. A full cross match consists of incubating the patient's serum with the donor red cells and then performing a direct agglutination and indirect Coomb's test as above. In an emergency, if the patient has no atypical antibodies a rapid cross match can be performed by briefly incubating the patient's serum with the donor cells and examining for agglutination.

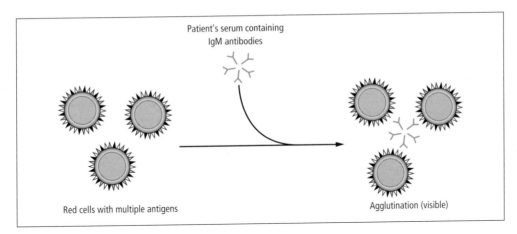

Figure 12.13 IgM antibody screening.

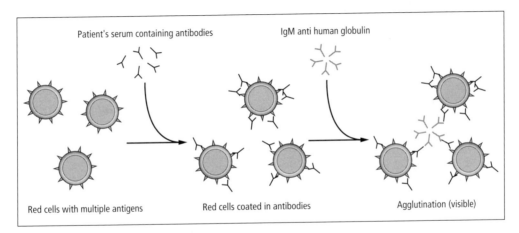

Figure 12.14 IgG antibody screening (Indirect Coomb's Test).

Table 12.10 Complications of blood transfusions

Immunological	Red cells	Immediate haemolytic transfusion reactions
		Delayed haemolytic transfusion reactions
	White cells/platelets	Non-haemolytic (febrile) transfusion reactions
		Post-transfusion purpura
		Graft-versus-host disease
	Plasma proteins	Urticaria and anaphylactic reactions
Non-immunological	Transmission of infection	Hepatitis, HIV, CMV, EBV, HTLV-1, Bacterial contaminants
		Cardiac failure due to volume overload
		Iron overload due to excessive transfusion

Transfusion complications

Complications to blood transfusions can be divided into immunological complications and other problems (see Table 12.10).

- Immediate haemolytic transfusion reaction is the most serious and is usually due to ABO incompatibility. There is intravascular haemolysis and coagulation. Patients become acutely unwell and shocked within a few minutes of commencing the transfusion.

- Delayed haemolytic reactions occur in patients previously sensitised to minor blood group antigens (eg Duffy, Kell, Kidd) by previous transfusion or pregnancy. Patient may develop anaemia and jaundice about a week after the transfusion.
- Urticarial transfusion reactions are of unknown aetiology but possibly result from antibodies reacting with plasma proteins in the transfusion. The transfusion should be slowed or stopped and an antihistamine given (e.g. chlorpheniramine).
- Non-haemolytic or febrile transfusion reactions are due to the presence of antibodies to leucocytes in the transfusion. Patients typically develop flushing, tachycardia, fever and rigors towards the end of transfusion.
- Anaphylactic transfusion reactions can occur in IgA deficient individuals (1 in 600 individuals) mediated by histamine and other vasoactive mediators (see below). Patients develop vasodilation, hypotension, bronchoconstriction and laryngeal constriction. It is treated as for anaphylaxis (see page 499). Any future transfusions should be with washed red cells, autologous blood or blood from IgA deficient donors.

If a transfusion reaction is suspected any ongoing transfusion should be stopped. The remaining blood unit and a sample of the patient's blood should be sent to the laboratory for repeat cross match. Other supportive treatments may be required.

Problems of massive transfusion

Transfusion equivalent to replacing the entire circulating volume within a 24 hour period is defined as a massive transfusion. This may be required following trauma, gastrointestinal or obstetric haemorrhage.

- Thrombocytopenia may result from the underlying bleeding and because there are no platelets in packed red cells. In severe cases platelet transfusion may also be required.
- Coagulation factor deficiency results from the dilution effect of massive fluid transfusion as there is a lack of factors in packed red cells. There may also be a consumptive coagulopathy due to ongoing bleeding. Patients may require fresh frozen plasma and/or cryoprecipitate.
- Hypocalcaemia results from the sodium citrate (which chelates calcium) used as an anti-coagulant

in blood products. If the ECG shows a prolonged QT interval i.v. calcium gluconate is required.
- Hyperkalaemia from degeneration of red cells within stored blood particularly if there is associated renal failure.
- Hypothermia from infusion of cold blood may precipitate a cardiac arrest.
- Acute respiratory distress syndrome may occur due to hypovolaemia, poor tissue perfusion or if patients are over-transfused.

Clinical immunology

Allergy

Hypersensitivity reactions

There are five basic types of hypersensitivity reactions (see Table 12.11)

Type I hypersensitivity (allergy)

On the first encounter with an antigen IgE antibodies are formed. These bind to a receptor on the surface of mast cells. On subsequent contacts with the antigen there is cross-linking of IgE on the mast cells which triggers them to degranulate releasing histamine and other preformed mediators (see Fig. 12.15). The reaction also triggers arachadonic acid metabolism leading to the production of leukotrienes, prostaglandins, prostacyclins and thromboxane. The clinical reaction is characterised by vasodilation, bronchoconstriction, and localised tissue oedema (see also anaphylaxis page 499).

Type II hypersensitivity (antibody dependent cytotoxic hypersensitivity)

Type II hypersensitivity is mediated by antibodies, these may be directed at:

Table 12.11 Hypersensitivity reactions

Type I	IgE and mast cells-mediator release and secondary inflammation.
Type II	IgG directed against self-antigens.
Type III	Immune complex mediated damage.
Type IV	Damage caused by activated T cells.
Type V	Stimulatory antibody mimics the action of a hormone.

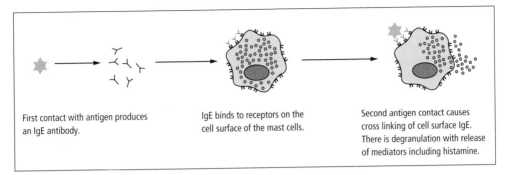

First contact with antigen produces an IgE antibody.

IgE binds to receptors on the cell surface of the mast cells.

Second antigen contact causes cross linking of cell surface IgE. There is degranulation with release of mediators including histamine.

Figure 12.15 Type I hypersensitivity.

- A normal 'self' antigen, e.g. Goodpasture syndrome, myasthenia gravis, or autoimmune haemolytic anaemia.
- A novel self-antigen may also become immunogenic e.g. α methyldopa (an antihypertensive) causes haemolysis by altering the cell membrane of red blood cells resulting in the expression of a red cell hidden antigen.
- Alternatively either the antibody (e.g. haemolytic disease of the newborn) or the antigen (e.g. transfusion reactions) may be foreign.

The cell becomes coated (opsonised) with antibody, which then activates the complement system leading to local tissue damage. An antibody coated target is also open to attack by phagocytes and killer cells (antibody dependent cellular cytotoxicity or ADCC).

Type III hypersensitivity (immune complexes)

Immune complexes are formed of antibodies bound to antigens. These are normally cleared from the tissues and the circulation. If they persist they result in local inflammation, cell accumulation, complement fixation and cellular damage. Immune complex mediated hypersensitivity can be divided into:

- External systemic which manifests as serum sickness, in which there is immune complex formation within the circulation, then tissue deposition resulting in local inflammation, cell accumulation, complement fixation and damage. Other examples include penicillin allergy and infective endocarditis.
- External local such as extrinsic allergic alveolitis in which there is local IgG production and cellular infiltration within the lung.
- Endogenous such as systemic lupus erythematosus and rheumatoid arthritis.

Type IV hypersensitivity (T cell mediated delayed type hypersensitivity)

This type of hypersensitivity reaction occurs when an antigen interacts with antigen-specific CD8 cytotoxic and CD4 helper T-cells. This results in the release pro inflammatory cytokines and causes the recruitment of multiple cells amplifying a small specific response into a large non-specific reaction. This is the basis of granuloma formation. Examples of type IV hypersensitivity include:

- Contact hypersensitivity: An epidermal reaction at the site of contact with the antigen often elicited by small molecules called haptens. Exposure to an agent such as nickel through the skin results in sensitisation of CD4+ T cells. Re-exposure to nickel results in T cell activation, activation of macrophages and release of local cytokines.
- Tuberculin hypersensitivity in which soluble antigens from mycobacteria administered subcutaneously results in fever, general unwellness, and an area of red, hard swelling at the site of injection.

Type V stimulatory

In type V hypersensitivity reactions an autoantibody is directly stimulatory via a target receptor. An example of this class is the antibody to the TSH receptor seen in Grave's disease, which stimulates the thyroid gland causing hyperthyroidism.

Urticaria (see page 390)

Anaphylaxis

Definition

Anaphylaxis is a severe allergic reaction consisting of urticaria and angioedema, hypotension and bronchospasm.

Aetiology/pathophysiology

Anaphylaxis is a type I hypersensitivity reaction (see page 498). On exposure to the allergen pre-sensitised mast cells secrete histamine, leukotrienes, prostaglandins and other mediators which increase bronchial smooth muscle tone, cause vasodilation and increase capillary permeability. Common allergens include foods (such as peanuts, eggs, shellfish and many others), antibiotics and bee/wasp stings.

Clinical features

Patients develop rapid onset of urticaria, erythema, pruritus and/or localised tissue swelling due to increased vascular permeability (angioedema). Bronchoconstriction and upper airway oedema may lead to severe airway obstruction. Patients may also develop vomiting and/or diarrhoea. On examination there may be tachypnoea, tachycardia, hypotension, wheeze and stridor. In severe cases vasodilation leads to severe hypotension, cardiovascular collapse and, if untreated, may be fatal.

Management

Anaphylaxis is an acute medical emergency. Patients require a rapid assessment of their airway, breathing and circulation:

- Airway/breathing: Patients with airway compromise including significant stridor should be treated with intramuscular adrenaline. Intubation may be difficult due to oedema and even with airway compromise bag & mask ventilation may be effective whilst awaiting response to adrenaline. Surgical airway by cricothyroidotomy may be necessary. Wheezing may be treated with nebulised β agonists, wheeze and mild stridor can treated by nebulised adrenaline.
- Circulation: If there is hypotension patients require intramuscular adrenaline. Large volume fluid resuscitation with crystalloids may also be required in refractory hypotension. Intravenous adrenaline is not used unless cardiovascular collapse and cardiac arrest have occurred.

H_1 antihistamines (e.g. chlorpheniramine) and corticosteroids are also given intravenously to all patients with anaphylaxis.

Subsequent events may be prevented by allergen avoidance, this may require referral to an allergy specialist for allergen testing (see page 467). Following an episode of anaphylaxis with hypotension and/or bronchospasm patients should carry at least a self-administration adrenaline device and in many cases a full anapylaxis kit including chlorpheniramine and steroids.

Hereditary angioedema

Definition

Inherited complement disorder resulting in episodic angioedema .

Age

Hereditary but may present in adulthood.

Aetiology

Inherited in an autosomal dominant pattern. Acute episodes may be triggered by trauma, exercise, menses or emotional stress.

Pathophysiology

Associated with C1 esterase inhibitor deficiency, which may be quantitative or qualitative. C1 esterase is a non competitive protease inhibitor that inactivates C1. In absence or low levels there is uncontrolled C1 activity with consumption of C4 and C2, C2a fragments cause oedema of the epiglottis and extremities due to release of vasoactive compounds (see Fig. 12.16).

Clinical features

Patients complain of recurrent episodes of swelling in the arms, legs, lips, eyes, tongue or throat. Intestinal swelling can be severe and result in abdominal pain, vomiting, and dehydration. Oedema of the upper airway may result in airway obstruction.

Investigations

C1 esterase levels are low.

Management

- Stanozolol and danazol may be used in an attempt to raise serum levels of C1 esterase inhibitor for long term treatment but their use in females leads to menstrual irregularities, fluid retention and androgenicity.
- Acute attacks may require treatment with fresh frozen plasma or purified inhibitor.

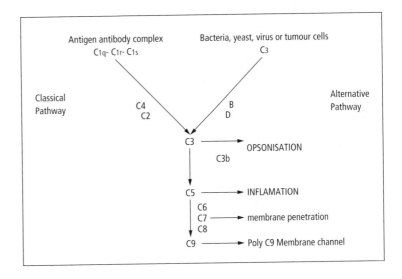

Figure 12.16 The complement pathway.

HIV

Human immunodeficiency virus and AIDS

Definition

AIDS or acquired immunodeficiency syndrome was first described in 1981 following the recognition of a group of homosexual males suffering from pneumocystis pneumonia and Kaposi's sarcoma. Two years later the causative human immunodeficiency virus (HIV) was isolated. Rapid advances in therapy have changed the natural history of the disease however various clinical states are recognised:

- Primary HIV infection/acute HIV infection/acute seroconversion
- Clinical latency, +/− persistent generalised lymphadenopathy (PGL)
- Early symptomatic infection/AIDS-related complex/"B symptoms"
- AIDS (criteria include a CD4 cell count below count $<0.2 \times 10^9/$ L)
- Advanced HIV infection

Centre for Disease Control in the United States (1993). In the developed world due to combination antiviral therapy, AIDS is very rarely seen except in undiagnosed patients who present with an AIDS defining diagnosis. It is however still a major problem in the developing world.

Incidence/prevalence

Epidemiological data collated by the World Health Organisation suggests that around 34,000 people in the United Kingdom were living with HIV in 2001. In the same year HIV accounted for 460 UK deaths. Worldwide however it is estimated that in 2002 42 million people were living with HIV, almost 35 million of whom live in Sub-Saharan Africa and South & South East Asia. 3.1 million people worldwide died of HIV and related illnesses in 2002.

Aetiology/pathophysiology

HIV is a retrovirus, an RNA virus that uses a reverse transcriptase enzyme to create a double stranded DNA copy of its genome, which then integrates into the host's genome. At present two virus families are recognised, HIV-1 and HIV-2 with 40% homology (see Fig. 12.17).

- HIV-1 varies with three genetic groups (M – Major, O – Outlier, N – non-M non-O). The M group is further divided into 10 subgroups (A–J).
- HIV-2 is endemic in West Africa.

HIV gains access to cells via a viral surface glycoprotein termed gp120 which interacts with CD4 on helper T lymphocytes and macrophages.

A co-receptor for T-cells and macrophages has been identified as chemokine receptor (CCR5), mutations in which may prevent cell entry and hence give some resistance to viral infection. A similar co-receptor on all lymphoid cells (CXCR4) has also been identified.

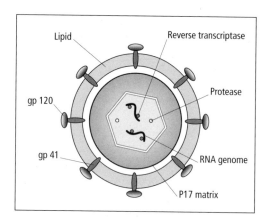

Figure 12.17 Schematic representation of HIV-1.

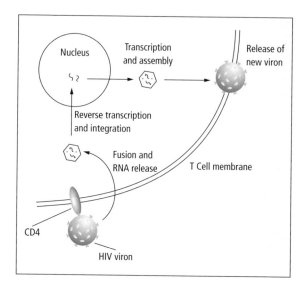

Figure 12.18 The HIV replication cycle.

Replication cycle

Human infection is usually with macrophage tropic (R5) viruses. HIV infected macrophages then fuse with CD4+ lymphocytes allowing the virus to spread. Once in the blood stream widespread dissemination occurs. An immune response to the virus results in a decrease in detectable viraemia followed by a prolonged period of clinical latency. The CD4+T cell count gradually decreases during this clinical latency, until levels fall to a critical level below which there is a significant risk of opportunist infections.

Following binding between gp120 and CD4 HIV is uncoated and its RNA is released into the cell cytoplasm. The action of viral reverse transcriptase converts the single stranded RNA genome to double stranded DNA, which is then transported to the cell nucleus and integrates into the host's chromosomal DNA. The pro-viral DNA is then transcribed, translated and the product assembled as if it were a normal cell constituent.

The resulting new viron is then released from the T-cell (see Fig. 12.18).

Transmission is by sexual intercourse (vaginal/anal), vertical transmission, blood products, intravenous drug use or by needle stick injury. Transmission co-factors include viral load, intercurrent sexually transmitted disease, exposure intensity, sexual practices and drug injecting practices.

Clinical features

- **Primary HIV infection/acute HIV infection/acute seroconversion:** Many patients are asymptomatic but may develop symptoms 2–8 weeks after exposure with fever, generalised lymphadenopathy, pharyngitis, rash, arthralgia, myalgia, diarrhoea, headache, nausea and vomiting. This illness is clinically difficult to distinguish from glandular fever. Rarely a neuropathy or an acute reversible encephalopathy (disorientation, loss of memory, altered personality and conscious level) may occur. These manifestations are self-limiting lasting up to 2 weeks from onset.

- **Clinical latency:** Following seroconversion the viral load and CD4 count varies until 6 months when it stabilises at a level correlating with prognosis. During this latent period most patients are asymptomatic, although the majority have symptomless persistent generalised lymphadenopathy (PGL) defined as enlarged lymph nodes involving two or more non-contiguous sites other than the inguinal nodes.

- **Symptomatic HIV infection and AIDS:**
  The Centre for Disease Control in the United States has produced a classification for HIV infection based on clinical state and the absolute CD4+ve T cell count (see Table 12.12). The patient's clinical state is divided into
  A. Acute seroconversion/asymptomatic/persistent generalised lymphadenopathy (PGL).
  B. Presence of 1 or more B symptoms (see Table 12.13).
  C. Presence of an AIDS defining illness (see Table 12.14).

Table 12.12 Clinical categories

CD4 count	Clinical State		
>500/mm³	A1	B1	C1*
200–499 /mm³	A2	B2	C2*
<200/mm³	A3*	B3*	C3*

*Patients defined as having AIDS.

Table 12.13 Examples of B symptoms/conditions

Bacillary angiomatosis
Cervical dysplasia / carcinoma in situ
Constitutional symptoms (fever >38.5°, diarrhoea)
   lasting >1 month
Herpes zoster that is recurrent or affecting more than 1
   dermatome
Idiopathic thrombocytopenia purpura
Listerosis
Oral hairy leucoplakia
Pelvic inflammatory disease with tubo-ovarian abscess
Peripheral neuropathy
Persistent, recurrent or refractory vaginal candidiasis

Table 12.14 AIDS defining illnesses 1993

Candidiasis of oesophagus or lower respiratory tract
Invasive cervical carcinoma
Extrapulmonary coccidiomycosis, crytococcosis
Chronic cryptosporidiosis or isosporosis with diarrhoea
Cytomegalovirus other than affecting reticuloendothelial
   system
HIV associated dementia
HIV associated generalised wasting
Kaposi's sarcoma
Lymphoma Burkitt's, immunoblastic or brain lymphoma
Mycobacterial infection (tuberculosis, avium, kansasii)
Pneumocystis jirovecii pneumonia
Recurrent bacterial pneumonia
Progressive multifocal lymphadenopathy
Recurrent salmonella septicaemia
Toxoplasmosis of internal organs

Infections and HIV

- Candidiasis: The commonest appearance is of pseudo-membranous creamy plaques which may be wiped off (distinguishes from leukoplakia) to reveal a bleeding surface. Infection of the distal oesophagus may cause retrosternal chest pain and dysphagia, or may be asymptomatic. Diagnosis is made on barium swallow or endoscopy. Treatment is with systemic anti-fungals such as fluconazole.

- Oral hairy leukoplakia is due to an opportunistic infection with Epstein Barr virus within the oral mucosa. It appears as unilateral whitish plaques on the side of the tongue. In the majority of cases no treatment is required, any coexistent candida should be treated, aciclovir may help although invariably it recurs.

- Toxoplasmosis causes encephalitis and abscesses in immunodeficient patients. Infections are due to reactivation of previously acquired infection. Patients present with headache, confusion, personality change, focal neurological signs, seizures and reduced consciousness. Fever may be absent. CT/ MRI shows multiple masses, often with ring enhancement and surrounding oedema. Treatment is with pyrimethamine and sulphadiazine.

- *Cryptosporidium parvum* is transmitted by the faecal oral route and causes watery diarrhoea, colic, nausea, vomiting and a severe fluid/electrolyte loss with severe weight loss. Stool microscopy shows cysts, stained with Ziehl Neelsen stain. Patients require rehydration. There is no satisfactory treatment.

- Cryptococcus fungal infection in HIV presents most commonly with meningitis. Patients present with headache, fever, impaired conscious level and abnormal affect. The classical neck stiffness and photophobia are rarely seen. A CT scan should be performed to exclude space occupying lesion prior to lumbar puncture. CSF is stained with Indian ink, serum and CSF antigen titre can be measured, cryptococci may be cultured from CSF and/or blood. Treatment is with iv amphotericin B or fluconazole.

- Cytomegalovirus can cause retinitis, colitis, oesophagitis, encephalitis and pneumonitis in HIV infected individuals. Colitis presents as abdominal pain and tenderness often in the left iliac fossa, profuse bloody diarrhoea and low grade fever. Stool culture is used to exclude other causes, endoscopy reveals an inflamed appearance of patchy colitis and vasculitis. Biopsy shows non-specific inflammatory changes, dense round (Owl's eye) intra-nuclear inclusion bodies in swollen cells. Retinitis may cause blindness and may present as loss of vision, field defect, acuity problems or pain. Eye disease is treated with ganciclovir (myelosupressive) or foscarnet (nephrotoxic) and must be followed by maintenance therapy.

- *Mycobacterium tuberculosis* infections are usually due to reactivation of latent infection in the context of

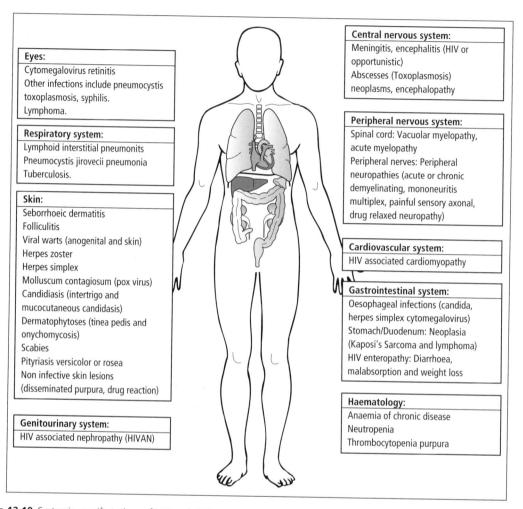

Figure 12.19 Systemic manifestations of HIV and AIDS.

progressive immunodeficiency. Symptoms may be less specific with fever, weight loss, fatigue and cough. Patients with low CD4 counts frequently have extrapulmonary disease, e.g. bone marrow, lymph nodes, CNS or liver. Drug resistance (often multiple) is a growing problem.

- *Mycobacterium avium intracellulare* causes infection via the respiratory or GI tract and causes fever, night sweats, weight loss, anorexia and malaise, hepatomegaly, chronic diarrhoea and abdominal pain. Anaemia is common. Treatment is with a four drug combination such as ethambutol, rifabutin, clarithromycin and amikacin.

- Patients are at risk of developing lymphomas most commonly non-Hodgkin's large B cell lymphoma in extranodal sites. These may result from reactivated or latent Epstein Barr virus. Gastrointestinal lymphoma is the commonest site. Presentation is variable (dysphagia in oesophageal, haematemesis in the gastric, obstruction or perforation in the colon, altered bowel habit and bleeding in rectal lymphomas). Intrathoracic lymphomas cause pleural effusion, mediastinal lymphadenopathy and reticulonodular pulmonary infiltrates. Oral lymphomas may present in the tonsils, alveolus, palate, or cheek regions. Cerebral lymphomas present with encephalopathy, brain stem abnormalities or cranial neuropathy. CT is used for diagnosis. Lymphomas are often refractory to radiotherapy and chemotherapy.

- *Pneumocystis jirovecii* and Kaposi's sarcoma associated with HIV are covered separately (see below).

Investigations

The detection of IgG antibody against envelope components of the virus is the most commonly used diagnostic test and PCR can be used to detect the virus. The disease is followed using quantitative PCR to determine the viral load, and by the CD4 T cell count.

Management

At present, there is no consensus on whether patients with primary HIV infection should be treated. Antiretrovirals are only of proven benefit in advanced symptomatic disease. In general treatment is commenced if the patient is symptomatic, there is a rapidly falling CD4 count or a high viral load. Three classes of drugs are available:

- Nucleoside-analogue reverse transcriptase inhibitors such as zidovudine, didanosine, zalcitabine and lamivudine.
- Non-nucleoside reverse transcriptase inhibitors such as nevirapine.
- Protease inhibitors such as ritonavir, indinavir.

In general two nucleoside-analogue reverse transcriptase inhibitors with one drug from either of the other two classes are used as first line treatment. Treatment is tailored according to compliance, side effects and the response to treatment.

Prevention strategies include safer sexual practice (reducing the number of sexual partners, use of barrier contraception), needle exchange programmes, screening of donor blood, semen and organs. Strategies to reduce vertical transmission include screening, caesarean delivery, maternal and neonatal anti-retroviral treatment and avoidance of breast-feeding. Health-care workers also require education, careful disposal of sharps and prophylaxis following needle stick injuries.

Prognosis

Untreated the life expectancy of an HIV infected individual is approximately 10 years. A few individuals are classified as long-term non-progressors with normal CD4 counts and low viral load in the absence of treatment. Prognosis has been dramatically improved by combination antiretroviral therapy, and life expectancy is likely to be more than doubled by this treatment.

Kaposi's sarcoma

Definition

A multi-focal disease caused malignant by proliferation of vascular endothelial cells.

Aetiology/pathophysiology

Kaposi's sarcoma in AIDS patients is particularly common in sexually transmitted HIV suggesting a sexually transmitted cofactor such as human herpes virus 8. Kaposi's sarcoma affects the skin, lung, lymphatic system and gastrointestinal system.

Clinical features

Skin lesions occur most commonly on the lower limbs and appear in various colours from pale pink, through violet to dark brown due to their vascularity. They may appear as plaques especially on the soles of the feet or dome shaped firm papules, which may ulcerate. Gastrointestinal Kaposi's sarcoma is usually asymptomatic but may cause perforation, obstruction, haemorrhage, jaundice from biliary obstruction, or protein losing enteropathy due to mesenteric lymphatic obstruction. Dissemination to the lungs and brain may occur.

Investigations

A clinical diagnosis, however biopsy reveals endothelial lined spaces interspersed by proliferating spindle cells.

Management

Localised or cutaneous lesions may respond to radiotherapy. Dissemination or visceral lesions require systemic chemotherapy.

Prognosis

Cutaneous Kaposi's sarcoma may be non-aggressive, however visceral and disseminated disease can be serious and life threatening.

Pneumocystis pneumonia (PCP)

Definition

Pneumocystis jirovecii (previously known as *Pneumocystis carinii*) causes pneumonia and disseminated illness in imunocompromised patients.

Aetiology/pathophysiology

Pneumocystis jirovecii is described as a fungus however it was originally thought to be a protozoan due to its existence as cysts, sporozoites and trophozoites. The reservoir for infection is thought to be animals, with aerosol spread. Clinical pneumonia is thought to be a reactivation of latent infection. The risk of pneumonia increases as the CD4 count falls, it is rare until the count drops below 200 cells/mm^3.

Clinical features

Gradual onset of non-specific symptoms of anorexia and fatigue followed by dyspnoea, non-productive cough, low-grade fever and tachypnoea. On auscultation there may be fine crackles or breath sounds may be normal.

Investigations

- Chest X-ray: The typical features are diffuse bilateral ground glass infiltrates progressing to widespread consolidation in severe cases (sparing of the costophrenic angles and apices).
- Bronchoalveolar lavage reveals trophozoites & cysts on silver stain or immunofluorescence.

Management

Intravenous high dose co-trimoxazole (3 week regimen). In significant hypoxia steroids are used, patients may require CPAP or mechanical ventilation. Patients with HIV require prophylaxis with co-trimoxazole or monthly nebulised pentamidine if they have a CD4 count of less than 0.2×10^9/L, an AIDS defining illness or following an previous episode of PCP.

Prognosis

90% of patients with a first episode respond to treatment and survive. Failure to respond or development of respiratory failure has significant mortality.

Nutritional and metabolic disorders

13

Nutritional disorders

Obesity

Definition
The World Health Organisation defines overweight and obesity in terms of the body mass index (weight in kilograms divided by the square of height in metres (kg/m^2)). A BMI over $25\ kg/m^2$ is defined as overweight and a BMI of over $30\ kg/m^2$ as obese. Although these definitions are useful, the risk of disease in populations increases progressively from lower BMI levels. A full consideration of obesity including prevention, identification, evaluation, treatment and weight maintenance of overweight and obesity in adults is being conducted by the National Institute for Clinical Excellence (NICE) with a proposed publication in 2006.

Prevalence
Worldwide more than 1 billion adults are overweight and 300 million of these are clinically obese. In England in 1998, 18–19% of individuals were clinically obese, a rate increasing dramatically. Prevalence increases by social class (15% in class I to 30% in class V).

Age
Prevalence increases by age up to 60–65 years.

Sex
F > M

Aetiology
Most patients have simple obesity. Some conditions associated with obesity are as follows:
- Drug-induced weight gain: Antipsychotic drugs, anticonvulsant drugs, antidiabetic drugs and steroids.
- Endocrine disorders may be associated with the development of obesity, such as Cushing's syndrome, hypothyroidism and polycystic ovary syndrome.
- Obesity is characteristic of some congenital disorders associated with hypogonadism, such as Prader–Willi syndrome and Laurence–Moon–Bardet–Biedl syndrome.

Simple obesity is likely to be a combination of genetic and enviromental factors:
- Genetic factors: Studies of twins, adoption studies and family studies all suggest the existence of genetic factors in human obesity. Animal studies particularly in mice have identified several gene defects inherited in both dominant and recessive fashions that can cause obesity. Some correlates with human obesity have been identified, although the exact genetic basis remains unclear.
- Prenatal influences and breast-feeding may influence obesity in childhood. Obesity in adolescence rather than earlier in childhood is a better predictor of adult obesity.

Several factors that are associated with a high risk of obesity have been identified:
- Low metabolic rate, increased carbohydrate oxidation, insulin resistance and low sympathetic activity.
- Lower socioeconomic class, lower education level and cessation of smoking.

Pathophysiology

The mechanisms of obesity are poorly understood. At a simplistic level weight gain results when the energy intake exceeds expenditure; however, both intake and expenditure are controlled in complex physiological systems. Women tend to gain excess weight after puberty, precipitated by events such as pregnancy, use of the oral contraceptive therapy and the menopause. Changes in lifestyle in men during the third and fourth decade lead to reduced physical activity and hence weight gain, which continues until the sixth decade. The quantity, type and pattern of food intake have all been implicated in the development of obesity. Both the appetite and the sensation of satiety (fullness) are implicated. Central adiposity (waist-to-hip ratio measurements >0.9 in men and >0.84 in women) increases the risk of many health problems such as diabetes and hyperinsulinaemia.

The control system is complex, it is regulated by a control centre thought to be located in the hypothalamus. Afferent signals to the control centre may include nerves, hormones and nutrients:

- Leptin production correlates with body fat mass; a leptin receptor has been identified in the ventromedial region of the hypothalamus.
- Gastric distention signals satiety.
- Hormonal signals including cholecystokinin and glucagon-related peptides inhibit food intake; neuropeptide Y is a potent stimulus for appetite. Monoamines, including noradrenaline and serotonin, also modulate the hypothalamic control centre.

The efferent of the control is energy expenditure. Approximately 70% of energy expenditure is for resting metabolic processes such as temperature control and physiological function. A further 10% of energy expenditure is related to the thermic responses to food. Catecholamine-stimulated lipolysis is mediated via β_3 receptors, and low receptor activity decreases thermogenesis. The remaining 20% of energy expenditure is due to physical activity and exercise.

Clinical features

Evaluation of obese or overweight patients requires aetiological factors and co-morbid conditions to be identified. Blood pressure, cardiovascular risk factors and diabetes should all be reviewed. Smoking cessation may lead to increase in weight; however, the health benefits of smoking cessation override the weight increase. The BMI should be calculated and the fat distribution documented by measurements of skin fold thickness, and waist and hip circumference ratio calculated.

Management

It is important to use goal setting in the management of obesity. Initially the aim is to maintain weight prior to establishing a realistic weight loss (average of 0.5–1 kg/week). Patients should be aware that weight loss induces a reduction in energy expenditure and therefore makes further weight loss more difficult. Techniques used include the following:

- Behaviour modification including examining the background of the individual, the eating behaviour and the consequences of the behaviour, usually conducted by psychologists.
- Dietary manipulation: Reducing the calorie intake to below expenditure results in weight loss; however, food diaries are recognised to be inaccurate as all patients underestimate their intake. Diets include balanced low-calorie diets, low-fat diets and low-carbohydrate diets, which are ketogenic possibly inducing calcium loss and tend to be high in saturated fat.
- Medications have a limited role in the treatment of obesity. Their use falls under guidelines issued by NICE.
  1 Sibutramine is a noradrenaline and serotonin re-uptake inhibitor and promotes a feeling of satiety. It should be prescribed only as part of an overall treatment plan for management of obesity in patients aged 18–65 years who have a BMI of 27.0 kg/m^2 or more in the presence of significant co-morbidities or a BMI of 30.0 kg/m^2.
  2 Orlistat inhibits pancreatic lipases so that ingested fat is not completely hydrolysed or absorbed. NICE guidelines dictate that Orlistat should only be prescribed for patients aged 18–75 years who have lost at least 2.5 kg in weight by dietary control and increased physical activity in the month prior to the first prescription. They must have a BMI of 28 kg/m^2 or more in the presence of significant co-morbidities or a BMI of 30 kg/m^2. Treatment is reviewed at 4 and 6 months to confirm that weight continues to be lost and should stop at 12 months.
- The use of surgery is also covered by guidelines issued by NICE. Its use is confined to patients with

morbid obesity, i.e. BMI of 40 kg/m^2 or more or be-tween 35 and 40 kg/m^2 in the presence of significant co-morbid conditions. Surgery is considered only if a patient has been receiving intensive management in a specialised hospital or obesity clinic, is over 18 and all available non-surgical techniques have been tried and failed. Previously jejunoileal and gastric bypass proce-dures were performed, which despite being effective were associated with significant side effects. Vertical banded gastroplasty either by laparoscopic surgery or open procedure is the usual procedure of choice.

Prognosis
The greater the BMI, the higher the risk for morbidity and mortality from diabetic-related illness and cardio-vascular, coronary artery and cerebrovascular diseases.

Malnutrition (including kwashiorkor and marasmus)

Definition
Protein–energy malnutrition results in severe weight loss in adults and can result in two syndromes in chil-dren: kwashiorkor characterised by oedema or maras-mus characterised by wrinkled skin due to loss of lean tissue and subcutaneous fat.

Aetiology
Many countries in the developing world are on the verge of malnutrition. Drought, crop failure, severe illness and war often precipitate malnutrition in epidemics.

Pathophysiology
It is unclear why insufficient energy and protein in-take causes marasmus in some cases and kwashiorkor in others, but both are syndromes of severe malnutri-tion. The oedema seen in kwashiorkor results from in-creased permeability of capillaries and low colloid on-cotic pressure (low serum albumin). Oncotic pressure is produced by the large molecules within the blood (albumin, haemoglobin), and it draws tissue water os-motically back into blood vessels.

Clinical features
- Adults and children with marasmus have loss of mus-cle and subcutaneous fat with wrinkled overlying skin.

Patients appear apathetic and complain of cold and weakness.
- Children with kwashiorkor develop oedema, conceal-ing the loss of fat and soft tissues, the hair may be discoloured and an enlarged liver may be found.

Complications
Malnutrition greatly increases the susceptibility to infec-tion. In children it has been shown to affect brain growth and development.

Management
Treat associated dehydration, if present, and any coex-isting infection. Often oral rehydration is safest, fol-lowed by nutritional replacement therapy. A gradual refeeding policy is essential initially 100 kcal/kg/day with 3 g protein/kg/day together with vitamins and minerals. Nutritional replacement is gradually increased until 200 kcal/kg/day.

Hyperlipidaemia

Definition
Increased concentration of specific lipoproteins in the plasma. Although 'normal' reference ranges exist even within this range, there is still a risk of developing com-plications.

Aetiology/pathophysiology
Lipids are found in dietary fat and are an important en-ergy source as well as provide essential vitamins and fatty acids. The two main lipids are triglycerides and choles-terol, which are found in dietary fat and may also be synthesised in the liver and adipose tissue (see Fig. 13.1).
- Lipids are insoluble; they are absorbed from the small intestine as chylomicrons (a combination of triglyc-eride, cholesterol and apoproteins). These are then transported to the liver where the triglyceride is re-moved and the remaining cholesterol-containing par-ticle is also taken up by the liver.
- The liver synthesises very-low-density lipoproteins (VLDL), containing lipoproteins, triglyceride and cholesterol, these circulate allowing trigyceride to be removed and utilised. The end product, deplete of triglyceride, is termed an intermediate-density lipoprotein (IDL).

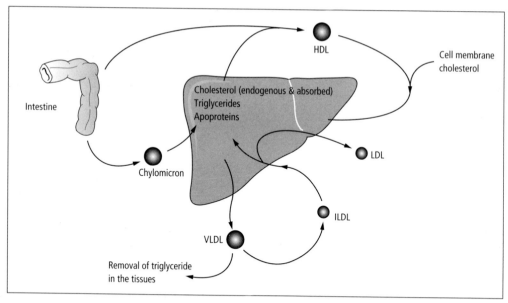

Figure 13.1 Cholesterol and triglyceride transport.

- Most of these are broken down in the liver. Some are further depleted of triglyceride and are released as low-density lipoproteins (LDL) – the main cholesterol carrier.
- High-density lipoproteins (HDL) from the intestine and the liver collect cholesterol from cell membranes in the tissue and transport it back to the liver.

Hyperlipidaemias are classified as primary and secondary (see Table 13.1).

Primary hyperlipidaemia is a group of inherited conditions subdivided into those that cause hypertriglyceridaemia, hypercholesterolaemia and combined hyperlipidaemia.

- Hypertriglyceridaemia: Familial hypertriglyceridaemia, lipoprotein lipase deficiency, apoprotein C-II deficiency.

Table 13.1 Causes of secondary hyperlipdaemia

Hormonal	Pregnancy, diabetes mellitus, hypothyroidism
Liver disease	Primary biliary cirrhosis, extrahepatic biliary obstruction
Nutritional disorders	Obesity, anorexia nervosa, alcohol abuse
Drug induced	High dose thiazides, corticosteroids, sex hormones
Renal dysfunction	Nephrotic syndrome, chronic renal failure

- Hypercholesterolaemia: Heterozygous familial hypercholestrolaemia (LDL receptor deficiency), homozygous familial hypercholesterolaemia, defects in apoprotein B.
- Combined hyperlipidaemia: Familial combined hyperlipidaemia, remnant hyperlipidaemia.

Clinical features

The clinical signs of hypercholesterolaemia are premature corneal arcus, xanthelasmata and tendon xanthomata. Acute pancreatitis and eruptive xanthomata are features of hypertriglyceridaemia. More commonly it is diagnosed through targeted screening of high-risk patients (family history of hyperlipidaemia or coronary heart disease, hypertensive, diabetic and obese patients.

Complications

Atherosclerosis leads to coronary heart disease, cerebrovascular disease and peripheral vascular disease. Hypertriglyceridaemia can cause acute pancreatitis.

Investigations

Random, non-fasting plasma cholesterol is used as a screen in low-risk populations. Full fasting lipid profile, including total, LDL and HDL cholesterol and triglyceride, is used if high cholesterol is found or in high-risk patients.

Management

The management of hyperlipidaemia is based on an assessment of overall cardiovascular risk and current cardiovascular status.

- General measures include weight loss, lipid-lowering diets, reduction of alcohol intake, stopping smoking and increasing exercise.
- Control of hypertension is important preferably avoiding drugs that raise lipid or glucose levels.
- Lipid-lowering drugs include the following:
  1 Cholesterol-lowering drugs include resins, which sequestrate bile salts such as cholestyramine.
  2 Cholesterol and triglyceride lowering drugs such as HMG CoA reductase inhibitors (statins), fibrates, nicotinic acid and analogues.
  3 Triglyceride-lowering drugs such as fish oils (omega-3 marine triglycerides) may be required.

Vitamin deficiencies

Vitamin A deficiency

Definition

Deficiency of vitamin A, a fat-soluble vitamin, is a major cause of blindness in many areas of the world.

Aetiology

Insufficient intake of carotenoids, especially β-carotene found in carrots and dark green leafy vegetables and retinol found in fish oils, liver, eggs butter and cheese. Dietary vitamin A deficiency is generally seen in the developing world. Occasionally it can be seen in disorders of fat malabsorption, such as cystic fibrosis, cholestatic liver disease and inflammatory bowel disease.

Pathophysiology

Vitamin A is required for maintenance of mucosal surfaces, the formation of epithelium and production of mucus. It also plays a role in normal immune function. Retinal function is dependent on retinol, a constituent of the retinal pigment rhodopsin.

Clinical features

Xerophthalmia begins with night blindness and conjunctival xerosis. Bitot's spots, which are flecks caused by heaped up desquamated cells occur and progress to corneal xerosis, and eventually corneal clouding ulceration and scaring. Patients are at risk of secondary infection.

Management

- Prevention of eye disease with adequate diet and supplementation in patients with disorders of fat metabolism. In pregnant women, vitamin A but not β carotene is teratogenic.
- Xerophthalmia should be treated with oral or intramuscular retinol. Corneal transplant may be required for irreversible corneal ulceration.

Prognosis

Night blindness is easily reversible. Signs of a dry conjunctiva and Bitot's spots precede irreversible corneal ulceration unless rapidly treated.

Vitamin B$_1$ (thiamine) deficiency

See also Wernicke–Korsakoff syndrome in Chapter 7 (Nervous System; page 317)

Definition

Deficiency of thiamine (vitamin B$_1$).

Aetiology

Insufficient intake of thiamine, which is present in fortified wheat flour (the natural thiamine is removed by milling, so it is replaced in most countries), fortified breakfast cereals, milk, eggs, yeast extract and fruit. Alcoholics are most commonly affected in the United Kingdom, because of malnutrition.

Pathophysiology

Thiamine is an essential factor for the maintenance of the peripheral nervous system and the heart. It is also involved in glycolytic pathways, mediating carbohydrate metabolism.

Clinical features

Dry beriberi is an endemic form of polyneuritis resulting from a diet consisting of polished rice deficient in thiamine. The neuropathy predominantly affects the legs with weakness, parasthesia and loss of ankle jerks. Cerebral involvement causes Wernicke–Korsakoff's syndrome (see page 317). Wet beriberi is the high output heart failure caused by thiamine deficiency resulting in oedema. Wet beriberi is rare in alcoholics.

Investigations
Diagnosis is usually clinical and on response to thiamine. Erythrocyte transketolase activity and blood pyruvate are increased.

Management
Thiamine is replaced orally, intravenously or intramuscularly. The cardiac failure usually responds rapidly, but neuropathies may only partially resolve if they are long-standing.

Niacin deficiency (pellagra)

Definition
Niacin (vitamin B_3) has two principle forms: nicotinic acid and nicotinamide. Deficiency of niacin causes pellagra.

Aetiology
Niacin is found in plants, meat and fish. It can also be synthesised from tryptophan. Pellagra is seen in people with a predominantly maize diet, low in tryptophan. Other causes include increased tryptophan consumption in the carcinoid syndrome, prolonged use of isoniazid and Hartnup disease, an autosomal recessive congenital disorder with reduced absorption of tryptophan from the gut and reduced amino acid re-uptake in the renal tubules.

Pathophysiology
Nicotinic acid is involved in energy utilisation. It is a precursor of nicotinamide, as in NAD and NADP, which are essential to glycolysis and oxidative phosphorylation. It is also used in maintaining skin, especially in sun-exposed areas. Deficiency also causes villus atrophy in the small intestine.

Clinical features
Pellagra is due to lack of nicotinic acid, it often occurs as part of a more general nutritional deficiency. Pellagra presents with dermatitis, diarrhoea and dementia. Se-

vere, chronic deficiency may lead to encephalopathy and spasticity.

Management
Supplementation with nicotinic acid and treatment of other coexisting deficiencies.

Vitamin B_6 (pyridoxine) deficiency

Definition
Deficiency of pyridoxine is rarely a primary disorder, but it does occur as a secondary disorder.

Aetiology
Important sources of Vitamin B_6 are similar to those of the other B vitamins: liver, meat, whole grain cereals, vegetables and nuts. Deficiency may occur with malabsorption such as coeliac disease, dietary lack in alcoholism and drug toxicity especially isoniazid.

Pathophysiology
Pyridoxine is important in the metabolism of amino acids, especially tryptophan to nicotinic acid. In some rare metabolic disorders, pyridoxine deficiency is associated with infantile convulsions and sideroblastic anaemia.

Clinical features
Marginal deficiency may cause stomatitis, glossitis, dry lips, irritability and confusion. Deficiency causes mental confusion, glossitis, dry skin lesions and peripheral neuropathy.

Management
Oral replacement; however, high doses may cause neurotoxicity.

Vitamin B_{12} deficiency

See page 471.

Vitamin C deficiency

Definition
Vitamin C deficiency causes scurvy, which was first described by Lind in the eighteenth century.

Aetiology/pathophysiology

Occurs in the poor, pregnant or those on a peculiar diet. Young children have a high requirement. Vitamin C (ascorbic acid) is found in citrus fruits, potatoes, green vegetables and fortified fruit drinks. Vitamin C is involved in the hydroxylation of proline to hydroxyproline necessary for collagen synthesis.

Clinical features

Patients develop listlessness, anorexia, cachexia, gingivitis, loose teeth, petechial haemorrhages and bleeding.

Management

Ascorbic acid supplementation is rapidly effective.

Vitamin D deficiency

See page 374.

Vitamin K deficiency

See page 494.

Metabolic disorders

Amyloidosis

Definition

Amyloidosis refers to the extracellular deposition of fibrils composed of low-molecular-weight proteins, many of which circulate as constituents of plasma.

Aetiology/pathophysiology

At least 21 different protein precursors of amyloid fibrils are now known (see Table 13.2).

Besides systemic amyloid deposition, organ specific amyloid may occur in the skin or heart and most notably in the brain in Alzheimer's disease. Genetic factors may be involved in predisposing to the development of fibrillogenesis and amyloidosis:

- Genetic mutations resulting in proteins with increased propensity to form fibrils.
- Genetic polymorphisms in protein subunits and cofactors.
- Inherited disorders with chronic inflammation.

Clinical features

The precursor protein, the tissue distribution and the amount of amyloid deposited affect the clinical presentation. The kidneys, heart and liver are often affected.

- Renal amyloid deposition: asymptomatic proteinuria or nephrotic syndrome, deposition in blood vessels or tubules causes renal failure.
- Cardiac amyloid deposition leads to disorders of contractility and heart failure, arrhythmia and heart block. Deposition in the coronary arteries can lead to ischaemic heart disease.
- Gastrointestinal system: hepatomegaly, splenomegaly, gastrointestinal bleeding and dysmotility.
- Nervous system: various peripheral and autonomic neuropathies may occur. Central nervous system deposition is rare in systemic amyloid; however, organ specific CNS deposition is seen in Alzheimer's disease.
- Musculoskeletal system deposition may cause muscle pseudohypertrophy, macroglossia, arthropathy, spondyloarthropathy, bone disease and carpal tunnel syndrome. This form of deposition is particularly seen in dialysis-associated amyloid.
- Skin deposition causes a waxy thickening and easy bruising.

Investigations

Where possible biopsy and histology is used to confirm clinical suspicion. Amyloid appears as homogenous

Table 13.2 Classification of amyloidosis

Precursor	Amyloid type	Clinical associations
Serum amyloid	AA	Acquired disorder, serum amyloid A is an acute phase protein, related to chronic inflammation and infection.
Immunoglobulin chains	AL	Associated with lymphoproliferative disorders such as multiple myeloma, Waldenstrom's macroglobulinaemia and non-Hodgkins lymphoma.
	$\beta2$ microglobulin	Dialysis-associated amyloid.
Familial amyloidosis	Various	Autosomal dominant inherited, including familial transthyretin-associated amyloidosis.

substance that stains pink on haematoxylin and eosin and stains red with Congo red.

Management

Therapy is aimed at the underlying cause where possible such as inflammation, infection or blood dyscrasia. Differing manifestations such as renal failure require support. In the hereditary amyloidoses where the precursor protein is produced by the liver, liver transplantation is curative.

Porphyria

Definition

The porphyrias are genetic or acquired deficiencies in the activity of enzymes in the heme biosynthetic pathway.

Aetiology/pathophysiology

Heme is synthesised from succinyl Co A and glycine (see Fig 13.2); differing enzyme deficiencies cause different patterns of disease.

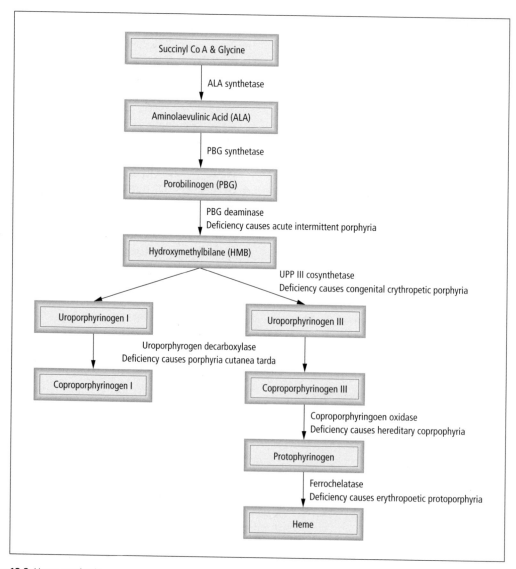

Figure 13.2 Heme synthesis.

The first enzyme, ALA synthetase is the rate-limiting step. Enzyme deficiencies result in increases in metabolic intermediates, which are excreted and accumulate in tissues. This results in neurological, visceral symptoms and photocutaneous manifestations. Pophyrias may manifest as acute or chronic disease, the excess porphyrins deposit either in the liver (hepatic porphyrias) or in the bone marrow (erythropoetic porphyrias).

Clinical features/management

- Acute intermittent porphyria is inherited in an autosomal dominant fashion. It presents in adult life with abdominal pain, vomiting and constipation, polyneuropathy, hypertension and tachycardia. Acute episodes are precipitated by alcohol and drugs. Diagnosis is suggested by leaving the urine to stand, which turns red brown.
- Porphyria cutanea tarda presents with a bullous photodermatitis precipitated by alcohol. Urinary levels of uroporphyrinogen (the substrate for the deficient enzyme) are raised. Remission is induced by venesection.
- Congenital erythropoietic porphyria is inherited in an autosomal recessive fashion. It causes an extreme photosensitivity with dystrophy and scarring.
- Erythropoietic protoporphyria is inherited in an autosomal dominant fashion. The photosensitivity that results can be controlled with β-carotene by an unknown mechanism.

Hyperhomocysteinaemia

Definition

Raised levels of homocysteine (an amino acid formed by the conversion of methionine to cysteine) have been associated with premature atherosclerotic disease.

Aetiology

1 Severe hyperhomocysteinaemia with raised homocysteine levels in the urine is due to a rare autosomal recessive disorder called homocystinuria.
2 Moderate homocysteinaemia occurs in approximately 5–7% of the population. Causes include the following:
   - Genetic defects in enzymes involved in homocysteine metabolism. The enzyme affected most commonly (approximately 10% of the population) is a variant of methylene tetrahydrofolate reductase,

which converts homocysteine into methionine, using folic acid as a co-factor.
- Vitamin deficiencies (folate, and to a lesser extent vitamin B_6 or vitamin B_{12}).
- Smoking and chronic illnesses, e.g. renal failure.

Pathophysiology

There are several postulated mechanisms by which homocysteine may have its atherogenic and prothrombotic effects, including increased uptake of LDL cholesterol into the arterial intima (to form foam cells), smooth muscle cell proliferation, activation of clotting factors and a pro-aggregatory effect on platelets. There may also be a pro-inflammatory effect by upregulating neutrophils through increased expression of cytokines such as IL-8, and oxidative stress caused by free radicals produced during the oxidation of homocysteine.

Clinical features

1 Homocystinuria presents in childhood with developmental delay. Other features include a Marfan's like syndrome, ocular abnormalities, thromboembolic disease and severe premature atherosclerosis.
2 Hyperhomocysteinaemia without the other features of homocystinuria has been found to be associated with ischaemic heart disease and stroke, although the effects are less strong than those of, e.g. hypertension, diabetes mellitus and smoking. It is more strongly associated with an increased risk of pulmonary embolism and deep vein thrombosis.

Investigations

Homocysteine levels can be measured (normal being 5–15 μmol/L, moderate 15–30 μmol/L and severe >100 μmol/L). A methionine challenge can be given to induce a rise in homocysteine levels in those with normal fasting levels, but the clinical significance of this is unknown.

Management

Increased folic acid intake reduces homocysteine levels. Vitamin supplementation with folic acid, vitamin B_6 and vitamin B_{12} is advocated by some for those with premature cardiovascular disease and recurrent venous thromboembolism. There is as yet no clear evidence that supplements should be given to all those with ischaemic heart disease, although several trials are in progress.

Patterns of inheritance

Autosomal dominant: Mendelian pattern of inheritance where the presence of a single abnormal allele is able to produce the disease. There may be reduced expression of the condition if the condition does not have full penetrance (see Fig. 14.1 and Table 14.1).

Autosomal recessive: Mendelian pattern in which both genes must be defective to produce the clinical phenotype (see Fig. 14.2 and Table 14.2).

X linked conditions are those that appear on the X chromosome, i.e. are linked to the sex of an individual. There is no male-to-male transmission, daughters of an affected male will be obligate carriers. In X linked dominant conditions, females may also demonstrate the clinical phenotype, and may also demonstrate mosaicism as a result of random X inactivation (see Fig. 14.3 and Table 14.3).

Mitochondrial: A number of conditions that do not follow normal Mendelian patterns of inheritance. In this set of conditions males and females may be affected, but only the offspring of female sufferers may be affected. These conditions result from the maternally inherited mitochondrial DNA, which code for at least 37 mitochondrial enzymes (see Table 14.4).

Down syndrome

Definition

Down syndrome is the clinical condition usually resulting from a trisomy of chromosome 21 first described by Langdon Down in 1865.

Incidence

Rises with increasing maternal age (1 in 3000 when mother is less than 30 years to 1 in 300 when mother is 35–40 years and 1 in 30 in women above 45 years). Because of the high birth rate in mothers below 35, half of all Down syndrome children are born to mothers below 35.

Age

Congenital.

Sex

M = F

Geography

All ethnic communities.

Aetiology

75% of cases result in spontaneous abortions in the first trimester. The additional chromosome 21 is usually (94% of cases) the result of non-disjunction of chromosome 21 during the formation of the maternal ovum. In rare cases there may be a maternal translocation (3%) involving chromosome 21 with the extra 21 attached to another chromosome, e.g. Robertson translocation between 21q and 14 or 22. In about 3% of cases there is mosaicism with some cells demonstrating a normal karyotype.

Pathophysiology

The Alzheimer's disease seen with Down syndrome is thought to be due to the presence of three copies of the amyloid protein gene on chromosome 21.

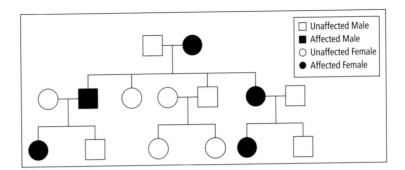

Figure 14.1 Autosomal dominant inheritance.

Table 14.1 Examples of autosomal dominant inherited conditions

Disease	Locus	Gene	
Achondroplasia	4p	FGFR3	Mutation in a fibroblast growth factor receptor causes dwarfism (90% new mutations)
Adult polycystic kidney	16p 4q	PKD1 PKD2	Abnormal membrane proteins (polycystin) cause development of cysts in kidney and other organs
Familial retinoblastoma	13q	RB1	Loss of tumour suppressor gene causing a retinoblastoma
Gilbert syndrome	2q	UGT1A1	Disorder of glucoronidation causing jaundice
Hereditary spherocytosis	8p	ANK1 SPTB EPB42 BND3	Disordered interaction between red cell cytoskeleton and membrane causing osmotic fragility of red cells and haemolysis
Huntington disease	4p	Huntingtin	Trinucleotide repeat (CAG) within the gene causing adult onset chorea and dementia.
Marfan syndrome	15q	Fibrillin 1	Disordered microfibrils in connective tissue
Myotonic dystrophy I	19q	DMPK	Cataracts, frontal balding, myotonia and proximal muscle weakness.
Myotonic dystrophy II	3q	ZNF9	
Neurofibromatosis I	17q	NF1	Loss of a tumour suppressor gene results in café au lait spots and multiple neural tumours
Peutz–Jeghers syndrome	19p	STK11	Tumour supressor gene causing mucocutaneous pigmentation, multiple hamartomas
Tuberose sclerosis	9q 16p	TSC1 TSC2	Hamartin – a growth inhibitory protein Tuberin – a tumour suppressor gene

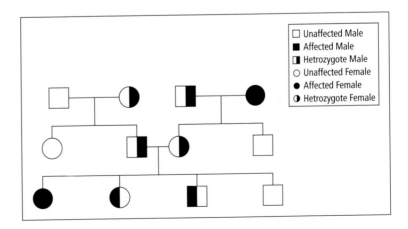

Figure 14.2 Autosomal recessive inheritance.

Table 14.2 Examples of autosomal dominant inherited conditions

Disease	Locus	Gene	
Congenital adrenal hyperplasia (21-OH)	6p	Multiple	21-hydroxylase deficiency results in virilisation, and renal salt wasting in severe cases
Phenylketonuria	12q	PKU1	Deficiency phenylalanine hydroxylase causing mental retardation if untreated
Sickle cell disease	11p	Hbβ	Sickling of red blood cells in hypoxia
Cystic fibrosis	7q	CFTR	Abnormalities in chloride channel results in thickened secretions in multiple organs
Gaucher disease I	1q	GBA	Mutations in the acid-β glucosidase gene results in hypersplenism, and bone lesions. Particularly common in Ashkenazi Jews
Tay Sachs disease	15q	Hexa	Lysosomal storage disease causing accumulation in GM2 ganglioside and progressive neurodegeneration
Galactosaemia	9p	GALT	Galactose-1-phosphate uridylyl-transferase mutation causing jaundice, hepatomegaly and mental retardation if untreated
Wilson disease	13q	ATP7B	Abnormal copper transporting protein causing Kayser–Fleischer rings, cirrhosis, hepatomegaly, tremor and dementia if left untreated

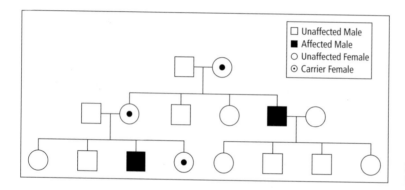

Figure 14.3 X-linked recessive inheritance.

Table 14.3 X-linked conditions

Disease	Inheritance	Gene	
Bruton agammaglobulinaemia	Recessive	BTK	Mutations in Bruton agammaglobulinaemia tyrosine kinase gene leads to absent B and plasma cells.
Chronic granulomatous disease	Recessive	Cytochrome b245	Neutrophils can phagocytose material, but are unable to generate respiratory burst and hence kill bacteria.
Duchenne muscular dystrophy	Recessive	Dystrophin	Progressive proximal muscle weakness with calf psuedohypertrophy. Dystrophin is a cytoskeletal protein found in muscle cells, which normally acts to anchor the cell membrane to the ECM.
Glucose-6-phosphate dehydrogenase deficiency	Recessive	G6PD	Highly polymorphic gene, so females may inherit 2 genes with low activity and hence be affected; causes congenital non-spherocytic haemolytic anaemia.
Fragile X syndrome	Female 'carriers' may also be affected	FMR1	Expanded (CGG)n repeat in the fragile X mental retardation 1 gene; unstable if > 52 repeats; symptomatic if > 200 repeats. Exhibits genetic anticipation.
X linked hypophosphataemia	Dominant	PHEX	Hypophosphataemic vitamin D resistant rickets.
Rett syndrome	Dominant	MECP2	Females only affected, thought to be lethal in-utero to males. Causes progressive intellectual deterioration, loss of purposeful use of hands and jerky truncal ataxia.

Table 14.4 Mitochondrial inherited conditions

Disease	Gene	
Kearns–Sayre syndrome	MTTL1	Mutations in mitochondrial tRNA (leucine)-1-gene or deletions of multiple genes. Ophthalmoplegia, ptosis, retinal degeneration, diabetes, ataxia, cardiomyopathy.
Leber optic atrophy	Multiple loci	Sudden onset adult blindness, cardiomyopathy, cardiac conduction defects.
Myoclonic epilepsy and ragged red fibre (MERRF)	MTTK1, MTTL1	Can be produced by mutations in more than one mitochondrial gene. Causes myoclonus, optic atrophy, retinopathy, deafness and ataxia.
Mitochondrial encephalomyopathy, lactic acidosis and stroke like episodes (MELAS)	MTTL1, MTND6, MTTQ	Can be produced by mutations in more than one mitochondrial gene. Causes headaches, seizures, hemiparesis, stroke like episodes, deafness, dementia, short stature, lactic acidosis.

Clinical features

- Neonatal features include hypotonia, poor Moro reflex, joint hyperflexibility, excess skin at the nape of the neck and flat facies.
- Characteristic facies with a small midface, low bridged upturned nose, oblique palpebral fissures, epicanthal folds and enlarged protruding tongue.
- Short stature (long bones of limbs are short). Short middle phalynx of little finger, single horizontal palmar crease in broad hands, increased space between the fist and second toe. Lax joints with risk of atlantoaxial dislocation.
- Congenital heart disease in 30%, most commonly atrioventricular septal defects.
- Tracheo-oesophageal fistula, duodenal atresia, annular pancreas, Hirschsprung's disease.
- Mental retardation, hypotonia, Alzheimer's disease by age 40 (cortical atrophy, ventricular dilation, neurofibrillary tangles).

Complications

Fifteenfold increased risk in developing leukaemia (ALL and AML), hypothyroidism.

Investigations

- Prenatal: Reduced maternal serum α feto protein and oestriol, and increased maternal serum βHCG indicates an increased risk of Down syndrome (triple test). Increased nuchal fold thickness on ultrasound at 12–14 weeks has been shown to be as sensitive and specific a test. Definitive diagnosis is made by chorionic villus sampling at 10–11 weeks or amniocentesis early in the second trimester (15–16 weeks). Indications for testing include maternal age and a Down

sibling (recurrence risk is 1% overall, higher if a balanced translocation).
- Postnatal chromosome analysis is diagnostic.

Prognosis

15–20% die before age 5, usually as a result of severe inoperative heart disease. The remainder survive well into adult life, but by 40 almost all have Alzheimer's disease.

Klinefelter syndrome

Definition

Chromosomal abnormality with a genotype 47XXY.

Incidence

1 in 1000 males.

Age

Congenital.

Sex

Phenotypically males.

Aetiology/pathophysiology

In 80–90% there is a 47XXY karyotype, the extra X coming from the mother. 48XXXY and 49XXXXY karyotypes are usually associated with mental retardation, i.e. the more X chromosomes the more severe the phenotype. Many cases go undetected as patients are generally normal. All appear normal until puberty when hypogonadism becomes prominent.

Clinical features

Tall, with long arms and legs, hypogonadism, female pubic hair profile, high-pitched voice, reduced facial and body hair. Other features that may be present include gynaecomastia. There is greatly reduced fertility, slight but significant reduction in IQ.

Investigations

Karyotype analysis.

Management

Testosterone replacement should be given during adolescence for psychosexual development and prevention of osteoporosis.

Turner syndrome

Definition

Loss of a sex chromosome resulting in a 45,XO genotype.

Incidence

1 in 5000 live births.

Age

Congenital.

Sex

Phenotypically female.

Aetiology/pathophysiology

The commonest underlying karyotype is 45,X; however, many females are mosaics: 45,X/46,XY (other mosaics include 45,X/47,XXX or 45,X/46,XY). There is no increase in incidence with advancing maternal age. Most cases of Turner syndrome spontaneously abort during pregnancy.

Clinical features

- During pregnancy there may be generalised hydrops or localised swelling on ultrasound due to late maturation of the lymphatic system. Intrauterine growth retardation is common.
- Neonates are phenotypically female, neck webbing, puffy hands, low posterior hairline, large carrying angles (cubitus valgus), wide spaced nipples, and carpal/pedal oedema.
- Adults present with infantile genitalia, short stature (<150 cm), wide spaced nipples, neck webbing, micrognathia and prominent ears, wide carrying angle.
- Increased frequency of renal (horseshoe kidney) and cardiovascular anomalies (coarctation of aorta) plus mild mental retardation in ~10%. As there is normally only one copy of the X chromosome, females suffer from X linked recessive conditions such as haemophilia.
- Usually normal intelligence and life expectancy, but deficient spatial perception, perceptual motor organisation or fine motor execution.

Investigations

Genetic karyotyping will confirm the clinical diagnosis.

Management

Growth hormone in childhood and oestrogen at puberty allows better growth and the development of secondary sexual characteristics but has no effect on fertility.

Alcohol and drugs of abuse

Alcohol abuse and dependence

Definition
Regular or binge consumption of alcohol sufficient to cause physical, neuropsychiatric or social damage.

Incidence/prevalence
3–4% of the population report alcohol-related problems.

Sex
2M : 1F

Aetiology
Various factors have been implicated:
- Genetic factors: Evidence includes variation across racial groups and twin studies.
- Psychiatric factors: Family history of depression, increased risk in the presence of chronic psychiatric and physical illness especially pain.
- Social factors: Occupation, cultural and peer group pressure.

Clinical features
Alcohol abuse and alcohol dependence are classified as recognisable entities.
- Alcohol abuse is a drinking pattern associated with social compromise such as work or school absenteeism, legal problems related to alcohol use, or continued alcohol use despite causing social or relationship problems.
- Alcohol dependence is defined as a maladaptive pattern of use associated with tolerance and withdrawal syndrome despite significant physical and psychological problems. Patients often exhibit a stereotyped drinking pattern with alcohol consumption taking preference over other activities.

A history of alcohol consumption should be taken from all patients with consideration given to the aforementioned social consequences of heavy drinking. In addition signs of chronic liver disease and other complications may be evident.

Complications
- Medical complications include gastritis, peptic ulcer disease, pancreatitis, hepatitis, cirrhosis, portal hypertension with oesophageal varices, cardiomyopathy, hypertension.
- Neuropsychiatric complications: Acute withdrawal (also known as delirium tremens) within 48 hours may result in malaise, nausea, autonomic hyperactivity, tremulousness, lability, insomnia, and transient hallucinations, illusions especially visual (e.g. spiders), frequent seizures. Serious delirium tremens has a significant mortality.
- Chronic dependence causes Wernicke–Korsakoff psychosis (see page 317).
- Other neuropsychiatric complications include dementia, peripheral neuropathy, cerebellar degeneration, alcoholic hallucinations, symptoms of depression and/or anxiety.
- Social problems include job loss, marital difficulties, criminal activity and alcohol-related accidents.

Investigations

Blood alcohol levels are of limited value, a persistently raised MCV or γGT are suggestive of continued alcohol use.

Management

1 Identification and advice at an early stage may be enough to avert serious medical, neuropsychiatric and social consequences of alcohol. Precipitating factors should be identified and psychological support/therapy instituted as appropriate.
2 Abstinence, individuals may require general support (rehydration, correction of electrolyte imbalance, complex intravenous vitamin preparations) and treatment to avoid specific complications, e.g. chlordiazepoxide in the treatment of delirium tremens and diazepam or lorazepam in the treatment of seizures.
3 Disulfiram (Antabuse) blocks metabolism resulting in acetaldehyde accumulation resulting in flushing, headache, anxiety and nausea. This may be implanted to give 6 months of treatment.

Prognosis

15% die by suicide, 30% continue to have life-long alcohol-related problems.

Opiate abuse and dependence

Definition

Opiate dependence or addiction is defined as the continued use of opiates, despite these causing significant problems, which may be physical, neuropsychiatric and social.

Opiates are all drugs derived from opium, i.e. the milk of the opium poppy. Opium contains morphine and codeine. Natural and synthetic derivatives of these drugs are useful, effective analgesics, but opiates also have the potential to become drugs of abuse.

Heroin (a derivative of morphine) is a popular opiate of abuse, but other drugs including morphine, pethidine, codeine and dihydrocodeine are also commonly abused. In its pure form, heroin is a white powder, but on the streets it is bought as an off-white or brown powder, and is known by many street names including 'H, gear, smack,

junk, skag, white stuff, sugar'. Health care professionals with access to opiates may abuse drugs like fentanyl.

Incidence/prevalence

Heroin abuse fell during the late 1990s, but rose again rapidly in 2000 and 2001. A fall in use since then has been attributed to the fall in supply after the Taliban banned production in Afghanistan. Despite the fall in numbers of users, the number of heroin-induced deaths has remained static. Heroin and morphine account for ~40% of drug-abuse-related deaths in the United Kingdom.

Pathophysiology

Opiates have central nervous system depressant effects, and they act as analgesics and cause euphoria. Abusers repeatedly take the drug to achieve the euphoric effect; however, this results in opiate tolerance, i.e. increased doses are required to achieve the same effect. Withdrawal symptoms also occur, and so further doses are taken to avoid the withdrawal.

Heroin can be smoked ('chasing the dragon'), snorted, or injected into a vein ('shooting up' or 'mainlining'), or subcutaneously ('skin popping') or intramuscularly. It acts rapidly, within 10–20 seconds, if injected, and within 20–30 seconds, if snorted. Snorting is the most common method of use, as it does not require any special preparation. The effects last 4–6 hours.

Clinical features

Following use of heroin, side effects include nausea and vomiting (usually only on first few uses), drowsiness, sedation, constricted pupils and dry, itchy skin.

Long-term users generally have constipation, features of self-neglect, weight loss, there may be needle-tracks and evidence of complications.

A history should be taken of recent and previous heroin use, including methods of administration, use of other drugs such as benzodiazepines, alcohol intake, previous attempted rehabilitation and any previous heroin-related problems. A close social history should be taken, as well as a medical history and examination.

Complications

- The most serious complications are associated with intravenous use. Use of non-sterile equipment and water used to mix the powder lead to cellulitis, thrombophlebitis, skin and organ (e.g. cerebral) abscesses and infective endocarditis. Sharing of needles means that hepatitis B and C, and HIV can be transmitted. Deep vein thromboses and pulmonary emboli occur. Other problems include acute pulmonary oedema, anaphylaxis and aspiration pneumonia.

- With excessive doses, coma and death from respiratory failure occur. The variability in the purity of street heroin means that with every use there is a risk of accidental overdose, especially after a break from use when tolerance is reduced, or if other drugs or alcohol increase the sedative effect.
- Withdrawal leads to nausea, vomiting, abdominal cramps, diarrhoea, watery eyes and nose and muscle twitching. Seizures may occur.
- Social problems include loss of job, deterioration in relationships and criminal activities to obtain money to buy drugs, including stealing, prostitution and drug dealing.

Investigations

These depend on the presentation of the individual. Investigations may be needed for possible complications such as infective endocarditis, HIV, hepatitis and DVT, depending on the history and clinical diagnosis.

Management

Heroin intoxication is treated by ensuring airway protection, and giving the opiate antagonist naloxone. This rapidly reverses the opiate action, but is short-acting, so the patient requires further monitoring for 24 hours and may need a naloxone infusion.

Heroin abusers should be referred to a drug rehabilitation counsellor or centre, and considered for rehabilitation. Methadone, a long-acting opiate, which does not cause euphoria, is used as a method of programmed withdrawal, to ameliorate the withdrawal symptoms. Supportive therapy is needed to prevent the patient from seeking increased doses (either of heroin, other drugs or even methadone) elsewhere, and relapse is common. In some cases, patients stay on long-term methadone at a low maintenance dose. Although they remain dependant on methadone, they are less likely to relapse, less likely to have an overdose, and are not at risk from HIV infection.

Cocaine abuse and dependence

Definition

Cocaine abuse is defined as the continued use of cocaine/crack despite it causing significant problems, which may be social, neuropsychiatric or physical.

Cocaine hydrochloride (HCl) is made from the leaves of the coca shrub. It is normally bought as a white powder, which is usually snorted or smoked. Freebasing is where cocaine HCl (the salt) is dissolved in water and heated with baking soda, ether or ammonia to free the cocaine alkaloid base. This combusts more readily making the cocaine more potent. Crack is a form of freebase cocaine made by using baking soda, which looks like little lumps ('rocks') and makes a crackling sound when burnt.

Street names for cocaine include 'C, charlie, coke, dust and white', and for crack include 'base, freebase and rock'. The street term 'freebasing' means smoking cocaine, either as the salt or base. Cocaine and crack can also be injected, although this is far less common.

Incidence/prevalence

7% of 20–24 year olds have tried cocaine, mainly snorting. About 10–15% of those who try snorting cocaine become abusers. Crack is less commonly used, but addiction occurs faster. Crack is linked with areas of social deprivation, whereas cocaine HCl tends to be associated with an expensive lifestyle. Cocaine HCl and crack abuse is rising.

Pathophysiology

Cocaine HCl and crack are strong, short-acting stimulant drugs. They are not physically addictive in the same way as opiates, but cocaine addicts will compulsively take doses in a 'binge' in order to keep experiencing the highs and to avoid the depression and fatigue that occur when the drug wears off. Tolerance does seem to occur to some extent. Snorting cocaine HCl leads to effects within minutes, which last about half an hour. Base forms of cocaine, including crack, have a more rapid onset but a much shorter duration of action. When cocaine is taken with alcohol, its effects are increased by an active metabolite, which only forms in the presence of alcohol.

Clinical features

After taking cocaine, the user feels intense euphoria. Physical side effects include dilated pupils, dry mouth, sweating, tachycardia and loss of appetite. Within half an hour of the last dose of a binge, there is a 'crash' when the user feels intense cravings, depression and anxiety. After a further 1–4 hours, they usually sleep for hours to days, intermittently waking up with hunger ('the munchies'). After a few days, the user becomes low in mood, with lack of motivation, impairment of memory and intermittent anxiety, even suicidal ideation. Long-term users may become persistently restless, with anorexia, weight loss and insomnia.

A history should be taken of recent and previous cocaine use, including methods of administration, use of other drugs, alcohol intake, previous rehabilitation and any problems associated with drug use. A close social history should be taken, as well as a medical history and examination.

Complications

- Physical: Snorting cocaine repeatedly causes damage to the nasal mucous membranes with septal perforation, cribiform plate damage and CSF rhinitis. Smoking can cause granulomas and pulmonary oedema. Injecting carries risks of abscesses, infective endocarditis, HIV and hepatitis infection. Other medical complications include hypertension, myocardial infarction (MI) due to coronary artery spasm, arrhythmias, seizures, stroke and cardiorespiratory arrest.
- Neuropsychiatric: Anxiety, paranoia, depression and hallucinations.
- Social: The most common reason for a cocaine addict to present for treatment of dependency is running out of money, as a cocaine or crack binge can cost hundreds to thousands of pounds. Other problems include loss of job and criminal activities such as stealing, prostitution and drug dealing.

Investigations

These depend on the presentation of the individual. Cocaine use can be tested for using a urine screen. Investigations may be needed for possible complications such as MI, arrhythmias, stroke and infections.

Management

Cocaine intoxication: Initial management includes ensuring a clear airway and ventilation if needed.

1 Seizures are treated with diazepam or lorazepam. Phenytoin may be needed.

2 Agitation and hypertension often respond to diazepam. Haloperidol and phenothiazines should be avoided, as they increase the risk of seizures.

3 Persisting hypertension should be treated with intravenous glyceryl trinitrate (GTN), with calcium antagonists as second line therapy. β-blockers should be avoided (may cause paradoxical hypertension and coronary vasoconstriction due to unopposed alpha effects).

4 Aspirin, sublingual GTN and diazepam should be given to all patients who have chest pain. If pain continues, intravenous GTN should be commenced and if despite this, the ECG shows an acute MI, thrombolytic therapy as for a conventional MI should be given, unless there are any contraindications.

5 Cardiac arrhythmias require specialist advice, for example from the National Poisons Information Service (NPIS).

6 Cocaine abusers should be referred to a drug rehabilitation counsellor or centre. There are no serious physical effects from withdrawal so sedatives or a replacement drug are not needed. Propanolol may help anxiety (but may exacerbate cocaine-induced hypertension or myocardial ischaemia) and antidepressants may be indicated.

Amphetamine abuse

Definition

Amphetamines were originally widely used for medical reasons such as appetite suppressants and for insomnia, but are now recreationally used. Medical use of amphetamine (and derivatives) is now limited to selected cases of narcolepsy and attention deficit hyperactivity disorder.

There are several derivatives of amphetamine, such as methamphetamine, which can be smoked, and therefore became popular for their increased speed of onset and intense effect. Amphetamines can be taken orally, intranasally, smoked or injected. Street names for amphetamine include 'speed, whizz, sulphate', and for methamphetamine 'meth, ice'.

Incidence/prevalence

Amphetamine and derivatives (including ecstasy) are the second most common class of illegal drug used after cannabis.

Pathophysiology

Amphetamines are stimulant drugs with cardiovascular, neuropsychiatric and other physiological effects. Multiple doses, taken to maintain euphoria, can lead to intoxication, and feelings of anxiety and paranoia. Tolerance to amphetamines can take place with increased doses or a different method of administration, e.g. smoking or injecting rather than oral. In psychological dependence withdrawal can cause depression, profound lethargy and hunger. Street amphetamine usually only contains ~5% of the drug, mixed with other substances including baby milk powder, lead, caffeine and paracetamol or codeine. This makes it particularly dangerous to inject. The excretion of amphetamine depends on urine pH – acid urine increases its clearance.

Clinical features

Physical effects of an amphetamine-intoxicated state include tachypnoea, tachycardia, decreased appetite and increased motor activity. A history should be taken of recent and previous recreational drug use, including methods of administration, and alcohol intake. A psychiatric and social history should be taken, as well as a medical history and examination.

Complications

Medical complications include seizures, coma, tachyarrhythmias, hyperthermia and hypertension. Acute hepatic failure has been reported. Psychiatric complications include paranoia, eating disorders, hallucinations and panic attacks. Loss of judgement, e.g. when car driving or a bad trip can lead individuals to become uncharacteristically aggressive and violent, causing harm to themselves or others.

Investigations

If the individual is euphoric, but with no physical side-effects, there is no need for specific investigations and should be monitored for 4 hours. If physical side-effects are present, U&Es, liver function tests, creatine kinase and an ECG should be performed. The core temperature should be checked.

Management

In more than mild toxicity, patients should have cardiac monitoring.

1 Seizures and agitation are treated with diazepam or lorazepam.
2 Hypertension should be treated with diazepam or if this is ineffective, intravenous glyceryl trinitrate (GTN).
3 Hypovolaemia should be treated with fluid resuscitation, consider inotropes, and treat metabolic acidosis with sodium bicarbonate as necessary.
4 Cardiac arrhythmias or refractory hypertension require specialist advice, for example from the NPIS.
5 Amphetamine abusers should be offered drug rehabilitation counselling.

Ecstasy abuse

Definition

Ecstasy is a semi-synthetic derivative of amphetamine with hallucinogenic properties. Its full name is 3,4-methylenedioxymethamphetamine (MDMA). Ecstasy usually comes in tablets or capsules, which may have logos or pictures on them. Street names include 'doves, E, M and Ms, sweeties, X, brownies'. Occasionally it is found in a powder form that is smoked or snorted.

Incidence/prevalence

Ecstasy use continues to rise, doubling in the last 5 years. Now 2.2% of the population aged 16–59 years take ecstasy, with rates approaching 30% in university students. There have been over 200 deaths from the drug in 15 years.

Pathophysiology

MDMA causes the release of serotonin and dopamine in the brain, and both central and peripheral catecholamine release. The pills can contain from 30 to 300 mg of MDMA, and in some cases the drug is replaced or mixed with other substances such as amphetamine, caffeine or toxic substances. The effects of taking a dose are therefore highly variable, but in addition idiosyncratic responses appear to occur, both in naïve and chronic users.

Clinical features

● Effects begin within an hour and usually last 4–6 hours, but may persist for 48 hours with very high doses. Common physical effects include tachycardia, mild hypertension, dry mouth, reduced appetite, sweating. Increased thirst can be marked, such that excessive water intake occurs, leading to hyponatraemia.

- Occasionally transient gastrointestinal upset, confusion, dizziness and ataxia may occur. Mood effects are of euphoria, and ecstasy is unique in its ability to make users feel 'in tune' with their surroundings and other people, which is why it is so popular in the clubbing world.
- Severe toxicity (usually an idiosyncratic response, rather than dose-related) includes cardiac arrhythmias, hypotension and shock, hyponatraemia, seizures, increasing confusion and loss of consciousness.
- A history should be taken of recent and previous recreational drug use, including methods of administration, alcohol intake. A psychiatric and social history should be taken, as well as a medical history and examination.

Complications

Deaths: These appear to be due to cardiac arrhythmias, fulminant liver failure and neuroleptic malignant syndrome, which may cause acute renal failure, disseminated intravascular coagulation and metabolic acidosis. Neuropsychiatric complications include memory and concentration loss, insomnia, hallucinations and flashbacks.

Investigations

In all cases, ECG, U&Es, LFTS and creatine kinase (CK) should be performed. In severe cases a coagulation screen and arterial blood gases should be performed.

Management

In severe toxicity, initial management includes ensuring a clear airway, and ventilation if needed.

1 All patients should have cardiac, pulse, blood pressure and temperature monitoring.
2 Diazepam for agitation, anxiety, significant hypertension and seizures.
3 Continued hypertension is treated with intravenous glyceryl trinitrate, but in refractory hypertension contact the NPIS.
4 Symptomatic hyponatraemia is usually treated with water restriction; however, in coexisting hypotension normal saline infusion may be required.

5 Metabolic acidosis should be corrected with sodium bicarbonate intravenously, with rapid correction if there is prolongation of the QT interval on ECG.
6 Narrow complex tachycardias are treated with intravenous β-blockers.
7 Hyperthermia is initially treated with sedation and cooling, but if it is persistently >39°C, ice baths and dantrolene may be used.
8 In severe liver failure seek advice from a liver unit, liver transplantation has been used.

Overdose and poisoning

Overview of acute poisoning

Definition

Acute poisoning may result from accidental self-ingestion, deliberate self-harm or medical error.

Incidence/prevalence

Common presentation to A&E, commonest cause of medical admission of teenagers.

Age

Any, accidental ingestion most common in age 2–3 years.

Sex

Deliberate self-harm is more common in females.

Aetiology

Many different substances are involved in poisoning, especially in children (see Table 15.1).

Clinical features

Acute poisoning should be considered in any patient presenting with altered levels of consciousness; however, the vast majority of patients who present are conscious. The patient or carers may be able to give a history and bring the containers or tablets. A full physical examination should be made.

- Central nervous system: Impaired consciousness, this can rapidly be assessed using the AVPU (Alert, responds to Voice, responds to Pain, Unresponsive) system or more formally using the Glasgow Coma scale.

Table 15.1 Common causes of acute poisoning

Type	Examples
Over the counter medicines	Salicylates, paracetamol, ibuprofen
Psychotropic drugs	Benzodiazepines, lithium, tricyclic antidepressants
Drugs of abuse	Opiates, cocaine, ecstasy, amphetamines, ketamine
Metals	Iron, lead
Household	Alcohol, detergent, bleach, solvents
Garden	Plants, seeds, mushrooms, insecticides, organophosphates
Central heating systems	Carbon monoxide

Other neurological features include altered behaviour, seizures, hallucinations, motor disturbances.
- Respiratory system: Altered respiration, halitosis.
- Cardiovascular system: Altered heart rate, arrhythmias, blood pressure instability.
- Gastrointestinal tract: Dry mouth, salivation, jaundice, vomiting and diarrhoea, alcohol may be smelt on the patient's breath.
- Eyes: Miosis (constriction of the pupil is seen with opiates and organophosphates) or mydriasis (dilation of the pupil is seen with amphetamines, cocaine and tricyclic antidepressants), nystagmus.
- Ears: Tinnitus.
- Core temperature should be checked in unconscious patients.

Investigations
These will depend on the presentation and the availability of a reliable history. If this is not available the patient may have to be investigated and managed as an acute confusional state or coma. Appropriate investigations may include
- plasma paracetamol and salicylate levels.
- blood glucose.
- urine toxicology screen, there are immediate bedside urine screening tests available for opiates, amphetamines, cocaine and cannabis.
- blood gases to detect respiratory failure or metabolic acidosis.

Complications
These depend on cause and clinical state but may include hypothermia, rhabdomyolysis and convulsions.

Table 15.2 Some specific antidotes used in the treatment of acute poisoning

Drug	Antidotes
Benzodiazepines	Flumazenil
Paracetamol	N-acetylcysteine
Opiates	Naloxone
β-blockers	Atropine and glucagon
Digoxin	Digoxin specific antibody

Management
If the patient is conscious, management is directed at the overdose itself. Specific information is available from the NPIS by phone or computer database available to NHS staff on the Internet (see also Table 15.2).

Principles of management:
- Reduction of absorption by emptying the stomach (vomiting or gastric lavage), if large quantities of drugs have been taken within the last hour. However, lavage or induced emesis is contraindicated following ingestion of corrosives, hydrocarbons or lipoid substances. The patient must have an intact cough reflex or a cuffed endotracheal tube to protect the airway. Alternatively activated charcoal is useful for certain drugs, ideally within 4 hours of ingestion dependent on the drug.
- Active elimination may be used for certain poisons such as forced diuresis, exchange transfusion, peritoneal dialysis, haemodialysis, haemoperfusion.
- Care of the patient not only involves acute medical management, but also an investigation into the circumstances of the poisoning. Following an accidental overdose social circumstances need to be considered with regard to level of care. Patients presenting following deliberate ingestion require a psychiatric evaluation prior to discharge in order to assess their risk of further self-harm and to identify and manage any underlying precipitants for the overdose.

Paracetamol poisoning

Definition
Accidental or deliberate overdose of paracetamol, causing liver damage.

Incidence
Currently the commonest drug used for deliberate overdose.

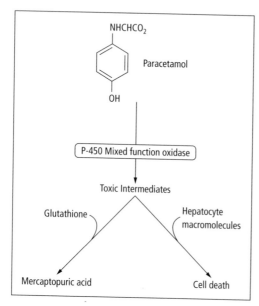

Figure 15.1 Paracetamol metabolism.

Aetiology

Overdose is generally accidental in toddlers. In older patients it is usually a form of deliberate self-harm; however, it may be accidental due to combination drug use.

Pathophysiology

Paracetamol in overdose causes hepatocellular necrosis. Normally toxic metabolites are inactivated by conjugation with glutathione. When glutathione and other conjugating substances become depleted, the metabolites (e.g. epoxides) bind to intracellular proteins and cause hepatocyte damage (see Fig. 15.1). Liver failure leads to encephalopathy, haemorrhage, hypoglycaemia, cerebral oedema and death. Paracetamol can also cause renal failure.

Clinical features

There are often no early symptoms following paracetamol overdose, patients may present with nausea, vomiting and pallor, which usually settle within 24 hours. Right subcostal pain and tenderness may then develop, and after 48 hours jaundice and a large, tender liver are apparent, indicating hepatic necrosis. Other features include hypotension, arrhythmias, excitement, delirium and coma.

Investigations

Serum paracetamol levels are taken 4 hours after ingestion and plotted to demonstrate if treatment is required (see Fig. 15.2). Patients on liver enzyme inducing drugs, malnourished patients or those who consume alcohol above recommended limits require treatment if levels are above the high-risk treatment line. In significant overdose a prothrombin time, liver and renal function tests and a lactate should be checked and repeated at 24 hours. Prothrombin time measured 24 hours post ingestion is the best marker for liver damage.

Management

- Activated charcoal is given if the patient presents within 1 hour of ingestion and >12 g (6 g in the high risk treatment group) or ≥ 150 mg/kg have been ingested, whichever is the smaller.
- *N*-acetylcysteine (a glutathione precursor) is given by intravenous infusion if the plasma paracetamol level is higher than the appropriate treatment line. It is maximally effective before 8 hours following ingestion but may be of value up to and beyond 24 hours. It may be appropriate to start *N*-acetylcysteine prior to blood levels are known if very high doses have been taken or if presentation is delayed.
- Severe hepatotoxicity may necessitate liver transplantation.

Prognosis

If acute hepatic failure occurs, mortality is $<50\%$ with good management.

Salicylate poisoning

Definition

Accidental or deliberate overdose of salicylate (aspirin).

Aetiology

Ingestion of salicylates is usually accidental in toddlers; it is now rare as paracetamol and ibuprofen have become the household analgesic and antipyretic agents of choice. Deliberate self-harm with aspirin is also unusual.

Pathophysiology

Salicylates have a direct effect on the central respiratory drive increasing both the rate and depth of

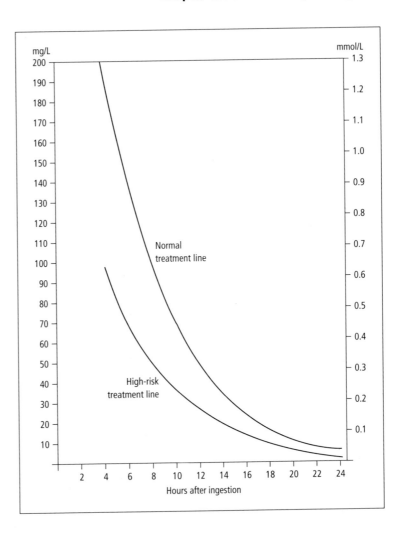

Figure 15.2 Paracetamol treatment lines.

ventilation. This hyperventilation leads to respiratory alkalosis, which is compensated for by renal excretion of bicarbonate and potassium. Salicylates also uncouple oxidative phosphorylation in skeletal muscle with consequent accumulation of pyruvic, lactic and aceto-acetic acids. The combination of the metabolic and renal effects result in a metabolic acidosis. The increase in metabolic rate can lead to hyperpyrexia and the antiplatelet effects of salicylate increases the risk of bleeding.

Clinical features

Patients may appear asymptomatic even in the presence of significant overdose. In moderate overdose patients may present with deep respiratory movements and tinnitus as early signs, and later with, deafness,

hyperpyrexia, vasodilation and tachycardia. In severe overdose disorders of consciousness occur progressing to coma especially in children.

Complications

Cerebral oedema and pulmonary oedema, which may be exacerbated by forced diuresis.

Investigations

Blood glucose, blood gases, U&Es, prothrombin time and bicarbonate levels should be measured. Treatment is based on plasma salicylate levels (>500 mg/L (3.6 mmol/L) in adults, >300 mg/L (2.2 mmol/L) in children) taken 2 hours in symptomatic patients and 4 hours in asymptomatic patients following ingestion.

Management

Activated charcoal may be considered in conscious patients within 1 hour of ingestion and consumption above 120 mg/kg. Patients may require protection of the airway, correction of hypoglycaemia and hypokalaemia, and then any metabolic acidosis with intravenous sodium bicarbonate.

Haemodialysis is used if plasma salicylate level is 700 mg/L (5.1 mmol/L), renal or cardiac failure, convulsions or if there is severe metabolic acidosis.

Iron overdose

Definition

Accidental or deliberate overdose of iron salts.

Aetiology

Iron poisoning is usually seen in childhood and results from accidental ingestion of iron-containing medications such as vitamin preparations mistaken for sweets.

Clinical features

Iron causes acute necrotising gastritis. Patients may develop nausea, vomiting, abdominal pain and diarrhoea. In severe poisoning acute upper gastrointestinal bleeding, convulsions and metabolic acidosis may occur. Late signs in severe overdose include hypotension, coma, hypoglycaemia and hepatocellular necrosis.

Investigations

A serum iron level (ideally at 4 hours after ingestion) is the best laboratory measure of severity. Abdominal X-ray may show radio-opaque tablets present in the stomach or small bowel if taken within 2 hours of ingestion. A raised neutrophil count and serum glucose suggests toxicity. LFTs and blood gas measurements should be performed.

Complications

Gastrointestinal perforation or infarction.

Management

- In severe poisoning (unconscious or hypotension) intravenous fluids and desferrioxamine (a chelating agent for iron) should be commenced immediately before waiting for serum iron levels. Gastrointestinal haemorrhage may require blood replacement and metabolic acidosis should be corrected. Liver and renal support may be required.
- In absence of symptoms, serum levels are monitored every 2 hours until levels fall or symptoms develop. Symptomatic patients with moderate (3–5 mg/L or 55–90 μmol/L) or severe (>5 mg/L or 90 μmol/L) poisoning may require treatment with i.v. desferrioxamine. Patients who have not developed symptoms by 6 hours following ingestion are unlikely to have had a significant overdose and do not require further monitoring.
- Within an hour of ingestion of large doses of iron, gastric lavage or endoscopic removal of tablets may be performed.

Tricyclic antidepressant overdose

Definition

Accidental or deliberate overdose of tricyclic antidepressant drugs.

Incidence/prevalence

Almost 1.8% of poisoning cases, but 18% of all deaths by poisoning.

Pathophysiology

Tricyclic antidepressants have anticholinergic, alpha-adrenergic blocking, and adrenergic uptake inhibiting properties. They also have a quinidine like effect on the myocardium. Alcohol and other psychotropic drugs increase the toxicity.

Clinical features

- Common features include hot, dry skin, dry mouth, dilated pupils and urinary retention.
- Cardiovascular consequences include sinus tachycardia, vasodilation, hypotension and cardiac arrhythmias.
- Neurological consequences include ataxia, nystagmus and altered levels of consciousness including coma, hypothermia and respiratory depression. There may be increased tone, increased deep tendon reflexes and extensor plantar responses. If the patient is comatose, all reflexes may be absent.

- Convulsions occur in over 5%.
- Confusion, agitation and visual hallucinations may occur during recovery.

Complications
Pulmonary oedema due to decreased cardiac contractility and fluid overload.

Investigations
Arterial blood gases to check both pH and bicarbonate levels. ECG may reveal prolonged PR interval and QRS complexes or bizarre changes in severe toxicity. Continuous ECG monitoring is essential. U&Es and urine output should be monitored.

Management
- Patients should be stabilised with management of airway, breathing and circulation as required. Acidosis should also be corrected.
- Gastric emptying is only of use up to 1 hour after ingestion. Activated charcoal should be given within 1 hour of ingestion; however, multiple doses may be considered if a modified release preparation has been ingested.
- Cardiac arrhythmias do not respond to conventional anti-arrhythmic treatments many of which may make toxicity worse. Sodium bicarbonate reverses QRS prolongation, and may correct arrhythmias even in the absence of acidosis. Intravenous lidocaine may be of benefit in treatment of cardiac arrhythmias; however, it may precipitate seizures.
- Convulsions are treated with intravenous diazepam or lorazepam. Phenytoin is contraindicated, as it may increase the risk of cardiac arrhythmias. Refractory seizures require intubation, ventilation, paralysis and other anticonvulsant medication.
- Persisting hypotension may require intravenous fluids, glucagon bolus and infusion (corrects myocardial depression) and in severe cases inotropes.

Prognosis
Tricyclic antidepressant overdose carries a high morbidity and mortality; however, prolonged resuscitation following cardiac arrest may be successful. In surviving patients most cardiac complications resolve within 12 hours and consciousness returns within 24 hours.

Lithium overdose

Definition
Lithium poisoning usually results from chronic drug accumulation, accidental or deliberate overdose of lithium carbonate.

Aetiology/pathophysiology
Lithium has a narrow therapeutic index (the levels at which it becomes toxic are only marginally higher than those needed to be therapeutic). Impaired renal excretion such as with dehydration or renal failure may induce toxicity, as may concomitant use of nonsteroidal anti-inflammatory drugs or ACE-inhibitors.

Clinical features
There is good correlation between symptoms and plasma concentration.
- Mild toxicity: Nausea, diarrhoea, blurred vision, polyuria, fine resting tremor, muscle weakness and drowsiness.
- Moderate toxicity: Confusion, faints, muscle fasciculation, hyperreflexia, myoclonus, incontinence, restlessness or decreased consciousness.
- Severe toxicity: Depressed conscious level, convulsions, arrhythmias including conduction block, hypotension and renal failure.

Investigations
Serum lithium levels should be measured if chronic toxicity is suspected. Therapeutic concentration between 0.4 and 1 mmol/L. Serious toxicity and significant mortality in levels above 2 mmol/L. In acute overdose, levels should be taken 6 hours post-ingestion and 6–12 hourly thereafter. Symptomatic patients require ECG monitoring.

Management
In chronic accumulation, stopping lithium is often all that is needed to alleviate symptoms; however, patients may require other treatments for bipolar disorder.
- In acute severe toxicity, airway and ventilatory support may be required if unconscious. All patients should be observed for a minimum of 24 hours post-ingestion. Ensure adequate hydration and correct any electrolyte imbalance. In refractory hypotension, inotropes may

be required. Convulsions are treated with intravenous diazepam.

- In severe poisoning the treatment of choice is haemodialysis which is considered if there are any neurological features or if very high plasma levels are detected.

Prognosis

The mortality in chronic poisoning is 9%, but as high as 25% in acute overdose. Clinical symptoms may persist after the serum lithium levels have fallen and 10% of patients with chronic poisoning have long-term neurological sequelae.

Index

Note: page numbers in *italics* refer to figures, those in **bold** refer to tables.